# CANCER 1

A COMPREHENSIVE TREATISE

**ETIOLOGY:** Chemical and Physical Carcinogenesis

# CANCER 1

## A COMPREHENSIVE TREATISE

## ETIOLOGY: Chemical and Physical Carcinogenesis

FREDERICK F. BECKER, EDITOR

*New York University School of Medicine*

PLENUM PRESS • NEW YORK AND LONDON

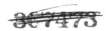

Library of Congress Cataloging in Publication Data

Becker, Frederick F.
   Etiology—chemical and physical carcinogenesis.

   (His *Cancer, a comprehensive treatise;* v. 1)
   Includes bibliographies and index.
   1. Carcinogenesis. I. Title.
[DNLM: 1. Neoplasms. QZ200 B397c]
RC261.B42 vol. 1. [RC268.5]   616.9'94'008s
ISBN 0-306-35201-X       [616.9'94'071]       74-31195

# To Mary Ellen Becker

without whose encouragement and support
this treatise would not have been completed.

# Contributors

## to Volume 1

ROBERT W. BALDWIN, Cancer Research Campaign Laboratories, University of Nottingham, Nottingham, England

ISAAC BERENBLUM, The Weizmann Institute of Science, Rehovot, Israel

K. GERHARD BRAND, Department of Microbiology, University of Minnesota Medical School, Minneapolis, Minnesota

EMMANUEL FARBER, Fels Research Institute and Department of Pathology, Temple University School of Medicine, Philadelphia, Pennsylvania

JACOB FURTH, Institute of Cancer Research and Department of Pathology, Columbia University College of Physicians and Surgeons, New York, New York

W. E. HESTON, Laboratory of Biology, National Cancer Institute, National Institutes of Health, Bethesda, Maryland

ALBRECHT M. KELLERER, Department of Radiology, Columbia University College of Physicians and Surgeons, New York, New York

ALFRED G. KNUDSON, JR., The University of Texas Health Science Center at Houston, Graduate School of Biomedical Sciences, Houston, Texas

CORNELIS J. M. MELIEF, Hematology Service, New England Medical Center Hospital, and the Department of Medicine, Tufts University School of Medicine, Boston, Massachusetts

PETER C. NOWELL, University of Pennsylvania, Philadelphia, Pennsylvania

MICHAEL POTTER, National Cancer Institute, Leukemia Studies Section, Bethesda, Maryland

MICHAEL R. PRICE, Cancer Research Campaign Laboratories, University of Nottingham, Nottingham, England

S. RAJALAKSHMI, Fels Research Institute and Department of Biochemistry, Temple University School of Medicine, Philadelphia, Pennsylvania

viii

CONTRIBUTORS

JANARDAN REDDY, Department of Pathology, University of Kansas Medical Center, Kansas City, Kansas

HARALD H. ROSSI, Department of Radiology, Columbia University College of Physicians and Surgeons, New York, New York

D. S. R. SARMA, Fels Research Institute and Department of Pathology, Temple University School of Medicine, Philadelphia, Pennsylvania

ROBERT S. SCHWARTZ, Hematology Service, New England Medical Center Hospital, and the Department of Medicine, Tufts University School of Medicine, Boston, Massachusetts

JOHN B. STORER, Biology Division, Oak Ridge National Laboratory, Oak Ridge, Tennessee

DONALD SVOBODA, Department of Pathology, University of Kansas Medical Center, Kansas City, Kansas

GEORGE W. TEEBOR, Department of Pathology, New York University School of Medicine, New York, New York

ARTHUR C. UPTON, Health Sciences Center, State University of New York at Stony Brook, Stony Brook, New York

FREDERICK URBACH, Temple University Health Sciences Center, Skin and Cancer Hospital, Philadelphia, Pennsylvania

J. H. WEISBURGER, Naylor Dana Institute for Disease Prevention, American Health Foundation, New York, New York

G. M. WILLIAMS, Fels Research Institute, Temple University School of Medicine, Philadelphia, Pennsylvania

# Preface

This series of books attempts to present, in a comprehensive manner, the field of oncology divided into three major areas; etiology, biology, and therapy. These books should serve as landmarks in the rapidly expanding experimental and clinical "universe" of this field. To some, they will be introductory; to others, a summary; for all, critical comments on the future of research. In recognition of the difficulties inherent in attempting to pause and reflect while experimental data emerge with ever-increasing rapidity, the presentations take the form of *overviews* rather than *reviews*. Where possible, an historical perspective on observations and experimentation which led to our present understanding is presented, the state of the art in technique and approach is reviewed, and the gaps in knowledge and in technique are indicated. The aim throughout is integration—using the findings from one approach for comparison with others.

The tremendous expansion of interest in oncology as a medical–biological discipline stimulated the publication of these volumes. This expansion, well warranted in terms of the impact of oncology on human morbidity, has been characterized by at least three phenomena. First, there has been an enormous increase in money and manpower devoted to the investigation and treatment of malignancy. That the research has become more and more "directed" or program-oriented signals the interest of those beyond the scientific community in the management of the effort. Second, increasing numbers of students are entering the field of oncology as their major training program. Third, public awareness of these activities has increased greatly, marked positively by large-scale support and negatively by hurried release of findings.

Nonetheless, one major problem continues to diminish the immediate importance of the results of every experiment and casts a shadow of doubt on the relevance of every observation. That problem is *our inability to define the malignant cell*. A vast amount of information exists that describes what this cell *does* and—to a lesser extent—*how* it does what it does; but the *why* evades us. Until now the malignant cell has been defined only in comparison with its normal version. We temporize, using the excuse that it is similar to its normal progenitor. Ultimately, our understanding of the malignant cell will rest on our ability to define the benign cell, within the study of cell biology. Once we acquire that knowledge, the pattern of phenotypic schizophrenia which is typical of malignancy may assume real meaning. Until we grasp its definition, we will be able to describe the malignant cell only in the most general way, as a cell whose sense of order is defective—a cell which has lost its sense of belonging to a larger community. One might suggest then that the malignant cell is one which attempts to break free from its metazoan community and return to the primeval condition of individuality.

The impact of basic research on oncology has been particularly impressive in the recent search for the etiology of malignancy. Equally impressive is the contribution of clinical observation. For over a century, the association between exposure to specific substances or participation in particular occupations and an exceptional incidence of specific forms of tumors has been recognized. The epidemiological approach remains as pertinent today as ever in studying etiology, whether it relates to the ingestion of "natural" substances in the instance of hepatocarcinogenic aflatoxin or to the suspected relationship of vinyl chloride and malignancy. It is therefore in the study of etiology that the dual disciplines of laboratory investigation and clinical observation best demonstrate a harmony of effort.

The search for the effects of carcinogenic agents cannot be separated from the search for the etiology of malignancy. Without an appreciation of the nature of malignant development, we are helpless to define the key macromolecular events induced by such agents. We cannot differentiate between obligatory alterations and the broad spectrum of unrelated effects produced by oncogens. The strategy is clear: (1) We must identify carcinogenic agents, and by an analysis of their "nature," e.g., structure and physical characteristics, we may better understand their mechanism of action. (2) We must identify crucial interactions between these carcinogens and important macromolecules within the cell, distinguishing those which relate to carcinogenesis from those which are extraneous. (3) We must examine the alterations of cell function induced by these reactions, for it is with an understanding of phenotypic variation that we may know why malignant cells escape from normal homeostatic control. (4) Last, and perhaps of greatest importance, we must define malignancy—define those characteristics of cellular activity that permit the malignant cell to compete so effectively with the normal constituent, which ultimately leads to such destructive events.

The purpose of the first volume in this treatise is to present the progress that has been made toward these goals and to delineate the vast as yet unknown areas.

F.F.B.

*New York*

# Contents

## General Concepts

# Genetic Influences in Human Tumors    3

Alfred G. Knudson, Jr.

# Hormones as Etiological Agents in Neoplasia     4

JACOB FURTH

# Immunocompetence and Malignancy     5

CORNELIS J. M. MELIEF AND ROBERT S. SCHWARTZ

## Pathogenesis of Plasmacytomas in Mice 6

MICHAEL POTTER

# Chemical Carcinogenesis

## Metabolism of Chemical Carcinogens 7

J. H. WEISBURGER AND G. M. WILLIAMS

# Chemical Carcinogenesis: Interactions of Carcinogens with Nucleic Acids        8

D. S. R. SARMA, S. RAJALAKSHMI, AND EMMANUEL FARBER

# Some Effects of Chemical Carcinogens on Cell Organelles 9

DONALD SVOBODA AND JANARDAN REDDY

# Sequential Aspects of Chemical Carcinogenesis: Skin 10

ISAAC BERENBLUM

# Sequential Aspects of Liver Carcinogenesis 11

GEORGE TEEBOR

# Neoantigen Expression in Chemical Carcinogenesis 12

ROBERT W. BALDWIN AND MICHAEL R. PRICE

# Physical Carcinogenesis

# Physical Carcinogenesis: Radiation—History and Sources 13

ARTHUR C. UPTON

# Biophysical Aspects of Radiation Carcinogenesis 14

ALBRECHT M. KELLERER AND HARALD H. ROSSI

## Ultraviolet Radiation: Interaction with Biological Molecules   15

FREDERICK URBACH

## Radiation Carcinogenesis   16

JOHN B. STORER

# Foreign Body Induced Sarcomas     17

K. GERHARD BRAND

# General Concepts

# Cytogenetics

Peter C. Nowell

## 1. Introduction

The relationship between chromosome abnormalities and neoplasia has been the subject of investigation and speculation for many years. It was noted very early that mitotic irregularities were common in routine sections prepared from many human tumors, and these observations were extended by workers such as von Hansemann (1890) and Boveri (1914) near the turn of the century, to suggest a causal relationship between chromosome alterations and cancer. With the development of modern techniques of mammalian cytogenetics in the late 1950s, interest in chromosome studies of tumors was reawakened, and subsequently a wide variety of human and animal neoplasms were studied. This work has received additional impetus recently from the introduction of "banding" methods which permit the identification of individual chromosomes and of alterations in smaller segments of chromosomes than was possible by previous methods. These newest techniques have not yet been fully exploited, but it must also be recognized that even with the "banding" procedures there may still remain significant genetic alterations in neoplastic cells which are below the level of visual detection.

Nonetheless, the data which have been accumulated on chromosome alterations in tumor cells do provide some significant evidence on the role of genetic change in neoplasia and also have proved to be of some practical clinical value. It is the purpose of this chapter to summarize present knowledge in this field and to speculate briefly on its significance. No attempt has been made to present an exhaustive review, rather, the purpose is to illustrate with pertinent data such generalizations as can be made and to emphasize those findings which appear to have the greatest theoretical or practical interest at this time.

*Technical Considerations:* Before discussing the chromosome findings in various types of neoplasms, it is appropriate to comment on some of the technical

Peter C. Nowell ● University of Pennsylvania, Philadelphia, Pennsylvania.

problems associated with these studies, as they significantly influence the quality and quantity of data available. First, it must be reiterated that the chromosome alterations under consideration are limited to the neoplastic cells and do not represent constitutional changes affecting all of the tissues of the individual. Hence dividing *tumor* cells must be obtained, and the usual sources of normal cells for chromosome study, lymphocytes from peripheral blood cultures and fibroblasts from skin cultures, are not appropriate. For investigation of the cytogenetic changes in the leukemias, both in man and in animals, suspensions of proliferating neoplastic cells frequently have been obtainable from blood or bone marrow. With solid tumors, however, it has been necessary to apply various mechanical and chemical means of disaggregation in order to prepare suspensions of cells suitable for chromosome study. With small early tumors and precancerous lesions in which mitoses are few, it has been particularly difficult to obtain preparations with adequate numbers of mitotic figures, and there has been much debate concerning the relative merits of direct vs. tissue culture methods. Opponents of the use of short-term culture as a source of dividing cells, both with the solid tumors and with the leukemias, have shown that under some circumstances the cells which proliferate *in vitro* are not representative of those dividing *in vivo*. On the other hand, if direct preparative techniques are used, many of the abnormal metaphases observed may represent cells incapable of completing mitosis successfully in the body, and the normal metaphases seen may be proliferating inflammatory cells rather than tumor cells.

With respect to the last possibility, it has been generally recognized, both with the leukemias and with solid neoplasms, that most tumor chromosome preparations contain a mixture of normal and neoplastic cells and, more importantly, that the tumor metaphases are often of much poorer technical quality than the normal cells (Nowell and Hungerford, 1964; Sandberg, 1966). Individual chromosomes are fuzzy and overlapping, with poorly defined centromeres, and the neoplastic metaphases can easily be overlooked in favor of the technically more satisfactory chromosomes present in the normal cells. The problem may become even more troublesome as the new banding techniques are more widely applied to tumor studies. These methods require technically good material for the recognition of alterations in small segments of individual chromosomes (Miller *et al.*, 1973), and one should be aware of these special problems in assessing the results of cytogenetic studies on neoplastic material.

## 2. Human Leukemias

### 2.1. Chronic Granulocytic Leukemia and the Philadelphia Chromosome

Chronic granulocytic leukemia (CGL) is unique in that it is, at present, the only well-documented example of a neoplasm in which nearly every typical case is characterized by the same chromosome change. This characteristic abnormality, the Philadelphia chromosome (Ph), is a small acrocentric chromosome derived from one of the group-G autosomes by the loss of approximately one-half of its long arm (Fig. 1). Fluorescent banding studies indicate that the involved chromosome is a No. 22, rather than a No. 21 as had been concluded with earlier techniques. Thus different chromosomes are involved in CGL and in Down's

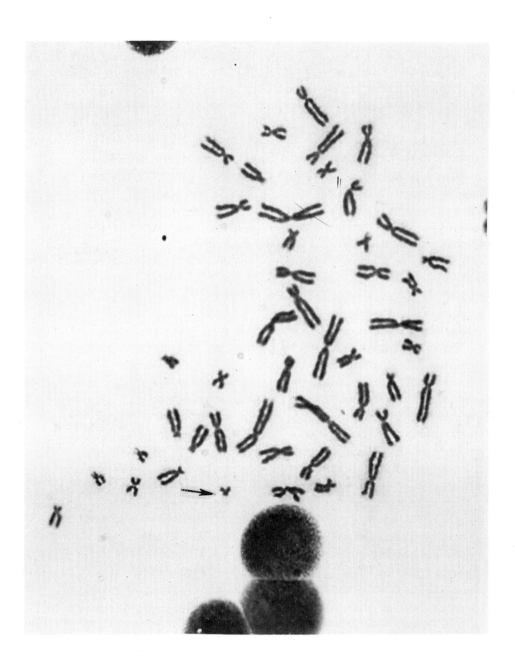

FIGURE 1. Dividing marrow cell arrested in metaphase from a patient with chronic granulocytic leukemia (CGL). The smallest of the 46 chromosomes is the abnormal Philadelphia chromosome, found in the neoplastic cells in nearly every typical case of CGL.

syndrome (trisomy 21), and the increased incidence of leukemia in the latter disease cannot be attributed to the same genetic locus as is altered in CGL. A recent study by Rowley (1973), using banding methods, indicates that the missing chromosome segment in CGL may not be lost from the cell but rather translocated onto chromosome No. 9, one of the C-group chromosomes in the human complement.

There is considerable evidence that the Ph abnormality is an acquired phenomenon rather than an inborn defect. It is apparently limited to the neoplastic cells of affected individuals, including megakaryocytic and erythroid precursors as well as those of the myeloid series, but it is not found in other cell types such as lymphocytes and cells cultured from the skin (Trujillo and Ohno, 1963; Whang et al., 1963). In addition, the Ph chromosome has been found to be absent in monozygotic twins of six patients with Ph$^+$ CGL, and it is also not observed in children whose parents have the disease (Woodliff, 1971).

These data have led to the suggestion that CGL is induced by the production, in a marrow stem cell, of this specific aberration by one or another of the mutagenic agents known to break chromosomes. The fact that ionizing radiation has been shown to produce a similar chromosome change in occasional cells of otherwise normal individuals lends support to this hypothesis.

It seems a reasonable assumption that the presence of the Ph chromosome confers a selective advantage on the mutant stem cell, and that this results in leukemia. Proliferation of the mutant cell leads to a clone of Ph$^+$ hematopoietic precursors which overgrow the normal marrow and produce the clinical disease. While the foregoing process has not been defined in terms of a specific advantageous metabolic alteration in the leukemic cells, it is noteworthy that CGL is characterized by an unusually constant biochemical change, markedly reduced levels of alkaline phosphatase in the neoplastic granulocytes. This observation suggests that there may be a genetic locus on chromosome 22 which influences in some fashion the quantity of this enzyme in the leukemic cells (Pedersen and Hayhoe, 1971). There is, however, no obvious association between this demonstrable enzyme change (which is useful diagnostically) and the undefined alteration which provides the leukemic cells with their neoplastic growth characteristics.

With successful treatment of CGL, immature cells normally disappear from the peripheral blood, but even in remission the abnormal clone persists in the marrow, and chromosome studies on dividing marrow cells usually show the Ph chromosome in all or nearly all metaphases. There have been occasional case reports of unusual sensitivity to chemotherapy, with marked marrow depression and a concomitant marked reduction in the size of the neoplastic clone as judged by the percentage of Ph$^+$ cells. In several instances, this response to therapy has been associated with prolonged remission, and this observation has raised the question of whether survival time in this disease could be improved if a more vigorous effort were generally made to deplete or eliminate the Ph$^+$ clone from the patient's marrow (Finney et al., 1972).

When CGL progresses to the blast cell crisis, which usually characterizes the terminal stages of the disease, chromosome studies frequently reveal the presence in the neoplastic cells of one or more chromosome abnormalities in addition to the Ph chromosome. These normally vary from case to case, but a second Ph has been perhaps the most commonly observed. It has been suggested that these additional alterations represent evidence of further significant genetic change in the neoplastic cells, producing greater deviation from normal patterns of differentiation (Pedersen, 1973). The further selective advantages conferred by these new characteristics may permit the cells with supplementary chromosome changes to overgrow not only normal elements but also the original Ph+ clone. It has been noted in some instances that the emergence of such a new clone may precede clinical evidence of the terminal phase of the disease and prove a useful prognostic indicator of its imminence (Sandberg and Hossfeld, 1970).

The Ph chromosome is not present in a small proportion of adult patients with CGL. The percentage varies from less than 10% to approximately 15% in different series, and apparently depends to some extent on the clinical criteria used for establishing the diagnosis. There is general agreement that Ph⁻ CGL usually occurs in patients over 60, and frequently one or more aspects of the disease is clinically atypical. These individuals generally do not respond well to therapy and have a survival time significantly shorter than that of patients with the Ph chromosome in their neoplastic cells (Whang-Peng *et al.,* 1968; Woodliff, 1971).

Two forms of CGL occur in childhood. The "adult" form is very similar to the typical disease in the adult. The Ph chromosome is present, and the response to therapy is usually good. In the "infantile" or "juvenile" form, there is usually a more subacute clinical picture, the Ph chromosome is absent (although there may be other chromosome changes), and the response to therapy is usually not favorable. Since the "adult" form can occur in children as young as 2 years of age, chromosome studies may be prognostically valuable, particularly so because leukocyte alkaline phosphatase levels may be low in both of the childhood forms of CGL (Nowell, 1967).

This latest point illustrates the occasional lack of correlation between the presence of the Ph chromosome and reduced leukocyte alkaline phosphatase, a lack of correspondence that has been reported in a few cases in adults as well. There have also been rare instances in which the Ph chromosome has been observed in marrow cells in the absence of CGL, usually in association with another myeloproliferative disorder such as polycythemia vera or megakaryocytic myelosis; but in at least one instance, the patient's disorder was diagnosed as lymphoblastic leukemia (Propp and Lizzi, 1970). Several of the myeloproliferative cases eventually evolved into CGL, and in other instances the small abnormal chromosome observed may have been mislabeled, having been derived from a chromosome 21 or from the Y chromosome rather than from chromosome 22. This problem can now be definitely resolved through the use of banding techniques, which should provide a more accurate assessment of how frequently, if ever, the Ph chromosome is present in disorders other than CGL.

Despite the few exceptions noted, the Philadelphia chromosome remains the most constant cytogenetic change in human neoplastic disorders, and as such can be of clinical as well as theoretical importance.

2.2. *Other Myeloproliferative Disorders and "Preleukemia"*

PETER C.
NOWELL

As just discussed, typical chronic granulocytic leukemia is normally distinguishable, by the presence of the Ph chromosome, from other disorders which comprise the so-called myeloproliferative syndrome and are characterized by abnormal proliferation of marrow elements. These other dyscrasias, which include such entities as polycythemia vera, myelofibrosis, and myeloid metaplasia, frequently have no chromosome abnormality at all in the bone marrow in the early stages of the disease. When cytogenetic changes are present, they have not proved to be constant from case to case, although involvement of one or more chromosomes in group C (chromosomes 6–12 and the X) may occur with more than random frequency. For example, in one series of 26 untreated cases of polycythemia vera, an extra C-group chromosome was present, in varying proportions of the marrow cells, in five patients (Millard *et al.,* 1968).

There is some indication in our own small series (see Table 1), as well as in the reports of others, that marrow chromosome abnormalities are more common in the early stages of polycythemia vera than in the other, less well-defined myeloproliferative variants. In some instances, the cytogenetic alterations in polycythemia vera appear to be radiation induced (by therapy with $^{32}$P), but in other cases they have been present prior to treatment (Millard *et al.,* 1968; Nowell, 1971). It is of interest that follow-up studies on patients treated with $^{32}$P, as well as comparable investigations in experimental animals, have indicated that chromosomally abnormal clones in the bone marrow, induced by radiation, may be functionally normal and not have any neoplastic propensity. No characteristic chromosome change has been consistently noted in these radiation-induced

TABLE 1

*Relation between Marrow Chromosome Findings and Clinical Course in Preleukemia*

| Original diagnosis | Total patients | Patients who developed leukemia | |
|---|---|---|---|
| | | With marrow chromosome abnormality | Without marrow chromosome abnormality |
| Myeloproliferative syndrome | | | |
|   Polycythemia vera | 11 | 0/6[a] | 0/5 |
|   Other | 21 | 5/7[b] | 5/14 |
| Pancytopenia | 25 | 8/9 | 4/16 |
| Miscellaneous | 13 | — | 0/13 |
| Total | 70 | 13/22[c] | 9/48[d] |

[a] 3 patients treated with $^{32}$P.
[b] 1 patient with 45,XY⁻ clone.
[c] 13/16 if polycythemia vera excluded (81%); all within 6 months.
[d] 9/43 if polycythemia vera excluded (21%); 6/9 within 6 months.

clones in man, although in one series several patients treated with $^{32}$P showed a similar abnormality involving group F (chromosomes 19 and 20) (Lawler *et al.*, 1970).

The myeloproliferative disorders, including polycythemia vera, are considered "preleukemic" on the basis that a significant proportion of affected individuals ultimately progress to acute or subacute granulocytic leukemia. Some sort of chromosome change is almost always present in the neoplastic cells at this time, but these abnormalities do not include the Philadelphia chromosome, nor are they of any constant type. As in the earlier stages of these disorders, aberrations involving one or more of the chromosomes in group C have been most frequently observed (Sandberg and Hossfeld, 1970; Woodliff, 1971). However, since this is the largest of the groups of chromosomes in the human complement, and since its members have been difficult to distinguish until the recent development of banding techniques, earlier reports of group-C chromosome involvement in the myeloproliferative disorders have been difficult to evaluate. It will be of interest to see whether the new methods indicate that it is the same group-C chromosome which is frequently involved in these disorders.

Some effort has been made in recent years to determine whether in the myeloproliferative disorders and in other "preleukemic" blood dyscrasias chromosome studies of marrow cells have any value in determining which patients will soon progress to a definitely leukemic state. The patients studied have included, in addition to those with polycythemia vera, myelofibrosis, and myeloid metaplasia, others with pancytopenia of indeterminant etiology, sideroblastic anemia, and other unexplained alterations in circulating leukocyte levels which suggested to the examining hematologist the possibility of an incipient leukemic process.

Our own study, which has extended over a number of years (Nowell, 1971), is summarized in Table 1. In this series, now encompassing 70 patients, there appears to be a definite correlation between the presence of a chromosome abnormality in the marrow and the subsequent prompt appearance of frank leukemia. Thirteen of 16 patients with myeloproliferative disorders (other than polycythemia vera) or with pancytopenia who had a cytogenetically abnormal clone in the marrow progressed to definite leukemia within 6 months; only 9 of 30 patients with the same disorders but without a marrow chromosome change followed a similar course. It is interesting that in polycythemia vera marrow chromosome changes have not appeared to be of the same grave prognostic significance as in the other myeloproliferative disorders, whether or not the chromosome alterations were considered to be radiation induced.

Other workers with comparable series have reported generally similar findings to those summarized in Table 1 (Rowley, 1970; Jensen and Philip, 1970). The data suggest that in clinical "preleukemia" the finding of a clone of cytogenetically abnormal cells in the bone marrow is a strong indication that a leukemic population is already proliferating and will become clinically manifest within the next few months. The results also make it clear, however, that some patients will progress to frank leukemia without ever demonstrating a marrow change in the neoplastic cells, and this correlates with the cytogenetic findings in patients who present initially with acute leukemia, as will be discussed in the next section.

It should be pointed out that one of the two patients in Table 1 with a myeloproliferative disorder and a marrow chromosome abnormality who did not progress to clinical leukemia had a clone of cells with 45 chromosomes, minus the Y. This is an example of what is currently recognized as probably the only type of aneuploidy that can occur in human somatic cells without significant alteration in function. The loss of the second X from a female cell or of the Y from a male cell seems not to confer a significant disadvantage in many somatic tissues, and 45,X,− clones, apparently spontaneously developed, have been observed among both peripheral blood lymphocytes and marrow cells in a number of elderly humans. Although such clones have in some cases been associated with marrow dysfunction, as in our patient, in other instances there has been no indication of related hemic disorder and even evidence for normal immunological function of 45X,− cells (Nowell, 1965a; O'Riordan *et al.*, 1970). To date, marrow clones with other types of chromosome change have not been identified in man in the absence of a history of irradiation or blood disorder, but few chromosome studies have been done on marrow from normal individuals.

## 2.3. Acute Leukemias

Cytogenetic studies in human acute leukemias have been of particular interest, because in a significantly large proportion of cases these disorders do not exhibit any demonstrable chromosome change throughout the course of the disease, a phenomenon not observed with any other major type of mammalian neoplasm. In some early studies, technical problems undoubtedly accounted for some "false negative" results. It is frequently difficult to obtain dividing neoplastic cells from cultures of peripheral blood in the acute leukemias, and when direct marrow preparations are employed the neoplastic metaphases are of technically poor quality and may be overlooked. However, even after these problems were recognized and avoided in recent years, results have indicated that approximately half of the patients with acute leukemia show no chromosome change by standard technique (Fitzgerald *et al.*, 1973). It is possible that if the newer banding techniques can be successfully applied some of these negative cases may prove to be "pseudodiploid" (i.e., a normal chromosome number, but with minor rearrangements of chromosome segments).

In some series, cases of acute leukemia without demonstrable chromosome changes are more common among adults than in children, and in the myeloblastic rather than the lymphoblastic varieties. However, some negative cases have been described for every type of acute leukemia, including the rarer forms such as erythroleukemia; thus from a diagnostic standpoint the presence of a chromosome change in a suspected case may help substantiate the clinical impression of acute leukemia, but the absence of such abnormalities cannot be accepted as strong evidence against the presence of the disease.

Those cases of acute leukemia with cytogenetic alterations show considerable variation, ranging from translocations within the diploid chromosome set to extensive departures from normal in both chromosome number and morphology. Perhaps the most extreme aberrations have been observed in some of the acute lymphoblastic leukemias of childhood and in some cases of erythroleukemia, with chromosome numbers markedly hypodiploid in some cases and near-tetraploid in others (Sandberg and Hossfeld, 1970; Woodliff, 1971) (Fig. 2). From the

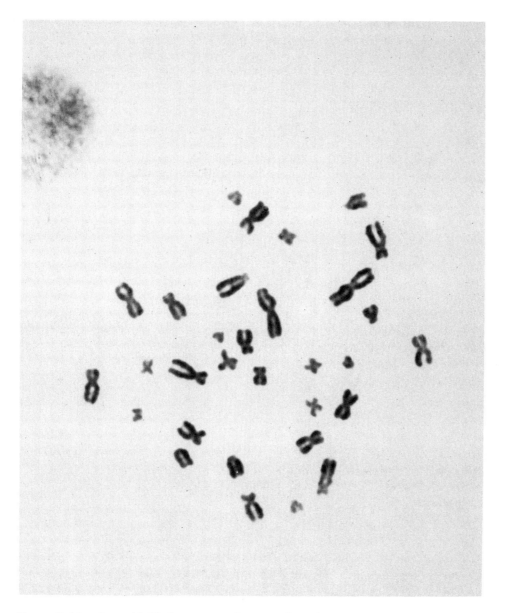

FIGURE 2. Metaphase with 31 chromosomes from a patient with acute leukemia. This degree of hypoploidy is highly unusual, but was characteristic of one neoplastic clone in this patient's marrow; a related cell clone with chromosome numbers in the 60s was also present.

standpoint of prognosis, it appears that neither the presence nor the type of chromosome change is of value in predicting clinical course or response to therapy (Fitzgerald *et al.*, 1973).

When chromosome abnormalities are present, they have generally indicated a clonal pattern of growth of the neoplastic cells. Commonly, all of the dividing leukemic cells examined from a patient's blood and marrow show the same karyotypic alteration, or related changes, suggesting evolution of the entire neoplastic population from a single progenitor cell. Unlike in CGL, however, the abnormal pattern observed in one patient has generally been different from that in others with the same disease. Although there has been some indication that certain chromosome groups are more commonly involved than others, particularly group C, it has been unusual to find more than two or three patients in any series of cases of acute leukemia with the same chromosome change.

The abnormal karyotype in acute leukemia appears to be quite stable in most instances, with the same aberration persisting in a given individual throughout the course of his disease. During remissions, dividing cells with the abnormal pattern may not be demonstrable either in the peripheral blood or in the bone marrow; however, this does not represent the reversion of leukemic cells to normal, but simply the depression of the neoplastic clone to such small size as to be undetectable among regenerating normal elements. With subsequent exacerbation of the disease and recurrence of large numbers of neoplastic cells in the marrow and peripheral blood, cells with the same aberrant karyotype are again readily demonstrable. Although evolutional changes in the chromosome pattern may occur as the disease progresses, this appears to be much less common than in chronic granulocytic leukemia (Fitzgerald *et al.*, 1973).

### 2.4. Lymphoproliferative Disorders

Chronic lymphocytic leukemia (CLL) has not been adequately studied cytogenetically because it has been extremely difficult to obtain sufficient numbers of dividing neoplastic cells. The proliferating elements in direct preparations of bone marrow are undoubtedly mostly normal cells, and few mitoses occur in standard peripheral blood cultures stimulated with phytohemagglutinin (PHA). Recent studies suggest that in most cases the circulating lymphocytes in CLL are neoplastic B lymphocytes which do not respond to the T-cell mitogen PHA, and the few dividing cells observed in PHA cultures of CLL lymphocytes probably represent residual normal T-cells in the circulation. For these reasons, it seems probable that some reports of normal chromosome findings in CLL may not, in fact, have involved study of leukemic metaphases (Peckham, 1972). It may be possible to obtain adequate chromosome preparations in CLL through the use of mitogens which stimulate B cells (i.e., pokeweed, anti-immunoglobulins, lipopolysaccharides), but to date there have been no such reports.

An apparent association between familial chronic lymphocytic leukemia and a specific inherited chromosome aberration (a G-group chromosome, probably No.

21, missing its short arm) now appears to be coincidental, as the relationship has
not been consistent (Fitzgerald *et al.*, 1966). A number of families with familial CLL have now been described in which no chromosome change was noted, and, conversely, this alteration (the so-called Christchurch chromosome) has been reported in association with a number of other diseases and in normal individuals. This aberrant chromosome may be an example of one of the several small karyotypic variations which have been observed occasionally in man without apparent phenotypic effect. Similarly, a suggestion that there is a statistically significant difference in the total length of the group-G chromosomes (Nos. 21 and 22) in lymphocytes of males with chronic lymphocytic leukemia, as compared with normal controls, remains to be evaluated critically (Fitzgerald, 1965). Until adequate numbers of dividing neoplastic cells can be consistently obtained in this disease, it will be difficult to assess the frequency and significance of chromosome alterations in CLL.

It has also been difficult to obtain cytogenetic data on the *solid lymphomas,* but some information has been acquired, primarily from direct lymph node preparations or short-term culture of cells from neoplastic nodes. Abnormalities have been observed in nearly all cases where adequate material has been obtained, and the findings have generally indicated a clonal type of neoplastic growth. No specific chromosome aberration has been consistently correlated with a particular histological pattern or clinical course (Millard, 1968).

In Hodgkin's disease, cells with abnormal chromosome numbers in the hypo-tetraploid range have been observed, and these presumably represent Sternberg–Reed cells in division. On the other hand, metaphases with chromosome numbers in the diploid range obtained from nodes involved in this disease have usually had a normal karyotype, and these may well represent proliferating normal cells involved in an inflammatory or immune host response rather than actual constituents of the neoplasm. In several cases of Hodgkin's disease, as well as some of the other solid lymphomas, an abnormal group-E chromosome (probably a No. 18) has been described, and this may represent a "marker" of lymphoma in that it has not yet been described in association with any other type of neoplasm (Miles *et al.*, 1966; Millard, 1968).

Chromosome changes of particular interest have been reported in three of the less common lymphoproliferative disorders: multiple myeloma, Waldenström's macroglobulinemia, and Burkitt's lymphoma. In a significant proportion of multiple myeloma patients, abnormal chromosomes have been observed in some of the dividing cells of the bone marrow, presumably derived from a chromosome in group D (chromosomes 13–15) in some cases and resembling a large group-A member in others. Similarly, a number of cases of Waldenström's macroglobulinemia have been described in which the karyotype was characterized by a large marker chromosome, again apparently derived from one of the group-A chromosomes (Nos. 1–3), although the marker was not identical in all instances. Attempts have been made in both of these disorders to relate the particular chromosome alteration observed to the specific abnormal protein being produced by the neoplastic cells, but no correlation has thus far been demonstrable (Bottura *et al.*, 1961; Tassoni *et al.*, 1967). There appear to be some well-documented instances in which these dyscrasias can occur without demonstrable chromosome change (Woodliff, 1971), although the possibility of "false negatives" on technical grounds, similar to those obtained in CLL, must be considered. In any event, present data suggest that for the paraproteinemias, as with acute leukemia, the presence of a chromosome change may help to establish the neoplastic character of a case under study, but the absence of cytogenetic alterations does not definitely indicate a benign process.

The Burkitt tumor is being extensively investigated from many standpoints because of the strong possibility of a viral etiology. Direct cytogenetic preparations from several primary African tumors revealed a large abnormal chromosome, somewhat similar to that observed in a few cases of Waldenström's macroglobulinemia (Jacobs *et al.*, 1963). More recently, Manolov and Manolova (1971), using banding techniques, reported an extra terminal bright band on chromosome 14 in biopsies and cell cultures from ten of 12 patients.

A different chromosome aberration has been observed in chromosome studies of several Burkitt tumor cell lines carried in tissue culture: a secondary constriction near the end of the long arms of a group-C chromosome. It has been suggested that this lesion is the specific result of infection of these cultures by the Epstein–Barr virus (EBV), although the association has not been completely consistent (Kohn *et al.*, 1967; Huang *et al.*, 1970). This question is of some interest, as EBV, which has now been identified as the causative agent of infectious mononucleosis, may also be involved in the etiology of Burkitt's lymphoma. The possibility that some viruses may damage specific chromosomal sites (unlike the random damage of radiation and most chemicals) has been suggested by several experimental studies (McDougall, 1970), and the EBV-induced abnormality, if confirmed, might thus identify a specific virus-induced carcinogenic lesion in the human genome.

## 3. Human Solid Tumors

Many of the generalizations made concerning the leukemias also apply to solid human tumors. Because of greater technical difficulties in preparing material for chromosome study, most of the early investigations were on far-advanced lesions, including cells from malignant effusions. More recently, some data have been obtained, by direct and culture methods, on earlier stages of malignancy and on some benign and "premalignant" lesions of the cervix, bowel, breast, and other organs.

### 3.1. Malignant Tumors

Nearly all human malignant solid tumors studied to date have shown chromosome abnormalities; there are only a very few cases reported in which the karyotype appeared normal (Sandberg and Hossfeld, 1970; Koller, 1972). In many instances, particularly in the far-advanced tumors and malignant effusions, extensive alterations have been observed, with chromosome numbers varying widely and major structural rearrangements producing distinctive "marker" chromosomes (Fig. 3). There has frequently been, in these cases, correlation between the extent of chromosome change and the stage of progression of the tumor, the most advanced tumors showing the most extensive cytogenetic alterations. There has also been observed, however, some relationship between the chromosome pattern and the particular organ involved, tumors at some sites tending to have chromosome numbers with a diploid mode (e.g., cervix) while in other organs the tetraploid range is more common (e.g., colon, bladder).

As with the leukemias, a clonal type of growth is commonly indicated by a characteristic chromosome number or the presence of a distinctive abnormal marker within most cells of a particular tumor. In some instances, the same marker chromosome present in cells with different chromosome numbers has suggested the possible sequence of evolutionary events occurring during the development of the neoplasm (Atkin and Baker, 1966). However, the clonal pattern of growth in human solid malignancies has been generally much less clear than in the leukemias, and, particularly in those solid tumors examined by direct preparative techniques, considerable variation in chromosome number and morphology within the same tumor has been common (Koller, 1972). More than in the leukemias, it appears that instability of the mitotic apparatus permits constant production of additionally aberrant cells within the proliferating population. Most of these presumably do not survive, but some provide the basis for continual selection of more and more deviant clones superimposed on earlier ones. Similar conclusions may be drawn from the few chromosome studies which have been done on metastatic human tumors. The karyotype of the metastasis has generally been similar to that of the primary neoplasm, but frequently with additional superimposed cytogenetic alterations, tending toward higher ploidy and more variation in chromosome number (Sandberg and Hossfeld, 1970).

With this degree of variability, it is not surprising that specific cytogenetic alterations associated with particular solid neoplasms have been difficult to demonstrate in man. No chromosome change comparable in consistency to the Philadelphia chromosome in CGL has been observed in human solid tumors. As with several of the malignant lymphomas, however, there have been a few types of epithelial and mesenchymal neoplasms in which distinctive chromosome abnormalities appear to occur with greater than random frequency. In several series of ovarian tumors and testicular tumors, for instance, a large abnormal chromosome, similar from case to case, has been observed (Atkin, 1971; Martineau, 1966). Also, a large submetacentric marker chromosome replacing a chromosome of group A has been described in several cases of carcinoma of the cervix, and an abnormal medium-sized acrocentric chromosome in several colon tumors (Sandberg and Hossfeld, 1970).

An unusually consistent finding has been the absence of a G-group chromosome, recently identified by banding methods as a No. 22, in human meningiomas, some of which were considered clinically benign (Mark *et al.*, 1972).

PETER C.
NOWELL

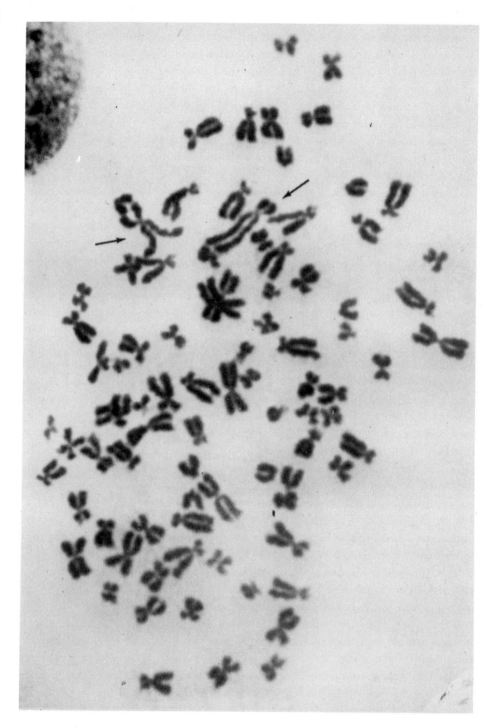

FIGURE 3. Metaphase from a squamous cell carcinoma of the skin. There are 87 chromosomes including two large abnormal "marker" chromosomes (arrows) which helped characterize the predominant cell clone in this tumor. This degree of hyperploidy is not uncommon in solid malignancies.

Additional cytogenetic alterations were also present in a number of the meningiomas studied, and it has been suggested that the extent of these further changes, as with CGL, may indicate progression of the neoplasm to a definitely malignant state (Benedict *et al.*, 1970).

## 3.2. Benign and Precancerous Lesions

In agreement with the meningioma data, chromosome studies on other human benign and "premalignant" lesions have also revealed a rough correlation between degree of histological abnormality and the extent of cytogenetic change. Data are relatively sparse, in part because of the scarcity of mitoses available for study in small early lesions and in slow-growing benign tumors, but some results have been obtained from lesions of the colon, cervix, breast, bladder, and ovary (Auersperg *et al.*, 1967; Enterline and Arvan, 1967; Koller, 1972). Those bowel polyps diagnosed as benign or hyperplastic by the pathologist have generally shown less alteration in karyotype than those considered premalignant. Similarly, "dysplasias" of the cervix have been less abnormal cytogenetically than "carcinoma *in situ*." Comparable results have been obtained at the other sites mentioned, but it is also clear that the relationship among the pattern of cytogenetic change, the degree of histological alteration, and subsequent malignant behavior does vary from one organ to another.

Even in very early lesions, marker chromosomes frequently indicate a clonal type of neoplastic growth. However, considerable random variation is frequently also present, as well as numbers of diploid metaphases which may or may not represent neoplastic elements. These difficulties, coupled with the relative paucity of mitotic figures for study, indicate that laborious collection of additional data will be needed before it can be decided whether the demonstration of aneuploidy or of a specific marker chromosome in a given "premalignant" lesion is of practical value in predicting its subsequent course.

## 4. Animal Tumors

Chromosome studies of tumors in animals have provided the opportunity to investigate in detail the relationship between cytogenetic change and various stages of neoplastic development. The results have generally paralleled the findings in man, but it has been possible with animal systems to study much more closely the very early steps in neoplastic transformation, both *in vivo* and *in vitro*, as well as later events in tumor progression.

## 4.1. Viral Tumors and Transformed Cells

Only in animals can one investigate chromosome patterns in neoplasms known to be caused by oncogenic viruses, and the results indicate that a significant number of virus–induced tumors, at least in their early stages, show no demonstrable cytogenetic alterations. This has been particularly true of those neoplasms induced by RNA viruses, such as the Rous sarcoma and the murine leukemias of Moloney, Friend, and Rauscher, but several studies on tumors induced by DNA viruses (SV40, polyoma, and the Shope rabbit papilloma virus) have also demonstrated a diploid chromosome constitution in a proportion of early lesions (Nowell, 1965b; Mark, 1969; Mitelman, 1971; Koller, 1972).

When it has been possible to follow such experimental neoplasms over time, it has been common to find chromosome alterations in the later stages of tumor progression (Mark, 1969; Mitelman, 1971), but it is clear that developing virus-induced tumors have generally had much less karyotypic abnormality than similar tumors induced by radiation or by chemicals. This difference may suggest that most mechanisms of viral oncogenesis do not require direct damage to the host cell genome, while actual chromosome breakage may be important in the production of neoplasms by ionizing radiation and some carcinogenic chemicals.

One approach to this question has been made through studies of cellular transformation *in vitro* by oncogenic viruses and by other agents. Unfortunately, the results do not provide a clear answer about the importance of direct chromosome damage in the initiation of cancer. Viral transformation of mammalian cells in tissue culture to a malignant state, as indicated by their capacity to form tumors when transplanted into animal hosts, is usually associated with major cytogenetic alterations, but not always. Also, a number of aneuploid tissue culture lines do not form tumors *in vivo,* and some cytogenetically abnormal "transformed" cell lines, having biological characteristics of neoplasia *in vitro,* may be caused to revert to a "nonneoplastic" state in culture without change in their aneuploid status (Moorhead and Weinstein, 1966; MacPherson, 1970; Freeman and Huebner, 1973).

Cell hybridization techniques may eventually provide more precise information on the role of specific chromosome alterations in the initiation and maintenance of malignant characteristics in tissue culture lines. Several experiments have suggested that "malignancy" acts as a "recessive" trait, with hybrids of malignant and nonmalignant cell lines losing their malignant properties (Harris *et al.,* 1969). However, the results have not been totally consistent, and it has thus far not been possible to identify the acquisition or maintenance of neoplastic characteristics with a particular chromosome in either the human complement or the complement of other mammalian species. Further studies with hybridization methods may ultimately permit both identification and chromosomal mapping of one or more gene loci which when present in the cell repress its unlimited growth potential and hence prevent expression of a "neoplastic" character. The *in vitro* studies have made it clear already, however, that significant genetic change which is not visible at the chromosome level can occur in cells in conjunction with neoplastic "transformation." Even with the newer banding techniques, the problem of correlating specific chromosome alterations with carcinogenic mutations remains formidable.

Cytogenetic studies in animal systems have not only permitted investigation of the earliest stages of neoplastic growth, but have also provided some of the strongest evidence in support of the concept of clonal evolution in tumor progression. Although human malignancies have provided "snapshots" of what has been interpreted as an evolutionary process of neoplastic development, it has been possible with animal tumors to biopsy sequentially individual neoplasms or study serial generations of a transplantable tumor line and thus follow in detail the progression of a particular malignant cell population.

In a number of *primary* sarcomas induced in rodents by the Rous virus, as shown both by Mark (1969) and by Mitelman (1971), the karyotype was initially normal. Serial biopsies of individual tumors revealed the subsequent appearance of predominant cell clones, identified by abnormalities in chromosome number and morphology, overgrowing and replacing the original diploid tumor population. With time and progression of the neoplasm, more divergent stem lines appeared, with a different cytogenetic pattern evolving in each individual tumor. These involved chromosome changes in addition to those first observed, presumably reflecting further selective growth advantages over the earlier tumor cells, both diploid and aneuploid. There have been similar observations with other induced primary tumors in animals, although, as has already been noted with some human leukemias and "premalignant" lesions, results have differed from one study to another, in terms of both the variation around the modal chromosome number in a particular tumor and the stability of the basic cytogenetic alteration with time (Koller, 1972).

Studies with *transplantable* tumors have shed additional light on the concept of clonal evolution within neoplastic cell populations. In general, transplanted solid tumors have been aneuploid, with a single stemline predominating in a particular transplant generation (Hsu, 1961; Al-Saadi and Beierwaltes, 1967). Frequently, particularly in early passages, it has been possible to demonstrate the appearance over several generations of progressively more abnormal predominant clones, with cytogenetic changes in addition to those first seen. In some cases, very stable chromosome patterns have emerged after a number of passages and subsequently persisted for years; in other tumor lines, variants have continued to appear.

These phenomena have been well illustrated in cytogenetic studies of the Morris hepatomas, a series of transplantable rat liver tumors induced by chemical agents and generally selected for their high degree of differentiation and slow growth. In a few of these neoplasms, the cells were diploid when first studied, and the development of predominant aneuploid clones was not observed until later generations. Most of the tumors were already aneuploid when first investigated, however, and a number have subsequently developed additional chromosome changes, often accompanied by an increase in growth rate and other indications of greater "malignancy" (Nowell *et al.*, 1967; Nowell and Morris, 1969). The fact that there has been a conscious effort with these hepatomas to retard progression by selection for the slowest-growing neoplasms in each generation probably accounts for the relatively high degree of both phenotypic and karyotypic stability in the Morris tumors. This view is supported by the chromosome findings in an exceptional subline which was isolated because of a sudden change to an unusually rapid growth rate. This subline demonstrated marked cytogenetic and histological deviation in its second transplant generation as compared to the normal diploid karyotype of the well-differentiated slow-growing parental line.

Finally, one further example of cytogenetic evidence for clonal growth in an animal solid tumor deserves special mention. Canine venereal sarcoma is a malignancy of dogs which occurs with a worldwide distribution. Chromosome studies of this sarcoma from widely separated geographical locations in the United States and in Japan have consistently revealed highly aneuploid but very similar karyotypes (Makino, 1963; Weber *et al.*, 1965). The findings strongly suggest that the tumors seen in different countries are not separate primary neoplasms but instead are evidence of a spontaneously transplantable malignancy, not requiring human intervention for passage, which in spreading throughout the world has maintained a highly abnormal but very stable basic stemline over a long period of time and extensive geographical distribution.

This explanation of the surprising chromosome findings in canine venereal sarcoma as reflecting spontaneous transplantation permits the general statement that no study of animal tumors has revealed a characteristic chromosome abnormality consistently associated with a particular type of *primary* neoplasm. As in some human tumors, however, certain alterations have been observed with greater than random frequency in occasional investigations. Wald *et al.* (1964) described an abnormal marker chromosome in a number of RF mice carrying a radiation-induced myeloid leukemia transmitted by cell-free filtrates, and Stich (1960) found 41 chromosomes (vs. a normal number of 40) in 13 of 14 chemically induced mouse leukemias in one series. Similarly, an extra chromosome, an acrocentric, has been reported in a significant proportion of chemically induced rat leukemias (Sugiyama *et al.*, 1967), and a missing metacentric chromosome in rat thyroid tumors produced by iodine depletion and repletion (Al-Saadi and Beierwaltes, 1967). Since it has not been possible, with repeated investigations, to demonstrate that a particular type of induced neoplasm in experimental animals is always or nearly always associated with a specific chromosome abnormality, it has remained difficult to assess the significance of these apparently nonrandom aberrations.

## 5. Chromosome Breakage and Cancer

There have been observed a number of circumstances in which increased numbers of chromosome and chromatid breaks and rearrangements occur in human somatic cells in association with an increased incidence of cancer. Although these are attributable in most instances to the action of exogenous agents (e.g., ionizing radiation, "radiomimetic" and other chemicals, infectious viruses), a number of relatively rare congenital disorders have been described which confer on affected individuals an increased propensity for spontaneous chromosome breakage. These subjects are discussed in more detail elsewhere in this volume, and will be considered only briefly here.

## 5.1. Genetic Disorders

There are at least four rare genetically determined syndromes in man associated with excessive chromosome breakage and increased tumor incidence (German, 1972). These are Bloom's syndrome, Fanconi's anemia, ataxia-telangiectasia (Louis–Bar syndrome), and xeroderma pigmentosum. Each of the first three syndromes appears to be determined by a single recessive gene, and chromosomal instability has been demonstrated in peripheral blood lymphocyte cultures, where metaphases commonly demonstrate various kinds of chromatid aberrations, including gaps, breaks, and multiradial products of complex exchanges. Each of these congenital disorders is characterized by a somewhat different cluster of clinical abnormalities, but each involves some degree of immunological deficiency, and also an associated increased incidence of malignant tumors, particularly of the reticuloendothelial system.

The frequency with which chromosome aberrations occur spontaneously in the body in these three disorders is not known, nor is the mechanism, but it is presumed that chromosome breaks *in vivo* could initiate the frequent evolution of cell clones with abnormal karyotype, some presumably neoplastic. Such a clone, in this case "pseudodiploid" with a balanced D-group translocation, has been described among the lymphocytes of a patient with ataxia-telangiectasia (Hecht *et al.*, 1973). Whether these clones ultimately appear as a malignancy may depend not only on their increased frequency but also on whether they are eliminated by the immune system, and one can imagine this function impaired by spontaneous chromosome breakage in dividing cells of the lymphoid system.

Another postulated mechanism for tumor induction in patients with these disorders involves the increased susceptibility of their cells to neoplastic "transformation" by oncogenic viruses. Todaro *et al.* (1966) have demonstrated that fibroblast cultures from patients with Fanconi's anemia are more susceptible to transformation by the SV40 virus than are cells from normal individuals. Interestingly, this type of observation has also been extended to cell lines from individuals with constitutional chromosomal "imbalance" (e.g., XXY cells from Klinefelter's syndrome, trisomic cells from Down's syndrome) (Miller and Todaro, 1969). Thus various mechanisms may operate at several levels to produce the increased numbers of tumors observed in individuals with Bloom's syndrome, ataxia-telangiectasia, and Fanconi's anemia.

The fourth genetic disorder associated with chromosome breakage, xeroderma pigmentosum, is better understood in terms of the specific metabolic abnormality involved. In these individuals, an enzyme defect results in inadequate repair mechanisms for the DNA damage continually being produced in skin cells by the ultraviolet radiation in sunlight. The repair deficiency leads to persistent chromosome aberrations, cytogenetically abnormal clones in the skin cell population, and an extremely high incidence of skin cancer. Whether similar specific metabolic defects will be identified in conjunction with the other three syndromes described remains to be determined, but at least for Fanconi's anemia and ataxia-telangiectasia it appears that DNA repair is not involved (German, 1972).

These syndromes in which a genetically determined propensity for random chromosome breakage is associated with a general increase in tumor incidence should be contrasted with the few congenital syndromes due to a specific *constitutional* cytogenetic abnormality which include high frequency of a particular neoplasm (Knudson *et al.*, 1973). Perhaps most striking in this category is the syndrome resulting from deletion of a portion of the long arm of chromosome 13, characterized by mental retardation, various physical defects, and a 25% incidence of retinoblastoma (Wilson *et al.*, 1973). Also well documented is the increased frequency of childhood leukemia in Down's syndrome (trisomy 21). The mechanism of neoplasia induction in these states is not known, but the possibility of increased susceptibility to cellular transformation by oncogenic viruses has already been mentioned.

## 5.2. Exogenous Agents—Radiation, Chemicals, Viruses

It is clear from a number of experimental and clinical studies that many exogenous agents can produce breakage in mammalian chromosomes. The data have been largely qualitative in nature, restricted to the enumeration of those agents which produce damage and the types of aberrations produced (e.g., chromatid vs. chromosome lesions). Additional investigations are now going forward, however, in an attempt to obtain quantitative data on the cytogenetic effects produced by exposure to various agents and the relationship to subsequent tumor development.

Ionizing radiation has long been known to produce chromosome breakage in many different organisms, and it has even become possible recently, by enumerating chromosome lesions in cultured lymphocytes from the peripheral blood, to make rough estimates of radiation dose in some exposed humans. Ionizing radiation is also a potent carcinogen, and it has been suggested that in some instances tumor induction may be mediated through direct damage to the genome, as indicated by visible chromosome lesions. However, there have been few attempts to establish a precise quantitative relationship among a given radiation exposure, the resultant chromosome aberration yield, and the number and kind of tumors subsequently observed to occur. In one preliminary study (Nowell and Cole, 1965), comparing the effects on the mouse liver of high and low dose rate radiation, the chromosome aberration yield was *higher* but the subsequent incidence of hepatomas *lower* after exposure to radiation at a high dose rate than after exposure at a low dose rate. It was postulated that a cell-killing effect of the high dose rate radiation, associated with visible chromosome aberrations, may have removed potentially neoplastic cells from the surviving population. It seems clear that until there is a somewhat better understanding of the specific mechanisms of carcinogenesis in various circumstances it will be difficult to relate the number or type of radiation-induced chromosome abnormalities observed in a mammalian system to the incidence or kind of neoplasms which subsequently appear.

Similar statements can be made concerning those chemicals known to produce mammalian chromosome damage and their potential carcinogenicity. A variety of drugs and chemicals are capable of producing chromosome lesions in human and other mammalian cells both *in vivo* and *in vitro*. Very few of these agents, however, have been clearly shown to be carcinogenic in man, and thus it is difficult to demonstrate a direct relationship (Shaw, 1970). Benzene is one of the few agents known to produce neoplasia (leukemia) in man as well as chromosome aberrations *in vivo* (Forni and Moreo, 1967). Testing programs, now being introduced, which will investigate the ability of new drugs to produce mammalian chromosome damage *in vivo,* as well as their carcinogenicity, may well provide additional examples in the near future of chemical agents in which these two capacities are related.

The fact that both RNA and DNA viruses can also break chromosomes in mammalian cells has already been mentioned. This was first observed with nononcogenic viruses, but has subsequently been demonstrated, both *in vivo* and *in vitro,* with a wide spectrum of oncogenic agents as well (Nichols, 1966). At the present time, no general statement is possible concerning differences between the cytogenetic effects of carcinogenic and noncarcinogenic viruses, but it is of interest that the Schmidt–Ruppin strain of the Rous virus causes chromatid abnormalities in human leukocyte cultures, and tumors in experimental animals, but the Bryan strain of the Rous virus, under similar circumstances, produces neither chromosome changes nor neoplasms (Nichols *et al.,* 1964). Such correlations have not been universal, but they do indicate the need for additional investigation of the possible significance, both for mutagenesis and for carcinogenesis, of virus-induced chromosome abnormalities in mammalian cells.

It has also been previously noted that some viruses, particularly RNA viruses, can produce malignant tumors without visible chromosome change, presumably through more subtle interaction with the host cell genome. It may be of additional significance that in the case of viruses, and most of the chemical mutagens which have been studied to date, only chromatid-type lesions are observed in the first mitoses following exposure of cells *in vitro*. Damage by these agents is produced, apparently, only in the course of DNA synthesis, and cells in the $G_1$ (presynthetic) stage of the cell cycle are left unscathed. Exposure to ionizing radiation, on the other hand, produces chromosome-type aberrations as well as chromatid lesions in the first postexposure division, indicating damage to cells in the presynthetic stage of the cycle as well as during DNA synthesis. Thus ionizing radiation, but not most viruses or chemicals, can produce genetic alterations in a mitotically inactive cell population such as the liver, kidney, or circulating lymphocytes, alterations which will be expressed as chromosome lesions whenever these cells subsequently proliferate. Although such "resting" cells may repair chromosome damage to a varying degree during the period prior to cell division, these differences between the action of ionizing radiation and most viruses and chemicals must be considered in assessing their carcinogenic potential (Nowell, 1969).

In general, ionizing radiation may have more severe effects *in vivo* than the other exogenous agents mentioned, but the latter may have the more likely propensity to damage specific chromosome sites. Although the exact mechanism of carcinogenesis for any of these agents remains unsolved, there is clearly a correlation between the capacity to produce chromosome aberrations and that to induce neoplasia. Meaningful estimates of the risks of tumor production from exposure to these exogenous agents, however, will require additional chromosome data, supplemented by use of more precise methods for assessing the effects of point mutations and other interactions with the genome which are not visible at the chromosome level.

## 6. Conclusions and Speculations

The data summarized in the preceding sections indicate that most mammalian neoplasms are associated with demonstrable cytogenetic abnormalities and that many carcinogenic agents have the capacity to break chromosomes. In attempting to assess the significance of these observations, one may first consider chromosome change in relation to the initiation of neoplasia, and secondly its role in tumor progression.

The fact that some mammalian malignancies show no visible cytogenetic alteration clearly indicates that chromosome change is not a requirement for the neoplastic state. This does not rule out the possibility that neoplasia may always involve genetic change at some level, but the absence of demonstrable chromosome aberrations in some of the human acute leukemias and experimental solid tumors in animals demonstrates that if genetic alteration is present in all neoplasms it is sometimes submicroscopic. The late appearance of chromosome changes in some animal tumors studied sequentially which were originally diploid further supports the view that the cytogenetic alterations seen in many fully developed cancers were not present at the outset.

It has also been difficult to associate specific chromosomal sites with the initiation of neoplasia, either *in vivo* or *in vitro,* or, for that matter, with any of the early metabolic abnormalities observed in transformed cells. With the exception of the Philadelphia chromosome in chronic granulocytic leukemia, it has not been possible to relate any characteristic chromosome alteration consistently to a specific type of tumor, although we have noted a number of other tumors in which certain individual chromosomes appear to be involved with greater than random frequency. It remains to be seen whether wider application of modern banding techniques will lead to the identification of any other chromosomal sites associated with particular tumors in the same degree of consistency as the Ph chromosome in CGL.

One cannot then point to specific chromosomes as clearly involved in the initiation of most mammalian neoplasms, but there is considerable evidence relating chromosomal changes in a nonspecific fashion to the malignant state. Perhaps, in these circumstances, the chromosome lesions represent only the visible evidence of genetic damage occurring at several levels, and the critical alterations in the genome involved in tumor initiation are submicroscopic. Thus in the congenital disorders associated with increased chromosome damage, as well as following exposure to those exogenous agents which break human chromosomes, the incidence of neoplasia is significantly increased, and the resulting tumors generally have demonstrable, although variable, chromosome alterations. Similarly, although some tumors may come to macroscopic size without visible chromosome change, in many instances the very early stages on neoplasia are associated with cytogenetic alterations. In a number of studies, such as those of Stich (1963) on the liver, there is evidence that application of a carcinogen produces a whole spectrum of potentially neoplastic cells with chromosome alterations from which one or more clones eventually emerge as a macroscopic tumor.

Taken together, these data suggest that direct involvement of the host cell genome is a necessary concomitant in the initiation of essentially all forms of neoplasia, and that in many instances, but not all, this involvement is indicated by demonstrable chromosome change. The exact nature of the critical genetic lesion, or the resulting "initial" alteration in cell function, is, of course, not known, and remains the key mystery in defining the primary carcinogenic event.

This difficulty in associating the initiation of neoplasia with specific chromosome alterations, or their gene products, has led some authors to invoke a more nonspecific concept, "chromosomal imbalance," to explain carcinogenesis. Von Hansemann (1890) and subsequently Boveri (1914) envisioned cancer as caused by "asymmetrical mitosis" with resulting chromosomal imbalance in daughter cells and subsequent failure of normal differentiation. Later theories (Rabinowitz and Sachs, 1970) have extended such concepts to a postulated balance between specific factors localized to certain sites in the genome. Thus gain or loss of particular chromosomes would alter the balance, lead to expression or suppression of the "transformed" state in tissue culture, and determine whether the cells involved would demonstrate neoplastic characteristics. Preliminary supportive evidence has been obtained (Hitotsumachi et al., 1971), but the general applicability of this hypothesis remains to be proved. Ohno (1971) has suggested that the loss of genetic material represented by the Philadelphia chromosome in CGL may permit expression of a critical recessive gene on the homologous No. 22 chromosome, initiating the disease through this type of imbalance. In this connection, it may be of interest that clones of cells proliferating in vivo with radiation-induced chromosome aberrations tend to be neoplastic if the cytogenetic abnormality is "unbalanced," with gain or loss of centromeres and chromosome segments, but usually function normally if the rearrangement is a balanced translocation (Ford, 1966). At present, however, it must be considered unresolved as to whether initial expression of the neoplastic state depends on one or more highly specific genetic alterations or can result from the action of a variety of genes under conditions of significant "imbalance."

Furthermore, the concept of genetic balance may have greater relevance in considering progression of neoplasia rather than its initiation. When one examines the relationship of chromosome change to *tumor progression,* two general phenomena seem apparent: an evolutionary process in which one or a few clones of cells predominate at each stage of the disease, and sufficient mitotic instability to frequently produce cells with additional chromosome alterations, permitting sequential development of increasingly aberrant clones superimposed on earlier ones.

One may view the natural history of tumor progression as a microevolutionary process with the continuing production of variant cells (Makino, 1956; Levan and Biesele, 1958; Hauschka, 1961). Among these variants is an occasional mutant with growth advantage over the parental line, permitting it to overgrow not only normal cells in the area but the parental tumor line as well. Demonstrable chromosome changes may appear early or late in this process, but once present they permit easy identification of the sequential nature of genetic alterations taking place. Prior to the appearance of karyotype changes, evolutionary stages in the tumor cell population may be difficult to distinguish from one another and, in some cases, from adjacent normal cells.

Although there is no direct evidence to indicate that the same mechanism(s) which operates to initiate and maintain the biological characteristics which we call "tumor progression" is also important in the production of sequential chromosome changes, it is clear that the two phenomena proceed in parallel. This has led to speculation that an early step in carcinogenesis is the activation of a genetic locus for nondisjunction or other mitotic dysfunction (Nichols, 1963). If one or more such loci are active in most evolving neoplasms, they could be responsible for repeated genetic alterations, explaining both the frequency of new chromosome rearrangements, with opportunity for selection of more variant stemlines, and the progressive functional deviation of the neoplastic cells. This concept of "flexible aneuploidy" (Ohno, 1971), particularly through the maintenance of useful recessive mutations by duplication of affected chromosomes, may help to explain the remarkable ability of neoplastic cells to sustain themselves and progress in a variety of different environments. It has also been suggested, however, that these very altered environmental conditions (Freed and Schatz, 1969), or perhaps the persistence of carcinogen, might account for the observed mitotic instability in tumor cell populations rather than the postulated specific gene activation.

Whatever the mechanism, continuous chromosome alterations do frequently occur in evolving tumor cell populations, and as one observes this phenomenon sequentially in experimental tumors the trend with respect to chromosome number is usually toward an increase. Commonly, the first demonstrable change may be the gain of a single chromosome (Mitelman, 1971). Ohno (1971) has discussed the deleterious effects of monosomy and the potential advantages to the tumor cell, particularly with respect to both lethal and useful recessive mutations, of chromosome duplication. He has used these concepts to explain why tumors with a hypodiploid DNA content are uncommon, and why later steps in the progression of many mammalian solid malignancies may be toward a near-triploid or near-tetraploid karyotype.

One important corollary of these concepts of tumor progression derived from chromosomal evidence is the clear suggestion of a unicellular origin for most cancers (Atkin, 1970; Fialkow, 1970). This conclusion does not rule out the possibility that application of a carcinogen to an organ or an area of skin can produce many potentially neoplastic cells; it simply indicates that as a tumor evolves from such an area the progeny of one or at most a very few cells ultimately overgrow the site and account for the macroscopic neoplasm.

Another significant concern raised by the chromosome findings in advanced tumors is the indication that neoplastic growth is ordinarily at an irreversible stage when first observed in man. If the aneuploid karyotype which we find in most fully developed cancers is the result of a multistep evolutionary process, in which mutants have been repeatedly selected for their increasingly efficient capacity to function as malignant cells, the possibility of restoring this population to normal seems extremely remote. Introducing a normal karyotype, by some trick of genetic engineering, into a proportion of the tumor cells would not be helpful, in that any remaining aberrant cells, retaining their selective advantages, would once again overgrow the normal elements and reestablish the malignancy. Nor does it seem likely that manipulation of the internal environment of the host might somehow induce highly aneuploid neoplastic cells to differentiate and function normally, even though most, if not all, of the normal genetic information presumably remains within the aneuploid genome. There have been a few experiments which suggest that under specialized circumstances aneuploid neoplastic cells or nuclei can be induced to differentiate *in vivo* (DiBerardino and King, 1965; Johnson *et al.*, 1971; Prasad, 1972). but there seems little likelihood that *in vivo* conditions can be provided to a growing tumor which would cause an aneuploid cell population to undergo such a developmental course. Nevertheless, this possibility deserves further study, particularly if it is shown that those human cancers such as neuroblastoma, Ewing's tumor, and Wilms' tumor which occasionally undergo differentiation and loss of malignant characteristics *in vivo* or *in vitro* can do so even when the tumor cell population is predominantly aneuploid (Braun, 1969; Gellhorn, 1973).

From all of these considerations, one may finally ask what is the practical value, for diagnosis or prognosis, of chromosome studies in human tumors. Some aspects have already been considered earlier in the text, as well as possibilities for further development. The use of cytogenetic data in the classification and prognosis of some cases of human leukemia and preleukemia has been mentioned, as well as the occasional differentiation of benign vs. malignant solid lesions and effusions by these techniques.

The practical results with respect to therapy have been less encouraging. To date, neither particular chromosome alterations nor the range of chromosome numbers has been consistently of predictive value in gauging response to therapy of particular types of human cancer. With additional cytogenetic data obtained by the newer banding techniques, it is possible that useful prognostic information of this type may emerge.

More importantly, however, in considering the general problem of cancer therapy, one must acknowledge the chromosomal evidence which indicates that most malignancies, as seen clinically, are highly individual and highly abnormal from a genetic standpoint. There are a few diploid neoplasms, notably many cases of acute leukemia, which because of their less altered genetic makeup may prove more consistent in their response to various types of therapeutic manipulation. The vast majority of cancers, however, are aneuploid and in addition to having highly individualized genetic patterns also demonstrate the capacity to readily generate new predominant variants if their environment is altered. These characteristics must be recognized by the cancer therapist, and they provide a profound challenge to his ingenuity.

## 7. References

AL-SAADI, A. A., AND BEIERWALTES, W. H., 1967, Sequential cytogenetic changes in the evolution of transplanted thyroid tumors to metastatic carcinoma in the Fischer rat, *Cancer Res.* **27**:1831.

ATKIN, N. B., 1970, Cytogenetic studies on human tumors and premalignant lesions, in: *Genetic concepts and Neoplasia* (M. D. Anderson Hospital Symposium), pp. 36–56, Williams and Wilkins, Baltimore.

ATKIN, N. B., 1971, Modal DNA value and chromosome number in ovarian neoplasia, *Cancer* **27**:1064.

ATKIN, N. B., AND BAKER, M. C., 1966, Chromosome abnormalities as primary events in human malignant disease; evidence from marker chromosomes, *J. Natl. Cancer Inst.* **36**:539.

AUERSPERG, N., COREY, M. J., AND WORTH, A., 1967, Chromosomes in preinvasive lesions of the human uterine cervix, *Cancer Res.* **27**:1394.

BENEDICT, W. F., PORTER, I. H., BROWN, C. D., AND FLORENTIN, R. A., 1970, Cytogenetic diagnosis of malignancy in recurrent meningioma, *Lancet* **1**:971.

BOTTURA, C., FERRARI, I., AND VEIGA, A. A., 1961, Chromosome abnormalities in Waldenström's macroglobulinemia, *Lancet* **1**:1170.

BOVERI, T., 1914, *Zur Frage der Entstehung maligner Tumoren*, Vol. 1, Gustav Fischer Verlag, Jena.

BRAUN, A. C., 1969, *The Cancer Problem*, Columbia University Press, New York.

DIBERARDINO, M. A., AND KING, T. J., 1965, Transplantation of nuclei from the frog renal adenocarcinoma. II. Chromosomal and histologic analysis of tumor nuclear-transplant embryos, *Develop. Biol.* **11**:217.

ENTERLINE, H. T., AND ARVAN, D. A., 1967, Chromosome constitution of adenoma and adenocarcinoma of the colon, *Cancer* **20**:1746.

FIALKOW, P. J., 1970, Genetic marker studies in neoplasia, in: *Genetic Concepts and Neoplasia* (M. D. Anderson Hospital Symposium), pp. 112–137, Williams and Wilkins, Baltimore.

FINNEY, R., MCDONALD, G. A., BAIKIE, A. G., AND DOUGLAS, A. S., 1972, Chronic granulocytic leukemia with Ph negative cells in bone marrow and a ten year remission after Busulphan hypoplasia, *Brit. J. Haematol.* **23**:283.

FITZGERALD, P. H., 1965, Abnormal length of the small acrocentric chromosomes in chronic lymphocytic leukemia, *Cancer Res.* **25**:1094

FITZGERALD, P. H., CROSSEN, P. E., ADAMS, A. C., SHARMAN, C. V., AND GUNZ, F. W., 1966, Chromosome studies in familial leukemia, *J. Med. Genet.* **3**:96.

FITZGERALD, P. H., CROSSEN, P. E., AND HAMER, J. W., 1973, Abnormal karyotypic clones in human acute leukemia: Their nature and significance, *Cancer* **31**:1069.

FORD, C. E., 1966, The use of chromosome markers, in: *Tissue Grafting and Radiation* (H. Micklem and J. Loutit, eds.), pp. 197–206, Academic Press, New York and London.

FORNI, A., AND MOREO, L., 1967, Cytogenetic studies in a case of benzene leukemia, *Europ. J. Cancer* **3**:251.

FREED, J. J., AND SCHATZ, S. A., 1969, Chromosome aberrations in cultured cells deprived of single essential amino acids, *Exp. Cell Res.* **55**:393.

FREEMAN, A. E., AND HUEBNER, R. J., 1973, Problems in interpretation of experimental evidence of cell transformation, *J. Natl. Cancer Inst.* **50**:303.

GELLHORN, A., 1973, The background and promise of tumor virology, immunology, and chemotherapy and a challenge to radiotherapy, *Am. J. Roentgenol. Radium Ther. Nucl. Med.* **117**:489.

GERMAN, J., 1972, Genes which increase chromosomal instability in somatic cells and predispose to cancer, *Prog. Med. Genet.* **8**:61.

HARRIS, H., MILLER, O. J., KLEIN, G., WORST, P., AND TACHIBANA, T., 1969, Suppression of malignancy by cell fusion, *Nature (Lond.)* **223**:363.

HAUSCHKA, T. S., 1961, The chromosome in ontogeny and oncogeny, *Cancer Res.* **21**:957.

HECHT, F., McCAW, B. K., AND KOLER, R. D., 1973, Ataxia-telangiectasia—Clonal growth of translocation lymphocytes, *New Engl. J. Med.* **289**:286.

HITOTSUMACHI, S., RABINOWITZ, Z., AND SACHS, L., 1971, Chromosomal control of reversion in transformed cells, *Nature (Lond.)* **231**:511.

HSU, T. C., 1961, Chromosomal evolution in cell populations, *Int. Rev. Cytol.* **12**:69.

HUANG, C. C., MINOWADA, J., SMITH, R. T., AND OSUNKOYA, B. O., 1970, Revaluation of relationship between C chromosome marker and Epstein–Barr virus, *J. Natl. Cancer Inst.* **45**:815.

JACOBS, P., TOUGH, I. M., AND WRIGHT, D. H., 1963, Cytogenetic studies in Burkitt's lymphoma, *Lancet* **2**:1144.

JENSEN, M. K., AND PHILIP, P., 1970, Cytogenetic studies in potentially leukemic myeloid disorders, in: *Proceedings of the XIII International Congress of Hematology, Munich,* p. 20 (abst.).

JOHNSON, A. S., FRIEDMAN, R. M., AND PASTAN, I., 1971, Restoration of general morphological characteristics of normal fibroblasts in sarcoma cells treated with adenosine 3':5'-cyclic monophosphate and its derivatives, *Proc. Natl. Acad. Sci.* **68**:425.

KNUDSON, A. G., STRONG, L. C., AND ANDERSON, D. E., 1973, Heredity and cancer in man, *Prog. Med. Genet.* **9**:113.

KOHN, G., MELLMAN, W. J., MOORHEAD, P. S., LOFTUS, J., AND HENLE, G., 1967, Involvement of C-group chromosomes in five Burkitt lymphoma cell lines, *J. Natl. Cancer Inst.* **38**:209.

KOLLER, P. C., 1972, *The Role of Chromosomes in Cancer Biology,* Springer, New York.

LAWLER, S. D., MILLARD, R. E., AND KAY, H. E. M., 1970, Further cytogenetical investigations in polycythemia vera, *Europ. J. Cancer* **6**:223.

LEVAN, A., AND BIESELE, J. J., 1958, Role of chromosomes in cancerogenesis as studied in serial tissue culture of mammal cells, *Ann. N.Y. Acad. Sci.* **71**:1022.

MACPHERSON, I., 1970, Characteristics of animal cells transformed *in vitro, Advan. Cancer Res.* **13**:169.

MAKINO, S., 1956, Further evidence favoring the concept of the stem cell in ascites tumors of rats, *Ann. N.Y. Acad. Sci.* **14**:818.

MAKINO, S., 1963, Some epidemiologic aspects of venereal tumors of dogs as revealed by chromosome and DNA studies, *Ann. N.Y. Acad. Sci.* **108**:1106.

MANOLOV, G., AND MANOLOVA, Y., 1971, A marker band in one chromosome No. 14 in biopsies and cultures from Burkitt lymphomas, *Hereditas* **69**:300.

MARK, J., 1969, Rous sarcoma in mice: The chromosomal progression in primary tumors, *Europ. J. Cancer* **5**:307.

MARK, J., LEVAN, G., AND MITELMAN, F., 1972, Identification by fluorescence of the G chromosome lost in human meningiomas, *Hereditas* **71**:163.

MARTINEAU, M., 1966, A similar marker chromosome in testicular tumors, *Lancet* **1**:839.

McDOUGALL, J. K., 1970, Effects of adenoviruses on the chromosomes of normal human cells and cells trisomic for an E chromosome, *Nature (Lond.)* **225**:456.

MILES, C. P., GELLER, W., AND O'NEILL, F., 1966, Chromosomes in Hodgkin's disease and other malignant lymphomas, *Cancer* **19**:1103.

MILLARD, R. E., 1968, Chromosome abnormalities in the malignant lymphomas, *Europ. J. Cancer* **4**:97.

MILLARD, R. E., LAWLER, S. D., KAY, H. E. M., AND CAMERON, C. B., 1968, Further observations on patients with a chromosomal abnormality associated with polycythemia vera, *Brit. J. Haematol.* **14**:363.

MILLER, O. J., MILLER, D. A., AND WARBURTON, D., 1973, Application of new staining techniques to the study of human chromosomes, *Prog. Med. Genet.* **9**:1.

MILLER, R. W., AND TODARO, G. J., 1969, Viral transformation of cells from persons at high risk of cancer, *Lancet* **1**:81.

MITELMAN, F., 1971, The chromosomes of fifty primary Rous rat sarcomas, *Hereditas* **69**:155.

MOORHEAD, P. S., AND WEINSTEIN, D., 1966, Cytogenetic alterations during malignant transformation, in: *Recent Results in Cancer Research,* Vol. VI: *Malignant Transformation by Viruses* (W. Kirsten, ed.), pp. 104–111, Springer, New York.

NICHOLS, W. W., 1963, Relationships of viruses, chromosomes, and carcinogenesis, *Hereditas* **50**:53.

NICHOLS, W. W., 1966, The role of viruses in the etiology of chromosome aberrations, *Am. J. Hum. Genet.* **18**:81.

NICHOLS, W. W., LEVAN, A., CORIELL, L. L., GOLDNER, H., AND AHLSTRÖM, C. G., 1964, Chromosome abnormalities *in vitro* in human leukocytes associated with Schmidt–Ruppin Rous sarcoma virus, *Science* **146**:248.

NOWELL, P. C., 1965*a*, Unstable chromosome changes in tuberculin-stimulated leukocyte cultures from irradiated patients, *Blood* **26**:798.

NOWELL, P. C., 1965*b*, Chromosome changes in primary tumors, *Prog. Exp. Tumor Res.* **7**:83.

NOWELL, P. C., 1967, Chromosome abnormalities in the childhood leukemias, in: *The Clinical Pathology of Infancy* (F. Sunderman and F. Sunderman Jr., eds.), pp. 447–482, Thomas, Springfield, Ill.

NOWELL, P. C., 1969, Biological significance of induced human chromosome aberrations, *Fed. Proc.* **28**:1797.

NOWELL, P. C., 1971, Marrow chromosome studies in "preleukemia": Further correlation with clinical course, *Cancer* **28**:513.

NOWELL, P. C., AND COLE, L. J., 1965, Hepatomas in mice: Incidence increased after gamma irradiation at low dose rates, *Science* **148**:96.

NOWELL, P. C., AND HUNGERFORD, D. A., 1964, Chromosome changes in human leukemia and a tentative assessment of their significance, *J. Natl. Cancer Inst.* **27**:1013.

NOWELL, P. C., AND MORRIS, H. P., 1969, Chromosomes of "minimal deviation hepatomas": A further report on diploid tumors, *Cancer Res.* **29**:969.

NOWELL, P. C., MORRIS, H. P., AND POTTER, V. R., 1967, Chromosomes of "minimal deviation" hepatomas and some other transplantable rat tumors, *Cancer Res.* **27**:1565.

OHNO, S., 1971, Genetic implication of karyological instability of malignant somatic cells, *Physiol. Rev.* **51**:496.

O'RIORDAN, M.L., BERRY, E., AND TOUGH, I., 1970, Chromosome studies on bone marrow from a male control population, *Brit. J. Haematol.* **19**:83.

PECKHAM, M. J., 1972, Lymphocyte transformation in chronic lymphocytic leukemia, *Lancet* **1**:1127.

PEDERSEN, B., 1973, The blastic crisis of chronic myeloid leukemia: Acute transformation of a preleukemic condition? *Brit. J. Haematol.* **25**:141.

PEDERSEN, B., AND HAYHOE, F. G. J., 1971, Cellular changes in chronic myeliod leukemia, *Brit. J. Haemetol.* **21**:251.

PRASAD, K. N., 1972, Morphological differentiation induced by prostaglandin in mouse neuroblastoma cells in culture, *Nature (Lond.)* **236**:49.

PROPP, S., AND LIZZI, F. A., 1970, Philadelphia chromosome in acute lymphocytic leukemia, *Blood* **36**:353.

RABINOWITZ, Z., AND SACHS, L., 1970, Control of the reversion of properties in transformed cells, *Nature (Lond.)* **225**:136.

ROWLEY, J. D., 1970, The chromosomes in the myelodysplasias, in: *Myeloproliferative Disorders of Animals and Man* (W. Clark, ed.), pp. 556–569, US AEC, Washington.

ROWLEY, J. D., 1973, A new consistent chromosomal abnormality in chronic myelogenous leukemia identified by quinacrine fluorescence and Giemsa staining, *Nature (Lond.)* **243**:290.

SANDBERG, A. A., 1966, The chromosomes and causation of human cancer and leukemia, *Cancer Res.* **26**:2064.

SANDBERG, A. A., AND HOSSFELD, D. K., 1970, Chromosomal abnormalities in human neoplasia, *Ann. Rev. Med.* **21**:379.

SHAW, M. W., 1970, Human chromosome damage by chemical agents, *Ann. Rev. Med.* **21**:409.

STICH, H. F., 1960, Chromosomes of tumor cells. I. Murine leukemias induced by one or two injections of 7,12-dimethylbenz[a]anthracene, *J. Natl. Cancer Inst.* **25**:649.

STICH, H. F., 1963, Chromosome and carcinogenesis, *Canad. Cancer Conf.* **5**:99.

SUGIYAMA, T., KURITA, Y., AND NISHIZUKA, Y., 1967, Chromosome abnormality in rat leukemia induced by 7,12-dimethylbenz[a]anthracene, *Science* **158**:1058.

TASSONI, E. M., DURANT, J. R., BECKER, S., AND KRAVITZ, B., 1967, Cytogenetic studies in multiple myeloma: A study of fourteen cases, *Cancer Res.* **27**:806.

TODARO, G. J., GREEN, H., AND SWIFT, M. R., 1966, Human diploid fibroblasts transformed with SV40 or hybrid Adeno-7× SV40, *Science* **153:**1252.

TRUJILLO, J. M., AND OHNO, S., 1963, Chromosomal alteration of erythropoietic cells in chronic myeloid leukemia, *Acta Haematol.* **29:**311.

VON HANSEMANN, D., 1890 Über asymmetrische Zellteilung in Epithelkrebsen und deren biologische Bedeutung, *Virchows Arch. Pathol. Anat. Physiol.* **119:**298.

WALD, N., UPTON, A. C., JENKINS, V. K., AND BORGES, W. H., 1964, Mouse post-irradiation leukemia: Consistent occurrence of an extra and a marker chromosome, *Science* **143:**810.

WEBER, W. T., NOWELL, P. C., AND HARE, W. C. D., 1965, Chromosome studies of a transplanted and a primary canine venereal sarcoma, *J. Natl. Cancer Inst.* **35:**537.

WHANG, J., FREI, E., TJIO, J. H., CARBONE, P. P., AND BRECHER, G., 1963, The distribution of the Philadelphia chromosome in patients with chronic myelogenous leukemia, *Blood* **22:**664.

WHANG-PENG, J., CANELLOS, G. P., CARBONE, P. P., AND TJIO, J. H., 1968, Clinical implications of cytogenetic variants in chronic myelocytic leukemia (CML), *Blood* **32:**755.

WILSON, M. G., TOWNER, J. W., AND FUJIMOTO, A., 1973, Retinoblastoma and D-chromosome deletion, *Am. J. Hum. Genet.* **25:**57.

WOODLIFF, H. J., 1971, *Leukemia Cytogenetics,* Lloyd-Luke, London.

# 2

# Genetics: Animal Tumors

W. E. HESTON

## 1. Introduction

The development of our knowledge of the role of genes in the physiology and biochemistry of the cell during the past three-quarters of a century has erased any doubt that cancer is in some way genetic. It is inconceivable that anything so closely related to the physiology of the organism and the differentiation of the cell could be otherwise.

During the first decade of the century, Tyzzer, Haaland, Loeb, Murray, and Bashford had individually observed in mice that mammary cancer, the one so easily observed, occurred in certain families more than in others. Bashford (1909) and Murray (1911) kept pedigrees of their mice and noted that females in whose ancestry mammary cancer occurred not further back than grandmothers were more liable to develop cancer than those in whose ancestry it was more remote. During the second decade, Slye (1926) collected extensive pedigree data on her mice. She appears to have been motivated by the hope of demonstrating a simple mode of inheritance and the possibility of eradicating cancer through eugenics. Indeed, she concluded from her early data that cancer was inherited as a simple recessive gene. During subsequent decades, the problem of cancer has not been solved by eugenics, but genetics has had a very significant role in our continuing search for a complete understanding of the disease.

Genetics has given us the inbred strains with which to do cancer research. Genetics has helped us to understand that cancer is not a single disease but a group of different diseases, separate entities genetically. Genetics has contributed to our appreciation of the complexity of the problem, for few cancers are inherited as single genes; in fact, in the mouse most have been shown to behave as threshold characters influenced by multiple genetic and nongenetic factors. Genetics has

---

W. E. HESTON ● Laboratory of Biology, National Cancer Institute, National Institutes of Health, Bethesda, Maryland.

integrated the approaches to the problem, for each approach has had to take into account the genetic elements. The genetics of cancer has thus evolved as an integral part of all cancer research, helping us to understand the occurrence and nature of cancer, supplying us with the proper genetic material for the research, establishing the foundation for the immunological and immunogenetic studies of cancer, and leading to the identification of some of the cancer viruses. A major role in the immediate future will be in advancing our understanding of the transmission of these viruses.

## 2. Speciation and Tumor Formation

If the occurrence of cancer, even a specific kind of cancer, is influenced by genes, one would expect that in the course of evolution there would be established certain gene patterns which would tend to produce specific kinds of tumors in the different species. This has occurred. Tumors have been observed in practically all species of multicellular animals. Even plants have neoplasms, as any naturalist can tell you who has walked among the spruce trees on Mt. Desert Island in Maine and observed their huge tumors. It is particularly significant that some form of tumor occurs in the most lowly multicellular organism with little normal cell differentiation. This indicates that the basic neoplastic change involves a very primitive physiological process.

### 2.1. Invertebrates

Without becoming involved in the question of how far back in phylogeny one can rightfully call disorganized growth a true neoplasm, it can be accepted that such uncontrolled growth does occur, and from it certain basic information on neoplasia can be gained.

Neoplasms have not been described in sponges, possibly because they cannot be recognized in the primitive growth and differentiation of these forms, but abnormal growth structures do occur in the diploblastic coelenterates. Many who have worked with *Hydra* have observed the phenomenon described by Brien (1961). *Hydra pirardi* goes into a sexual phase when cultured at low temperatures, developing testes and ovaries. If the temperature is then raised, the testes involute and in their place sprouts of disorganized heads and other parts of the *Hydra* occur. This has sometimes been compared with teratogenesis in man, where a higher incidence of teratomas has occurred in undescended testes maintained at higher temperatures than that of the testes in the scrotal sac. It is also inconceivable that some of the genes of this primitive animal are not involved in the occurrence of these growths. Could these genetic mechanisms be comparable in some way to those controlling the occurrence of the genetic teratomas of the testes of strain 129 mice studied extensively by Stevens (1970)? If segregating differences could be demonstrated in *Hydra*, they might be analyzed more easily there than in the more complex mammal.

Higher up the evolutionary scale, spontaneous tumors have been described by Lange (1966) in two species of *Planaria*. These apparently are derived from the neoplasts, and they grow progressively and lead to lysis of the host. Tumors induced with carcinogens in other species of *Planaria* are also derived from this cell type (Foster, 1969), suggesting that in this lower organism any gene action involved may well be the same for the spontaneous and the induced neoplasms. Cooper (1969) believes that the earthworm may be an excellent species for investigating primitive neoplastic processes. Myoblastomas occur in *Lumbricus* spontaneously. They can be transplanted and studied immunologically. Fontaine (1969) has described in the echinoderm *Ophiocomina nigra* a pigmental tumor the growth and invasiveness of which suggest that it may be a true neoplasm. Neoplasms have been described in mollusks, but as Pauley (1969) points out in his review of these lesions, it is difficult to distinguish among neoplasia, hyperplasia, and injury response in them. These and other examples that could be given indicate that these primitive species of invertebrates can inherit genes that not only cause abnormal growths that in many cases could be called neoplasms, but also determine the type of neoplasm and the cell of origin.

It is in the insects where we first encounter significant genetic studies of neoplasia. Tumors or tumorlike lesions have been observed in crustaceans and have been studied in the cockroach, but the tumor that has received greatest genetic attention in the arthropods has been the small melanoma in *Drosophila*. This is not because it is a highly progressed neoplasm—in fact, there are those who still doubt that it is a true neoplasm—but it happens to occur in a species long a model for genetic studies. The tumors appear in the late larvae as rounded masses of cells that become surrounded by shells of melanin. They are transplantable but apparently not malignant, since they do not kill the host, probably because pupation stops their growth.

These tumors in *Drosophila* were first described by Bridges (1916) as being inherited as sex-linked lethals in a stock designated as *l(1)7*. Russell (1940) later attributed the lethality in this stock to an accompanying abnormality of the gut causing complete obliteration of the lumen so that the larvae die of starvation. She concluded that all the melanotic tumors in *Drosophila* were similar and that none was malignant. Russell's (1942) genetic analysis showed that the tumor factor in the *tu-36a* strain was located on chromosome II with modifiers on I and III. Hartung (1950) in his analysis of the inbred strain *bu tu* confirmed the presence of a recessive tumor factor on chromosome II and estimated the locus at 83.9. There was limited penetrance, however, in that his strain although inbred had a tumor incidence of only 40%. Nongenetic factors such as temperature, nutrition, and crowding could affect the incidence.

Some investigators have discounted the value of studies on these tumors since it can be questioned whether they represent true neoplasms. However, Burdette (1951) has found them of value in his attempted correlation between carcinogenesis and mutagenesis, since tests for both can be made in the same organism.

An inherited abnormality designated as "tumorous head" has been described in *Drosophila* (Gardner and Woolf, 1949; Gardner, 1959). The trait is caused by two interacting genes, *tu-1* on chromosome I and *tu-3* on chromosome III. Expression is influenced by modifying genes and also by temperature. Reciprocal crosses have revealed a maternal effect controlled by *tu-1*. There is no genetic relationship between tumorous head and the internal malanotic tumors, and there is no evidence that these irregular growths of the head are neoplastic.

## 2.2. Vertebrates

There is equal evidence among the vertebrates as among the invertebrates that in the evolution of the species certain gene complexes have been sorted out to give rise to specific tumors in specific species. This has been confirmed in the development of the inbred strains of mice and rats, where man has hastened selection of such gene patterns, as will be discussed later. Along with this process, oncogenic viruses have also been selected, and these or at least most of them have undoubtedly been transmitted genetically.

The melanoma of the platyfish–swordtail hybrid offers clear evidence of such selection of tumor genes. This neoplasm results from a complex of genes, some of which are contributed by each of the parent species. The genetics of this tumor will be discussed in a subsequent section along with that of other tumors resulting from hybridization.

Other tumors possibly also of genetic origin occur in fish. Schlumberger (1952) extensively studied a colonly of goldfish in the lily pond in front of the Art Museum on the campus of Case-Western Reserve University in Cleveland, Ohio, because these fish had a high incidence of neurilemomas and neurofibromas. It would appear that these neoplasms were due to genes or oncogenic viruses selected not only in this species but in this specific colony. No exogenous carcinogen could be identified, and bluegills and largemouthed black bass in the pool did not have these neoplasms. Recently, attention has been focused on the epidemic of hepatomas in rainbow trout from fish hatcheries (Halver and Mitchell, 1967). While it is now well established that these hepatomas were caused by aflatoxin contamination in the food, the fact that, in contrast to the highly susceptible rainbow trout, channel catfish were very resistant and coho salmon intermediate indicated the influence of genetic factors (Halver, 1969; Halver *et al.*, 1969).

Among the amphibians, attention has been focused on the Lucké adenocarcinoma of the kidney of leopard frogs, reviewed by Mizell (1969). This occurs naturally in a high proportion of frogs from certain geographical areas. Present evidence indicates that it is caused by a herpes-type virus, but the geographical restriction (McKinnell, 1969) suggests that genes for susceptibility are isolated in animals of those areas. The fact that in man herpes viruses appear to be associated with Burkitt's lymphoma and in chickens with Mareck's disease further suggests the establishment in the leopard frog of a gene complex limiting the neoplastic action of the virus to the kidney. Also, the viral information may yet be shown to be transmitted genetically in this species.

The predominant tumors of the domestic fowl belong to the group of
lymphomas and related neoplasms caused by the avian tumor viruses. These neoplasms have been a model for extensive, fruitful genetic studies integrated with studies of the viruses. In his summary of work in this area, Payne (1972) points out that host genes, sometimes single loci, have been identified which control virus infection, neoplastic transformation of the infected cell, and progressive growth of the neoplasm. There is also evidence of integration of this viral genetic material with the genome of the host, a discussion of which is beyond the scope of this chapter.

Schlumberger (1954) reported a large number of spontaneous chromophobe adenomas of the hypophysis in parakeets. No etiological factors were identified. If a virus was involved, it was not transmitted in unsuccessful attempts to transplant the neoplasm. Schlumberger pointed out that he had no evidence of a genetic factor in the induction of the tumors, yet the fact that this appears to be the most frequently occurring tumor in this species and that it occurs in this species probably more frequently that in any other species would certainly suggest that in the evolution of the parakeet a certain genetic complex favoring the development of this neoplasm had been established.

Progressing to mammals, certain tumors characteristic of species stand out. The tumor most often found in cattle surprisingly is not a mammary tumor—neoplasms of the udder are rare—but rather the ocular squamous carcinoma commonly known as "cancer eye." This is of great economic importance for the ranchers of the southwestern states with Hereford herds. From 3 to 10% of the animals must be removed each year because of the disease. Etiological agents include both nongenetic factors, particularly sunlight, and genetic factors. The genetic factors are of two groups, those controlling the amount of pigment of the eyelid—the greater the amount of pigment the less chance for cancer when it involves the eyelid—and those controlling susceptibility (Anderson, 1959). The gene loci for susceptibility and the loci for pigmentation do not appear to be the same. Although the possibility of a viral factor in the etiology is presently stressed in approaches to control of the disease, breeding systems have been outlined which undoubtedly would eliminate it (J. L. Lush, personal communication). However, it has been difficult to get a rancher to follow these breeding systems. He hesitates to eliminate a bull for which he may have paid several thousand dollars.

As the most typical tumor of the rat, one would probably have to name the induced sarcoma, although many other tumors can be induced. *Induced* denotes action of a carcinogen, but the fact that these sarcomas are so easily induced indicates the establishment of certain genetic complexes for susceptibility in this species.

Most striking about guinea pigs is their apparent resistance to neoplasms. Rogers (1951), who kept guinea pigs to very old age, observed a few spontaneous tumors, but they are rare in this species. It is interesting to speculate that this resistance may be the result of artificial genetic drift. From what one can ascertain, laboratory stocks of guinea pigs in this country were derived from European stocks, but it seems highly likely that they were originally derived from a relatively few animals brought from their native South America.

Lung tumors and subcutaneous tumors can be induced with the polycyclic hydrocarbons in guinea pigs, but unlike those in other species most of the induced subcutaneous tumors are liposarcomas (Shimkin and Mider, 1941; Russell and Ortega, 1952; Heston and Deringer, 1952b). This is a genetic characteristic of the guinea pig.

The widest spectrum of tumors outside the human species occurs in the laboratory mouse, undoubtedly because of the multitude of inbred strains in which genes for specific kinds of neoplasms have been purposely or unintentionally selected. This has led to the mouse being used more extensively in cancer research than any other species, which in turn has led to description of more tumors in the species (see Heston, 1960). When all strains are considered, probably leukemia and other reticulum cell neoplasms are the most prevalent tumors of the mouse. It appears now that C-type viruses are involved in the etiology of most of these neoplasms, but they are transmitted vertically, apparently as genes are transmitted, and thus may have become fixed during the evolution of the species much as gene complexes are fixed.

## 3. Hybridization and Tumor Formation

### 3.1. Hybridization of Species

Since cancer must be a negative selective factor in the evolution of species, there must have been some selection against certain complexes of genes or genes and viruses favoring the development of cancer which could be restored through hybridization of species. That this has in fact occurred is beautifully illustrated in the melanomas of platyfish–swordtail hybrids extensively studied by Gordon (1958).

The melanomas of these small fish result from stimulation of macromelanophores by certain modifying genes. The neoplasms are so invasive that it is hard to conceive of a species surviving with them. The platyfish (*Xiphophorus maculatus*) that Gordon collected in southeastern Mexico had the macromelanophores, which he showed are controlled by five dominant sex-linked genes, but within this species these cells do not become neoplastic. Of 9000 adults collected, 1879 had macromelanophores but in not one had they progressed to melanoma. The swordtail (*Xiphophorus helleri*) has the modifying genes which could cause the malignant change but they are balanced in this species by the recessive allele of the dominant genes for the macromelanophores. When Gordon hybridized the two species, bringing together the genes for the macromalanophores and the modifying genes in the $F_1$ hybrid, these large pigment cells developed into melanomas. A recent interpretation by Anders *et al.* (1974) is that the melanomas result from a loss in the hybrids of controller genes on chromosomes other than that with the macromelanophore genes.

Gordon also hybridized geographically distinct populations of the platyfish, but in these hybrids progression of the atypical growth was not as great as in the interspecies hybrids, indicating that the modifiers are not as divergent in the isolated populations of the same species as in the different species.

Alleles of the macromelanophore gene established the site of spotting, e.g., dorsal fin spotting or belly spotting. In the outcross, these alleles thus in turn established the location in which the melanoma would develop.

Melanin itself was not an important factor in the neoplastic process. When platyfish with macromelanophores were outcrossed to albino swordtails, the hybrids developed melanotic melanomas, but when these hybrids with melanomas were backcrossed to the albino swordtail parent, some of the backcross hybrids developed amelanotic melanomas. These had certain cellular characteristics of even a higher degree of malignancy than the pigmented neoplasms.

Diagnosis of malignancy was justified in that these melanomas eventually led to the death of the fish. However, transplantation was not possible because the fish were not inbred. Tissue culture of the melanotic tumors could be maintained, providing systems for biochemical studies of this form of neoplasia (Grand *et al.*, 1941).

Little (1939) recorded an increase in tumors resulting from hybridization of mammalian species. When he crossed the common laboratory mouse, *Mus musculus*, of strain C57BL, with the little Asiatic mouse, *Mus bactrianus*, he observed a higher incidence and greater variety of tumors in the $F_1$ than in either the C57BL strain or the stock of the small Asiatic species. Whereas nonepithelial tumors occurred in none of the *Mus bactrianus* mice and in only 13% of the C57BL, they occurred in 40% of the $F_1$ hybrids. Furthermore, multiple tumors were found more frequently in the $F_1$ hybrids.

## 3.2. Hybridization of Strains

Anyone who has hybridized inbred strains of mice and observed the $F_1$ generation for occurrence of tumors generally has found not only a higher incidence of tumors but also a greater variety of tumors in the $F_1$ than in either parent strain. This can be the result of bringing together more genes favoring tumor development, introduction of specific genes having a general positive effect on tumor development, or even production of new virus–gene combinations that cause tumors. In a cross between strains C3HfB (then called C3Hb) and C57BL, we noted a greater variety of tumors in the $F_1$ than in either parent strain, including some tumors not found in either strain (Heston and Deringer, 1952a). Yellow $F_1$ mice resulting from crossing various strains with the low tumor strain YBR usually had more tumors than either parent strain because of the $A^y$ gene introduced from YBR (Heston and Vlahakis, 1961). When one crosses strain BALB/c with a strain having a medium incidence of mammary tumors and having the mammary tumor virus (MTV), the resultant $F_1$ has a higher mammary tumor incidence than either parent strain because of combining the high genetic susceptibility of BALB/c with the MTV.

Two other reasons, both of which are basically genetic, for an increase of tumors in the $F_1$ are that $F_1$ mice tend to grow faster and live longer than either parent strain. Both of these factors tend to increase tumor incidence and a greater variety of tumors.

It is interesting to speculate whether hybridization in the people of the United States, in contrast to the more homogeneous populations of other countries, may have increased the occurrence of certain cancers. While this possibility exists, the degree of hybrid effect in the people of the United States cannot be expected to be comparable to that in a cross between two inbred strains of mice.

## 4. Inbreeding and Occurrence of Tumors

### 4.1. Development of Inbred Strains

With the early research on effects of inbreeding, from which Johannsen in 1903 postulated his pure-line theory as background, C. C. Little as early as 1909 could foresee that to make an adequate study of tumors genetically or otherwise it would be necessary to have genetically controlled strains of experimental animals. It was in that year that he started inbreeding strain DBA mice. Inbreeding increases the percentage of gene pairs that are homozygous, the rate of increase depending on the mating system used. An inbred strain has been defined as one in which brother and sister inbreeding has been performed for 20 or more generations. With that number of inbred generations, the percentage of homozygous genes would theoretically exceed 99%.

Origins and relationships of the inbred strains are of importance. In 1921, Little started the C57 strains and strain C58 from mice received from Miss Lathrop. Two females, 57 and 58, were mated to littermate male 52. Offspring from female 57 segregated as black and brown, and these segregants when inbred gave rise to strains C57BL and C57BR. Strain C57L was derived from a leaden mutation that later arose in C57BR. MacDowell inbred the offspring of female 58, developing strain C58.

A second family of strains is that derived from strain DBA that Little had started from a stock with the three coat color mutations dilution (*d*), brown (*b*), and nonagouti (*a*) and from the Bagg albino mice. Dr. Halsey Bagg started the Bagg albinos from some albino mice he obtained in 1913 from a dealer in Ohio. In 1920, Dr. L. C. Strong crossed the Bagg albinos with Little's strain DBA and from the hybrids inbred several strains including the well-known C3H and CBA. In 1921, Strong crossed a Bagg albino mouse with one from an albino stock that Little had and from these hybrids inbred strain A. About a year later, MacDowell started inbreeding some Bagg albinos, giving rise to strain BALB/c.

Other strains have been derived elsewhere such as two originated in Europe, RIII started by Dr. Dobrovolskaia-Zavadskaia and GR inbred more recently by Mühlbock, but the major part of cancer research throughout the world has been done with mice of these two families of strains that were started in the first quarter

of the century by Little and by Strong. Since then, many geneticists have
contributed to the inbreeding of these strains, developing the various sublines we
have today, but the origins of the strains have continued to be of extreme
importance in understanding observations made on them.

41
GENETICS:
ANIMAL
TUMORS

## 4.2. Tumor Characteristics of Inbred Strains of Mice

Certain of these strains were developed as high tumor strains not as a result of the
inbreeding *per se* but by the selection during inbreeding of susceptibility genes and
related oncogenic viruses. Little selected for mammary tumors in strain DBA, but
the Bagg albinos also must have had susceptibility genes and the mammary tumor
virus (MTV), for strain BAGG was a high mammary tumor strain, as was strain A.
In the process of inbreeding strain BALB/c from the Bagg albinos, the virus must
have been lost, for BALB/c has the susceptibility genes but not the MTV. It was
also from the DBA and Bagg albino source that C3H received susceptibility genes
and the MTV. Probably all lines of MTV have come from this narrow source
except the lines in strains RIII, GR, and DD, which may be a third family of strains.
Although strain DD was developed in Japan, it originally came from Central
Europe, where RIII and GR were derived, and all three have the same coat color
genes and all develop premalignant hormone-responsive plaques from which at
least some of their mammary tumors originate. In contrast, in the American-
derived strains the mammary tumors appear to originate in hyperplastic nodules.

The DBA–Bagg albino family also contains the high lung tumor strains A and
BALB/c and the high hepatoma strains C3H and CBA. Selection for these tumors
was done without anyone being aware of it, for these strains were discovered as
being high lung tumor and high hepatoma strains after they were inbred.

Except for C58, which is a high leukemia strain, the strains in the Lathrop
family of strains have generally been used as low tumor strains. It is interesting,
however, that all the C57 strains related to the high leukemia strain C58 have a
relatively high incidence of other reticulum cell neoplasms.

## 4.3. Role of Inbred Strains and Their Hybrids in Cancer Research

These inbred strains of mice, and to a lesser degree inbred strains of rats, guinea
pigs, and now rabbits, hamsters, and chickens, have supplied the tumors for basic
cancer research. They also have supplied groups of experimental animals that are
genetically identical in which response is uniform and from which repeatable
results can be obtained with smaller numbers.

Wide use has likewise been made of the $F_1$ hybrid between two inbred strains.
Like animals of the parent inbred strains, the $F_1$ hybrids are genetically uniform,
although heterogeneity occurs with any further matings. There are several
advantages offered by the $F_1$. Deleterious genes tend to be recessive but their
effects are often suppressed in the $F_1$, resulting in more vigorous, longer-lived
animals than those of either parental inbred strain. Furthermore, by proper

choice of parental strains, one can get many desirable gene–gene, gene–virus, or gene–absence of virus combinations. Today, there are approximately 200 inbred strains of mice, and from 200 one could get 39,800 kinds of reciprocal hybrids. In addition, by systems of backcross matings, as Snell (1958) originally demonstrated, isogenic lines can be developed. These are two lines of an inbred strain that differ only at one gene locus and possibly closely linked loci. If the concept of an oncogene or provirus proves to be a reality with respect to oncogenic viruses, it presumably will be possible through a similar mating system to develop two lines exactly alike except that one has the genetically transmitted virus and the other does not. In all these ways, genetics has amply provided the animal material with which to do cancer research.

## 5. Genetics of Spontaneous Tumors

### 5.1. The Threshold Concept in the Inheritance of Cancer

The development of the inbred strains in itself yielded significant data on the inheritance of cancer. The fact that through inbreeding with selection strains were produced that developed specific kinds of cancer of specific incidences generation after generation was good evidence that genes were involved. We have since come to realize that in addition to genes certain viruses also were selected, the most recent concept being that they were selected as a segment of the host genome—the provirus as conceived by Bentvelzen (1972) or the oncogene as conceived by Huebner (see Huebner and Gilden, 1972).

Of special significance was the fact that the incidence of a specific kind of spontaneous tumor in an inbred strain, although relatively constant from generation to generation, usually fell someplace between zero and 100%. At the time, the genetics of lung tumors in the mouse was being studied extensively (Lynch, 1940; Heston, 1942a, b); the incidence in strain A was 90% instead of 100% and the incidence in strains C57BL and C57L was less than 5% but not zero. Yet the incidence in BALB/c was 20% and the incidence in Lynch's SWR was approximately 40%. The same picture prevailed even when a virus was involved, as in mammary tumors in the mouse.

In this regard, tumors fell in line with other so-called threshold characters. In working with otocephaly and polydactyly in inbred strains of guinea pigs, Wright (1934a, b) had first described this kind of character as one influenced by multiple genetic and nongenetic factors, the character appearing when the total effect of these factors surpassed certain physiological thresholds. The factors leading to the occurrence of such a trait can encompass inherited genes, inherited or introduced viruses, endogenous or exogenous hormones, physical or chemical carcinogens, or even ordinary nutritional factors. Deficiencies in one set of factors can be overcome by introduction of others. Time can be a factor, and thus latency as well as incidence can be a measure of response.

But what is this threshold? Obviously, it is the neoplastic change in the cell, and in certain tumors where there are well-defined preneoplastic stages there is more than one threshold. Early attempts to define this change or these changes gave birth to the somatic mutation hypothesis, the concept that the malignant change involves a mutation in the genetic material of the somatic cell. No hypothesis concerning cancer has through the years stimulated more discussion than this one, and in the end resolution depends on just how one defines mutation, but some change in the genetic material of the cell is indicated.

In the past, approaches to confirmation of the hypothesis had to be indirect, because it was not possible to hybridize somatic cells. One approach was to look for a positive correlation between mutagenicity and carcinogenicity, and within certain limits there was a positive correlation. The alkylating agents that were shown to induce mutations in *Drosophila* (Auerbach, 1949) induced lung tumors in mice when injected intravenously or inhaled and induced sarcomas when injected subcutaneously (Heston, 1953). But a detailed review by Burdette (1955) of data on all agents tested for mutagenicity and carcinogenicity did not establish a 100% positive correlation. Burdette tested for both carcinogenicity and mutagenicity in *Drosophila* using the induction of the melanomas as his measure of carcinogenicity and the induction of lethal mutations in the special stocks as his measure of mutagenicity. Even these tests in the same species did not give an absolute answer, and the plaguing question was whether these melanomas in *Drosophila* are true neoplasms. Yet the hypothesis continued to stimulate research. For example, when it was shown that increased oxygen increased the mutation rate in lower organisms, strain A mice were exposed to various oxygen levels. It was found that oxygen concentration greater than that in air increased the number of methylcholanthrene-induced lung tumors and concentrations less than that of air decreased the number (Heston and Pratt, 1959).

Another approach to information relative to the somatic mutation hypothesis has been through an analysis of the dose–response curve in induced tumors. In their analysis of the number of papillomas induced in mice with repeated paintings with benzpyrene, Charles and Luce-Clauson (1942) noted a linear relationship between the square root of the number of papillomas and the elapsed time, which would be proportional to the cumulative dose of carcinogen. This indicates the necessity of two events in the neoplastic change, which would be expected with a recessive gene mutation. In contrast, Heston and Schneiderman (1953) observed a straight-line relationship between the number of induced pulmonary tumors in mice and the dose of the carcinogen dibenz[*a,h*]anthracene above a certain low threshold. This indicated the necessity of only a single event, which if a gene mutation would be dominant.

Today the somatic mutation hypothesis is finding supporting evidence in viral carcinogenesis. It is generally assumed that in the cell neoplastically transformed by a DNA virus the viral genetic material has been integrated in the cell genome as a provirus. Furthermore, it now appears that with the recently demonstrated

RNA-dependent DNA polymerase DNA copies of RNA oncornaviruses are made which then serve as a template for further RNA synthesis, resulting in the neoplastic conversion. It is suggested that this synthesized DNA provirus is integrated in the host genome. Bentvelzen and Daams (1972) have pointed out that this would be a form of somatic mutation, a concept suggested earlier but without the present substantiating evidence (Heston, 1963).

## 6. Genetics of Chemically Induced Tumors

### 6.1. Pulmonary Tumors in Mice

Chemically induced pulmonary tumors of the mouse offered a great advantage for genetic analysis in that by counting the induced nodules one obtained a quantitative measure of response. Responses measured in this way of susceptible strain A and resistant strain C57L and their hybrids to intravenous injection of dibenz[$a,h$]anthracene were typical of characters with multiple-factor quantitative inheritance (Heston, 1942$a$). $F_1$ hybrids were intermediate between the parent strains, as were the $F_2$s, but the distribution curve of the $F_2$ showed a greater spread than that of the $F_1$, indicating segregation of genes. From a comparison of the variance of the $F_2$ with that of the $F_1$, it was estimated that the parent strains differed by at least four pairs of genes controlling susceptibility.

An analysis of the genetics of induced pulmonary tumors was then made using latent period as a measure of response, and again the results indicated multiple gene inheritance. Then the carcinogen was omitted and response was measured in incidence and latent period. The results indicated that spontaneous pulmonary tumors, like the induced tumors, were controlled by multiple genes (Heston, 1942$b$).

One advantage in working with the induced pulmonary tumors was that the latent period was greatly reduced, which along with the quantitative measure of response has greatly facilitated linkage studies. Lethal yellow ($A^y$) on chromosome 1 was associated with an increase in lung tumors. Vestigial tail ($vt$), shaker-2 ($sh$-$2$), and waved-2 ($w$-$2$) on chromosome 11, obese ($ob$) on chromosome 6, flexed-tail ($f$) on chromosome 13, hairless ($hr$) on chromosome 14, and fused ($fu$) on chromosome 17 all were associated with a decrease in lung tumors. Dwarf ($dw$) inhibited lung tumors (Heston, 1957; Burdette, 1952). It would appear, however, that these results represented the effect of the genes themselves rather than true linkage, that they were in some way related to the effect of the genes on normal growth. Each gene affected normal growth in the same direction as it affected the number of induced tumors, or in the case of spontaneous tumors the incidence of tumors.

Tatchell (1961) obtained similar results in her test for linkage with the genes $wa$-$2$, $sh$-$2$, and $vt$ on chromsome 11. She interpreted her results as indicating true linkage with a tumor gene that she designated as $tu$. Her observations, however, were based on coupling data and were not confirmed by repulsion data. From results of crosses between strains A and C57BL, Bloom and Falconer (1964) postulated a pulmonary tumor resistant gene *ptr*, but this proposed gene has not been located in a linkage group.

## 6.2. Subcutaneous Sarcomas in Mice

In general, the genetics of chemically induced subcutaneous sarcomas in mice is similar to that of pulmonary tumors. The fact that the inbred strains differed in their response to subcutaneous injection of a carcinogen indicated the influence of genetic factors. Andervont (1938) mated susceptible strain C3H with resistant strains I and Y and noted that the susceptibility of the $F_1$ hybrids to induced subcutaneous tumors was intermediate between that of the parent strains. He concluded that if there were genetic factors involved they probably were multiple. Later, Burdette (1943) measured the susceptibility of strains C3H and JK mice and their $F_1$ hybrids to methylcholanthrene-induced subcutaneous sarcomas and observed that the $F_1$s were intermediate between the susceptible C3H and the resistant JK. He concluded that these observations were compatible with the existence of more than one gene controlling susceptibility, at least one of which was dominant and at least one recessive.

## 6.3. Selection of Appropriate Strain for Testing Carcinogens

This concept of multiple-factor inheritance involving a threshold assists in the selection of the genetically appropriate strain for testing a suspected carcinogen. Any population of experimental animals when plotted according to the total genetic and nongenetic susceptibility factors of each would have a bell-shaped distribution, with a few relatively susceptible animals, a few relatively resistant animals, and most of the animals in between these extremes. For the inbred strain with reduced genetic variation, this distribution would be narrowed. With constant nongenetic factors, the genotype of the inbred strain would determine the tumor incidence by determining where this distribution fell with respect to the tumor threshold. The role of the carcinogen could be viewed as that of shifting the distribution of the population to the right, bringing a greater percentage of the individuals beyond the threshold and thus increasing the incidence of tumors. When the genetic susceptibility of the strain is relatively weak so that only the outer edge of the bell-shaped distribution is beyond the threshold, the shift in this distribution by a carcinogen, especially if it is a weak carcinogen, may not bring enough of the whole population beyond the threshold to make a significant increase in incidence. When the genetic susceptibility is very strong so that all except the lower tail of the distribution is above the threshold, the shift in the population by the same carcinogen also may not make a significant change in incidence. However, when the genetic susceptibility of the strain approximately equally distributes the population above and below the threshold the same shift to the right in the population distribution by this carcinogen will bring a much greater portion of the total population beyond the threshold, giving a significant increase in tumor incidence. Thus the appropriate inbred strain for testing whether a substance is carcinogenic is neither one that has a high genetic susceptibility nor one that has a low genetic susceptibility but a strain with an intermediate susceptibility.

Carbon tetrachloride could not be shown to be carcinogenic in C3H mice. In this highly susceptible strain, it did not increase the occurrence of hepatomas above the spontaneous incidence. Its hepatic carcinogenicity was discovered in the less susceptible strain A. Dibenz[a,h]anthracene probably would not have been shown to be carcinogenic for pulmonary tumors had it been tested only in the genetically very resistant strain C57L. Only a very long time after administration of the carcinogen did any pulmonary tumors appear, and then they were so few and so small that they would have been overlooked in a casual examination. Yet the same dose of dibenz[a,h]anthracene induces multiple lung tumors in 100% of the more susceptible strain BALB/c mice.

A carcinogen should not be considered only as a substance that will induce tumors in a strain of mouse that otherwise never gets tumors. Such a strain in which a certain kind of tumor never occurs is probably nonexistent. Furthermore, by selecting very resistant strains one would probably miss many potential carcinogens. The aim in carcinogenic testing is to ascertain whether or not the substance to be tested will cause tumors to arise in any animals that would not have gotten them without the substance.

With the bell-shaped distribution in mind, one can visualize the argument for using an inbred strain rather than a heterogeneous population of test animals. The object is not to duplicate the heterogeneous population of human beings but to get an established, repeatable result. This can be done best by selecting an inbred strain the distribution of which falls in proper relation to the threshold so that an increase in tumors can be noted. Since it is inbred, with a narrower distribution, a significant increase in incidence can be shown with fewer animals, and since the inbred strain is genetically uniform the result is repeatable.

Of course, the results of testing for carcinogenesis in an inbred strain of mice or rats cannot necessarily be applied to a particular human being. Results of testing in one human being might not be applicable to a second human being, for they would probably differ in genetic susceptibility. If a substance can be shown to be carcinogenic in a mammal such as the mouse or rat, it is highly probable that some human beings would have the degree of susceptibility for the substance to induce tumors in them. It is these susceptible individuals about whom we are concerned.


## 7. Genetics of Hormonally Induced Tumors

### 7.1. Mammary Tumors

Even before the discovery of the mammary tumor virus, it was known that hormones were influential in the induction of mammary tumors in mice. Castration reduced the occurrence of mammary tumors in female mice, and

stilbestrol induced mammary tumors in castrated males. In practically all mouse
strains, parity increased the incidence of mammary tumors or lowered the tumor
age in proportion to the number of litters born.

This effect of parity was much more noticeable in strains with a median
susceptibility than in either the very susceptible or the very resistant strains. Both
breeding and virgin females of the highly susceptible strain C3H have a mammary
tumor incidence of 100%, but the tumors arise about 2 months later in the virgins
than in the breeders. But in strain C3HfB, with a lower mammary tumor
incidence because of the absence of the milk-borne MTV, the incidence is
significantly higher in breeders than in virgins. In the highly resistant strain
C57BL, in which few mammary tumors occur, breeding does not significantly
increase their occurrence. Yet in strain A, in which with MTV the incidence in
breeders is around 70%, the incidence in virgins is about 5 or 10%.

In reciprocal crosses between the highly susceptible strain C3H, in which the
effect of parity was expressed only as a 2-months' difference in tumor age, and
strain A, in which parity greatly increased the mammary tumor incidence, both
groups of $F_1$ females had a high mammary tumor incidence (Bittner et al., 1944;
Heston and Andervont, 1944). This indicated that the difference in effect of parity
of these two strains was basically a genetic difference that could be expressed
through control over hormonal production or over response of the mammary cell
to hormonal stimulation. The fact that both conditions prevailed was evident from
results of Huseby and Bittner (1948), who transplanted ovaries between the
parent strains C3H and A and their $F_1$ hybrids. Spayed (C3H × A)$F_1$ females
bearing C3H and (C3H × A) $F_1$ transplanted ovaries had a higher tumor
incidence than did those $F_1$ females with A ovaries, suggesting, since the hosts
were the same and the ovaries were different, that genic action was controlling
amount of hormone produced by the ovary. However, $F_1$ females bearing A
ovaries had a higher tumor incidence than spayed A females bearing transplanted
A ovaries, indicating that some genic action was controlling response of the
mammary cell to the hormonal stimulation from the ovary since in this case the
ovaries were the same but the hosts were different.

## 7.2. Hypophyseal Tumors

The usual tumor of the hypophysis of the mouse is the chromophobe adenoma,
and it occurs rarely except in the C57 strains. In a recent tabulation in this
laboratory (Heston et al., 1973) of 151 untreated C57BL virgin females, 49 had
chromophobe adenomas of the hypophysis and one had a tumor of the pars
intermedia.

Prolonged treatment with estrogenic hormones induces these chromophobe
adenomas, particularly in the susceptible C57 strains. In the study referred to
above, there were 149 C57BL females continuously fed the antifertility drug
Enovid, which contains estrogen, and of these 89 developed chromophobe
adenomas, a significant increase over the untreated mice. Yet the Enovid did not
produce a significant increase in the other four strains used in the study.

Gardner and Strong (1940) had observed induction of hypophyseal tumors in C57BL mice with prolonged estrogen treatment but not in strains A, C3H, CBA, C12I, N, and JK similarly treated. When Gardner (1954) crossed C57BL with the resistant strains CBA and C3H, he observed a high incidence in the estrogen-treated $F_1$ hybrids approaching that in the C57BL, and this high incidence was maintained in the backcross generation of the $F_1$ to the C57BL, but greatly reduced in the backcross to the CBA. Similar results were observed in this laboratory (Heston, unpublished data). The strain differences in occurrence of tumors of the hypophysis suggest the influence of genetic factors on this tumor, and these results from the $F_1$ and backcross hybrids indicate segregation of such genes.

## 7.3. Adrenocortical Tumors

Spontaneous adrenocortical tumors occur in the mouse, particularly in certain strains. Accurate incidences were obtained for five strains in a study mentioned above (Heston *et al.*, 1973) in which the adrenals were routinely fixed and sectioned from control virgin females permitted to live their natural life span. Strain BALB/c was the susceptible strain, with these tumors found in 43 of 163 mice. In contrast, one of 55 C3H females and seven of 156 C3HfB females had adrenocortical tumors, but none occurred in 169 strain A and 151 strain C57BL females. Such strain differences indicate the influence of genetic factors.

However, genetic influences have been much more clearly shown in studies by Woolley *et al.* (1941, 1953) on the occurrence of the adrenocortical tumors in various strains of mice by neonatal gonadectomy. The most susceptible strain was CE/Wy, in which all the mice developed adrenocortical carcinomas following early gonadectomy. The adrenal glands of strain DBA/2Wy also responded to early gonadectomy, but the lesion progressed only to hyperplasia of the cortex. With the same treatment, hybrids of the two strains always developed adrenocortical carcinomas, indicating dominance of the carcinoma.

An interesting hybrid effect was noted in some crosses (Dickie, 1954). When strain A/Wy, which showed little change in the adrenal gland following gonadectomy, was crossed with C3H/Di, which responded with nodular hyperplasia, the $F_1$ hybrids after gonadectomy responded with adrenocortical carcinomas. The same response was also observed in $F_1$ hybrids between DBA, which responded with nodular hyperplasia, and DE/Wy, which gave little response in the adrenal glands. These results can be compared with those of Gordon (1958) reviewed earlier on the production of melanomas in the platyfish hybrids. It would appear that the neoplastic response of the adrenal gland to neonatal gonadectomy in the mouse was due to multiple genes controlling the degree of response, and in certain crosses genes that were contributed from both parents could result in carcinoma in the hybrid whereas in neither parent strain did progression extend beyond hyperplasia.

## 8. Genetics of Virally-Induced Tumors

### 8.1. Inheritance of Susceptibility to the Mammary Tumor Virus

Following their development of high and low mammary tumor strains of mice, geneticists made one of the signal discoveries of cancer research—the discovery of the mouse mammary tumor virus. The original observation was made simultaneously by the staff of the Jackson Laboratory (1933), where many of these strains were being inbred, and by Korteweg (1934) at the Netherlands Cancer Institute with strains he had obtained from the Jackson Laboratory. In crossing their high and low strains, both groups had the good fortune to make reciprocal crosses. The observation was that the $F_1$ females tended to develop mammary cancer when their mothers were of the high tumor strain but not when their fathers were of the high tumor strain. This indicated that some causative factor was being transmitted from the mother, and since the reciprocal $F_1$ females were genetically identical it had to be some extrachromosomal factor. The sequence of events that followed is well known. Through his foster-nursing experiments, Bittner (1939) showed that this extrachromosomal factor was passed through the milk; he referred to it as the "milk agent." Later, the agent was shown to be filtrable, a particle was seen, and this agent became accepted as a mammary tumor virus which in the mature virion is now referred to as the "B particle."

Evidence that this virus was under genetic control accumulated. It was only in certain strains that this virus replicated and was transmitted well. Strain C3H had the virus and it caused a high mammary tumor incidence, but when the virus was removed by foster-nursing C3H on C57BL, the C3HfB, as it was now designated, had a greatly reduced mammary tumor incidence with an increased latent period, and remained thusly through successive generations. When the virus was reintroduced, the picture in the original C3H was immediately restored. Strain BALB/c did not have the milk-transmitted virus and had a low mammary tumor incidence, but it was obviously genetically susceptible to the virus because when infected with C3H virus BALB/c immediately became a high mammary tumor strain and remained so generation after generation. In contrast, when C3H MTV was introduced into C57BL, although some of the originally infected females developed mammary tumors the virus died out in a generation or two, indicating that C57BL was genetically resistant to it (Andervont, 1945).

Proof that segregating genes did in fact control the replication of the virus came from a hybridization study by Heston *et al.* (1945). High tumor strain C3H females with MTV were mated to low tumor strain C57BL males. The resulting $F_1$ females, also with MTV which caused a high mammary tumor incidence in them, were then backcrossed on the one hand to strain C3H males and on the other to C57BL males. That the resulting C3H backcross females could replicate and transmit the agent better than the C57BL backcross females was shown by a higher tumor incidence in test females foster-nursed by the C3H backcross females than in the same kind of test females foster-nursed by the C57BL backcross females. This difference in degree of replication and transmission had to be the result of the difference between the C3H genes and the C57BL genes in these two groups of backcross females.

Later studies (Heston *et al.*, 1956) showed that in further backcrosses to the C57BL males the MTV was completely eliminated, and this was done as early as the third backcross generation. This indicated that the virus was controlled by only a few genes and possibly only one. However, a later attempt (Heston, 1960) to show distinct backcross groups segregated as to their ability to transmit MTV failed, indicating that the influencing genes must be multiple.

Another significant observation in these backcross studies was that once the MTV was eliminated by eliminating the susceptibility genes it could not be caused to reappear by then backcrossing to C3H males to reintroduce the susceptibility genes. None of these genes was the more recently described provirus that will be discussed in a later section.

## 8.2. Inheritance of Susceptibility to Leukemia

In some respects, the genetics of leukemia has paralleled that of mammary tumors. Through selection, high and low leukemia inbred strains of mice were developed. These were then hybridized in attempts to observe patterns of segregation.

Cole and Furth (1941) crossed the high leukemia strain AKR with the low leukemia strain Rf and from the incidences of leukemia in the $F_1$, $F_2$, $F_3$, and backcross generations concluded that leukemia was probably inherited as a multiple-factor character. The common logarithm of the percent leukemia in the various crosses was a simple function of the percent heredity from the AKR strain.

Another attempt to ascertain whether single-gene segregation could be demonstrated in leukemia was carried out by MacDowell *et al.* (1945) in one of the most carefully executed genetic experiments in all of cancer research. The approach was through progeny tests of 50 backcross males that were the progeny of (susceptible C58 × resistant Sto-Li)$F_1$ females backcrossed to Sto-Li males. The question was whether the incidence of leukemia in the progeny of each of these males would show them to be intrinsically uniform or diverse in regard to the tendency to leukemia. Results showed that the males were diverse. The incidences of leukemia in the 50 backcross families varied from zero to 42.8%, which indicated the segregation of genes. However, instead of the families grouping as would be expected from segregation of a single pair or few pair of genes, the frequency distribution was fairly symmetrical with the modal class as 17–20%. Thus it was apparent that genes were influential in the causation of leukemia but that the number of such genes by which these two strains differed was multiple.

## 8.3. Genetic Transmission of Tumor Viruses

### 8.3.1. MuLV

Gross (1951) made cell-free filtrates from leukemic AKR mice and injected them into C3H mice, which later developed leukemia. He then noted that this leukemia

was transmitted from parent to offspring through future generations of the C3H
mice. He referred to this as "vertical" transmission of what experiments later proved to be a leukemia virus. There was, however, a clear distinction between this vertical transmission of leukemia and the vertical transmission of the mammary tumor virus that had been described earlier. The mammary tumor virus known at that time was transmitted maternally through the milk, but, as Gross rightfully noted, crosses involving AKR mice had shown that the leukemia was transmitted by the father as well as by the mother. He therefore considered that this vertical transmission of leukemia was through the embryo, presumably from the sperm and egg.

Stimulated by these earlier observations of vertical transmission of leukemia in mice now recognized as due to C-type RNA virus, Huebner and Todaro (1969) carried out seroepidemiological and cell culture studies from which they formulated the hypothesis that the cells of most or all vertebrate species have C-type RNA virus genome. They refer to this viral information as the "virogene," which would include that portion causing the normal cell to undergo the malignant transformation which they have termed the "oncogene" (see Huebner and Gilden, 1972). Physical and chemical carcinogens and other factors associated with the normal aging process would induce the leukemia through the activation or derepression of the oncogene. It is this viral information that is inherited, presumably as an integrated portion of the chromosome. Further discussion of the genetics of the virus and the mechanisms through which it induces the neoplasm is found in other chapters of this volume.

Genetic studies of the vertical transmission of the mouse leukemia virus have been carried out by Rowe and coworkers (Rowe, 1972; Rowe and Hartley, 1972; Rowe et al., 1972) through hybridization of high and low leukemia mouse strains. They used the high leukemia strain AKR, in which the virus is normally transmitted vertically and can be detected readily as appearance of virus infectivity. The bone of the tail was found to be high in virus, providing readily accessible tissue for viral assay in tissue culture by the technique they describe. The AKR virus is N-tropic; i.e., it replicates readily in the presence of a gene, $Fv-1^n$ that AKR carries. Strain AKR was outcrossed to five low leukemia mouse strains, all of which also carried the $Fv-1^n$ gene so that maximum opportunity should have been provided for replication of the virus in any hybrids that had inherited the virus inducing locus or loci which might actually be the viral information. $F_1$, $F_2$, and first and second backcross hybrids were produced and tested for virus in the tails at 2 wk of age and again at 6 wk.

Results with the $F_1$ hybrids indicated dominant inheritance with high penetrance of the AKR viruses contributed equally well by both sexes. Segregation ratios of the $F_2$ and first backcross generations, however, did not show single-gene or two-gene inheritance, but indicated that the virus resulted from the presence of either of two independently segregating genes, which initially were labeled $V_1$ and $V_2$. Tests of 19 second backcross generation families indicated that three (or four) of the first backcross parents carried two virus-inducing loci, 12 (or 13) carried one, and three carried none. This substantiated the two-locus model indicated by the $F_2$ and first backcross generations.

In an attempt to determine if the virus-inducing loci in AKR actually contain MuLV genetic determinants or are genes which promote the expression of the viral information located elsewhere (presumably Huebner's oncogene), strain AKR ($Fv-1^n$ genotype and with N-tropic virus) was outcrossed to four low leukemia strains of the $Fv-1^b$ genotype which are sensitive to B-tropic virus and relatively resistant to the N-tropic virus. Since the segregating hybrids could be $Fv-1^n$, $Fv-1^{nb}$, and $Fv-1^b$, one would expect all the hybrids to carry N-tropic AKR MuLV if the virus-inducing loci were genetic elements of the virus itself, whereas virus-positive hybrids should show virus of both parental types if the virus-inducing loci merely promoted the expression of the "oncogene" located elsewhere. The virus identified in the segregating hybrids was almost always of the AKR type, providing evidence that the $V_1$ and $V_2$ loci contain MuLV genetic determinants.

By utilization of the markers carried by the various strains, it was demonstrated that one of the virus-inducing loci ($V_1$) was linked with albinism (c) and the β-chain of hemoglobin locus (Hbb) in linkage group I with the probable gene order $V_1$–c–Hbb, and with $V_1$ about 30 units from the c–Hbb region. In a later cross (Rowe et al., 1973) involving the locus for the isozymes of glucose phosphate isomerase (Gpi-1) also in linkage group I, it was established that $V_1$ is about 12 units from Gpi-1, the order now being $V_1$–Gpi-1–c–Hbb. Other crosses have now located in linkage group VIII the $Fv-1$ locus, the major determinant of the sensitivity of mouse cells to infection with naturally occurring MuLV.

### 8.3.2. MTV

The mouse mammary tumor virus was originally observed to be transmitted through the milk, but over the past 25 years evidence has also been accumulating for genetic transmission of mouse MTV. Strain C3HfB/He, derived in this laboratory in 1945 by foster-nursing caesarean-derived C3H mice on C57BL to remove the milk-transmitted MTV, instead of having no mammary tumors as expected had an incidence among breeding females of approximately 40% (Heston et al., 1950). The tumors in these C3HfB females, however, arose at an average age of 18 months rather than the 7 months observed in the C3H. In contrast to the early crosses between high and low tumor lines in which maternal transmission was demonstrated, when C3HfB was crossed with C57BL no difference in tumor incidence was observed between the reciprocal hybrids, indicating that the factor or factors causing the mammary tumors in C3HfB were transmitted by the male parent as well as by the female parent (Heston and Deringer, 1952a).

A line of strain C3HfB was sent to the Cancer Research Genetics Laboratory at Berkeley, and the staff there examined the tumors that arose in the breeding females electron microscopically and in them found B particles indistinguishable from the B particles found in the high tumor strains with milk-transmitted MTV (Pitelka et al., 1964). This indicated that the mammary tumors of C3HfB were also caused by a virus, which was designated as the nodule-inducing virus (NIV) since the C3HfB, like C3H, developed the hyperplastic nodules from which the tumors arose (Nandi, 1966).

Later, another strain, C3H-A$^{vy}$fB, was developed by foster-nursing a litter of caesarean-derived C3H-A$^{vy}$ mice on C57BL (Vlahakis et al., 1970). Because of the presence of the A$^{vy}$ gene, strain C3H-A$^{vy}$ has a higher susceptibility to mammary tumors than C3H, which is expressed in earlier appearance of the tumors since the incidence in both strains is 100%. Also strain C3H-A$^{vy}$fB has a higher tumor response than C3HfB, the tumor incidence in C3H-A$^{vy}$fB being 90% with an average tumor age of 15 months. These C3H-A$^{vy}$fB tumors also contain B particles.

Although C3H-A$^{vy}$fB had a relatively high incidence of mammary tumors, its virus was not transmitted through the milk. BALB/c females foster-nursed on C3H-A$^{vy}$fB females had the same low tumor incidence normally seen in BALB/c. The virus of the C3H-A$^{vy}$fB was, however, readily transmitted through the germ cells. When reciprocal crosses were made between C3H-A$^{vy}$fB and BALB/c, both groups of reciprocal hybrid females had a high incidence of mammary tumors like that of C3H-A$^{vy}$fB. Furthermore, the tumors of these hybrid females also contained B particles. Thus this strain C3H-A$^{vy}$fB had a high incidence of mammary tumors caused by a virus indistinguishable morphologically from the usual MTV but instead of being transmitted in the milk was transmitted through the sperm and egg.

At the Netherlands Cancer Research Institute, Mühlbock (1965) had developed mouse strain GR that was to make a unique contribution to our understanding of the genetic transmission of the mammary tumor virus. This is a very high mammary tumor strain with an incidence of 100% at an average age of 4 months. Through a series of well-designed experiments, Mühlbock and his staff showed that the virus of this strain, which is also a B particle morphologically not unlike other lines of MTV, was transmitted through the sperm and egg, although it could also be transmitted in the milk. When this GR virus was transmitted to strain 020, it was no longer transmissible through the sperm but was transmitted maternally as the usual MTV. Thus it appeared that this male transmission of the GR virus was not a characteristic of the virus but of the GR strain of mice (for review, see Bentvelzen, 1968).

As a result of his analysis of hybridization studies, Bentvelzen concluded that the high susceptibility of the GR strain to mammary tumors was due to a single Mendelian factor. Furthermore, in an analysis of the male transmission, he concluded that the ability of the male to transmit MTV was also due to a single Mendelian factor, probably the same as the gene for the high susceptibility of the strain. It was from these and other observations that Bentvelzen (1972) formulated his provirus theory for the transmission of the GR mammary tumor virus and possibly other lines of MTV. He postulated that the viral information is transmitted as a provirus incorporated in the host genome, transcription of this DNA viral information to the RNA virus being controlled by a regulator gene and an operator gene.

In certain aspects, Bentvelzen's concept of the provirus parallels Huebner's concept of the oncogene. That the two are not the same is evidenced by the fact that they control different viruses. The virus that presumably arises from the oncogene in its mature form is a C particle. The mammary tumor viruses of the various lines are B particles, and thus far they have been found to produce only mammary tumors.

Proof of the MTV provirus, like proof of the oncogene, will come through segregation studies demonstrating that the viral information segregates as a genetic locus followed by linkage studies locating it on a certain chromosome. Early mammary tumor segregation studies were troubled by the fact that the expression of the MTV was the occurrence of the mammary tumor late in life after possible influence by any of a number of other factors. This difficulty can now be overcome by identification of the virus early in the life of the mouse. Van Nie *et al.* (1972) in Amsterdam have identified the presence of the virus by hormonal induction of early small mammary tumors in the GR strain. She can identify these approximately 3 wk after introduction of the first hormonal pellet. Ratios in hybrids resulting from their outcrossing strain GR to low tumor strains have indicated segregation of a single locus controlling production of the virus.

Using originally the immunofluorescent test and later the radioimmune test, Hilgers, also of the Amsterdam group, has likewise obtained evidence of single Mendelian segregation of the viral antigen. It is hoped that both observations can be extended and confirmed by establishing this gene, presumably the provirus in a linkage group.

These observations on the genetic transmission of mouse tumor viruses may be of significance in understanding the transmission of human cancer. Early studies on breast cancer in women showed that something transmitted from parent to daughter influenced the probability that breast cancer later would occur. Yet whatever was being transmitted was transmitted from the father as readily as from the mother. If there are human tumor viruses, as we suspect there are, they too will probably be found to be transmitted genetically.

## 9. References

ANDERS, A., ANDERS, F., and KLINKE, K., 1974, Regulation of gene expression in the Gordon–Kosswig melanoma system. I. The distribution of the controlling genes in the genome of the Xiphophorin fish, *Platypoecilus maculatus* and *Platypoecilus variatus*, in: *Genetics and Mutagenesis of Fish* (J. H. Schröder, ed.), pp. 34–52, Springer-Verlag, Berlin-Heidelberg-New York.

ANDERSON, D. E., 1959, Genetic aspects of bovine ocular carcinoma, in: *Genetics and Cancer* (Staff of University of Texas, M. D. Anderson Hospital and Tumor Institute, eds.), pp. 364–374, University of Texas Press, Austin.

ANDERVONT, H. B., 1938, The incidence of induced subcutaneous and pulmonary tumors and spontaneous mammary tumors in hybrid mice, *Publ Health Rep.* **53**:1665.

ANDERVONT, H. B., 1945, Fate of the C3H milk influence in mice of strains C and C57 black, *J. Natl. Cancer Inst.* **5**:383.

AUERBACH, C., 1949, Chemical mutagenesis, *Biol. Rev.* **24**:355.

BASHFORD, E. F., 1909, The influence of heredity on disease, with special reference to tuberculosis, cancer and diseases of the nervous system, *Proc. Roy. Soc. Med.* **2**:63.

BENTVELZEN, P., 1968, *Genetical Control of the Vertical Transmission of the Mühlbock Mammary Tumor Virus in the GR Mouse Strain*, pp. 35–40, Hollandia, Amsterdam.

BENTVELZEN, P., 1972, Hereditary infections with mammary tumor viruses in mice, in: *RNA Viruses and Host Genome in Oncogenesis* (P. Emmelot and P. Bentvelzen, eds.), pp. 309–337, North-Holland, Amsterdam and London.

BENTVELZEN, P., and DAAMS, J. H., 1972, Oncornaviruses and their proviruses, *Rev. Europ. Etudes Clin. Biol.* **17**:245.

BITTNER, J. J., 1939, Relation of nursing to the extra-chromosome theory of breast cancer in mice, *Am. J. Cancer* **97**:90.

BITTNER, J. J., HUSEBY, R. A., VISSCHER, M. B., BALL, Z. B., and SMITH, F., 1944, Mammary cancer and mammary structure in inbred stocks of mice and their hybrids, *Science* **99**:83.

BLOOM, J. L., and FALCONER, D. S., 1964, A gene with major effect on susceptibility to induced lung tumors in mice, *J. Natl. Cancer Inst.* **33**:607.

BRIDGES, C. B., 1916, Non-disjunction as proof of chromosome theory of heredity, *Genetics* **1**:1.

BRIEN, P., 1961, Étude d'*Hydra pirardi*. Origine et repartition des nematacystes. Gamétogènese. Involution postgamétique. Evolution reversible des cellules interstitielles, *Bull. Biol. France Belg.* **95**:301.

BURDETTE, W. J., 1943, The inheritance of susceptibility to tumors induced in mice. II. Tumors induced by methylcholanthrene in the progeny of C3H and JK mice, *Cancer Res.* **3**:318.

BURDETTE, W. J., 1951, A method for determining mutation rate and tumor incidence simultaneously, *Cancer Res.* **11**:552.

BURDETTE, W. J., 1952, Induced pulmonary tumors, *J. Thoracic Surg.* **24**:427.

BURDETTE, W. J., 1955, The significance of mutation in relation to the origin of tumors: A review, *Cancer Res.* **15**:201.

CHARLES, D. R., and LUCE-CLAUSEN, E. M., 1942, The kinetics of papilloma formation in benzpyrene-treated mice, *Cancer Res.* **2**:261.

COLE, R. K., and FURTH, J., 1941, Experimental studies on the genetics of spontaneous leukemia in mice, *Cancer Res.* **1**:957.

COOPER, E. L., 1969, Neoplasia and transplantation immunity in annelids, *J. Natl. Cancer Inst. Monogr.* **31**:655.

DICKIE, M. M., 1954, The use of $F_1$ hybrid and backcross generations to reveal new and/or uncommon tumor types, *J. Natl. Cancer Inst.* **15**:791.

FONTAINE, A. R., 1969, Pigmented tumor-like lesions in an ophiuroid echinoderm, *Natl. Cancer Inst. Monogr.* **31**:255.

FOSTER, J. A., 1969, Malformation and lethal growths in *Planaria* treated with carcinogens, *Natl. Cancer Inst. Monogr.* **31**:683.

GARDNER, E. J., 1959, Genetic mechanism of maternal effect for tumorous head in *Drosophila melanogaster*, *Genetics* **44**:471.

GARDNER, E. J., and WOOLF, C. M., 1949, Maternal effect involved in the inheritance of abnormal growths in the head region of *Drosophila melanogaster*, *Genetics* **34**:573.

GARDNER, W. U., 1954, Studies on ovarian and pituitary tumorigenesis, *J. Natl. Cancer Inst.* **15**:693.

GARDNER, W. U., and STRONG, L. C., 1940, The strain-limited development of tumors of the pituitary gland in mice receiving estrogens, *Yale J. Biol. Med.* **12**:543.

GORDON, M., 1858, A genetic concept for the origin of melanomas, *Ann. N.Y. Acad. Sci.* **71**:1213.

GRAND, C. G., GORDON, M., and CAMERON, G., 1941, Neoplasm studies. VIII. Cell types in tissue culture of fish melanotic tumors compared with mammalian melanomas, *Cancer Res.* **1**:660.

GROSS, L., 1951, Pathogenic properties, and vertical transmission of the mouse leukemia agent, *Proc. Soc. Exp. Biol. Med.* **78**:343.

HALVER, J. E., 1969, Aflatoxicosis and trout hepatoma, in *Aflatoxin—Scientific Background, Control, and Implications* (L. A. Goldblatt, ed.), pp. 265–306, Academic Press, New York.

HALVER, J. E., and MITCHELL, I. A. (eds.), 1967, Trout Hepatoma Research Conference Papers, Research Report no. 70, Bureau of Sport Fisheries and Wildlife, Government Printing Office, Washington, D.C.

HALVER, J. E., ASHLEY, L. M., and SMITH, R. R., 1969, Aflatoxicosis in coho salmon, *Natl. Cancer Inst. Monogr.* **31**:141.

HARTUNG, E. W., 1950, The inheritance of a tumor in *Drosophila melanogaster*, *J. Hered.* **41**:269,

HESTON, W. E., 1942a, Genetic analysis of susceptibility to induced pulmonary tumors in mice, *J. Natl. Cancer Inst.* **3**:69.

HESTON, W. E., 1942b, Inheritance of susceptibility to spontaneous pulmonary tumors in mice, *J. Natl. Cancer Inst.* **3**:79.

HESTON, W. E., 1953, Occurrence of tumors in mice injected subcutaneously with sulfur mustard and nitrogen mustard, *J. Natl. Cancer Inst.* **14**:131.

HESTON, W. E., 1957, Effects of genes located on chromosomes III, V, VII, IX, and XIV on the occurrence of pulmonary tumors in the mouse, in: *Proceedings of International Genetics Symposia, 1956, Cytologia,* Suppl. Vol. 219.

HESTON, W. E., 1960, The genetic concept of the etiology of cancer, in: *Proceedings of the 4th National Cancer Conference,* Lippincott, Philadelphia.

HESTON, W. E., 1963, Genetics of neoplasia, in: *Methodology in Mammalian Genetics* (W. J. Burdette, ed.), pp. 247–264, Holden-Day, San Francisco.

HESTON, W. E., and ANDERVONT, H. B., 1944, Importance of genetic influence on the occurrence of mammary tumors in virgin female mice, *J. Natl. Cancer Inst.* **4**:403.

HESTON, W. E., and DERINGER, M. K., 1952a, Test for a maternal influence in the development of mammary gland tumors in agent-free strain C3Hb mice, *J. Natl. Cancer Inst.* **13**:167.

HESTON, W. E., and DERINGER, M. K., 1952b, Induction of pulmonary tumors in guinea pigs by intravenous injection of methylcholanthrene and dibenzanthracene, *J. Natl. Cancer Inst,* **13**:705.

HESTON, W. E., and PRATT, A. W., 1959, Effect of concentration of oxygen on occurrence of pulmonary tumors in strain A mice, *J. Natl. Cancer Inst.* **22**:707.

HESTON, W. E., and SCHNEIDERMAN, M. A., 1953, Analysis of dose response in relation to mechanism of pulmonary tumor induction in mice, *Science* **117**:109.

HESTON, W. E., AND VLAHAKIS, G., 1961, Influence of the $A^{vy}$ gene on mammary-gland tumors, hepatomas, and normal growth in mice, *J. Natl. Cancer Inst.* **26**:969.

HESTON, W. E., DERINGER, M. K., AND ANDERVONT, H. B., 1945, Gene–milk agent relationship in mammary-tumor development, *J. Natl. Cancer Inst.* **5**:289.

HESTON, W. E., DERINGER, M. K., DUNN, T. B., AND LEVILLAIN, W. D., 1950, Factors in the development of spontaneous mammary gland tumors in agent-free strain C3Hb mice, *J. Natl. Cancer Inst.* **10**:1139.

HESTON, W. E., DERINGER, M. K., AND DUNN, T. P., 1956, Further studies on the relationship between the genotype and the mammary tumor agent in mice, *J. Natl. Cancer Inst.* **16**:1309.

HESTON, W. E., VLAHAKIS, G., AND DERINGER, M. K., 1960, Delayed effect of genetic segregation on the transmission of the mammary tumor agent in mice, *J. Natl. Cancer Inst.* **24**:721.

HESTON, W. E., VLAHAKIS, G., AND DESMUKES, B., 1973, Effects of the antifertility drug Enovid in five strains of mice, with particular regard to carcinogenesis, *J. Natl. Cancer Inst.* **51**:209.

HUEBNER, R. J., AND GILDEN, R. V., 1972, Inherited RNA viral genomes (virogenes and oncogenes) in the etiology of cancer, in: *RNA Viruses and Host Genome in Oncogenesis* (P. Emmelot and P. Bentvelzen, eds.), pp. 197–219, North-Holland, Amsterdam and London.

HUEBNER, R. J., AND TODARO, G. J., 1969, Oncogenes of RNA tumor viruses as determinants of cancer, *Proc. Natl. Acad. Sci.* **64**:1087.

HUSEBY, R. A., AND BITTNER, J. J., 1948, Studies on the inherited hormonal influence, *Acta Unio Int. Contra Cancrum* **6**:197.

JACKSON LABORATORY STAFF, 1933, The existence of nonchromosomal influence in the incidence of mammary tumors in mice, *Science* **78**:465.

KORTWEG, R., 1934, Proefondervindelijke onderzoekingen Aangaande Erfelijkhéid von Kanker, *Nederl. Tijdschr. Geneesk.* **78**:240.

LANGE, C. S., 1966, Observations on some tumors found in two species of planaria: *Dugesia etrusca* and *D. ilvana, J. Embryol. Exp. Morphol.* **15**:125.

LITTLE, C. C., 1939, Hybridization and tumor formation in mice, *Proc. Natl. Acad. Sci.* **25**:452.

LYNCH, C. J., 1940, Influence of heredity and environment upon the number of tumor nodules occurring in lungs of mice, *Proc. Soc. Exp. Biol. Med.* **43**:186.

MACDOWELL, E. C., POTTER, J. S., AND TAYLOR, M. J., 1945, Mouse leukemia. XII. The role of genes in spontaneous cases, *Cancer Res.* **5**:65.

MCKINNELL, R. G., 1969, Lucké renal adenocarcinoma: Epidemiological aspects, in: *Recent Results in Cancer Research,* Special Suppl.: *Biology of Amphibian Tumors* (M. Mizell, ed.), pp. 254–260, Springer, New York, Heidelberg, and Berlin.

MIZELL, M., 1969, State of the art: Lucké renal adenocarcinoma, in: *Recent Results in Cancer Research,* Special Suppl.: *Biology of Amphibian Tumors* (M. Mizell, ed.), pp. 1–25, Springer, New York, Heidelberg, and Berlin.

MÜHLBOCK, O., 1965, Note on a new inbred mouse strain GR/A, *Europ. J. Cancer* **1**:123.

MURRAY, J. A., 1911, Cancerous ancestry and the incidence in mice, *Proc. Roy. Soc. Lond.* **84**:42.

NANDI, S., 1966, Interactions among hormonal, viral, and genetic factors in mouse mammary tumorigenesis, *Canad. Cancer Conf.* **6**:69.

PAULEY, G. B., 1969, A critical review of neoplasia and tumor-like lesions in mollusks, *Natl. Cancer Inst. Monogr.* **31**:509.

PAYNE, L. N., 1972, Interaction between host genome and avian RNA tumor viruses, in: *RNA viruses and Host Genome in Oncogenesis* (P. E. Emmelot and P. Bentvelzen, eds.), pp. 93–115, North-Holland, Amsterdam and London.

PITELKA, D. R., BERN, H. A., NANDI, S., AND DE OME, K. B., 1964, On the significance of virus-like particles in mammary tissues of C3Hf mice, *J. Natl. Cancer Inst.* **33**:867.

ROGERS, J. B., 1951, Spontaneous tumors of senile guinea pigs, *J. Gerontol.* **6**(Supplement to No. 3): 142.

ROWE, W. P., 1972, Studies of genetic transmission of murine leukemia virus by AKR mice. I. Crosses with $Fv-1^n$ strains of mice, *J. Exp. Med.* **136**:1272.

ROWE, W. P., AND HARTLEY, J. W., 1972, Studies of genetic transmission of murine leukemia virus by AKR mice. II. Crosses with $Fv-1^b$ strains of mice, *J. Exp. Med.* **136**:1286.

ROWE, W. P., HARTLEY, J. W., AND BREMNAR, T., 1972, Genetic mapping of a murine leukemia virus–inducing locus of AKR mice, *Science,* **178**:860.

ROWE, W. P., HUMPHREY, J. B., AND LILLY, F., 1973, A major genetic locus affecting resistance to infection with murine leukemia viruses. III. Assignment of the *Fv-1* locus to linkage group VIII of the mouse, *J. Exp. Med.* **137**:850.

RUSSELL, E. S., 1940, A comparison of benign and "malignant" tumors in *Drosophila melanogaster, J. Exp. Zool.* **84**:363.

RUSSELL, E. S., 1942, The inheritance of tumors in *Drosophila melanogaster*, with special reference to an isogenic strain of *st sr* tumor 36a, *Genetics* **27**:612.

RUSSELL, W. O., AND ORTEGA, L. R., 1952, Methylcholanthrene induced tumors in guinea pigs, a review of the literature on tumors induced with polycyclic carcinogenic hydrocarbons in this species, *Arch. Pathol.* **53**:301.

SCHLUMBERGER, H. G., 1952, Nerve sheath tumors in an isolated goldfish population, *Cancer Res.* **12**:890.

SCHLUMBERGER, H. G., 1954, Neoplasia in the parakeet. I. Spontaneous chromophobe pituitary tumors, *Cancer Res.* **14**:237.

SHIMKIN, M. B., AND MIDER, G. B., 1941, Induction of tumors in guinea pigs with subcutaneously injected methylcholanthrene, *J. Natl. Cancer Inst.* **1**:707.

SLYE, M., 1926, The inheritance behavior of cancer as a simple mendelian recessive, *J. Cancer Res.* **10**:15.

SNELL, G. D., 1958, Histocompatability genes of the mouse. II. Production and analysis of isogenic resistant lines, *J. Natl. Cancer Inst.* **21**:843.

STEVENS, L. C., 1970, Experimental production of testicular teratomas in mice of strains 129, A/He, and their $F_1$ hybrids, *J. Natl. Cancer Inst.* **44**:923.

TATCHELL, J. A. H., 1961, Pulmonary tumors, group VII and sex in the house mouse, *Nature (Lond.)* **190**:837.

VAN NIE, R., HILGERS, J., AND LENSELINK, M., 1972, Genetical analysis of mammary tumor development and mammary tumor virus expression in the GR mouse strain, in: *Recherches Fondamentales sur les Tumeurs Mammaires*, pp. 21–29, Ministere de la Santa Publique, Paris.

VLAHAKIS, G., HESTON, W. E., AND SMITH, G. H., 1970, Strain C3H-A$^{vy}$fB mice: Ninety percent incidence of mammary tumors transmitted by either parent, *Science* **170**:185.

WOOLLEY, G. W., FEKETE, E., AND LITTLE, C. C., 1941, Effect of castration in the dilute brown strain of mice, *Endocrinology* **28**:341.

WOOLLEY, G. W., DICKIE, M. M., AND LITTLE, C. C., 1953, Adrenal tumors and other pathological changes in reciprocal crosses in mice. II. An introduction to results of four reciprocal crosses, *Cancer Res.* **13**:231.

WRIGHT, S., 1934*a*, The results of crosses between inbred strains of guinea pigs, differing in number of digits, *Genetics* **19**:537.

WRIGHT, S., 1934*b*, On the genetics of subnormal development of the head (otocephaly) in the guinea pig, *Genetics* **19**:471.

# 3

# Genetic Influences in Human Tumors

Alfred G. Knudson, Jr.

## 1. Introduction

Although the genetic analysis of cancer in animals has played a major role in the development of knowledge and new ideas about the etiology and pathogenesis of cancer, the genetic study of human cancer has played a very minor role. Part of this difference is attributable to the fact animal data have been provided to a great extent by experimental manipulation of selected species and genetic strains, whereas human data have been largely descriptive and not related either to animal data or to critical etiological hypotheses. Genetic analyses of human cancer have consisted primarily of population, family, and twin studies of tumor occurrence and cytogenetic analyses. The results of cytogenetic analyses of human tumors are thoroughly discussed elsewhere in this volume, and reference to them in this chapter will be confined largely to discussion of genetically predisposing conditions which involve chromosomal abnormality. It is the study of the occurrence of tumors that has contributed most significantly to the understanding of etiology.

The study of cancer in populations is of course not necessarily a study of the genetics of cancer. It has been repeatedly observed that population or subpopulation (e.g., occupational) differences are attributable to differences in environmental exposure. Nevertheless, it is still not known whether the gross ethnic differences in incidence of many specific cancers, such as those occurring in breast, stomach, and colon, are due to genetic or environmental factors. Support for a genetic basis for ethnic difference could be provided by evidence of correlation of

Alfred G. Knudson, Jr. ● The University of Texas Health Science Center at Houston, Graduate School of Biomedical Sciences, Houston, Texas. Supported in part by Medical Genetics Center Grant GM 19513 from the National Institute of General Medical Sciences.

cancer incidence with a specific genetic marker, as has been provided by the finding within the Caucasian population that cancer of the stomach shows some association with blood group A. Evidence may also be provided by comparing the incidence of a particular tumor in populations genetically alike but living in different environmental conditions. However, at present there is no conclusive evidence that any ethnic differences in cancer incidence are attributable to genetic difference.

Study of the families of cancer patients has revealed that most forms of cancer display an increased familial incidence, suggesting a genetic component to susceptibility. The patterns of inheritance are not generally those of single Mendelian genes, and broad surveys have therefore not shed any light on the origin of human cancer. On the other hand, detailed analysis of selected families in which there is a concentration of similar cases has clearly shown that cancer in some instances is inherited in Mendelian fashion. These examples will be discussed in further detail.

A unique category of family study is that of twins. Comparison of concordance in identical and in fraternal twins has often been employed as a measure for assessing the relative roles of heredity and environment in the causation of disease. For most cancers, the concordance is very low for both kinds of twins, suggesting that heredity plays a minor role. Exceptions include cancer of the breast, childhood cancer, and the tumors which demonstrate a Mendelian form of predisposition.

With these general observations in mind, it can only be concluded that the informative cancers of man are those in which predisposition occurs in individuals with well-defined genetic states or in which the tumor is inherited in Mendelian fashion.

## 2. Genetic States Predisposing to Cancer

### 2.1. Chromosomal Disorders

In Down's syndrome, or mongoloid idiocy, there is an extra chromosome 21. In most cases this appears in the form of trisomy 21, but in some it appears as an equivalent translocation. In both forms there is an increased risk of leukemia, estimated to be 10–20 times the risk in normal children (Miller, 1970). An increased susceptibility to solid tumors has also been reported (Young, 1971). Leukemia is found in children with Down's syndrome 2–3 yr earlier on the average than it is in normal children. An increased incidence of leukemia has also been observed in trisomy D and in Klinefelter's syndrome (Fraumeni, 1969). *In vitro* oncogenic transformation by the tumor virus SV40 is also increased in fibroblasts from trisomic individuals.

The enhanced risk of leukemia in these aneuploid states may not be attributable to the aneuploidy *per se*. There has also been reported an increased risk for leukemia in the sibs of subjects with Down's syndrome, raising the possibility that some causative factor may be common to both (Miller, 1963). Hecht *et al.* (1964) mention several possible mechanisms, including (1) underlying chromosomal rearrangement, (2) an autoimmune process, as has been suggested by Fialkow (1966) for aneuploidy, and (3) latent virus infection.

No other such highly significant relationship is known between aneuploidy and cancer. As far as structural abnormality and cancer are concerned, there is the very important example of the Philadelphia chromosome and chronic myeloid leukemia (Nowell and Hungerford, 1960, 1961). This is a deleted chromosome 22 (Caspersson *et al.*, 1970), which has been demonstrated to be associated with an apparently balanced translocation to chromosome 9 (Rowley, 1973). But the Philadelphia chromosome is found only in the hematopoietic system and is clearly a somatic rather than germinal change. This reduces any assurance that it *precedes* the development of leukemia. The problem of the relationship of cytogenetic change in somatic cells to the origin of cancer is discussed elsewhere in this volume.

One deletion which is definitely prezygotic and predisposing to a specific form of cancer is a deletion in the long arm of a D chromosome, chromosome 13 in verified cases. This deletion is often associated with a clinical syndrome of congenital defects known as the D deletion syndrome. Nine of some 40 affected individuals have also suffered from retinoblastoma, seven of these bilaterally (Wilson *et al.*, 1973). However, retinoblastoma is not usually accompanied by this deletion; in 12 cases, seven bilateral, no D chromosome deletion was found (Ladda *et al.*, 1973).

Although newer techniques for disclosing subtle chromosomal abnormality may yet prove the opposite, present evidence suggests that very few cases of cancer occur in individuals with visible chromosomal abnormalities in any significant number of noncancerous cells.

## 2.2. Mendelian Conditions

The syndromes of Fanconi and Bloom are both autosomal recessive disorders, both predispose to leukemia and cancer, and both are associated with increased rates of chromosome breakage *in vitro* and *in vivo* (German, 1972). Cells from patients with Fanconi's syndrome are also abnormal in their response to various environmental carcinogens; there is a greatly increased sensitivity to X-ray-induced chromosome breakage (Higurashi and Conen, 1971), an increased incidence of endoreduplication and tetraploidy *in vitro* in response to benzpyrene (Hirschhorn and Bloch-Shtacher, 1970), and a greatly increased rate of *in vitro* neoplastic transformation of fibroblasts in response to the tumor virus SV40 (Miller and Todaro, 1969).

Although leukemia is the only neoplastic condition reported excessively in patients with Fanconi's syndrome, it is not the only one in Bloom's syndrome. Three patients with the latter condition who have attained the age of 30 yr have each developed at least one cancer of the digestive tract (German, 1972). Since

Fanconi's syndrome is so often lethal, it should not be eliminated as a more generally predisposing disorder. Quite possibly the transformation of normal cells to cancer cells occurs at an increased rate in all tissues in these two diseases. Knowledge of the mechanisms which are defective in these diseases could obviously illuminate early steps in neoplastic transformation, possibly relating molecular change to the chromosomal changes so ubiquitous in cancer cells.

Ataxia-telangiectasia is another autosomal recessive disease associated with chromosomal abnormality and a strong predisposition to cancer, in this instance lymphoid neoplasia. In the majority of reported cases, lymphocytes respond poorly to mitogens *in vitro,* but the cells which do divide show increased rates of spontaneous chromosome breakage. The manner in which leukemia might develop in this disease has been suggested by Hecht *et al.* (1973), who studied the development of a clone of chromosomally abnormal cells in a patient over a 4-yr period. A population of cells containing a translocation, involving both chromosomes 14, grew from 1–2% to 56–78% of the patient's peripheral lymphocyte population. Although the patient died without leukemia, two of his sibs with the disease did die of leukemia. These authors report two other patients with ataxia–telangiectasia with translocation clones, one between chromosomes 7 and 14 and one between 14 and 1. The break occurred at the same point on chromosome 14 in all three cases.

Patients with ataxia-telangiectasia also commonly have a deficiency in the immune system, most often involving immunoglobulins A and E. The cause for this and its relation to chromosome breakage and leukemia are not known. Conceivably the immune deficiency could result from the emergence of a defective clone of lymphocytes, as noted above, suggesting that immune deficiency and leukemia are different end points of the same process.

Lymphoreticular neoplasms are also much more common than expected by chance among patients with any of several recessively inherited immune deficiency diseases. Gatti and Good (1971) have classified these according to autosomal or X-linked inheritance and to impairment of humoral and/or cellular immunity. The detailed features of these conditions will not be noted, except to observe that chromosomal abnormality and SV40 transformability are not features of cells from affected individuals (Kersey *et al.*, 1972). Predisposition to cancer in this case seems not to involve the process of transformation of a normal cell to a cancer cell but rather failure of the immunological surveillance mechanism which normally operates to interfere with cell proliferation. In this respect these conditions seem to differ from ataxia-telangiectasia.

Another recessively inherited disease which predisposes to cancer is also the one whose basic defect is best understood, namely, xeroderma pigmentosum. Photosensitivity and skin cancer are major features of this condition, an inborn error of metabolism in which there is a deficiency of an enzyme necessary for the repair of ultraviolet light-induced damage to DNA (Cleaver, 1968, 1969; Setlow *et al.*, 1969). Defective repair of damage induced by the chemical carcinogen N-acetoxy-2-acetylaminofluorene has also been observed (Setlow and Regan, 1972). Chromosomal abnormality is not a feature of the condition *in vivo,* but cultured fibroblasts show occasional pseudodiploid clones (German, 1972) and there is a great increase in ultraviolet light-induced chromosomal aberrations *in vitro* (Parrington *et al.*, 1971). On the other hand, SV40-induced transformation is not increased (Aaronson and Lytle, 1970; Parrington *et al.*, 1971). It is apparent that xeroderma pigmentosum is a genetic state which predisposes to environmentally induced skin cancer. This effect may be mediated via chromosome damage.

Some general conclusions emerge from a consideration of genetic states which predispose to cancer. None of these states invariably leads to cancer, with the exception of xeroderma pigmentosum. Several conditions are chromosomal abnormalities and some others predispose to the generation of chromosomal abnormality in somatic tissues. This observation, combined with the knowledge that most cancers have abnormal karyotypes, suggests that chromosomal damage may be a mediating event in the initiation of cancer cells. A different kind of predisposition is evidently provided by the immune deficiency diseases, in which initiation is not enhanced but tumor cell growth after initiation is.

## 3. Dominantly Inherited Tumors

As a group, the dominantly inherited tumors differ sharply from the genetic conditions discussed above in that tumor is a critical phenotypic feature and occurs with high penetrance. In some instances, a tumor is part of a syndrome, other manifestations of which are other kinds of tumors or nonneoplastic signs. In other instances, tumor occurs in just one tissue, although it may be multiple in that tissue.

### 3.1. Tumor Syndromes

#### 3.1.1. Polyposis of the Colon

Perhaps the best known and clinically most important dominant cancer syndrome is polyposis of the colon. Multiple benign polyps of the colon are an invariant feature in gene carriers by adulthood. What makes the disease serious is the also invariant occurrence of one or more adenocarcinomas, nearly always by the age of 50 yr. The average age at death is 40 yr (Neel, 1971); in contrast is the much later age at death for patients with carcinoma of the colon generally. Polyposis thus displays two features typical of dominantly inherited tumors: earlier onset than their nongenetic counterparts and multiplicity.

Some patients with polyposis develop tumors at other sites. The most common site is connective tissue, with such tumors as fibroma, fibrosarcoma, and osteoma. In some families, these tumors have so high an incidence that the name "Gardner's syndrome" is applied (Gardner and Richards, 1953). Whether such diversity of polyposis cases is attributable to alleles at the same genetic locus is not known.

### 3.1.2. Cancer Family Syndrome

Another dominant syndrome associated with cancer of the colon is the cancer family syndrome, or hereditary adenocarcinomatosis, made famous by the early report by Warthin (1913) of a large pedigree which has since been extended by Lynch and Krush (1971). In this family and similar ones, cancer has been reported at several sites, but two, colon and endometrium, are particularly common (Anderson, 1970). More than one tumor may occur in an organ, especially colon. Tumors frequently occur before the age of 40 yr, so this syndrome resembles polyposis with respect to both multiplicity in a given organ and early onset. Each syndrome accounts for only a small fraction of all cases of colon cancer, probably of the order of magnitude of 1% or less.

### 3.1.3. Basal Cell Nevus Syndrome

The basal cell nevus syndrome consists of a complex which includes multiple basal cell carcinomas of the skin, epidermoid cysts of the jaw, ectopic calcification of soft tissues, and various congenital skeletal anomalies. The jaw cysts are usually evident by adulthood and the carcinomas often by then, which is much earlier than these tumors appear in the population generally. Again, multiplicity and early onset characterize a dominant syndrome (Anderson, 1970).

As noted above, various cystic tumors appear excessively in this syndrome. In addition, there is a significant incidence of a very uncommon tumor, medulloblastoma, which has an incidence of less than one per 10,000 in the normal childhood population. All these syndromes noted so far therefore predispose to tumors in more than one tissue.

### 3.1.4. Multiple Endocrine Tumor Syndromes

There are two distinct multiple endocrine tumor syndromes. One of these, usually called "multiple endocrine adenomatosis," is very complex because so many tissues may be involved. These tissues include anterior pituitary, parathyroid, thyroid, pancreas (islet cells), and adrenal cortex. Carcinoid tumors of the bronchus and digestive tract have also been observed. The clinical expression of this syndrome is therefore understandably varied, depending on tumor site. In one instance, at least, the symptoms have given rise to the creation of a separate syndrome, the Zollinger–Ellison syndrome of peptic ulcer, excessive gastric secretion, and non-insulin-producing islet cell tumors. Penetrance for expression of some feature of the parent multiple endocrine syndrome is very high in early adulthood (Anderson, 1970), expression occurring at a much earlier age than when solitary tumors of these tissues occur in the general population.

The second syndrome has a narrower spectrum, producing two tumors, pheochromocytoma of the adrenal medulla and medullary carcinoma of the thyroid, with high penetrance, and parathyroid adenomas, with intermediate penetrance. A number of cases of the syndrome have been reported in children. Nearly all gene carriers attaining the age of 50 yr have developed at least one of

each of the first two tumor types, the mean number of tumors at each site being
estimated at four (Knudson and Strong, 1972a). When pheochromocytoma is found, it is bilateral in 75–80% of cases.

A significant fraction of patients with the syndrome of pheochromocytoma and medullary carcinoma of the thyroid do not have a family history of the disease. However, the offspring of such individuals are at a 50% risk, indicating that these sporadic cases result in fact from new mutations. Tumor multiplicity and age at expression are similar whether the family history is positive or not (Knudson and Strong, 1972a).

A variant of this syndrome involves other lesions, notably neuromas of the buccal mucosa and other selected areas. Known as the "mucosal neuroma syndrome," it displays the same features with respect to pheochromocytoma and medullary carcinoma of the thyroid. It may represent a different allele at the same genetic locus. The presence of café-au-lait spots has caused it to be confused with neurofibromatosis, from which it should be distinctly separated (Williams and Pollock, 1966; Gorlin et al., 1968).

Although these syndromes involve more than one endocrine tissue, they have readily separable specificities. Thus pheochromocytoma and medullary carcinoma of the thyroid are not found in the first syndrome. Both syndromes resemble other dominantly inherited syndromes in that only specific tissues are affected, tumor multiplicity is common, and age at onset is earlier than usual for solitary sporadic tumors.

### 3.1.5. Neurofibromatosis

Pheochromocytoma is also found in about 10% of cases of the syndrome of neurofibromatosis, the principal manifestations of which are café-au-lait spots and neurofibromas. The pheochromocytomas do not occur multiply in one patient, nor do they occur earlier than in unselected cases (Knudson and Strong, 1972a). The incidence of pheochromocytoma is not concentrated in certain pedigrees.

Neurofibromatosis is one of a group of dominant syndromes categorized as phacomatoses. Other entities are the von Hippel–Lindau syndrome and tuberous sclerosis. Each is associated with unusual tumors which in some respects resemble hyperplasia more than neoplasia. In this regard the phacomatoses depart from the other dominant tumor syndromes.

## 3.2. Specific Tumors

### 3.2.1. Childhood Tumors

The best-known example of a dominantly inherited tumor which is not a feature of a syndrome is retinoblastoma, a malignant eye tumor of young children with an incidence of more than one person 20,000 000 children in the United States. Since surgery and radiotherapy have been partially effective weapons for some time, a substantial number of patients have survived to reproduce, permitting the demonstration of dominant genetic transmission. However, a puzzling result was that, while essentially 50% of the offspring of bilaterally affected persons were also affected, only 10–15% of the offspring of unilaterally affected persons were also affected. Furthermore, while approximately 25–30% of all cases are bilateral, the frequency of bilaterality in the affected offspring of affected individuals, whether unilateral or bilateral, is approximately 70%. The conclusion has been reached that only some (about 40%) of all cases are germinal, or hereditary, and that the remainder are nonhereditary. Many of the hereditary cases result from new mutations and do not involve a family history. About 5% of those who carry the responsible mutation develop no tumor at all, about 30% develop tumor unilaterally, and the remainder have bilateral tumors. These observations fit the hypothesis that tumor development in gene carriers is a matter of chance, with a mean number of tumors of three per carrier (Knudson, 1971). Those who do not carry the gene have a probability of about one in 30,000 of developing one tumor and therefore a vanishingly small prospect of having bilateral disease.

The transformation of a retinoblast into a tumor cell is a rare event even in the gene carrier. The number of retinoblasts during early development can probably be numbered in the millions, suggesting that the rate of transformation is of the same order of magnitude as mutation itself. The hypothesis has been developed therefore that transformation is a mutational event occurring in somatic cells (Knudson, 1971). The initiation, or formation of the first tumor cell, of retinoblastoma is visualized as a two-step process in gene carriers; both are regarded as mutational, the first in germinal cells, the second in somatic cells. Nonhereditary cases presumably result from the same process, except that both mutations occur in somatic cells; since both of these events must occur postzygotically, it is anticipated that the age at onset would be later. It is not surprising then that hereditary and nonhereditary cases occur at mean ages of 15 and 30 months, respectively.

Retinoblastoma has been an uncommon disease because the incidence has been limited by mutation rates and because the disease until this century was probably always lethal. It should become more common as gene carriers survive and reproduce. It would also increase if mutation rates generally were increased.

Although most patients with germinal, or hereditary, retinoblastoma do not have an affected parent or other antecedent relative, a few percent have an affected sibling. This event is too frequent to be attributed to lack of penetrance, which is very high (95%) once the mutation is expressed in a pedigree. Some of these sibling cases probably result from mutation in early stages of gametogenesis and the subsequent gonadal mosaicism it produces. Others may be examples of "premutation" (Auerbach, 1956; Neel, 1962). In rare instances, the affected sibling is a twin. From the above considerations, an expectation can be created: the probability that a fraternal twin of an affected child would also be affected is slightly less than 0.5 if they have an affected parent and about 0.02 if they do not, giving an overall expectation for concordance of the order of magnitude of 0.05. Unfortunately, there have not been enough reports to test this expectation. On the other hand, since approximately 40% of all cases are germinal, the probability that the identical twin of an affected child would be a gene carrier is 0.4, which taken together with a penetrance of 0.95 leads to an expected probability of 0.38. The observed data, which are too sparse to be very reliable, suggest a fraction of 0.40–0.45.

Two other childhood tumors, Wilms' tumor of the kidney and neuroblastoma, have been examined for compatibility with this model (Knudson and Strong, 1972*a,b*). Again multiplicity of tumor and earlier age of patient are associated with hereditary cases. It is estimated that approximately 38% of Wilms' tumor cases and 22% of neuroblastoma cases are of the hereditary, or germinal, type. These tumors have not previously been regarded as similar in etiology to retinoblastoma because so few examples of generation-to-generation transmission exist. However, there are numerous cases of sib involvement. These results are presumed to be an expression of the fact that until very recently the mortality rates for Wilm's tumor and for neuroblastoma were far higher than for retinoblastoma. In addition, some survivors have undoubtedly been sterilized by irradiation. As survival and fertility increase, an increase in the number of examples of vertical transmission and an increasing resemblance to retinoblastoma can be expected. A survey of other childhood tumors suggests that other types exist in germinal and somatic forms, too, and that the phenomenon is a general one for childhood cancer.

### 3.2.2. Pheochromocytoma

Although pheochromocytoma is primarily an adult tumor, it also displays the main features of the childhood tumors. A number of pedigrees showing dominant inheritance have been presented. These are pedigrees that contain no cases of medullary carcinoma of the thyroid, so the two mutations are obviously different. They differ in other ways, too; pheochromocytoma alone may occur in any part of the sympathetic nervous system, it is often associated with sustained hypertension, and the principal amine produced is norepinephrine. In syndrome cases, pheochromocytoma is found only in the adrenal, sustained hypertension is not found, and the principal amine is epinephrine. In familial cases of simple pheochromocytoma, tumor is multiple in 50%, whereas only 12% of all cases are multiple. The modal age in multiple cases is approximately 20 yr, whether they are familial or not, while the modal age in nonfamilial cases is 35–40 yr. Again, familial cases are multiple and earlier in onset. The hereditary, or germinal, form of this tumor is estimated to comprise 22% of all cases (Knudson and Strong, 1972*a*). Approximately 90% of gene carriers will have at least one tumor by the age of 50 yr, the mean number per gene carrier being between two and three.

Syndrome cases of pheochromocytoma with medullary carcinoma of the thyroid account for about 30% of all familial cases of pheochromocytoma. Presumably the two familial forms result from mutation at two different genetic loci. It is visualized that tumor initiation proceeds by two steps in both, just as with the childhood tumors. In both forms, the first step can be a germinal mutation and produce a dominantly inherited tumor. All cases of the syndrome with medullary carcinoma of the thyroid are of this type because the probability that both of these tissues would have both steps occur in them is vanishingly small, just as is the probability of two tumors arising in one tissue by somatic change alone. Nonhereditary, or somatic, cases of pheochromocytoma could therefore represent first-step mutations at either locus.

Retrospective examination of the syndrome of multiple endocrine adenomatosis suggests that here too a mutation is inherited which affects a multiplicity of tissues. In any one of those tissues in which further change takes place a tumor cell will be initiated. Thus different affected members of the same pedigree may be affected in quite different ways, which are dependent on the tissue site of the second stochastic process (Knudson *et al.*, 1973).

### 3.2.3. Common Cancers

Although there are other accepted examples of dominantly inherited tumors and tumor syndromes, not enough details are available to complete the kind of analysis that has been performed on the examples above. Qualitatively, however, these heritable, or prezygotic, forms do show the pattern of multiplicity and earlier onset, in contrast to nonheritable, or postzygotic, forms. The difference between the syndromes and single tissue tumors is also maintained. The syndromes are always heritable, presumably because the probability of mimicry by somatic mutations is so small, while the single-tissue tumors exist in both heritable and nonheritable forms. The dualism of dominant (syndrome or single-tissue) and somatic forms appears to hold for childhood tumors, endocrine tumors, cancer of the colon, and basal cell carcinoma of the skin. Question then arises whether this is a general phenomenon for all cancers.

For the two most common forms of cancer, skin and colon, it is already apparent that dominant forms exist. For colon cancer, there are at least two, polyposis and the cancer family syndrome. For skin cancer, there is at least one, the basal cell nevus syndrome, and a dominant form of melanoma also probably exists (Anderson, 1971). The chief difference between these common cancers and the childhood cancers is that the dominant forms comprise a much smaller fraction, probably about 1–2%, of total cases of the former, and 20–40% of the latter.

Another of the common cancers, carcinoma of the breast, may also exist in a dominant form (Anderson, 1972). Numerous pedigrees displaying vertical transmission of the disease have been reported. Concordance in identical and fraternal twins is estimated to be 28 and 12%, respectively (Knudson *et al.*, 1973), again suggesting a strong genetic effect. Familial cases of breast cancer occur at significantly younger ages and are much more frequently bilateral. The hereditary form is primarily a premenopausal disease.

The small contribution of the cancer family syndrome to endometrial carcinoma has already been noted. In addition, this cancer frequently occurs alone in a familial, possibly dominant, form (Lynch *et al.*, 1966). This latter form is estimated by these investigators to contribute at least 13% of all endometrial cancer. Numerous examples of what may be dominantly inherited cancers of other sites in

the gastrointestinal and genitourinary systems have been reported (Knudson *et*
*al.*, 1973).

One tumor which does not follow this pattern with any measurable frequency is
bronchogenic carcinoma. Perhaps this is a result of environmental influences
which have greatly expanded any nonhereditary component in this century.
Heredity in some way does seem to be important, and evidently interacts with
cigarette smoking to produce a synergistic effect (Tokuhata, 1964). Further
details of the interaction of heredity and environment in this disease will be
discussed below.

It is quite clear that leukemia and lymphoma are associated with several
chromosomal abnormalities and recessively inherited disorders, but it is less clear
whether a dominant contribution exists. There are pedigrees with as many as four
generations of affected individuals. Concordance in twins is estimated to be
approximately 25% (MacMahon and Levy, 1964; Miller, 1968), which is too high
to be explained by the contribution of known predisposing recessive conditions. It
has been surmised on the basis of familial patterns and earlier onset of familial
cases that a dominant subgroup exists, although its contributions to the total
cannot be estimated (Knudson *et al.*, 1973).

Consideration of the common cancers leads then to the conclusion that it is
highly probable that all human cancers contain at least one dominantly inherited
subgroup of cases, even though its contribution to the total may vary from as high
as 40% for some childhood tumors to as low as 1% or less for some adult tumors.
Features that the dominant forms invariably share are earlier onset and tendency
to multiplicity,

## 4. A Mutation Model for Human Cancer

### 4.1. Initiation in Two or More Steps

A two-step mutation model has been created for retinoblastoma in which it is
assumed that initiation of cancer occurs by the transformation of a normal cell into
a cancer cell in two steps. The first step is thought to be a mutation because it can be
inherited; in nonhereditary, or postzygotic, cases it is thought to occur in somatic
cells. The second step always occurs in somatic cells and may also be a mutation.
The process is considered to be essentially the same in all cases. Tumor
development then proceeds by the proliferation of these initiated cells.

The possibility that all forms of cancer have a dominantly inherited subgroup
suggests that such a model may serve for cancer generally. Both two-stage and
multistage models have been constructed previously (Armitage and Doll, 1954,
1957; Ashley, 1969a). These models are based on consideration of the age-specific
incidence or mortality. A steep rise in incidence or mortality with age would
indicate more stages, or "hits." So many assumptions must go into these
estimates that they are very hazardous. In any case, however, more than one hit is
visualized. These hits have been considered as somatic mutations. Burch (1962,
1965) has surmised that one or more hits could be inherited, thus reducing the

necessary number of somatic mutations. A comparison has been made by Ashley (1969b) between colon cancer generally and polyposis of the colon in particular on this basis. It is concluded that the total number of hits is reduced by one or two in the latter. If mutant cells exhibit higher growth rates, the number would be placed at one. Since polyposis results from the heritable mutation, this may indeed be the case. A good possibility is that carcinoma of the colon arises in two or more steps and that in polyposis the number is reduced by one.

If, then, a model of two or more steps is tenable, question arises whether the second step is mutational. No direct evidence is available on this point, although support for the idea has been presented on the basis of an increased incidence of connective tissue tumors in hereditary cases of retinoblastoma and a still further increase in response to irradiation (Strong and Knudson, 1972; Knudson, 1973).

## 4.2. Genetic Consequences

A genetic initiation of cancer implies that individual cancers originate from a single cell. This prediction has been tested by the study of tumor-bearing females heterozygous for variant alleles at the X-linked locus for glucose-6-phosphate dehydrogenase. The evidence reviewed by Fialkow (1972) clearly supports the conclusion that cancer generally arises by clonal growth from a single cell. Contrary evidence is found in the case of neurofibromatosis and hereditary multiple trichoepitheliomas. Whether these tumors are relevant to cancer generally is not certain. If they are, this evidence argues against a second step being mutational. If hereditary tumors generally are derived clonally, then strong support is offered for the notion that any step beyond the first is also mutational. In any case, the available evidence gives strong support to the idea that the first step in nonhereditary tumors is a somatic mutation, even in viral-induced warts and in a tumor such as Burkitt's lymphoma, which is thought to be induced by a virus.

The initiation of cancer in two or more steps, at least one of which is mutational, creates no requirement for chromosomal change, yet the latter can be clearly associated with cancer. It was noted that in retinoblastoma visible chromosomal deletion can be associated, but is usually not. The term "mutation" should be used broadly here to signify heritable chromosomal change, be it deletion, rearrangement, point mutation, or other change. What relationship this mutation may have to the subsequent chromosomal abnormalities which characterize most cancers is not apparent. It is possible that these are only secondary changes having nothing to do with the process of initiation.

One consequence of this mutation hypothesis is that the mutational change in the first step is tissue(s) specific. All of the dominant tumors and tumor syndromes characteristically affect one or a few tissues and do not predispose to cancer generally. This may provide a clue to the physiological nature of the gene which is the site of the mutation. The most obvious type of candidate is a genetically specified cell-surface component, since cell surfaces are known to harbor tissue

specificity and to play a role in the normal cell-to-cell interactions which are
disturbed in cancer.

## 4.3. Role of Environmental Carcinogens

If mutation, either germinal or somatic, is an invariant phenomenon in the initiation of cancer, then what is the mechanism whereby environmental carcinogens act? Do they act as mutagens or do they operate in some basically different manner? A survey of principal carcinogens—viruses, radiation, and chemicals—suggests that all operate by changing the host genome, or, in the broadest sense, by acting as mutagens. Major sections of this volume are devoted to each of these environmental agents, so only those aspects related to the present discussion will be considered here.

Although there is no direct proof that viruses can cause cancer in man, it seems improbable that so many animal tumors could be caused by viruses without any human cancers being so caused. All that is known about mechanism must, however, come from animal tumor viruses. Tumor viruses in general, whether DNA- or RNA-containing, seem to interact with the host genome. Integration into host DNA is achieved by viral DNA, or, in the case of RNA viruses, a DNA transcript of viral RNA. Chromosomal breakage is characteristic of many tumor virus infections, and one, SV40, produces many more breaks in cells from individuals with Down's and Fanconi's syndromes than in normal cells (Miller and Todaro, 1969). Integrated tumor virus genomes can also be transmitted vertically and so resemble germinal mutations.

Point mutations and chromosome breaks could conceivably lead to cancer by providing tumor viruses with opportunity for integration; in this scheme, the viral genome might be considered as a necessary but not sufficient condition. Second, mutations or breaks might be caused by tumor viruses as well as by other agents; viruses would be sufficient but not necessary. Third, cancer mutations and integrated viral genomes—oncogenes (Todaro and Huebner, 1972)—or integrated precursors of viral genomes—protoviruses (Temin, 1972)—might be identical.

It has been repeatedly demonstrated that radiation can be a carcinogen in man. As noted above, recessively inherited xeroderma pigmentosum provides direct evidence that ultraviolet light is carcinogenic via damage to DNA. Increased sensitivity to X-ray-induced chromosome breakage occurs in Fanconi's syndrome (Higurashi and Conen, 1971), although the mechanism is not known. Such mutations do not provide tissue specificity in the sense that dominant mutations can, but are predisposing to damage by irradiation.

Xeroderma pigmentosum cells also exhibit defective repair of DNA lesions produced by a chemical carcinogen, $N$-acetoxy-2-acetylaminofluorene (Setlow and Regan, 1972). The carcinogenic metabolic derivatives of several polycyclic hydrocarbons have been shown to be mutagenic in a bacterial system (Ames *et al.*, 1973), making it now highly probable that the effects of chemical carcinogens are mediated via mutation. Of even greater consequence for human oncology is the observation that genetic predisposition to lung cancer is associated with a variant of an enzyme involved in the metabolic conversion of polycyclic hydrocarbons (of the type found in tobacco smoke) to active carcinogens. Kellermann *et al.* (1973) have studied the enzyme aryl hydrocarbon hydroxylase, an enzyme whose activity is greatly increased by various inducing agents. Approximately 50% of the population of the United states is homozygous for an allele associated with low inducibility. Among heavy smokers, these individuals are evidently less susceptible to lung cancer than are those who are homozygous for a "high inducibility" allele or those who are heterozygous for the two alleles. Among 50 patients with bronchogenic carcinoma, all heavy smokers, only two were found to be homozygous for low inducibility.

For all three classes of carcinogens evidence is mounting that their effects are produced by "mutation," using that term to include any transmissible change in the host genome.

## 5. Conclusions

The dominantly inherited tumors and tumor syndromes of man occur in all categories of cancer, where they comprise an estimated 1–40% of the total, depending on the tumor in question. More importantly, they suggest that a common mechanism, mutation in a tissue-specific gene, is a first step in the initiation of cancer. This step is not sufficient alone to produce cancer, and at least one more event must occur. Such another event may also be a mutation, although no direct evidence is available on that point.

Genetic predisposition to cancer is imparted by several chromosomal and recessively inherited conditions. The mechanisms whereby these genetic changes induce susceptibility are probably several, but for only one disease, xeroderma pigmentosum, is the mechanism known. There the genetic damage produced by ultraviolet light cannot be repaired, and it is reasonable to assume that mutations of the type found in the dominantly heritable tumors occur at an increased rate.

Environmental carcinogens seem to produce their effects via alterations in the host genome and are, in a broad sense, mutagenic. Tumor viruses present a special case in that integrated viral genomes or integrated precursors of viral genomes may be indistinguishable from mutations of the type which are dominantly inherited.

## 6. References

AARONSON, S. A., AND LYTLE, C. D., 1970, Decreased host cell reactivation of irradiated SV40 virus in xeroderma pigmentosum, *Nature (Lond.)* **228**:359.
AMES, B. N., DURSTON, W. E., YAMASAKI, E., AND LEE, F. D., 1973, Carcinogens are mutagens: A simple test system combining liver homogenates for activation and bacteria for detection, *Proc. Natl. Acad. Sci.* **70**:2281.

ANDERSON, D. E., 1970, Genetic varieties of neoplasia, in: *Genetic Concepts and Neoplasia* (M. D. Anderson Hospital Symposium), pp. 85–109, Williams and Wilkins, Baltimore.

ANDERSON, D. E., 1971, Clinical characteristics of the genetic variety of cutaneous melanoma in man, *Cancer* **28**:721.

ANDERSON, D. E., 1972, A genetic study of human breast cancer, *J. Natl. Cancer Inst.* **48**:1029.

ARMITAGE, P., AND DOLL, R., 1954, The age distribution of cancer and a multi-stage theory of carcinogenesis, *Brit. J. Cancer* **8**:1.

ARMITAGE, P., AND DOLL, R., 1957, A two-stage theory of carcinogenesis in relation to the age distribution of human cancer, *Brit. J. Cancer* **11**:161.

ASHLEY, D. J. B., 1969a, The two "hit" and multiple "hit" theories of carcinogenesis, *Brit. J. Cancer* **23**:313.

ASHLEY, D. J. B., 1969b, Colonic cancer arising in polyposis coli, *J. Med. Genet.* **6**:376.

AUERBACH, C., 1956, A possible case of delayed mutation in man. *Ann. Hum. Genet.* **20**:266.

BURCH, P. R. J., 1962, A biological principle and its converse: Some implications for carcinogenesis, *Nature (Lond.)* **195**:241.

BURCH, P. R. J., 1965, Natural and radiation carcinogenesis in man. II. Natural leukemogenesis: initiation, *Proc. Roy. Soc. Lond. Ser. B* **162**:240.

CASPERSSON, T., GAHRTON, G., LINDSTEN, J., AND ZECH, L., 1970, Identification of the Philadelphia chromosome as a number 22 by quinacrine mustard fluorescence analysis, *Exp. Cell Res.* **63**:238.

CLEAVER, J. E., 1968, Defective repair replication of DNA in xeroderma pigmentosum, *Nature (Lond.)* **218**:652.

CLEAVER, J. E., 1969, Xeroderma pigmentosum: A human disease in which an initial stage of DNA repair is defective, *Proc. Natl. Acad. Sci.* **63**:428.

FIALKOW, P. J., 1966, Autoimmunity and chromosomal aberrations, *Am. J. Hum. Genet.* **18**:93.

FIALKOW, P. J., 1972, Use of genetic markers to study cellular origin and development of tumors in human females, *Advan. Cancer Res.* **15**:191.

FRAUMENI, J. F., 1969, Constitutional disorders of man predisposing to leukemia and lymphoma, *Natl. Cancer Inst. Monogr.* **32**:221.

GARDNER, E. J., AND RICHARDS, R. C., 1953, Multiple cutaneous and subcutaneous lesions occurring simultaneously with hereditary polyposis and osteomatosis, *Am. J. Hum. Genet.* **5**:139.

GATTI, R. A., AND GOOD, R. A., 1971, Occurrence of malignancy in immunodeficiency diseases: A literature review, *Cancer* **28**:89.

GERMAN, J., 1972, Genes which increase chromosomal instability in somatic cells and predispose to cancer, *Prog. Med. Genet.* **8**:61.

GORLIN, R. J., SEDANO, H. O., VICKERS, R. A., AND CERVENKA, J., 1968, Multiple mucosal neuromas, pheochromocytoma and medullary carcinoma of the thyroid—A syndrome, *Cancer* **22**;293.

HECHT, F., BRYANT, J. S., GRUBER, D., AND TOWNES, P. L., 1964, The nonrandomness of chromosomal abnormalities: Association of trisomy 18 and Down's syndrome, *New Engl. J. Med.* **271**:1081.

HECHT, F., McCAW, B. K., AND KOLER, R. D., 1973, Ataxia-telangiectasia—Clonal growth of translocation lymphocytes, *New Engl. J. Med.* **289**:286.

HIGURASHI, M., AND CONEN, P. E., 1971, *In vitro* chromosomal radiosensitivity in Fanconi's anemia, *Blood* **38**:336.

HIRSCHHORN, K., AND BLOCH-SHTACHER, N., 1970, Transformation of genetically abnormal cells, in: *Genetic Concepts and Neoplasia* (M. D., Anderson Hospital Symposium), pp. 191–202, Williams and Wilkins, Baltimore.

KELLERMANN, G., SHAW, C. R., AND LUYTEN-KELLERMANN, M., 1973, Aryl hydrocarbon hydroxylase inducibility and bronchogenic carcinoma, *New Engl. J. Med.* **289**:934.

KERSEY, J. H., GATTI, R. A., GOOD, R. A., AARONSON, S. A., AND TODARO, G. J., 1972, Susceptibility of cells from patients with primary immunodeficiency diseases to transformation by simian virus 40, *Proc. Natl. Acad. Sci.* **69**:980.

KNUDSON, A. G., 1971, Mutation and cancer: Statistical study of retinoblastoma, *Proc. Natl. Acad. Sci.* **68**:820.

KNUDSON, A. G., 1973, Mutation and human cancer, *Advan. Cancer Res.* **17**:317.

KNUDSON, A. G., AND STRONG, L. C., 1972a, Mutation and cancer: Neuroblastoma and pheochromocytoma, *Am. J. Hum. Genet.* **24**:514.

KNUDSON, A. G., AND STRONG, L. C., 1972b, Mutation and cancer: A model for Wilms' tumor of the kidney, *J. Natl. Cancer Inst.* **48**:313.

KNUDSON, A. G., STRONG, L. C., AND ANDERSON, D. E., 1973, Heredity and cancer in man, *Prog. Med. Genet.* **9**:113.

LADDA, R., ATKINS, L., LITTLEFIELD, J., AND PRUETT, R., 1973, Retinoblastoma: Chromosome banding in patients with heritable tumor, *Lancet* **2**:506.

LYNCH, H. T., AND KRUSH, A. J., 1971, Cancer family "G" revisited: 1895–1970, *Cancer* **27**:1505.

LYNCH, H. T., KRUSH, A. J., LARSEN, A. L., AND MAGNUSON, C. W., 1966, Endometrial carcinoma: Multiple primary malignancies, constitutional factors, and hereditary, *Am. J. Med. Sci.* **252**:381.

MACMAHON, B., AND LEVY, M. A., 1964, Prenatal origin of childhood leukemia: Evidence from twins, *New Engl. J. Med.* **270**:1082.

MILLER, R. W., 1963, Down's syndrome (mongolism), other congenital malformations and cancer among the sibs of leukemic children, *New Engl. J. Med.* **268**:393.

MILLER, R. W., 1968, Deaths from childhood cancer in sibs, *New Engl. J. Med.* **279**:122.

MILLER, R. W., 1970, Neoplasia and Down's syndrome, *Ann. N.Y. Acad. Sci.* **171**:637.

MILLER, R. W., AND TODARO, G. J., 1969, Viral transformation of cells from persons at high risk of cancer, *Lancet* **1**:81.

NEEL, J. V., 1962, Mutations in the human population, in: *Methodology in Human Genetics* (W. J. Burdette, ed.), pp. 203–224, Holden-Day, San Francisco.

NEEL, J. V., 1971, Familial factors in adenocarcinoma of the colon, *Cancer* **28**:46.

NOWELL, P. C., AND HUNGERFORD, D. A., 1960, A minute chromosome in human chronic granulocytic leukemia, *Science* **132**:1497.

NOWELL, P. C., AND HUNGERFORD, D. A., 1961, Chromosome studies in human leukemia. ii. Chronic granulocytic leukemia, *J. Natl. Cancer Inst.* **27**:1013.

PARRINGTON, J. M., DELHANTY, J. D. A., AND BADEN, H. P., 1971, Unscheduled DNA synthesis, u.v.-induced chromosome aberrations and SV40 transformation in cultured cells from xeroderma pigmentosum, *Ann. Hum. Genet.* **35**:149.

ROWLEY, J. D., 1973, A new consistent chromosomal abnormality in chronic myelogenous leukemia identified by quinacrine fluorescence and Giemsa staining, *Nature (Lond.)* **243**:290.

SETLOW, R. B., AND REGAN, J. D., 1972, Defective repair of N-acetoxy-2-acetylaminofluorene-induced lesions in the DNA of xeroderma pigmentosum cells, *Biochem. Biophys. Res. Commun.* **46**:1019.

SETLOW, R. B., REGAN, J. D., GERMAN, J., AND CARRIER, W. L., 1969, Evidence that xeroderma pigmentosum cells do not perform the first step in the repair of ultraviolet damage to their DNA, *Proc. Natl. Acad. Sci.* **64**:1035.

STRONG, L. C., AND KNUDSON, A. G., 1972, Mutation and childhood cancer: A model and its implications, *Am. J. Hum. Genet.* **24**:48a.

TEMIN, H. M., 1972, The RNA tumor viruses—Background and foreground, *Proc. Natl. Acad. Sci.* **69**:1016.

TODARO, G. J., AND HUEBNER, R. J., 1972, The viral oncogene hypothesis: New evidence, *Proc. Natl. Acad. Sci.* **69**:1009.

TOKUHATA, G. K., 1964, Familial factors in human lung cancer and smoking, *Am. J. Pub. Health* **54**:24.

WARTHIN, A. S., 1913, Heredity with reference to carcinoma: As shown by the study of the cases examined in the pathological laboratory of the University of Michigan, 1895–1913, *Arch. Int. Med.* **12**:546.

WILLIAMS, E. D., AND POLLOCK, D. J., 1966, Multiple mucosal neuromata with endocrine tumours: A syndrome allied to von Recklinghausen's disease, *J. Pathol. Bacteriol.* **91**:71.

WILSON, M. G., TOWNER, J. W., AND FUJIMOTO, 1973, Retinoblastoma and D-chromosome deletions, *Am. J. Hum. Genet.* **25**:57.

YOUNG, D., 1971, The susceptibility to SV40 virus transformation of fibroblasts obtained from patients with Down's syndrome, *Europ. J. Cancer* **7**:337.

# 4

# Hormones as Etiological Agents in Neoplasia

JACOB FURTH

## 1. General Considerations

### 1.1. Historical

The hormonal concept of carcinogenesis was initiated by the intuitive studies of Beatson (1896) on the relation of breast cancer to the ovary. Epidemiological studies of mammary tumors of highly inbred strains of mice led Bittner and his associates (Bittner, 1946–1947) to the recognition of genetic, viral, and hormonal components in the development of breast cancer. Independently, Rous and Kidd (1941), on the basis of experimental studies on induction of skin cancers with carcinogens, advanced the multifactorial concept of tumorigenesis and postulated the existence of latent cancer cells. The recognition of "progression" during the course of neoplastic disease was best conceived by Foulds (cf. 1969). Finally, the recognition of immunosurveillance (Burnet, 1970; Jerne, 1973; Klein, 1973–1974) and of immunological and hormonal factors capable of restraining or enhancing tumor growth completed the picture of the complexity of forces involved in initiation and growth of tumors. The last of these—hormones—is reviewed here in light of all other forces.

### 1.2. Nomenclature and Abbreviations

Table 1 presents a simplified nomenclature (Furth et al., 1973d), slightly modified, with the many synonyms which are still widely used. Our nomenclature utilizes

JACOB FURTH ● Institute of Cancer Research and Department of Pathology, Columbia University College of Physicians and Surgeons, New York, New York. Supported by USPHS grant CA-02332 from the National Cancer Institute. Prepared with the technical and editorial assistance of Mrs. Judith Grauman.

TABLE 1
*Nomenclature and Abbreviations*

| Pituitary cell type | | Old nomenclature | Hormone | Class of Li (1972) | Pituitary tumor | End-organ tumor |
| Name | Abbreviation | | | | | |
| --- | --- | --- | --- | --- | --- | --- |
| Adrenotrope | At | Basophil (?) | AtH (ACTH) | I | AtT | AT |
| Mammotrope | Mt | Acidophil | MtH (prolactin, P[a], LtH[b]) | II | MtT | MT |
| Somatotrope | St | Acidophil | StH(growth hormone, GH[a]) | II | StT | |
| Thyrotrope | Tt | Basophil | TtH (TSH) | III | TtT | TT |
| Gonadotrope[c] | Gt | Basophil | GtH | III | GtT | OT, etc.[d] |
| Luteotrope | Lt | Basophil | LH[e] | III | LtT | |
| Folliculotrope | Ft | Basophil | FtH (FSH) | III | FtT | |

[a] Abbreviations such as these are helpful, but when first used they should be accompanied by the generally accepted synonym.
[b] The synonym LtH, for MtH (prolactin), is widely and, in my opinion, incorrectly used. Prolactin, as Li (1972) states, is involved in "growth, development and lactation of the mammary gland . . . ." Hence MtH is preferable.
[c] Recent studies favor the view that one cell, the gonadotrope, secretes both FtH and LH. Those who hold the opposite view can express it by the use of Ft and Lt.
[d] Since the gonads are composed of several different types of hormone-secreting cells, names of their tumors should be given in full and indicated according to the author's concept. For example, the ovarian tumors (OT) can be composed of granulosa cells secreting estrogens, lutein cells secreting predominantly progestins, and so on.
[e] The still common usage of LtH for prolactin made it inadvisable to adopt LtH for the luteinizing hormone.

three letters. The first is the initial of the target organ of the hormone; the second, a small "t," is for tropin (*tropos* = turning to; stimulating); the third is either H (hormone) or T (tumor). For example, TtH stands for thyrotropic hormone, TtT for thyrotropic tumor, and TT for thyroid tumor.

In historical sequence, the nomenclature of pituitary cells was first tinctorial, then morphological, and then "Greek lettered," combining the former two features. This terminology was rendered obsolete by great differences in staining properties of the same cell in different species and in different physiological states within a species, as well as by changes in techniques used. I recommend that the pituitary cells be named after the type of hormone they secrete. Presently, this scheme cannot be rigidly applied, as indicated in footnotes to Table 1. It remains for an international committee to arrive at a standard nomenclature based not on perpetuating the historical confusion but rather on sound current knowledge.

As to hypothalamic hormones, I recommend the suffix .RH (releasing) or .IH (inhibiting), preceded by the initial of the pituitary hormone, when the hormones have been isolated (or synthesized). When their existence is based on circumstantial evidence, the suffix .RF or .IF (F, factor) is preferable. Hormone release is probably a stimulus of hormone production, by virtue of hormonal homeostasis.

Hence the hypothalamic releasing hormones are analogous to the pituitary tropic
(or stimulating) hormones.

77
HORMONES AS
ETIOLOGICAL
AGENTS IN
NEOPLASIA

## 1.3. Neoplasia: Basic Defect and Types

Neoplasia is a multitude of diseases with one common denominator: failure of
homeostatic control to limit the number of differentiated cells. The neoplastic cells
are either hyperreactive to their physiological stimulant(s) or tardy in responding
to their physiological inhibitor(s), thus gaining a proliferative advantage in their
hosts. If the defect is complete, that is, if a cell fails to recognize its specific
restraining influences—hormones, in the broad sense—the resulting tumorous
growth is fully *autonomous*. If the defect is incomplete, the cell can be stimulated or
inhibited, but not fully arrested, by its specific regulators, and is best called
hormone *responsive*. The widely used mammary tumors (MT) induced in rats by
chemical carcinogens, as described by Huggins *et al.* (1959), belong in the latter
category. They are usually incorrectly labeled as hormone *dependent*. They grow
progressively in the presence of the ovary and normal prolactin levels (Nagasawa
*et al.*, 1973). Hence they are correctly labeled hormone responsive. Kim and Furth
(1960*a,b*) found that regression of these tumors following ablation of the pituitary
or ovaries (*cf.* Huggins and Yang, 1962) was incomplete and that the tumors could
be resuscitated by high levels of MtH (Kim *et al.*, 1960*a*) (Fig. 1). This was done by
grafting on these rats isologous, highly functional MtT, even several months after
apparently "complete" regression. Further, after such treatment many new
tumors appeared which can be considered hormone *dependent*. These studies were
confirmed by some (first by Sterental *et al.*, 1963) and challenged by others. The
controversy over the primacy of estrogens vs. proclactin is discussed in Section 3.

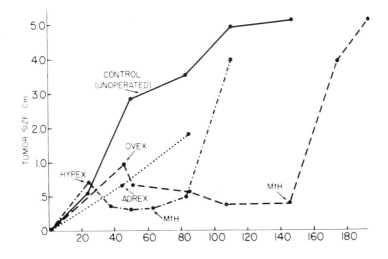

FIGURE 1. Induction, "extinction," and resuscitation of mammary tumors.
From Kim *et al.* (1960*a*).

In man, about one-third of all MT are hormone responsive, and hormone-dependent tumors are unknown. In rats, all three types are known, but among the spontaneous tumors the benign fibroadenomas represent the majority. In mice, most MT are autonomous; few are hormone responsive and fibroadenomas are extremely rare. Most, if not all, murine mammary carcinomas (autonomous or responsive) carry a virus (MTV of Bittner). This virus is homologous to that found in MT of other species, including man (*cf.* Spiegelman and Schlom, 1972; Schlom and Spiegelman, 1973). Some leukemia viruses bear a similar relation to thymic hormones.

Different species and different inbred strains of the same species have a characteristic range of spontaneous tumors and sensitivity to diverse inducing agents. For example, thyrotropic pituitary tumors can be induced in all mice by thyroid hormone (TH) deficiency, but not in any other species.

### 1.3.1. Inducers and Promoters

The popular two- or multistage concept of carcinogenesis was initiated by the work of Rous and Kidd (1941) and expanded by Berenblum and associates (Berenblum, 1947). The changes produced by inducers (initiators) are irreversible, while those produced by promoters are reversible. We conceive of initiation as akin to mutation, modifying the reproductive apparatus of somatic differentiated cells (DNA-protein). The three classes of inducers—chemicals, ionizing radiations, and viruses— can alone induce neoplastic transformation and do it more efficiently in cells stimulated to proliferation. In contrast, evanescence is a basic feature of the effect of hormonal promoters.

The three classes of carcinogens are essentially alike in their basic mode of action, all being chromatinophilic, but there are marked differences among them. Electromagnetic radiation can affect resting cells instantaneously; particulate irradiations are more slow acting. Chemicals differ widely in their mode of action. The nucleic acid of viruses can persist and multiply in the cytoplasm or become incorporated in the DNA of the host's cell in latent form until some secondary "factor" brings about neoplastic transformation of a host cell. By and large, the causative chemicals, unlike the viruses, are absent when the tumors are detected.

As a generalization, dividing the components of carcinogenesis into two categories, inducers and promoters, is didactically useful but not absolutely correct. There is suggestive evidence that sustained proliferation of cells, as induced by persisting hormonal derangement, is conducive to spontaneous mutations, even without the aid of a conventional carcinogen (see Section 6).

A unique feature of carcinogen-induced tumors is that they are usually autonomous at the start, while those initiated by homeostatic derangements are initially hormone responsive and then go through sequential transformation (mutation) toward autonomy. Notable exceptions are Huggin's dimethyl-benz[*a*]anthracene (DMBA) induced MT of rats (Huggins *et al.*, 1961), which begin as hormone-dependent tumors.

TABLE 2
*Breast Cancer Induction with Subcarcinogenic Doses
of Carcinogens Aided by Hormones*

| Carcinogen: | Radiation | Chemical[a] | Virus |
| --- | --- | --- | --- |
| Dose: | 50 R | 10 mg | 0.1 ml milk[b] |
| Species: | Rat | Rat | Mouse |
| Carcinogen alone: | 0 | 0 | 0 |
| MtH alone: | 0 | 0 | 0 |
| Carcinogen + MtH: | 58% | 85% | 40% |

[a] 3-Methylcholanthrene.
[b] Containing MTV.

Sustained, uninterrupted stimulation of a cell can be the determinant of whether a cell transformed by a carcinogen will develop into a tumor. This is illustrated in Table 2 (*cf.* Yokoro *et al.*, 1961; Yokoro and Furth, 1962; Kim and Furth, 1960*c*). The three classes of carcinogens were applied in subcarcinogenic doses. No tumors developed when either hormone or carcinogen alone was applied. The combination of the two caused many tumors.

Hormones promote carcinogenesis by enhancing cell replication. The consequences of enhanced replication of cells are (1) increasing the chance of error of DNA copying, (2) enhancing code-breaking action of subthreshold doses of mutagens (virus, chemicals, radiation), (3) unmasking latent DNA changes caused earlier by mutagens. (In this manner, hormones are procarcinogens.) Cell replication is enhanced *in vivo* by regenerative hyperplasia and in cell cultures by the absence of the cell-specific homeostatic inhibitors or by the addition of nonspecific growth factors. In cell cultures, neoplastic and nonneoplastic transformations are inevitable without a carcinogen. This can be explained as resulting from frantic replication of cells unchecked by homeostatic inhibitors and pushed by diverse growth factors.

The significance of the events sketched in Table 2 is apparent when one considers that small doses of carcinogens are invariably present in the human body and in its environment. The inducers can hit many cells and create mutants of various kinds (lethal or viable latent or overtly transformed cells). We propose to subdivide the mutants into metabolic and neoplastic types. The former are related to aging, the latter to neoplasia.

### 1.3.2. Progression

Foulds (*cf.* 1969) was the first to emphasize the concept of "progression" in neoplasia. The hormone-induced experimental cancers are the best models for demonstration of progression. Behind it lies the surveillance mechanism of the host (Burnet, 1970), which can act as a brake in progression, but it rarely brings about complete spontaneous arrest of spontaneous (unlike grafted) tumors.

Recent developments in knowledge of immunological deviations in spontaneous tumors promise significant therapeutic advancements.

### 1.3.3. Phanerosis

A rarely considered mode of hormonal action which can bring about expression of latent cancer may be termed "phanerosis." This has been best demonstrated by subjecting DMBA-treated, ovariectomized rats to large doses of MtH. It should be recalled that fully hormone-dependent MT grow only in MtH-enriched hosts. This is the mildest form of neoplastic transformation. It may explain the very late manifestation of some neoplasms due to changing hormonal environment with age—for example, MT of women in menopause or radiation-induced OT of mice.

### 1.4. Homeostasis (Cybernetics) and Neoplasia

The term "homeostasis," meaning the maintenance of the internal environment to attain a steady state, was introduced by Cannon (1932) following the ideas of Claude Bernard.

Hormones, in common usage, are substances produced by one type of cell that regulate the growth or function of another cell, which they reach by way of the bloodstream. Increase or decrease in function of cells regulated by hormones proceeds incessantly, as by a thermostat, without cytogenetic changes. Most hormones are pituitary related (hence the expression "master gland"). Until recently, neoplasia could be dealt with as a disturbance of feedback mechanisms (positive or negative) between a pituitary cell and its target organ. Neoplasia is now viewed as a derangement of a highly ordered communication system which limits the number of each cell type, assigning a quota to each, adjusting this quota to the shifting need (cf. Wiener, 1948; Furth, 1969). Mutation-like transformation of a cell is accepted as a common, but not the sole, event that can lead to neoplastic growth. Interruption of the communication system is another. Wiener (1948) pointed out that life in a pluricellular organism exists through a delicate integration of many regulatory centers possessing specialized functions. Integration is achieved by systems of communication, termed by him "cybernetics."

Recent developments have led to the recognition of four levels of communications—I, cerebral; II, hypothalamic; III, pituitary; and IV, visceral—the derangements of which play a major role in the origin and growth of neoplasms (Figs. 2 and 3). The basic defect can reside in either the regulating or the regulated cell or merely in disruption of their communication. Superimposed on this system are numerous nonspecific growth modulators. (For details on intercellular communications leading to loss of contact inhibition, see Lowenstein, 1968, and for details on the hypothetical substances acting by contact, named "chalones," see Iversen, 1970.)

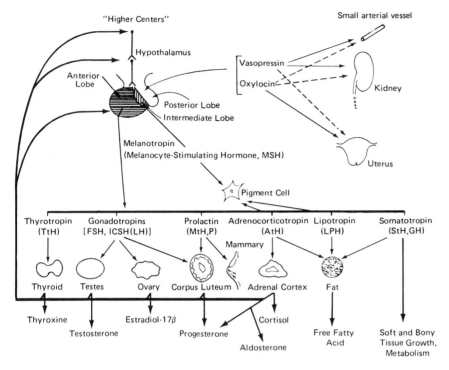

FIGURE 2. The classic scheme of Lyons and Li of pituitary cells, their hormones, and their major target organs, updated by Li (1972) and modified slightly by us.

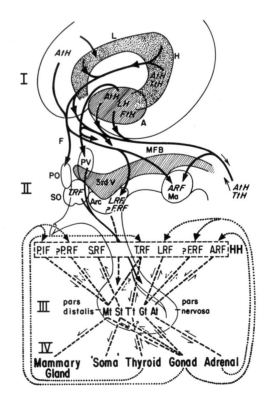

FIGURE 3. A cybernetic sketch indicating with arrows the four levels of communications. I. Cerebral and limbic; II, hypothalamic; III, pituitary; IV, peripheral target organs. Abbreviations: L, limbic system; H, hippocampus; A, amygdala; F, fornix; MFB, medial forebrain bundle; Ma, mammillary body; PV, paraventricular nucleus; PO, preoptic nucleus; SO, supraoptic nucleus; Arc, arcuate nucleus; HH, hypothalamic hormones. From Furth et al. (1973d).

The efficiency of procedures to induce tumorigenesis by hormonal derangement varies with different tumors. In general, the tumors so induced are benign, and there is a "fluid" transition between hyperplasia, conditioned neoplasia, and autonomous neoplasia. This is best exemplified by induction of TtT, in which events proceed in "slow motion." Neoplasms experimentally induced by carcinogens are often autonomous at the start. This may be a matter of the dose and may not hold for spontaneous neoplasms.

### 1.5.1. Ablation of an Endocrine Gland

Ablation of an endocrine gland, thereby removing the specific inhibitor of a pituitary tropic cell, is illustrated by induction of TtT by thyroidectomy (tumorigenesis by exaggeration of negative feedback) (Fig. 4) (*cf.* Furth *et al.*, 1973a). The induction of "basophilic" tumors of the anterior pituitary, estrogen-secreting adrenocortical tumors, and MT in neonatally gonadectomized mice was

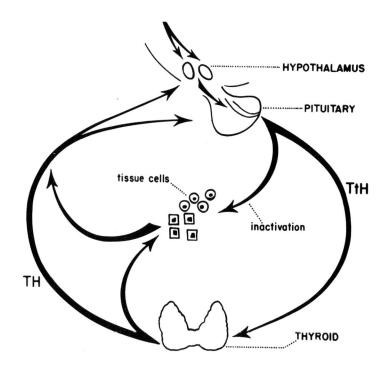

FIGURE 4. The original feedback scheme of the thyroid–thyrotrope axis. Disruption of TH pathway yields TtT by negative feedback; TtH excess yields TT by positive feedback. The routes of TH to peripheral (somatic) organs and the modulating routes of TH to the hypothalamic centers are indicated. From Furth (1969).

reported by Dickie and Woolley (1949) and Dickie and Lane (1956). Houssay *et al.* (1953, 1954) confirmed the induction of similar AT and pituitary tumors in gonadectomized rats and described the latter as GtT. Following similar procedures, Iglesias *et al.* (1969, 1972) reported the isolation of a GtT with very low potency. These observations are good examples of Claude Bernard's principle of determinism, illustrating how a single event (gonadectomy) sets in motion a sequence of changes: compensation by adrenal cortical cells for loss of ovarian estrogen secretion, formation of adrenal adenomas, and, finally, development of MT and pituitary adenomas of yet to be determined character (*cf.* Furth and Clifton, 1958).

### 1.5.2. Sustained Administration of a Specific Stimulant

Sustained administration of a specific stimulant, as induction of MtT with estrogens and of TT with TtH (Fig. 4), is an example of the reverse type of procedure: exaggeration of positive feedback (*cf.* Furth and Clifton, 1966). The induction of a pituitary tumor with estrogens was discovered almost simultaneously by several investigators in 1936. By 1953, Gardner *et al.* listed 24 articles on induction of pituitary tumors in animals by steroid hormones. The functional character and histological types of these tumors were disputed until transplantation studies, analysis of the secondary changes, and bioassays established that they have mammary gland stimulating and growth-promoting activities (*cf.* Furth and Clifton, 1966).

The convenient way to induce MtT in rats and mice is by administration of diethylstilbestrol (DES) pellets. The latency period of tumor development is in direct relation to the dose. Pellets of 5–10 mg are toxic in rats, causing early death of the animals with or without macroscopic MtT. Estradiol is more effective than estrone; estriol is ineffective. Androgens and progestins are antitumorigenic. Elevation of plasma MtH values is progressive during the course of estrogen treatment. Mammary gland hyperplasia with milk secretion documents the functional character of the primary tumors. On transplantation, MtH activity tends to decline; StH activity rises and occasionally becomes dominant.

MtT is the most common pituitary tumor in old rats of both sexes (*cf.* Ito *et al.*, 1972*a*). The high incidence of spontaneous MtT in male rats is puzzling.

Sustained hyperstimulation of GtH can be attained by grating ovaries in spleens of castrates. The gonadal hormones are inactivated in the liver, thereby raising the circulating GtH levels, as illustrated in Fig. 5 (more fully described in Section 2.3.1.).

Prolonged administration of StH (reported by Moon *et al.*, 1950*a,b,c*, 1951) causes an increase in development of several types of tumors.

### 1.5.3. Blocking Hormone Synthesis

Blocking hormone synthesis, as blocking TH synthesis by antithyroidal substances, can produce hyperstimulation of TtH, resulting in TtT and/or TT.

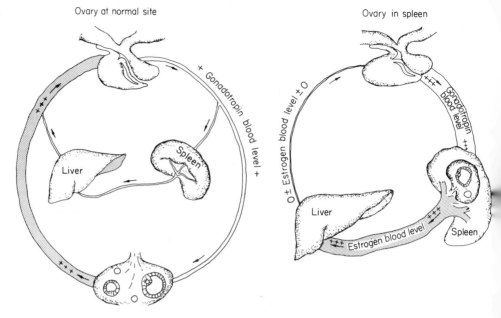

FIGURE 5. Ovarian tumor induction by intrasplenic grafts of ovaries in castrates, an example of neoplasia induction by misplacement of an organ. From Furth (1969).

### 1.5.4. Isografts of the Pituitary

Isografts of the pituitary (introduced by Loeb and Kirtz, 1939) in extrasellar locations result first in excessive discharge of MtH, causing MT and later MtT at the site of the graft. These and other related events have been reviewed elsewhere (Furth *et al.*, 1973*d,e*), including more recent studies with rats and the use of radioimmunoassays.

Hormone-responsive transplantable MT are best obtained by a *combination* of subthreshold doses of a carcinogen and high levels of MtH (Kim and Furth, 1960*b*).

### 1.5.5. Problems

The idea that low-dose irradiations and other carcinogens may lead to a technique for induction of as many types of transplantable pituitary tumors as there are hormone-producing pituitary cells has thus far not been adequately explored.

Although most findings reported are well documented the character and pathogenesis of the various tumors induced, notably pituitary tumors following gonadectomy and AtT induced by ionizing radiations, remain to be elucidated.

Tumorigenesis can probably be modified (promoted or inhibited), possibly even initiated, by drugs acting via the hypothalamus. This is another area yet to be fully explored.

For more detail on neoplasia induction by hormonal derangement, the reader is referred to the reviews or monographs of Gardner *et al.* (1953), Russfield (1966), Furth and Clifton (1966), Kwa (1961), and Furth *et al.* (1973*d, e*).

## 2. The Four Levels Of Communications

### 2.1. Neurohypothalamic Areas and Neoplasia

The existence of hypothalamic substances regulating anterior pituitary function was postulated by Green and Harris (1947) and demonstrated by Harris (cf. 1955) by tapping the hypophyseal portal veins. Subsequent developments led to the isolation of several low molecular weight polypeptides in the hypothalamus and to the recognition of neural influences on the hypothalamus. Hypothalamic factors (hormones) are now known to control production and release of the pituitary hormones AtH, TtH, LH, FtH, StH, and MtH. Two adenohypophyseal hormones, MtH and StH, are also under the influence of hypothalamic inhibitory factors (hormones).

Figure 2 is the classic diagram of Lyons and Li (updated by Li, 1972) on the levels of hormonal communications, including the target organ hormones. Figure 3 is our cybernetic sketch indicating lines of communications (Furth *et al.*, 1973*d*). The fulcrum of the four levels of the regulatory system is the pituitary gland. It receives impulses from both the visceral cells and the hypothalamus. The impulses or responses of the cerebral system are transmitted to the hypothalamus by neural routes, at the long terminals of which these messages are expressed by neurohormones. The hypothalamus is the transmitter of impulses received from the cerebral or visceral areas and acts by discharging hormones of its own into the hypophysis by way of the portal system.

Neoplasia can be initiated not only by a change in the four integrated areas but also by a mere disruption of communication among them (Fig. 3), resulting in an excess of "target cell" stimulating influences or a deficiency of its inhibiting influences. The role of hypothalamic hormones in neoplasia seems to be limited to modulation of pituitary hormones. Tumors do occur in the hypothalamic area (*cf.* Turkington, 1972), but none has been actually identified as a direct secretor of hypothalamic hormones. The pituitary can give rise to monomorphous tumors of perhaps all of its tropic cellular components. The differentiated neurons do not multiply. Tumors of neurons are likely to be congenital. The same applies to the neural lobe of the pituitary, which is a storage organ of oxytocin and vasopressin.

The hypothalamic hormones have been extensively studied from the standpoint of their physiological effects, but with the exception of P.IF little is known of their influence in tumorigenesis. The following are some illustrative examples: GH.IH (StH.IH) was isolated from ovine hypothalami by Brazeau *et al.* (1973). It strongly lowers GH levels in patients with acromegaly without affecting prolactin levels (Hall *et al.*, 1973), but also impairs the normal TtH and FtH responses to T.RH. T.RH is one of the best studied hypothalamic polypeptides. Administration of T.RH causes a sharp and marked rise of TtH within 3 min, with a slow dropping thereafter. Grant *et al.* (1973) found two binding sites on Tt cells, differing in intensity of affinity for T.RH and its analogues. However, Clifton (1963) has presented some suggestive evidence for the essentiality of hypothalamic connections in induction of TtT in mice and has suggested that T.RH plays some role in development of TT.

As concerns mammary neoplasia, P.IF and P.RF are highly important. Their discovery was "inevitable" following the studies of Harris (*cf.* 1955) on their presence in the hypophyseal portal vessels. The enhanced pituitary MtH secretion occurring as a sequel to pituitary isografts is due to lack of hypothalamic P.IF. This discovery of Everett and Nikitovich-Winer (1963) followed the analysis of the phenomenon that pituitary isografts were conducive to the development of MT (Loeb and Kirtz, 1939).

A great impetus in this area came from the recognition of drugs which act on the central nervous system via P.IF or P.RF. Flückiger (1972) names nine tranquilizers, two psychomotor stimulants, two antihistamines, two antihypertensives, and other drugs that influence prolactin secretion. Ten of these, tested for their influence on prolactin secretion, exhibited diverse unwanted side-effects, but some ergot alkaloids (Shelesnyak, 1954) have proved to be of practical value.

In his pioneer studies, Meites (*cf.* 1973) indicated that administration of drugs that decrease prolactin release (such as L-dopa, iproniazid, pargyline, and certain ergot drugs) results in reduced MT growth; while other drugs that increase prolactin release (as reserpine, haloperiodol, or methyldopa) accelerate growth of MT in rats. Incidentally, these findings lent further support to earlier biological studies indicating that prolactin is a major, often the essential, hormone for induction and growth of many MT.

The rapid advancement in this area is indicated by the proceedings of three international conferences on prolactin (Wolstenholme and Knight, 1972; Boyns and Griffiths, 1972; Pasteels and Robyn, 1973) and one monograph (Horrobin, 1973) containing a wealth of information on the biochemistry and physiology of prolactin, including its role in carcinogenesis.

The pivotal role of these hypothalamic factors in the growth of established hormone-sensitive carcinomas is attested to by the flood of current experimental and clinical observations (e.g., Minton and Dickey, 1973). Suppression of serum prolactin by L-dopa alone can produce clinical remissions in carcinoma of the breast and relieve the bone pain, presumably as a result of suppression of tumor growth, with no consistent changes in FtH, GH, LH, estradiol, estrone, estriol, and progesterone levels (Dickey and Minton, 1972*a,b*).

All known drugs exerting their effects by way of the hypothalamus are short-acting. The synthetic ergot alkaloid CB-154 (2-bromo-α-ergocryptine; Flückiger, 1972) can be injected daily over long periods of time. The development of long-acting prolactin inhibitors is required to attain a lasting depression of prolactin discharge with inhibition of tumor growth. Welsch and Gribler (1973) found that CB-154 is an effective inhibitor of the developmental phases of murine MT, but not of MT in mature multiparous mice. Welsch *et al.* (1973) found that the combined administration of ergocornine and reserpine (but neither drug alone) produced as prolonged and as good a regression of DMBA-induced MT of mice as did hyperphysectomy. Buckman and Peake (1973) found that stimulation of prolactin by perphenazine is augmented by prior estrogen treatment.

The hypothalamic hormones do not seem as specific as would be required for homeostasis of a target organ function. For example, several investigators have demonstrated elevated serum MtH following administration of T.RH. Mt cells

possess receptor sites for T.RH (*cf.* Grant *et al.*, 1973). Increase in the rate of synthesis of MtH produced by T.RH in cultures of rat pituitary cells was reported by Hinkle and Tashjiam (1973). However, no one, to our knowledge, has demonstrated biological MtH activity following administration of T.RH. To unravel the lack of specificity of these hormones is an intriguing problem. Mechanisms do exist to block biological activity by a circulating hormone. For example, in MtT F4-bearing rats, StH activity is blocked by adrenal corticoids. L-dopa has been reported to suppress T.RH-stimulated MtH release (Noel *et al.*, 1973). Dimethoxyphenylethylamine blocks the dopamine-inhibitory control of MtH secretion (Smythe and Lazarus, 1973). It is known that MtH and StH are related structurally and biologically, but Flückiger (*cf.* 1972) found that L-dopa and chlorpromazine have opposite actions on MtH and StH secretion. Competitive interaction can occur at hypothalamic, pituitary, or peripheral levels.

For more details on the rapidly evolving knowledge on neural and hypothalamic influences and other substances acting by way of the hypothalamus, the reader should see the respective mongraphs and reviews of Haymaker *et al.* (1969), Meites (1970), Knigge *et al.* (1972), Ganong and Martini (1973), Locke and Schally (1973) Vale *et al.* (1973), Schally *et al.* (1973), and Thomas and Mawhinney (1973).

Despite the problem of specificity, hypothalamic hormones hold considerable promise in cancer research, as either prophylactic or therapeutic agents, doing away with drastic surgical procedures in disease control (*cf.* Stoll, 1972).

## 2.2. Cell Types of the Adenohypophysis and Their Neoplasms

The adenohypophysis (pars distalis) is believed to be composed of five cell types secreting ten different hormones. On the basis of structural and biological effects, Li (1972) divides these hormones into three classes: I—AtH, melanocyte-stimulating hormones ($\alpha$- and $\beta$-MSH), lipotropic hormones ($\beta$- and $\gamma$-LPH); II—StH (GH) and MtH (P); III—LH (luteinizing and interstitial cell stimulating hormone = ICSH), FSH, TtH. The principal functions of the ten hormones are as follows: (1) *AtH* stimulates the adrenal cortex to produce steroid hormones as cortisol and corticosterone; (2, 3) *$\alpha$- and $\beta$-MSH* cause darkening of skin by melanogenesis in preexisting unpigmented melanocytes; (4, 5) *$\beta$- and $\gamma$-LPH* cause release of lipid from adipose tissue; (6) *StH (GH)* has an anabolic effect on various tissues of the body and affects fat, carbohydrate, and protein metabolism and general body growth; (7) *MtH(P)* is responsible for the growth, development, and lactation of the mammary gland; (8) *LH (ICSH)* in women, affects the development of interstitial cells in the ovaries and is related to reproduction and in men is responsible for development of interstitial cells in the testes and affects reproduction; (9) *FSH* in women induces the development of follicles in the ovaries and affects reproduction and in men stimulates seminiferous tubules and spermatogenesis; (10) *TtH* is responsible for the production and secretion of thyroid hormones. This schematic description, based mainly on Li's concepts, is given for general didactic purposes with the qualification that there are numerous "gray" areas concerning all unit systems of the adenohypophysis.

Structural relationships explain why one cell type can possess more than one hormonal potency. Although all hormones possess a high degree of specificity when used in physiological doses, they can exhibit several activities when their concentration is high, as is the case with various hormonal derangements. Classic examples of such structural relationships are those between StH and MtH and between TtH and GtH. The latter has been thoroughly analyzed (Canfield *et al.*, 1971; Pierce *et al.*, 1971; Rathnam and Saxena, 1971; Vaitukaitis and Ross, 1972; Furth *et al.*, 1973*b*).

A single macromolecular hormone such as TtH and LH can give rise to several antibodies. The cross-reactions can be analyzed by quantitative absorption or blocking tests. The type-specific antigenic groups are named "$\beta$," and the common subunit is "$\alpha$." The overlapping biological activities were first discovered years ago during the course of transplantation of TtT. The "built-in" MSH activity of AtT was similarly discovered during the course of transplantation studies by Steelman *et al.* (1956) and Bahn *et al.* (1957). According to more recent investigations (Nakane, 1970; Phifer *et al.*, 1972, 1973), the two gonadotropic hormones (FSH and LH) are secreted by the same cell, but what controls their secretion is obscure.

The physical properties of human MtH and StH are so close that separation was unsuccessful until Pasteels (*cf.* 1972) indicated the existence of a separate human MtH [subsequently purified by Friesen *et al.*, 1970 (*cf.* Friesen, 1972; Friesen and Hwang, 1973) and Lewis *et al.*, 1971]. The structural similarities of these two hormones are indicated by the following findings of Li (1973): For each milligram of human MtH there are 25 IU of lactogenic and 0.4 USP U of StH activity, while each milligram of human StH possesses 2 IU of lactogenic and 2 USP U of StH activity.

The "chromophobe" is a poorly secreting cell, a degranulated, functional differentiated cell, or a reserve undifferentiated cell. The term is now obsolete. The terms "acidophil" and "basophil" have some qualifying value (see Table 1).

Speculating on the evolution of pituitary hormones, Li (1972) considers AtH-MSH the ancestral molecule (see his Fig. 11). It is noteworthy in relation to his classification of hormones that when a pituitary cell becomes neoplastic the common change is usually a shift in its hormonal spectrum. For example, some MtT often exhibit more StH than MtH activity, to such an extent that three investigators independently described the transformation of the same MtT into an StT (MacLeod *et al.*, 1966; Tashjian *et al.*, 1968; Hollander and Hollander, 1971). Rare transplantable MtT strains appear to be predominantly AtH secreting and cause hypertension attributed to heightened adrenal cortical activity (Molteni *et al.*, 1972). Bates *et al.* (1966) and Martin *et al.* (1968) analyzed the relation of MStT of rats to diabetes. Similarly, when a TtT becomes autonomous it can exhibit greater gonadotropic than thyrotropic activity (Messier and Furth, 1962). Acquisition by one cell type of the biological activity of cells of another class of Li has also been reported (for example, StH activity of autonomous TtT; Furth *et al.*, 1973*c*).

When hormonal derangement is lasting, as is the case with neoplasms, secondary (minor) components may be expressed biologically (clinically) to such an extent that the primary (main) hormonal stimulation is obscured by secondary and tertiary derangements (see Section 5). This explains why the human (unlike the experimental) pituitary tumors are usually not named by the type of cell causing the initial change. For example, AtT is called Cushing's disease, MtT is known as Forbes–Albright syndrome, and StT as acromegaly or gigantism. Turkington (1972) identified MtH secretion in patients having tumors associated with Forbes–Albright syndrome, Chiari–Frommel syndrome, and Nelson's syndrome and in those having hypothalamic tumors.

Inasmuch as various hormone-secreting pituitary tumors (MtT, StT, MStT, AtT, FtT, and GtT) have been reviewed elsewhere (Furth *et al.*, 1973*d*), I have cited here only a few recent related reports.

Immunohistochemical staining can visualize the hormone content of all accepted pituitary cell types of man and experimental animals. The latter has been extensively illustrated in reviews of Baker (1970) and Nakane (1970) and in our own review (Furth *et al.*, 1973*e*). The two acidophils (Mt and St) are spherical (Fig. 6a, b). The characteristic feature of Mt is the "caplike" localization of the hormone about the nucleus, well illustrated in Fig. 6e. The Gt are somewhat larger and tend to be polyhedral (Fig. 6c). The At are highly angular, often resembling macrophages (Fig. 6d). In a human prolactin-secreting pituitary tumor (Fig. 6f), almost all cells have an affinity for antiprolactin, and for no other antihormone.

The counterpart of immunohistochemical staining is radioimmunoassay, which quantitates the discharged hormone in circulation at a given time. These two techniques are extremely useful tools in diagnosis and analysis of complex situations. For example, the half-life of various pituitary hormones can be studied by injecting labeled hormones and following their disappearance from the circulation. Storage and discharge can be ascertained by the rebound phenomenon (Furth *et al.*, 1973*a*). The character of a hormone-secreting tumor can be determined by immunohistochemical staining of the tumor for various hormones. The pharmacological effects of drugs can be similarly tested. For example, utilizing immunohistochemical staining Baker *et al.* (1972) found that treatment of adult female rats with a progestational compound (medroxyprogesterone acetate) caused a marked reduction in size of Mt cells and enlargement and increase in relative number of St cells. Gt cells responded variably and At cells were not affected significantly.

## 2.3. Neoplasia in Peripheral Endocrine-Related Organs

Neoplasia induced in peripheral organs by pituitary tumors and tumors arising in hormone-secreting organs outside the cranial cavity (such as hormone-related neoplasms of the parathyroid and insulinomas, medullary adrenal tumors,

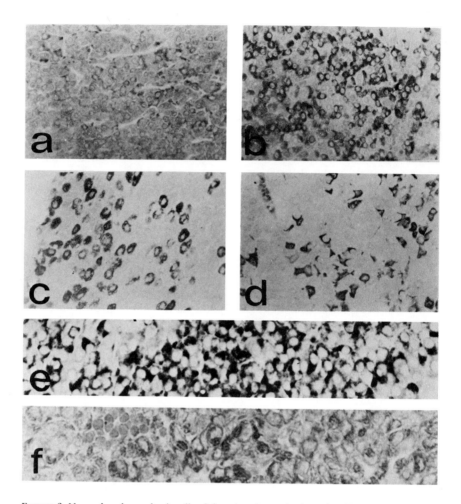

FIGURE 6. Normal and neoplastic cells of the adenohypophysis as visualized by immunohistochemical staining. (a) Normal female rat pituitary at 48 days of age, stained with anti-MtH. × 150. (b) Same, stained with anti-StH. × 150. (c) Same, stained with anti-LH. × 150. (d) Same, stained with anti-AtH. × 150. (e) Normal female rat pituitary at 124 days of age, stained with anti-MtH. × 350. (f) Human MtT stained with anti MtH. × 500. (Magnifications are approximate.)

melanomas, prostate tumors, and carcinoids) are omitted here. The following are brief general comments on tumors in peripheral areas illustrating the diversity of pathogenic mechanisms by which hormones can produce such tumors, notably those with which we have had personal experience. The character of hormone-related tumors varies with species, strain, tumor inducers, and the concentrations. For details on peripheral hormone-related tumors, the reader should see the comprehensive textbooks of Willis (1967) and Williams (1968) for general orientation, and subsequent volumes of this treatise.

Peripheral tumors are of two kinds: those affecting non-hormone-secreting organs, which do not feed back (as the mammary gland), and those affecting peripheral hormone-secreting organs, which do. The best example of the former is MT. Good examples of the second type are TT and OT. The latter are variously hormone secreting and can themselves induce tumors with different spectra. The male "analogy" of the mammary gland tumor is the prostate tumor. On clinical grounds, androgens are suspected of being the responsible hormone in the genesis of prostate tumors, but thus far attempts to develop a hormone-dependent prostatic carcinoma have been unsuccessful.

### 2.3.1. Ovarian Tumors

Experimental studies on induction of leukemias by X-rays led to the discovery of development of OT in most irradiated mice. Such tumors can arise from any cell of the ovary other than ova: from granulosa and lutein cells, which secrete characteristic steroid hormones, and from nonsecreting germinal, epithelial, stromal, and endothelial cells. By means of transplantation, monomorphous tumors can be obtained. The primary radiation-induced OT inevitably have a long latency; even if this inducer is applied very early in postnatal life, tumors will arise in the second half of the life span. Increasing the dose does not markedly hasten tumor induction. For references, see Bali and Furth (1949).

The identity of the GtH component in the mechanism of ovarian tumorigenesis was clarified following observations of Biskind and Biskind (1944) that mere transplantation of normal ovaries into the spleen of castrated rodents will also yield OT. This is attributed to (1) a break in the Gt–gonadal hormone feedback loop by diversion of the gonadal hormones to the liver, where they are inactivated as illustrated in Fig. 5 (Gardner *et al.*, 1959) (In cybernetics, this is said to "open the loop."), and (2) a consequential increase of GtH production. The primary tumors of ovarian grafts in the spleen are not autonomous—that is, transplantable into normal hosts—for about 9–12 months of the graft (Green, 1957). Numerous observations indicate the increase of GtH as one component of OT induction by radiation. The other is a direct injury to the ovary.

The transplanted granulosa cell tumors produce secondary changes indicative of estrogen secretion; those of luteomas point to progestin as the major steroid (Bali and Furth, 1949). Granulosa tumors produce a marked hypervolemia associated with anemia (Wish *et al.*, 1950), while the luteomas are associated with polycythemic hypervolemia and Cushing's syndrome (Gottschalk and Furth, 1951).

OT is one of the many tumors induced by the multipotent DMBA and other polycyclic aromatic hydrocarbons. The report of Howell *et al.* (1954) on the high incidence of granulosa cell OT in mice that had been repeatedly given oily solutions of DMBA was followed by numerous studies on the character and pathogenesis of those tumors. Jull and Phillips (1969) concluded that the carcinogenic effect of DMBA on mouse ovaries was direct but that it was modified by secretion of several pituitary hormones, notably gonadotropins. The tumors were autonomous, but gonadotropins accelerated tumorigenesis by DMBA (Orr, 1962). Some enzymatic and histochemical studies were made with such tumors by

Ueda *et al.* (1972), but the characterization of monomorphous OT from the standpoint of steroidogenesis and interrelationships and effects of serum and cell volumes remains to be fully explored. For further details on OT, the reader should consult Zuckerman (1962).

The most valuable technique for inducing OT is that of Biskind and Biskind (1944), because it is best suited for analysis of the sequential events from hyperplasia to dependent and this to autonomous OT.

### 2.3.2. Leydig Cell Tumors

Leydig cell tumors occur in small numbers of several strains of mice, rats, and dogs (*cf.* Gardner *et al.*, 1959; Russfield, 1966; Huseby, 1972). They are especially common in undescended testes and can be readily induced with estrogens. Experimental Leydig cell tumors were extensively studied by Huseby (1960) and Jacobs and Huseby (1972). The sequential changes from hyperplasia to neoplasia are similar to those of other estrogen-induced tumors (*cf.* Andervont *et al.*, 1957). The biological findings suggest that these tumors are usually androgen secreting, but the spectrum of steroids secreted by these tumors requires further study. Accumulation of $^3$H-estradiol in mouse testes following prolonged treatment with estrogen was reported by Bollengier *et al.* (1972). Our observations (Clifton *et al.*, 1956) suggest that some tumors may secrete both estrogens and androgens. The very problem of the source of estrogens in male rodents, usually related to Sertoli cells (*cf.* Huggins and Moulder, 1945), also requires further study.

Hormone-independent Leydig cell tumors in the mouse have been well maintained in organ cultures, whereas those that were hormone dependent were poorly maintained (Elias and Rivera, 1959).

### 2.3.3. Thyroid tumors

There are two features common to the development of "spontaneous" and induced TT: (1) presence of thyroid cells that are capable of multiplication but are imparied in synthesis of thyroid hormones, and (2) elevated TtH levels. TH synthesis begins with "capture" of iodine, followed by sequential enzymatic processes and culminating in formation of L-triiodothyronine (T3) and L-thyroxine (T4). Nature provides ample opportunities for insult to this normal sequence, including iodine deficiency and goiterogenic agents in the diet. To these have been added man-made injuries to the thyroid epithelium, such as by "fallout" or accidental irradiation of the newborn. This subject has been thoroughly reviewed at two international conferences on thyroid cancer (see Hedinger, 1969; Young and Inman, 1968).

The sequential events in the goiterogen-induced adenomas and carcinomas have been well analyzed and reproduced in the laboratory. The initial hyperplasia is usually nodular and diffuse (unlike Grave's disease, in which the hyperplasia is diffuse but not nodular and seems to be unrelated to TtH). The malignant neoplasia appears late and varies in frequency in relation to intensity and maintenance of the thyroid damage. We studied the sequential changes from hyperplasia to highly malignant carcinoma by long-continued, uninterrupted exposure of normal thyroid grafts to very high levels of TtH produced by cografts of an autonomous TtH-secreting pituitary tumor. Several years of sequential transplantations yielded "sarcomatoid carcinomas" which were indistinguishable from human sarcomatoid carcinomas (often called sarcomas), leaving unresolved the question of whether a carcinoma cell can turn into a sarcoma cell (Ueda and Furth, 1967).

### 2.3.4. Other Tumors

*a. Adrenal Tumors.* Adrenal tumors (AT) are unique in that they can give rise to four or more types of tumors—estrogen, androgen, glucocorticoid, and mineralocorticoid secreting—and in that they have different types of inductive mechanisms, of which some have already been discussed. The type of AT extensively studied by my associates is glucocorticoid secreting. It proved suitable for assay of AtH (Cohen *et al.*, 1957) and was used to first establish the high AtH serum level in a patient with Cushing's syndrome in whom bilateral adrenalectomy was followed by manifestations of Cushing's disease AtT with MSH activity (Cohen and Furth, 1959). This condition was later named "Nelson's syndrome" after the investigator who thoroughly studied this event in numerous patients. The steroidogenesis by our AT was well investigated by Bloch *et al.* (1960). This tumor was used to first study the mechanism of adrenal stimulation by labeled AtH (Lefkowitz *et al.*, 1970a). It produces corticoid *in vitro* (Buonassisi *et al.*, 1962).

*b. Renal Cortical Carcinomas.* Renal cortical carcinomas induced by estrogens in male hamsters (Kirkman and Bacon, 1950; Horning, 1954) are among the most puzzling estrogen-dependent tumors. They are malignant yet hormone dependent and seem "specific" to hamsters.

*c. Human Placental Lactogen.* Human placental lactogen (HPL), a hormone with both MtH and StH activity, stimulates carcinogenesis by DMBA in young rats. It promotes mammary tumorigenesis during pregnancy, both directly and indirectly, through its promotion of progesterone secretion by the ovary (Nagasawa and Yanai, 1973).

*d. Medullary Thyroid Carcinoma.* Thyrocalcitonin is the hypocalcemic polypeptide hormone secreted by the medullary cells of the thyroid. These cells can give rise to tumors (Munson *et al.*, 1968; Taylor and Foster, 1970).

*e. Ectopic Hormones.* The ectopic hormones are discussed in Section 4.

## 3.1. General Considerations

Hormonal stimulation or depression of an organ can be detected by clinical and anatomical changes. The criteria of malignancy are well defined in textbooks of pathological anatomy, but many hormone-dependent and responsive tumors do not possess such definitive identification marks as invasiveness and anaplasia, and masquerade as diffuse or nodular hyperplasia. Chromosomal abnormalities can be conspicuous in hyperplasia and, if marked, suggest cell transformation. However, the presence of transformed cells (commonly defined in tissue cultures by lack of contact inhibition) does not differentiate neoplastic from metabolic transformation. Both produce altered cells, either abnormally differentiated or mutated. Neoplastic cells possess a proliferative advantage over homeostatically controlled cells; metabolically altered cells usually do not. The latter are common in normal aging organs and may be a component of the aging process (*cf.* Furth, 1969). During sustained hyperplasia, as induced by hormonal derangement, an increasing number of cells undergo some transformation and exist intermingled with hyperplastic unaltered cells. Transformation of cells is hastened by chemical, viral, and radiation carcinogens. Depending on the dose of the carcinogen and other factors, the number of transformed cells may vary and some may be autonomous at the start. When neoplasia is rooted in a hormonal derangement, the initial phase is that of hyperplasia, which is usually followed by hormone-dependent and responsive neoplasia. Sustained hyperplasia may lead to neoplasia by means of spontaneous replication errors of the genetic apparatus (see Section 6).

It is likely that in their earlier (silent) phases, many tumors are hormone responsive or even hormone dependent—hence the importance of detecting such cells. For laboratory diagnosis of endocrine diseases, the reader should consult Sunderman and Sunderman (1971). For hormones in the blood, Gray and Bacharach (1967) should be consulted. Eckstein and Knowles (1963) have summarized the techniques in endocrine research. Some "footprints" of biochemical, histochemical, and immunological tests do exist; for evaluation of existing nodules of debatable character, transplantation assay is a useful tool.

Transplantation assays are suitable for both detection and characterization of neoplastic cells. They require the use of histocompatible strains of animals, and are therefore not feasible for assay of human tumors. As substitutes, techniques have been proposed which have one feature in common: the use of animals in which immunological antagonism is lacking or has been abolished. The older techniques are transplantation in the anterior chamber of the eye, or on the chorioallantoic membrane of the chick embryo, or in the cheek pouch of the hamster. These have been followed by the use of animals whose immunological capacity has been checked by administration of glucocorticoids, by neonatal thymectomy, or by cografts of transplantable AtT. Very recently, the congenital athymic nude mouse has become the host of choice. It is essential that the chosen method allow the expression of the hormonal effects of the grafts and of the added hormonal manipulations. No cell and organ culture method is known which faithfully imitates the homeostatic interplay of hormones *in vivo*.

In model animal systems using histocompatible hosts, the immunological antagonism of hosts, if at all expressed, is not much greater than that of the primary hosts. Histocompatible strains never have the 100% genetic identity of identical twins. Some genetic antagonism can be overcome by injection of large numbers of viable cells.*

## 3.2. Detection and Quantitation of Hormones

Three types of procedures for detection and quantitation of hormones are currently available: chemical assays and bioassays, radioimmunoassay, and immunohistochemical visualization of hormones by the use of fluorescent antibodies or immunohistochemical staining. None of these by itself is adequate for characterization of a given hormone-related neoplasm. The diverse techniques applied to hormone-related tumors have been reviewed by us (Furth *et al.*, 1973*d*). Listed below are other recent reviews and books. Utilization of these disciplines requires special expertise; the literature is replete with articles containing inconclusive reports and data due to lack of it. Problems requiring specialized techniques are best pursued by cooperative efforts of investigators majoring in the wanted areas.

Radioimmunoassay is now an indispensable tool in research in every area of endocrinology. The scope of its usefulness has rapidly expanded far beyond the quantitation of peptide hormones as introduced by Berson and Yalow (*cf.* 1973). Steroid hormones, enzymes, diverse antigens and antibodies, and many other substances of diagnostic and therapeutic value can now be measured in nanogram, some in picogram, quantities. Specific and group reactions can be estimated. As concerns hormone assays, it should be kept in mind that antigenic determinants, although related to biological activity are not identical with it. Conversely, biological activity can be expressed in the absence of detectable immunological reactivity. Consequently, purification by physicochemical procedures (such as gel filtration, electrophoresis, and ultracentrifugation) can yield immunologically active substances missed earlier, when purification was guided by bioassays. These substances may represent precursors or metabolic products of a biologically active hormone. Yalow (1974) reviewed the complex relationship of immunoreactive forms of five peptide hormones: parathormone, insulin, gastrin, AtH, and StH. Further, different antisera can detect different forms of the same peptide hormone, its precursor or metabolite, and relate them to its structure. Presently, the peptide hormones are named according to their molecular size: "big-big," "big," and "little." Goodman *et al.* (1972) demonstrated by Sephadex

---

* To make model systems available to qualified investigators, the National Cancer Institute has established a "bank" for hormone-related tumors. A word of warning: Because of the frequent changes occurring during the course of transplantations, one should not accept a studied tumor to be true to its name, but should verify its biological character.

G75 filtration that radioimmunoassayable StH in acromegalic and normal plasma contains a minor component (14–28%) of "big" StH, with molecular weight approximately 40,000, and a major component (67–86%) of "little" StH, with molecular weight approximately 21,000. Most original studies on heterogeneity were made on human hormone-related tumors; they have been extended recently to include experimental tumors. Studies along these lines will enhance our knowledge of the synthesis, storage, circulation time, and disposal of diverse hormones.

Immunohistochemical techniques (Nakane, 1970), by virtue of their great specificity, are increasingly replacing the chemical characterization of hormone-secreting cells. When coupled with electron microscopy, they visualize the organelles of cells and enable analysis of the synthesis, as well as disposal, of hormones in various physiological and pathological states. The techniques widely used have been reviewed and updated by Mazurkiewicz and Nakane (1972) and Moriarty (1973). Like radioimmunoassay, immunohistochemical staining is still subject to further refinements, but it is likewise sufficiently advanced for routine use. The appearance of the various types of pituitary hormone-secreting cells in rodents, as visualized by immunohistochemical staining, is characteristic for their identification (Fig. 6a–e).

The potentialities of electron microscopy in studies of the pathophysiology of the pituitary are well indicated by Farquhar (1971) and Hopkins and Farquhar (1973). These investigators also present excellent illustrations of the stages during the synthesis, intracellular transport, and excretion of synthesized hormones, and crinophagia. The various pituitary cell types have certain identifying features, of which the size and shape and location of the hormone are outstanding. The monograph of Benoit and DaLage (1963) and the abortive studies of Farquhar (personal communication) indicate the problems inherent in analysis of the neoplastic changes in the diverse pituitary tumors. Combining immunohistochemical staining with electron microscopy (Nakane, 1970) and other techniques (Hopkins and Farquhar, 1973) may be helpful in making some headway in this direction.

### 3.3. Steroid vs. Protein Hormones: Their Receptors and Translation of Their Messages

The disproportionate length of this section on steroid and protein hormones—with particular emphasis on estrogen and prolactin—is attributable to the temporal surge in establishing the pathogenesis of MT, the most common neoplasm in women, and the great promise of its control which followed the discovery of hypothalamic factors.

The discovery by Doisy et al. (1929) of the first neoplasia-related hormone (estrone) followed Beatson's intuitive studies (1896) on the relation of the ovary to human mammary cancers. This led to research on adrenal steroids and the disclosure that the adrenal is a reserve organ for production of gonadal steroids. Following their isolation, ovarian estrogens became the focal point in study of mammary carcinogenesis and the mouse the classic animal in MT research because of the high incidence of spontaneous MT in this species. Decades of thorough work led Bittner to formulate a triad in murine mammary carcinogenesis: genetics, estrogens, and his mammary tumor agent (MTA). He considered estrogen the basic carcinogen and his MTA a mere promoter (1946–1947, 1952). Subsequently, several investigators noted that natural and synthetic estrogens and certain nonsteroidal substances with estrogenic activity (as diethylstilbestrol) can induce pituitary tumors with high frequency in mice and rats. Furth and Clifton (*cf.* 1966) found that these tumors secreted prolactin and named them "mammotropic" (MtT). Transplanted MtT of rats and mice yield huge quantities of MtH. In our concept, prolactin is a major component in mammary tumorigenesis.

The recent discovery of hypothalamic P.IF and P.RF introduced a new set of factors which circumvent the gonads and operate via regulation of prolactin release. Thus there are three major types of hormones related to mammary tumorigenesis, but their relative roles and interrelationships remain to be fully clarified.

The discovery of Huggins *et al.* (1961) of the highly elevated sensitivity to DMBA of the mammary gland of female rats between the ages of 29 and 60 days (with a peak at about 55 days) has led many of us to investigate the hormonal status at this critical age. Beginning with immunohistochemical staining of the pituitaries, we found that at 5 and 10 days of age all pituitary hormones are present in the pituitary with the exception of prolactin, which begins to appear at about 15 days and becomes distinct at about 30 days (Furth *et al.*, 1974). Radioimmunoassays by Wuttke (1973) and Esber and Bogden (to be published) are in essential agreement with the results of immunohistochemical staining. (It should be noted that immunohistochemical staining represents storage of hormones, while radioimmunoassay detects their levels in the serum.)

Independent studies of Weisz and Gunsalus (1973) and Esber and Bogden (*cf.* Furth *et al.*, 1974) have shown that estrogens are present in the serum at birth and have a remarkable spurt at 19 days, that is, before ovarian follicular maturation. Their probable source is the adrenal. It is therefore reasonable to suppose that the primary factors in the differentiation of the mammary gland during the period of heightened susceptibility to carcinogens are estrogens, aided by other hormones, as will be discussed.

### 3.3.1. Steroid Hormones and Their Receptors

Jensen and his associates were among the first to investigate thoroughly the affinity of ovarian steroids for mammary and uterine tumors and the pathways of their actions (*cf.* Jensen and DeSombre, 1973). The gateways of hormone action are the receptors of their target organs. Jensen's team discovered that the estrogen receptor sites reside in the cytosol, where they combine with a specific 4S protein. The receptor–estrogen complex proceeds to the nucleus, where it interacts with DNA. How this interaction results in differentiation of primitive mammary tubules, proliferation of resting mammary gland during pregnancy, and the production of a functional lactating mammary gland or MT is the subject of much current research.

Advancing Jensen's findings, Bresciani *et al.* (1973) observed that the estrogen–receptor complex is modified by a proteolytic enzyme. The modified complex enters the nucleus and binds to a basic acceptor protein which is part of the chromatin; this is followed by "activation" of DNA synthesis and mitosis, especially when aided by oncogenic agents or viruses. However interesting, these findings have not yet lifted the veil surrounding the role of estrogens in cancer. The chain of events may be interrupted at some stage after fixation of the estrogen by its receptor. McCormick and Moon (1973) found that incremental doses of estradiol benzoate, either alone or in conjunction with progesterone, depressed tumor appearance in DMBA-treated female rats, but progesterone alone did not. Mešter *et al.* (1973) extracted an estrogen-binding protein from the nuclei of pituitary tumor cells (line $GH_3$) grown in culture. The nuclei contain an estradiol-binding system that functions independently of the presence or absence of cytosol in the incubation medium.

Most of the basic work of Jensen and associates was done with the uterus. Although estradiol is only mildly carcinogenic in the uterus, the sequence of events was found to be basically applicable to the mammary gland and its estrogen-responsive tumors. Estradiol reaches the nucleus unchanged. Agents such as nafoxidine, which inhibit its uptake *in vitro*, inhibit its growth effect *in vivo*. By means of dry-mount radioautography, Stumpf (1969) visualized in cells the intranuclear location of these steroids.

The estrogen-binding protein in rat MT is virtually indistinguishable from that in human MT. It has a high affinity for estradiol but does not bind nonestrogenic proteins such as hydrocortisone, progesterone, or testosterone (McGuire and DeLaGarza, 1973a).

The binding of steroid to a cell, or even its passage to nuclear DNA itself, is not adequate proof of carcinogenicity. The steroid–receptor–DNA complex may lead either to metabolic stimulation of a cell or to its growth. For example, cortisol uptake in the liver can lead to new formation of enzymes without neoplastic transformation, and estrogen uptake in the mammary gland to differentiation or milk secretion. Labeled estrogens are bound to several organs in varying grades of intensity. Corticoids are one of the factors known to stimulate milk production without being growth stimulating.

The estrogen receptors in human breast cancer are markedly labile under the conditions usually employed for assay. Significant increases in assay sensitivity can be achieved with the use of thiol reagents, such as dithiothreitol, at low temperatures. Such technical improvements may prevent misclassification of a tumor as being autonomous with regard to endocrine therapy (McGuire and DeLaGarza, 1973b).

The recent literature abounds in reports utilizing various methods to determine *in vitro* hormone responsiveness of experimental and human MT, correlating it with clinical progress. When tumors are cultured *in vitro* for hormone dependency, assays for DNA synthesis are the most useful parameter to explore; the site of

[3]H-thymidine uptake can be documented by radioautographs. Without the latter, the results may be paradoxical (Riley *et al.*, 1973). When model animal tumors are available, the results are best checked *in vivo* assays (*cf.* Takizawa *et al.*, 1970). Simultaneous receptor assays for steroids, MtH, and other agents which may affect the growth of MT are desirable (*cf.* Flaxman and Lasfargues, 1973). Flax (1973) maintained tumor cells *in vitro* cultures for 24 h in the presence of nearly physiological concentrations of 17 β-estradiol, testosterone, and prolactin. The results were determined by a histochemical reaction demonstrating total dehydrogenase activity of the pentose shunt, as well as by hematoxylin-eosin staining. The tumors were judged as hormone responsive by greater activity with a particular hormone. On this basis, 14% of 100 tumors were responsive to prolactin, 8% to estradiol, 10% to testosterone, 14% to both estradiol and prolactin, and 12% to prolactin and testosterone combined.

Much is yet to be learned about estrogen action. Even certain brain regions are known to stereospecifically bind estradiol, notably the hypothalamus-preoptic area–amygdala–midbrain. Nuclear uptake of estradiol rises in infancy through puberty (Plapinger and McEwen, 1973; Plapinger *et al.*, 1973). Kato (1970) demonstrated *in vitro* that estradiol is preferentially taken up by the anterior hypothalamus, as well as by the hypophysis, and is preferentially retained at these sites when the tissues are washed with estradiol-free medium. The precise location of the receptor sites in these organs is yet to be established. Eisenfeld (1970) studied the *in vitro* binding of [3]H-estradiol to sulfhydryl groups in macromolecules from the rat hypothalamus, pars distalis of the pituitary, and uterus. The macromolecular-bound radioactivity was separated by gel filtration. Higher concentrations of radioactive estradiol were found in the macromolecular fractions from the pituitary, uterus, and hypothalamus than from the cerebrum, cerebellum, heart, and plasma. By means of dry-mount radioautography, Keefer *et al.* (1973) demonstrated the topographical localization of estrogen-containing cells in the rat spinal cord following [3]H-estradiol administration.

Specific estradiol binding has been demonstrated in the mammary glands of the rat, the mouse, and man, and in experimental and spontaneous hormone-dependent MT of the rat. Tumors which do not regress after ovariectomy can be readily distinguished from the "hormone-dependent" tumors by both the magnitude of the estradiol uptake and the degree of sensitivity to inhibitors such as nafoxidine. The estradiol–receptor complex related to MT sediments at a well-defined 8S peak on sucrose density gradient ultracentrifugation. Tumors which do not regress after ovariectomy have only small 8S receptors (Jensen *et al.*, 1971). Of 84 primary human tumors investigated, 39 showed the presence of estrogen receptor. A Cooperative Breast Cancer Group (Engelsman *et al.*, 1973) studied 37 patients with progressive breast cancer. Two objective remissions were noted in 20 patients with estrogen receptor-negative tumors and 14 objective remissions in 17 patients with receptor-positive tumors. McGuire *et al.* (1973) found an estrogen receptor system in a mammotropic pituitary tumor corresponding to its biological activities. Neoplasia induction by estrogen seems to be maximum in the pituitary, next in the mammary gland, and greatly variable in different species. However, estrogen stimulates the synthesis and release of prolactin in the normal rat pituitary gland. Thus estrogen can act via the pituitary.

Watanabe *et al.* (1973) identified and partially characterized a receptor with specificity and high affinity for glucocorticoid hormones in the cytoplasmic fraction of a mouse adrenotropic pituitary tumor.

### 3.3.2. Protein Hormones and Their Receptors

The receptor sites and patterns of biochemical action of protein hormones were first demonstrated by the binding of AtH to cells of the adrenal cortex (Lefkowitz *et al.*, 1970*a,b*; Wolfsen *et al.*, 1972). Porcine $^{125}$I-AtH bound to the plasma membrane of the cells of the adrenal cortex initiated the events discovered by Sutherland and Robison (1966). The generalization followed that all peptide hormones react with membrane-bound nucleotide cyclase systems to stimulate the conversion of a nucleotide triphosphate, such as adenosine triphosphate (ATP), to the corresponding 3′,5′-monophosphate, for example, cyclic adenosine monophosphate (cAMP). In line with these observations, the specific receptor site for MtH was found by Turkington (1971) and Birkinshaw and Falconer (1972) to reside in the plasma membrane.

There are many gray areas concerning the relative roles of estrogen and prolactin in mammary gland neoplasia (*cf.* Kim, 1965). Investigators are divided into two factions. The faction championed by Jensen explains most events by steroid actions; the other presents evidence indicating the primacy of prolactin in stimulation of the differentiated mammary epithelium and of transformed latent or overt mammary cancer cells (*cf.* Kim and Furth, 1960*a,b*). Another challenge has come with the discovery of hypothalamic P.RF and P.IF, which can also circumvent the ovaries and influence the growth of MT in the presence of the ovaries. My impression is that estrogens play a major role in bringing about differentiation of the mammary gland, while prolactin exerts a dominant action on the differentiated mammary gland. Estrogens are inducers of prolactin and have receptor sites in both the mammary gland and the pituitary. Since the adrenal is a "reserve" organ for secretion of estrogens, it can influence the mammary gland even after menopause, directly or indirectly. It seems that estrogens are ever present and may be the sole inducers of prolactin. The hypothalamic factors may merely regulate prolactin release and secretory rates, and perhaps also the number of prolactin-secreting cells. Until these circuits are clearly defined, several critical questions remain unanswered.

Cortisol appears to play some permissive role in hormonal stimulation of diverse cells. Its role in mammary tumorigenesis is debatable. An elevated rate of cortisol production was found in patients with advanced breast cancer. After hypophysectomy, it was found to fall to one-sixth of the original level. The high preoperative cortisol production was attributed to stress-induced elevation of AtH (Lewis and Deshpande, 1973) This is a common feature of most advanced tumors. It is noteworthy that milk secretion is usual in stimulated mammary gland and mammary tumors of the rat, but not in human tumors. Adrenal corticoids are one essential component of milk production. The physiological pathway of their secretion and their relation to prolactin and estrogen require further clarification.

Failure to consider the fact that estrogen is a (or the) physiological inducer of prolactin is a common shortcoming of many experiments attributing to estrogens an absolute role in mammary tumorigenesis. Isolated prolactin preparations stimulate the mammary gland in gonadectomized-adrenalectomized-hypophysectomized rats and can resuscitate mammary cancers which regressed following ovariectomy of hypophysectomy. Correspondingly, P.IF can also inhibit "hormone-responsive" mammary cancers of man and experimental animals, as described above.

It is known that some MT can regress following treatment with pharmacological doses of estrogen. Several explanations given for these events have been reviewed by Stoll (1973). He offers a hypothesis of his own: "the effect of high-dosage oestrogen therapy in breast cancer may depend critically on the absolute and relative concentrations of prolactin and oestrogen actively available at the tumor . . . Differences in site sensitivity in the same patient may depend on tumoral factors such as the level of oestradiol and prolactin binding receptors in the tissue." A similar explanation is that the binding of the estrogens to MT does not leave enough estrogen free to stimulate the secretion of MtH by Mt. Others suggest that MtH levels are elevated in the pituitary but are not released.

There are no satisfactory analytical studies in which the presence of receptors for both estrogen and prolactin and their role in regression of a "certified" hormone-responsive experimental MT were compared. Experiments aimed at clarifying the estrogen vs. prolactin controversy should consider the following: (1) MtH has a very short half-life (less than 30 min). Injecting MtH is not equivalent to grafting on the animal a highly prolactin-secreting tumor, in which the MtH levels are continuously high (thousands of nanograms per milliliter of serum). (2) Such high levels cannot be attained by isografts of pituitaries in hypophysectomized animals. (3) Estrogens do have a double action—a direct one on the mammary gland and an indirect one on pituitary Mt cells; thus, in the presence of the pituitary (Mt cell), it is uncertain as to which of the two stimulates the mammary gland. (4) High estrogen levels inhibit the mammary gland and MT (hence the use of pharmacological doses of estrogens in treatment of MT). (5) The "Huggins tumors" are variously deviated from normal to highly autonomous types, are probably multiclonal, and are subject to "progression." Stating that the tumor used was a "DMBA-induced tumor" is not satisfactory. Each experimental situation requires assays for analysis of the various factors that influence the growth of the mammary gland. (Takizawa et al., 1970, used the sera of MtT-bearing rats, which contain such physiological costimulants as StH and insulin.) Whether injection of P.IF alone can inhibit and P.RF stimulate the mammary gland in the absence of the gonads and adrenals remains to be clarified.

Thus we face the apparent contradiction: Assays of Jensen for estrogen receptors suggest that they can predict almost all human hormone-responsive MT. In contrast, many others utilizing drugs which inhibit prolactin release claim the same results. Shall we conclude that hormone-responsive MT have receptors for both estrogens and prolactin?

Cell and organ cultures have been used extensively for the study of hormonal secretion and hormone responsiveness of neoplasms and for establishment of differentiated hormone-related cell lines (*cf.* Kruse and Patterson, 1973). An excellent compilation of articles written in this area from 1907 to 1971 is contained in *Readings in Mammalian Cell Culture* (Pollack and Sato, 1973).

## 4. Ectopic Hormones

The strongest argument in favor of the "dedifferentiation" theory of neoplasia is the finding that nonendocrine organs can give rise to tumors which secrete hormones (as AtH, insulin, TtH, GtH, and erythropoietin). Gellhorn (1966) gathered the evidence and stressed the association of ectopic hormone production with dedifferentiation. Certain tumors of infancy and childhood (such as neuroblastomas) may be linked to disturbance in differentiation, but as for the majority of tumors the relationship may be incidental to mutation.

The immunological relationship of ectopic AtH with that secreted by adrenotropes has been investigated by Yalow and associates. Gewirtz and Yalow (1973) found that ectopic AtH from all but one of 30 extracts of primary or metastatic carcinoma of the lung was immunoreactive with antinormal AtH. Its predominant reactive form was big AtH. About 7% of laboratory controls and hospital patients had elevated afternoon plasma levels of AtH (in excess of 150 pg/ml), with big AtH as the predominant component, compared to about half of 59 patients with carcinoma of the lung. Nevertheless, for screening procedures for detection of carcinoma of the lung and for evaluation of response to therapeutic procedures, this test may be useful (*cf.* Yalow, 1974).

Braunstein *et al.* (1973) demonstrated ectopic production of human chorionic gonadotropin in 113 out of 918 cancer patients, with a high incidence in those with cancer of the stomach (25.5%), liver (17.3%), and pancreas (50%). Ectopic hormone production in diverse human neoplasms has been reviewed by Omenn (1973).

## 5. Sequential Events: Multiglandular Syndromes

Decades of experimental studies on diverse types of carcinogenesis have given me the impression that neoplasia is rarely a single-step process. Each class of carcinogens has its own *modus operandi* of transforming normal into neoplastic cells. Now that many evidently environmental and occupational cancers are under control, anatomical studies rarely disclose a carcinogen. Man cannot escape living in a world containing low levels of carcinogens (such as radiations), and it is my impression that subtle neoplastic changes evolve and progress silently through the cooperation of some carcinogen and some promoter.

Among the hormone-related experimental tumors, those induced by ionizing radiations demonstrate best the inducer–promoter cooperation. Theoretically, ionizing radiations properly applied should be able to produce a neoplasm in all cells, the numbers of which are homeostatically regulated. The following are relevant well-documented examples: (1) Irradiation of mice often induces leukemias which originate in the thymus, can be prevented by thymectomy, and are restored by thymic grafts. (2) Irradiated mice frequently develop OT, but not when only one ovary is exposed to radiation or when the animals receive grafts of normal ovaries following irradiation. (3) Radiothyroidectomy induces pituitary tumors in all strains of mice. Originally, this was attributed to "stress" or to incidental pituitary irradiation, but subsequent studies have shown that these tumors are all thyrotropic, while most pituitary tumors induced by radiations are mammosomatotropic. Further, induction of TtT can also be achieved by surgical thyroidectomy (Dent *et al.*, 1956). Radiation brings about homeostatic derangements by virtue of its mutagenic effect. The transformed cell can be either the cell irradiated or its regulator cell.

Examples in which the sequence of events in neoplasia occurs in "slow motion" have already been mentioned. The insult can occur early in life, progresses slowly, and terminates fatally in old age. The sequential events from normal to fully autonomous neoplasms can occur in one host, but the complete spectrum of sequential changes is best disclosed by serial subpassages in histocompatible animals.

Progression from normal cells to autonomous cancers has been extensively studied in the gonadotrope–ovary, thyrotrope–thyroid, estrogen–Leydig cell, and estrogen/prolactin–mammary gland systems. The inducibility of tumors and the timetable of transformation vary with the strain of animal used. None is strictly applicable to corresponding human tumors, but analysis of the dynamics of events yields valuable information on the pathogenesis of corresponding human tumors. The following examples will amplify the observations sketched in Sections 1 and 2.

## 5.1. Neonatal Ovariectomy

Neonatal ovariectomy is an example of how a single insult can induce a variety of tumors evolving in sequence during the life span of an animal. Studies on induction of tumors by gonadectomy were begun in 1945 and have been thoroughly worked out morphologically by Woolley *et al.* (*cf.* Woolley, 1958). The end result was a multiglandular "syndrome": AT, MT, and pituitary tumors. The character of the last is still uncertain: Were they estrogen-induced MtT or gonadectomy-induced GtT? The incidental observation that the adrenal compensates with estrogen production in the absence of the gonads paid rich dividends years later by the introduction of adrenalectomy to control breast cancer in women in whom the compensatory estrogens of the adrenal lead to recurrence of MT after ovariectomy.

Houssay *et al.* (1955) have undertaken an analysis of the genesis of the "Woolley tumors." With the aid of parabiosis, staining reactions ("basophilia" and periodic acid–Schiff positivity), and electron microscopy, they demonstrated that the pituitary tumors were gonadotropic. My associates have not been able to confirm this. The pituitary tumors found in old gonadectomized rats were the MtT type, as were the overwhelming majority of the spontaneous pituitary tumors of the rat (Kim *et al.*, 1960*b*; Ito *et al.*, 1972*a*). In our experience, hyperplasia of Gt occurs rapidly after gonadectomy in both sexes. The majority of cells in the pituitary 242 days after gonadectomy were Gt cells in various stages of hypertrophy. They can be well stained by labeled anti-LH. The hyperplasia of Gt appears to plateau and persists without formation of tumors.

The work of Griesbach and Purves (1960), confirming that of Houssay and associates, is open to doubt because inadequate techniques were used to identify the tumors. However, some tumors isolated by Iglesias *et al.* (1969, 1972) in the course of studies on gonadal tumorigenesis in AxC rats appear to be transplantable GtT of low hormonal potency.

These observations on hormonal interrelationships in the gonadal–gonadotrope axis may explain the extreme rarity of GtT in man and laboratory animals.

### 5.2. Thyroidal Carcinogenesis

The first thoroughly studied hormone-related tumors were those of the thyroid. They can be produced by several different methods in rats and mice, and develop through a series of gradual changes which include (1) hyperplasia, (2) focal areas of proliferation of altered cells, (3) formation of multicentric adenomas, and finally (4) carcinomas. The techniques used to induce them have been well summarized and illustrated by Morris (1955).

Two monographs on thyroid cancer (Young and Inman, 1968; Hedinger, 1969) present a wealth of facts and opinions on this subject by endocrinologists, oncologists, and immunogeneticists. Once a major worldwide problem, the importance of nodular enlargement of the thyroid gland (goiter) and its relation to cancer has been greatly minimized by the discovery of the various causative agents of goiters, ranging from iodine deficiency to substances in food and drugs which block TH synthesis. Figure 4 illustrates the simple feedback mechanism of the TH–TtH "axis" (see Section 1.4).

Goiters and TT (spontaneous and experimental) can be induced by the following procedures: (1) *without carcinogen*—(a) by blocking TH synthesis with antithyroidal chemicals thereby producing a sustained elevation of TtH; (b) by $I_2$-deficient diet; (c) by sustained administration of TtH; (2) *with carcinogen*—by low dose of $^{131}I$ (*cf.* Lindsay, 1969) or certain chemicals such as acetylaminofluorene; (3) *combination* of procedures (1) and (2). Procedure (1) promotes tumorigenesis by (2).

The experimentally induced TT begin as hormone-responsive lesions and slowly acquire autonomy, usually after several consecutive animal passages. To verify the role of TtH in thyroidal tumorigenesis, my associates studied the induction of TT by sustained administration of homologous TtH (Haran-Ghera *et al.*, 1960; Sinha *et al.*, 1965; Ueda and Furth, 1967). The greatly hyperplastic thyroids so induced consisted of a conglomeration of follicular and papillary nodules which failed to grow in euthyroid animals for about 2 yr, during which they were carried in consecutive passages in animals rendered hyperthyroid with highly elevated TtH levels. They gave rise to autonomous, but hormone-responsive, tumors. After being carried in normal hosts for about another 2 yr, the tumors gradually lost their "organoid" structure completely, took up less and less $^{131}$I, and became less and less stimulated by TtH. Ultimately, they lost hormone responsiveness completely and became transformed into spindle- and giant-celled tumors as described by Russell (*cf.* Hedinger, 1969) in human TT. These sarcomatoid carcinomas were rapidly fatal. Why the nodularity of goiters in several species and the rarity of their giving rise to cancers is uncertain.

Thyroid cells in adults rarely multiply. Stimulation and inhibition are usually expressed by increased hormone production by the existing "resting" cells. Carcinogens, such as ionizing radiations, can readily induce tumors in immature, multiplying thyroid cells, but not in the adult thyroid. However, sustained elevation of TtH levels in adults can invariably induce the development of thyroid adenomas and the development of these into carcinomas, albeit very slowly, as our experiments indicate. We support the view that the first step in control of TT (benign or malignant) should be a trial of reduction of TtH levels (Astwood *et al.*, 1960).

Several ill-conceived notions, dogmatically held by many thyroidologists and not challenged by experimental observations, call for clarification:

1. Cold nodule formation (either adenomatoid or papillary) induced by goiterogens is not synonymous with cancer. We have failed to graft these in normal histocompatible hosts. Even such diagnostic points as presence of thyroid cells in venules do not unequivocally signify malignancy.
2. Chromosomal abnormalities may indicate mutations, but many mutants are not neoplastic. Thyroid remnants in mice given large does of $^{131}$I (and irradiated tissues in general) often contain such cells, which persist until death of the host without giving rise to tumors.
3. Electron microscopy is a good adjunct in the characterization of cells, but profound cellular changes induced by differentiation or hormonal stimulation may resemble alterations now considered by some workers to be indicative of neoplasia.
4. A fatal neoplasm is not necessarily an autonomous cancer. Many fully hormone-dependent neoplasms are known which are fatal unless the hormonal derangement is controlled, and they often metastasize to regional lymph nodes.

Immunological changes with nonneoplastic thyroid diseases are common; they are "autoimmune," not related to TT. It is a sound practice to characterize localized thyroid neoplasms by the therapeutic approach: administration of cold TH to reduce TtH levels.

## 5.3. Multiglandular Diseases

There are several mechanisms by which a multiglandular disease can be induced by a single hormone deficiency: (1) That encountered in female mice bearing TtT is attained by virtue of the structural relationship between TtH and GtH (Furth *et al.*, 1973*b*). A direct mechanism is also possible by virtue of MtH stimulation by T.RH. Grant *et al.* (1973) found that Mt cells possess membrane receptors for T.RH *in vitro*. The biological mammotropic effect by T.RH *in vivo* has yet to be demonstrated. Another example in this category is the "transformation" of an MtT into and StT (Ito *et al.*, 1972*b*) related to the structural relationship between MtH and StH. Yet another example of this is the syndrome of hypersomatotropism consisting of pituitary and pancreatic changes due to the StH–insulin relationship (Garay *et al.*, 1971; Bates and Garrison, 1973). (2) TtT is also a good example of acquisition of new hormonal capabilities when it becomes fully autonomous (Furth *et al.*, 1973*c*). The TtT syndrome has been fully described elsewhere (Furth *et al.*, 1973*a,d*) has been sketched in Section 2. (3) Evidence has been accumulated for the ability of a normal pituitary cell to produce more than one hormone when it becomes neoplastic. This has been summarized and illustrated by Ueda *et al.* (1973). The outstanding example is the acquisition by Mt of the ability to secrete three hormones, of which AtH is dominant (as in rat MtT strain F4). (For other examples, see Section 2.) The biological features of the AtH-secreting rat MtT/F4 are, in several respects, common with those of the purely AtH-secreting mouse AtT/20. Both are associated with marked hyperadrenolcorticoidism and thymic atrophy. While the mouse AtT also causes profound obesity similar to that of the genetically obese mouse (*cf.* Green, 1966), rats bearing MtT/F4 are not obese.

There are many human syndromes with multiple endocrine neoplasia (*cf.* Williams, 1968), the pathogenesis of which is subject to speculation. One of these, reported recently by Steiner *et al.* (1968), is a kindred with pheochromocytoma, medullary thyroid carcinoma, hyperparathyroidism, and Cushing's disease.

## 6. Problems and Prospects

### 6.1. The Basic Change in Neoplasia

Among the first attractive theories of neoplasia was that of somatic mutation (Boveri, 1929). Its first powerful opponent was Rous, who, following his excellent work with avian leukosis viruses, maintained that all tumors were caused by viruses (Rous, 1943). In the debates which followed, causation and basic nature were confused. The virus "theory" of cancer gained dominance until Rous himself, looking into the modes of chemical carcinogenesis, considered that viruses could not be the sole cause of cancer. A link between viruses and some genetic factor was demonstrated by the observations of the genetic inheritance of a leukemia factor in Ak mice (Cole and Furth, 1941), the isolation of a virus (Gross, 1953), and the association of viral RNA with the host cells' DNA by means of a reverse transcriptase (*cf.* Temin, 1972; Spiegelman and Schlom, 1972). The observation that thymectomy blocks the development of leukemia, but not the inheritance of leukemia virus, pointed to a thymus-related host factor essential for the expression of the somatic potentialities of this virus. Earlier, Bittner (1946–1947) discovered the presence of a similar causative agent in murine MT, calling it "milk factor" or "mammary tumor agent," now properly recognized as a virus.

Our present concept is based on the major discovery of Rous of the multifactorial concept of carcinogenesis (initiation, promotion, and the existence of latent cancers). The latter acquired solidity and popularity through subsequent studies of Berenblum (1947), Shubik, and others. The pathogenesis of neoplasia, the major roles of hormones, and other cybernetic forces (Wiener, 1948) became clarified, but the fundamental nature of neoplasia remained the subject of debates.

Mathematical analyses lent support to the hypothesis that sequential mutations were involved in the evolution of species (cf. Eigen, 1971) and probably also of neoplasia. As to the causative agents of mutations, three classes are generally accepted: radiations, certain chemicals, and viruses. All three are aided by some hormones. A fourth class of mutation, spontaneous DNA replication error, should, in my opinion, be included.

Promoters, by sustained enhancement of cell replication, increase the chances for spontaneous mutations. When the giant DNA molecule is replicating, it is indeed surprising that so few mistakes are made (or go unrepaired). Errors which do occur, spontaneous or induced, are now assumed to be more common than hitherto believed. Preferential replication of some mutants is conceived to be the basis of Darwinian evolution (Eigen, 1971). Mutants unable to recognize the homeostatic forces that limit the number of their normal ancestors, or defective in translating signals received by their receptors, gain a proliferative advantage over their normal ancestors. In his article "Cancer and the Evolution of Species: A Ransom," DeGrouchy (1973) states: "Evolution . . . is a direct consequence of chromosomal instability. At meiosis chromosomal instability is responsible for the occurrence of individuals carrying new karyotypes and liable to be at the origin of a new species. At mitosis, chromosomal instability produces cells carrying new karyotypes. According to the chromosomal theory of carcinogenesis these cells are potential ancestors of novel clones liable to become malignant tumors. Carcinogenesis therefore appears as inexorable as the evolution of species." Genetic instability leads to further modifications, hence the progression from dependent to autonomous tumors. The precise characterization of a human tumor soon after its discovery, with the aim of checking its promoters, should be a major task of cancer research.

Related to the mutation theory are those of abnormal differentiation and dedifferentiation. These gained prominence by the discovery of ectopic hormones (see Section 4).

Differentiation yields the many organs with their specific cell types. It is commonly conceived as being nearly as irreversible as mutation, but differentiation is not accompanied by changes in the *basic* DNA code. The irreversibility of tissue differentiation is not without challenge. DeCosse *et al.* (1973) have reported on induction of differentiation in MT by embryonic tissue. A mouse MT was maintained *in vitro*, separated from embryonic mammary mesenchyme by a Millipore filter. Tubules developed in the tumor, DNA synthesis declined, and a presumptive acid mucopolysaccharide matrix, not evident in the controls, appeared.

It is assumed that differentiation is achieved by repression of certain genes and derepression of others (*cf.* Wolstenholme, 1966). Following failure to clearly associate basic proteins (notably histones) with repression of DNA, research has recently turned to DNA-associated acidophilic proteins which may accomplish this basic function (see review by Stein *et al.*, 1974).

There is one reservation to the mutation hypothesis. It is conceivable that some neoplasms—notably, those fully hormone dependent—are not due to modification of DNA but to that of an associated protein repressor. It has been shown that the λ-phage repressor can block RNA polymerase (Ptashne, 1973–1974), and it is conceivable that such repressors are the agents causing differentiation of diverse organs without modification of the associated DNA. The requirement of a neoplastic "derepressed" cell is the acquisition of a proliferative advantage. Obviously, this hypothesis cannot apply to neoplasms with marked chromosomal alterations indicative of some DNA change. In this sense, one is tempted to hypothesize the existence of two types of neoplastic transformation of cells—one based on DNA modification, another on that of a DNA-associated protein repressor. The latter allows reversal of some neoplasms (such as the hormone-dependent ones), the former does not. Solid evidence for this concept will come from developments identifying nucleotide sequences in DNA and identifying the DNA repressor proteins and the loci of genes involved in the neoplastic change. (It should be noted that the modification of the repressor could itself be a consequence of a change in the DNA.)

### 6.2. Carcinogenesis without Extrinsic Carcinogens

Five lines of evidence support the hypothesis of carcinogenesis without extrinsic carcinogens:

1. Numerous observations suggested that sustained specific growth stimulation of a cell, initiated either by removal of its homeostatic growth inhibitor or by sustained application of its physiological growth stimulant, can induce tumors without extrinsic carcinogenic agents. Tumors so induced are specific for the hyperstimulated cell type and their transplantability is, at first, usually dependent on their inducer. However, successive transplantations usually elicit autonomous variants. Such hormone-specific tumors can be induced in practically any member of any strain of any species and in any geographic region. Although carcinogens are everywhere in the environment, it seems unlikely that the induction of such tumors is dependent on a ubiquitous carcinogen or on the cell's DNA-integrated specific viruses. Examples are given in Sections 1 and 2.

2. A recent observation supporting this hypothesis resulted from the search for an explanation of Huggins' finding (Huggins *et al.*, 1961) of the hypersensitivity of female rats to induction of MT by chemical carcinogens between the ages of about 20 and 60 days (with a peak at 50–60 days), dropping sharply thereafter (Furth, 1973). The most conspicuous histological change in the mammary gland during this period is a burst of mitoses at the terminal buds of the rudimentary ducts, reaching a climax at 50–60 days (Fig. 7) and sharply declining thereafter. The mature breast of virgin female rats subsequently becomes rather stationary after 70 days of age. Differentiation of the mammary gland is directly initiated by gonadotropin-induced estrogens, aided by other hormones such as StH, insulin, somatomedins, and MtH, which the estrogens induce. It is well on its way at 20 days of age, when all major pituitary hormones are present at about normal levels, with the exception of MtH. The presumed factors contributing to the heightened sensitivity to tumor induction are (a) an early spurt of estrogens (which are nucleophilic); (b) rapid replication of DNA, enhancing susceptibility to carcinogens; (c) errors in DNA synthesis (spontaneous mutation); and (d) increase in MtH, the specific stimulator of the mammary gland, and in other nonspecific growth factors. The difficulty in excluding the role of a latent genetically integrated virus in seemingly spontaneous neoplastic transformation is an obstacle to acceptance of the spontaneous mutation hypothesis. The now accepted sequence of events is RNA virus → integration with the cell's DNA → release of RNA virus (with or without associated neoplastic transformation of cells). However remote it may appear to be, the sequence DNA → RNA virus, as conceived by Temin (personal communication), is a possible explanation for the genesis of some tumor viruses, but not for the genesis of all tumors. The finding of electron microscopic particles in man and other species (*cf.* Moore *et al.*, 1971; Dmochowski, 1973), as well as biochemical evidence for the presence of a presumably causative MTV in several species including man (Schlom and Spiegelman, 1973), raises the question of whether or not all members of a neoplasia-prone species carry a latent neoplasia-inducing virus.

3. A survey of several epidemiological studies (*cf.* MacMahon *et al.*, 1973) indicates an initial sharp rise in the incidence of breast cancers in women at about 25–45 yr of age. These tumors may have been initiated during the estrogen-triggered differentiation and growth of the mammary epithelium at puberty. This sharp initial rise occurs in all parts of the globe where such epidemiological studies have been made, suggesting that neoplastic transformation at puberty (yet to be solidly documented) is not likely to be due to an extrinsic carcinogen. (The many speculative interpretations proposed to explain the changes in breast cancer incidence at later ages have been well reviewed by MacMahon *et al.*, 1973.) A closer analysis of events during the pubertal period in mice (now in progress in our laboratory) may clarify this problem. Success hinges on the accuracy of the view that there are mouse strains free from MTV.

4. Choh Hao Li (1972) isolated ten hormones from the anterior pituitary, each possessing specific functions. On the basis of amino acid sequences, he divided them into three classes in their presumed phylogenetic order of evolution. The

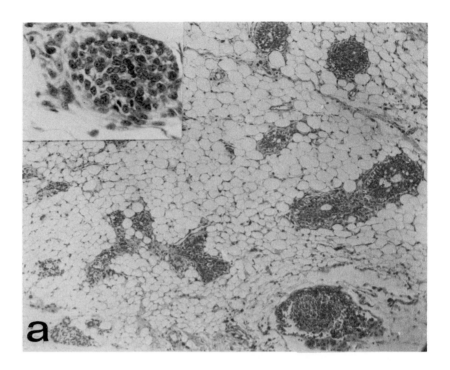

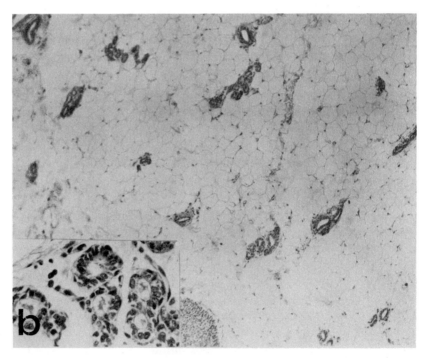

FIGURE 7. (a) The appearance of the female rat mammary gland at puberty. Note the bulbous growth of differentiating tubules containing numerous mitotic figures. Hematoxylin and eosin, × 75. Inset, × 400. (b) The fully differentiated ductal system of the virgin rat mammary gland at 87 days of age. Hematoxylin and eosin, × 75. Inset, × 400.

members of each class have strong common structural features and overlapping biological activities. During the past 20 yr, we have developed transplantable pituitary tumors of all three cell classes of Li, two of them by homeostatic derangement. The remarkable feature of the hormone-induced tumors is that they usually start as hyperplasia and only stepwise do they give rise to autonomous, fully hormone-independent tumors via fully hormone-dependent ones (see Section 5). A slight neoplastic code-change occurs within the class; marked derepression transgresses it. A single stable transplantable pituitary tumor cell can produce three separable hormones (Ueda *et al.*, 1973).

5. Indirect support to our hypothesis is given by the mathematical theories of Eigen (1971), solidified by DeGrouchy (1973). Recently, Macfarlane Burnet (1973) presented observations of his own supporting the spontaneous mutation hypothesis of neoplasia.

It is noteworthy that successive transplantation of normal cells *in vitro* often leads to transformation of the growth character of the cells, with acquisition of features known to characterize neoplastic cells. This occurs with or without acquisition of chromosomal abnormalities and with or without acquisition of transplantability. Because of the lack of homeostatic inhibitors *in vitro* and the oversupply of various nonspecific growth promoters, the opportunity for mutations is greatly enhanced. Possibly, the absence of a surveillance mechanism *in vitro* magnifies the chances for survival of many altered cells. It is surprising that despite decades of work on cell growth there has been no definitive study of the possibility of genetic and antigenetic modification of cells during the course of rapid replication without a carcinogen *in vitro* or *in vivo*.

## 6.3. Relation of Neoplasia to Aging

In Section 1.3, we postulated the existence of two types of mutations—metabolic and neoplastic—and related the former to aging. If one accepts the existence of mutations as an evolutionary force, one logically arrives at the conclusion that they can also be an involutionary force. If some transformed (mutated) cells have a proliferative advantage, they become cancer cells. Others, called metabolic mutants—that is, those disadvantaged in performing their physiological functions—may also slowly accumulate or may perish with age, depending on the existing homeostatic or immunological status. Cannon (1942), in his classical assay on homeostasis, writes: "The regulatory devices suffer a progressive impairment in most individuals as the decades pass after about the fortieth year." By "regulatory devices" he means homeostasis of temperature, salt, glucose, water, etc. To this we may add deterioration of immunosurveillance with age, which results in failure of the host to eliminate metabolically altered, as well as neoplastic, cells.

Chromosome analysis in relation to age sheds new light on the problem. Resting cells of the liver were studied at various ages and following exposure to mutagens. They were brought to division by subtotal resection of the organ (*cf.* Curtis, 1963,

1964). Curtis's findings indicate that the number of abnormal mitoses increases with age and that carcinogens administered early in life greatly enhance their number even late in life. Evidently, some of the transformed cells are compatible with life, some may even be functionally superior, but most of them seem inferior, hence senescence. Only a rare cell is a neoplastic mutant, and many of these may remain latent until some hormonal derangement or other homeostatic change induces them to multiply and form overt tumors (*cf.* Rous and Kidd, 1941; Kim and Furth, 1960*a*,*b*).

### 6.4. Prospects

Huggins (1967) lists seven hormone-responsive human cancers, three of which occur in both man and animals. None of the human tumors is surely curable by hormonal manipulation, although such treatment can produce lasting remissions. Many hormone-responsive tumors (including the three mentioned above) have been studied extensively in animals. Some were found to be curable because their pathogenesis was established, and they could be treated at the early phase of full hormone dependence.

Transformation of normal cells into cancer cells is, in our concept, no more preventable than evolution, senescence, and death. But with advancing knowledge in detecting liability to certain tumors, discovering latent tumors (from their "footprints"), and controlling the growth of frank neoplastic cells, an optimistic outlook of steady betterment of cancer control is well justified. As we have already learned, one can live with a highly carcinogenic, usually hidden, virus. The life span of the individual with cancer can be prolonged and made more comfortable. And the rare complete arrest of malignant growth (obtained by diverse therapeutic approaches) is, we believe, a portent of things to come.

ACKNOWLEDGMENTS

We gratefully acknowledge the assistance of our librarian, Ms. Betty Moore, in collecting the bibliography, and that of our photographer, Mr. Edward Hajjar. Special credit is due to numerous associates, whose dedicated work could not be adequately acknowledged in this review article.

### 7. References

ANDERVONT, H. B., SHIMKIN, M. B., AND CANTER, H. Y., 1957, Effect of discontinued estrogenic stimulation upon the development and growth of testicular tumors in mice, *J. Natl. Cancer Inst.* **18**:1.

ASTWOOD, E. B., CASSIDY, C. E., AND AURBACH, G. D., 1960, Treatment of goiter and thyroid nodules with thyroid, *J. Am. Med. Assoc.* **174**:459.

BAHN, R., FURTH, J., ANDERSON, E., AND GADSDEN, E., 1957, Morphologic and functional changes associated with transplantable ACTH-producing pituitary tumors of mice, *Am. J. Pathol.* **33**:1075.

BAKER, B. L., 1970, Studies on hormone localization with emphasis on the hypophysics, *J. Histochem. Cytochem.* **18**:1.

BAKER, B. L., ESKIN, T. A., AND CLAPP, H. W., 1972, The effect of medroxyprogesterone on cells of the pituitary pars distalis, *Proc. Soc. Exp. Biol. Med.* **140:**357.

BALI, T., AND FURTH, J., 1949, Morphological and biological characteristics of X-ray induced transplantable ovarian tumors, *Cancer Res.* **9:**449.

BATES, R. W., AND GARRISON, M. M., 1973, Synergism among growth hormone, ACTH, cortisol and dexamethasone in the hormonal induction of diabetes in rats and the diabetogenic effect of tolbutamide, *Endocrinology* **93:**1109.

BATES, R. W., SCOW, R. O., AND LACY, P. E., 1966, Induction of permanent diabetes in rats by pituitary hormones from a transplantable mammotropic tumor: Concomitant changes in organ weights and the effect of adrenalectomy, *Endocrinology* **78:**826.

BEATSON, G. T., 1896, On the treatment of inoperable cases of carcinoma of the mamma: Suggestions for a new method of treatment with illustrative cases, *Lancet* **2:**104.

BENOIT, J., AND DALAGE, C., eds., 1963, *Cytologie de l'Adénohypophyse*, Centre National de la Recherche Scientifique, No. 128, Paris.

BERENBLUM, I., 1947, Cocarcinogenesis, *Brit. Med. Bull.* **4:**343.

BERSON, S. A., AND YALOW, R. S., eds., 1973, *Methods in Investigative and Diagnostic Endocrinology*, Vol. 2: *Peptide Hormones*, American Elsevier, New York.

BIRKINSHAW, M., AND FALCONER, I. R., 1972, The localization of prolactin labelled with radioactive iodine in rabbit mammary tissue, *J. Endocrinol.* **55:**323.

BISKIND, M. S., AND BISKIND, G. R., 1944, Development of tumors in the rat ovary after transplantation into the spleen, *Proc. Soc. Exp. Biol. Med.* **55:**176.

BITTNER, J. J., 1946–1947, The causes and control of mammary cancer in mice, *Harvey Lect.* **42:**221.

BITTNER, J. J., 1952, The genesis of breast cancer in mice, *Texas Rep. Biol. Med.* **10:**160.

BLOCH, E., COHEN, A. I., AND FURTH, J., 1960, Steroid production *in vitro* by normal and adrenal tumor–bearing male mice, *J. Natl. Cancer Inst.* **24:**97.

BOLLENGIER, W. E., EISENFELD, A. J., AND GARDNER, W. U., 1972, Accumulation of ³H-estradiol in testes and pituitary glands of mice of strains differing in susceptibility to testicular interstitial cell and pituitary tumors after prolonged estrogen treatment, *J. Natl. Cancer Inst.* **49:**847.

BOVERI, T., 1929, *The Origin of Malignant Tumors* (trans. Marcella Boveri), Williams and Wilkins, Baltimore.

BOYNS, A. R., AND GRIFFITHS, K., eds., 1972, *Prolactin and Carcinogenesis*, Alpha Omega Alpha, Cardiff.

BRAUNSTEIN, G. D., VAITUKAITIS, J. L., CARBONE, P. P., AND ROSS, G. T., 1973, Ectopic production of human chorionic gonadotropin by neoplasms, *Ann. Int. Med.* **78:**39.

BRAZEAU, P., VALE, W., BURGUS, R., LING, N., BUTCHER, M., RIVIER, J., AND GUILLEMIN, R., 1973, Hypothalamic polypeptide that inhibits the secretion of immunoreactive pituitary growth hormone, *Science* **179:**77.

BRESCIANI, F., NOLA, E., SICA, V., AND PUCA, G. A., 1973, Early stages in estrogen control of gene expression and its derangement in cancer, *Fed. Proc.* **32:**2126.

BUCKMAN, M. T., AND PEAKE, G. T., 1973, Estrogen potentiation of phenothiazine-induced prolactin secretion in man, *J. Clin. Endocrinol. Metab.* **37:**977.

BUONASSISI, V., SATO, G., AND COHEN, A. I., 1962, Hormone-producing cultures of adrenal and pituitary tumor origin, *Proc. Natl. Acad. Sci.* **48:**1184.

BURNET, F. M., 1970, *Immunological Surveillance*, Pergamon Press, Sydney.

BURNET, F. M., 1973, A genetic interpretation of ageing, *Lancet* **2:**480.

CANFIELD, R., MORGAN, F., KAMMERMAN, S., BELL, J., AND AGOSTO, G., 1971, Studies of human chorionic gonadotropin, *Rec. Prog. Hormone Res.* **27:**121.

CANNON, W. B., 1932, Homeostasis, *Cycloped. Med.* **6:**861.

CANNON, W. B., 1942, Ageing of homeostatic mechanisms, in: *Problems of Ageing* (E. V. Cowdry, ed.), pp. 567–582, Williams and Wilkins, Baltimore.

CLIFTON, K. H., 1963, Tumor induction in hypophyseal grafts in radiothyroidectomized mice; hypothalamico-hypophyseal relationships, *Proc. Soc. Exp. Biol. Med.* **114:**559.

CLIFTON, K. H., BLOCH, E., UPTON, A. C., AND FURTH, J., 1956, Transplantable Leydig-cell tumors in mice, *Arch. Pathol.* **62:**354.

COHEN, A. I., AND FURTH, J., 1959, Corticotropin assay with transplantable adrenocortical tumor slices: Application to the assay of adrenotropic pituitary tumors, *Cancer Res.* **19:**72.

COHEN, A. I., BLOCH, E., AND CELOZZI, 1957, *In vitro* response of functional experimental adrenal tumors to corticotropin (ACTH), *Proc. Soc. Exp. Biol. Med.* **95:**304.

COLE, R. K., AND FURTH, J., 1941, Experimental studies on the genetics of spontaneous leukemia in mice, *Cancer Res.* **1:**957.

CURTIS, H. J., 1963, Biological mechanisms underlying the aging process, *Science* **141**:686.

CURTIS, H. J., 1964, The biology of aging, in:*Brookhaven National Laboratory Lecture Series No. 34*, pp. 1–11, Associated Universities, Upton, N.Y.

DECOSSE, J. J., GOSSENS, C. L., KUZMA, J. F., AND UNSWORTH, B. R., 1973, Breast cancer: Induction of differentiation by embryonic tissue, *Science* **181**:1057.

DEGROUCHY, J., 1973, Cancer and the evolution of species: A ransom, *Biomedicine* **18**:6.

DENT J. N., GADSDEN, E. L., AND FURTH, J., 1956, Further studies on induction and growth of thyrotropic pituitary tumors in mice, *Cancer Res.* **16**:171.

DICKEY, R. P., AND MINTON, J. P., 1972a, Levodopa relief of bone pain from breast cancer, *New Engl. J. Med.* **286**:843.

DICKEY, R. P., AND MINTON, J. P., 1972b, Levodopa effect on prolactin, follicle-stimulating hormone, and luteinizing hormone in women with advanced breast cancer, *Am. J. Obstet. Gynecol.* **114**:267.

DICKIE, M. M., AND LANE, P. W., 1956, Adrenal tumors, pituitary changes and other pathological changes in $F_1$ hybrids of strain DE × DBA, *Cancer Res.* **16**:48.

DICKIE, M. M., AND WOOLLEY, G. W., 1949, Spontaneous basophilic tumors of the pituitary glands in gonadectomized mice, *Cancer Res.* **9**:372.

DMOCHOWSKI, L., 1973, The viral factor in the genesis of breast cancer: Present evidence, *Triangle* **12**:37.

ECKSTEIN, P., AND KNOWLES, F., eds., 1963 *Techniques in Endocrine Research*, Academic Press, London.

EIGEN, M., 1971, Self-organization of matter and evolution of biological macromolecules, *Naturwissenschaften* **58**:465.

EISENFELD, A. J., 1970, $H^3$-estradiol: *In vitro* binding to macromolecules from the rat hypothalamus, anterior pituitary and uterus, *Endocrinology* **86**:1313.

ELIAS, J. J., AND RIVERA, E. M., 1959, Comparison of the responses of normal, precancerous, and neoplastic mouse mammary tissues to hormones *in vitro*, *Cancer Res.* **19**:505.

ENGELSMAN, E., PERSIJN, J. P., KORSTEN, C. B., AND CLETON, F. J., 1973, Oestrogen receptor in human breast cancer tissue and response to endocrine therapy, *Brit. Med. J.* **2**:750.

EVERETT, J. W., AND NIKITOVITCH-WINER, M., 1963, Physiology of the pituitary gland as affected by transplantation or stalk transection, in: *Advances in Neuroendrocrinology* (A. V. Nalbanov, ed.), pp. 289–304, University of Illinois Press, Urbana.

FARQUHAR, M. G., 1971, Processing of secretory products by cells of the anterior pituitary gland, in: *Subcellular Structure and Function in Endocrine Organs* (H. Heller and K. Lederis, eds.), *Mem. Soc. Endocrinol.* **19**:79.

FLAX, H., 1973, A new method of determining the hormone dependence of human breast cancer, *Brit. J. Surg.* **60**:317.

FLAXMAN, B. A., AND LASFARGUES, E. Y., 1973, Hormone-independent DNA synthesis by epithelial cells of adult human mammary gland in organ culture, *Proc. Soc. Exp. Biol. Med.* **143**:371.

FLÜCKIGER, E., 1972, Drugs and the control of prolactin secretion, in: *Prolactin and Carcinogenesis* (A. R. Boyns and K. Griffiths, eds.), pp. 162–171, Alpha Omega Alpha, Cardiff.

FOULDS, L., 1969, *Neoplastic Development*, Academic Press, New York.

FRIESEN, H. G., 1972, Prolactin: Its physiologic role and therapeutic potential, *Hosp. Prac.* **7**:123.

FRIESEN, H., AND HWANG, P., 1973, Human prolactin, *Ann. Rev. Med.* **24**:251.

FRIESEN, H., GUYDA, H., AND HARDY, J., 1970, Biosynthesis of human growth hormone and prolactin, *J. Clin. Endocrinol. Metab.* **31**:611.

FURTH, J., 1969, Pituitary cybernetics and neoplasia, *Harvey Lect.* **63**:47.

FURTH, J., 1973, The role of prolactin in mammary carcinogenesis, in: *Human Prolactin* (J. L. Pasteels and C. Robyn, eds.), pp. 232–248, Excerpta Medica, Amsterdam.

FURTH, J., AND CLIFTON, K. H., 1966, Experimental pituitary tumors, in: *The Pituitary Gland* (G. W. Harris and B. T. Donovan, eds.), pp. 460–497, Butterworths, London.

FURTH, J., MOY, P., HERSHMAN, J. M., AND UEDA, G., 1973a, Thyrotropic tumor syndrome: A multiglandular disease induced by sustained deficiency of thyroid hormones, *Arch. Pathol.* **96**:217.

FURTH, J., MOY, P., SCHALCH, D. S., AND UEDA G., 1973b, Gonadotropic activities of thyrotropic tumors: Demonstration by immunohistochemical staining, *Proc. Soc. Exp. Biol. Med.* **142**:1180.

FURTH, J., MARTIN, J. M., MOY, P., AND UEDA, G., 1973c, Growth hormonal activity of thyotropic pituitary tumors, *Proc. Soc. Exp. Biol. Med.* **142**:511.

FURTH, J., UEDA, G., AND CLIFTON, K. H., 1973d, Pathophysiology of pituitaries and their tumors: Methodological advances, in: *Methods in Cancer Research*, Vol. X (H. Busch, ed.), pp. 201–277, Academic Press, New York.

FURTH, J., UEDA, G., AND CLIFTON, K. H., 1973d, Pathophysiology of pituitaries and their tumors: Methodological advances, in: *Methods in Cancer Research*, Vol. X (H. Busch, ed.), pp. 201–277, Academic Press, New York.

FURTH, J., NAKANE, P. K., AND PASTEELS, J. L., 1973e, Pathology and pathogenesis of spontaneous and experimental pituitary tumors, in: *Pathology of Tumors in Laboratory Animals*, Vol. 1, Part 2: *The Rat* (V. Turusov, ed.), IARC Scientific Publication No. 6, International Agency for Research on Cancer, Lyon, France, in press.

FURTH, J., ESBER, H. J., BOGDEN, A. E., AND MOY, P., 1974, Evolution of pituitary tropic cells and estrogens in relation to differentiation of the mammary gland and mammary tumorigenesis, *Proc. Endocrine Soc.*, Abst. No. 366, p. A-238.

GANONG, W. F., AND MARTINI, L., eds., 1973, *Frontiers in Neuroendocrinology, 1973*, Oxford University Press, New York.

GARAY, G. L., ÅKERBLOM, H. K., AND MARTIN, J. M., 1971, Experimental hypersomatotropism: Serum growth hormone and insulin, and pituitary and pancreatic changes in MtT-W15 tumor-bearing rats before and after tumor removal, *Horm. Metab. Res.* **3**:82.

GARDNER, W. U., PFEIFFER, C. A., TRENTIN, J. J., AND WOLSTENHOLME, J. T., 1953, Hormonal factors in experimental carcinogenesis, in: *The Physiopathology of Cancer*, 1st ed. (F. Homburger and W. H. Fishman, eds.), pp. 225–297, Hoeber-Harper, New York.

GARDNER, W. U., PFEIFFER, C. A., AND TRENTIN, J. J., 1959, Hormonal factors in experimental carcinogenesis, in: *The Physiopathology of Cancer*, 2nd ed. (F. Homburger, ed.), pp. 152–237, Harper, New York.

GELLHORN, A., 1966, Editorial on cancer: Facts and theories. Clinical physiology, chemotherapy, fundamental nature and mechanism of gene control, *Sem. Hematol.* **3**:99.

GEWIRTZ, G., AND YALOW, R. S., 1973, Ectopic ACTH production: Big and little forms, *Endocrinology (Suppl.)* **92**:A-53.

GOODMAN, A. D., TANENBAUM, R., AND RABINOWITZ, D., 1972, Existence of two forms of immunoreactive growth hormone in human plasma, *J. Clin. Endocrinol. Metab.* **35**:868.

GOTTSCHALK, R. G., AND FURTH, J., 1951, Polycythemia with features of Cushing's syndrome produced by luteomas, *Acta Haematol.* **5**:101.

GRANT, G., VALE, W., AND GUILLEMIN, R., 1973, Characteristics of the pituitary binding sites of thyrotropin-releasing factor, *Endocrinology* **92**:1629.

GRAY, C. H., AND BACHARACH, A. L., eds., 1967, *Hormones in Blood*, Vol. 1, Academic Press, London.

GREEN, E. L., ed., 1966, *Biology of the Laboratory Mouse*, McGraw-Hill, New York.

GREEN, J. A., 1957, Morphology, secretion and transplantability of ten mouse ovarian neoplasms induced by intrasplenic ovarian grafting, *Cancer Res.* **17**:86.

GREEN, J. D., AND HARRIS, G. W., 1947, The neurovascular link between the neurohypophysis and adenohypophysis, *J. Endocrinol.* **5**:136.

GRIESBACH, W. E., AND PURVES, H. D., 1960, Basophil adenoma in the rat hypophysis after gonadectomy, *Brit. J. Cancer* **14**:49.

GROSS, L., 1953, A filterable agent, recovered from Ak leukemic extracts, causing salivary gland carcinomas in C3H mice, *Proc. Soc. Exp. Biol. Med.* **83**:414.

HALL, R., SCHALLY, A. V., EVERED, D., KASTIN, A. J., MORTIMER, C. H., TUNBRIDGE, W. M. G., BESSER, G. M., COY, D. H. GOLDIE, D. J., MCNEILLY, A. S., PHENEKOS, C., AND WEIGHTMAN, D., 1973, Action of growth-hormone-release inhibitory hormone in healthy men and in acromegaly, *Lancet* **2**:581.

HARAN-GHERA, N., PULLAR, P., AND FURTH, J., 1960, Induction of thyrotropin-dependent thyroid tumors by thyrotropes, *Endocrinology* **66**:694.

HARRIS, G. W., 1955, *Neural Control of the Pituitary Gland*, Arnold, London.

HAYMAKER, W., ANDERSON, E., AND NAUTA, W. J. H., eds., 1969, *The Hypothalamus*, Thomas, Springfield, Ill.

HEDINGER, C., ed., 1969, *Thyroid Cancer*, UICC Monograph Series, Vol. 12, Springer, Berlin.

HINKLE, P. M., AND TASHJIAN, A. H., JR., 1973, Receptors for thyrotropin-releasing hormone in prolactin-producing rat pituitary cells in culture, *J. Biol. Chem.* **248**:6180.

HOLLANDER, N., AND HOLLANDER, V. P., 1971, Development of a somatotropic variant of the mammosomatotropic tumor MtT/W5, *Proc. Soc. Exp. Biol. Med.* **137**:1157.

HOPKINS, C. R., AND FARQUHAR, M. G., 1973, Hormone secretion by cells dissociated from rat anterior pituitaries, *J. Cell Biol.* **59**:276 (Part 1).

HORNING, E. S., 1954, The influence of unilateral nephrectomy on the development of stilbestrol-induced renal tumors in the male hamster, *Brit. J. Cancer* **8**:627.

HORROBIN, D. F., 1973, *Prolactin: Physiology and Clinical Significance*, MTP Medical and Technical Publishing Co., London.

HOUSSAY, A. B., HOUSSAY, B. A., CARDEZA, A. F., PINTO, R. M., AND FOGLIA, V. G., 1954, Estrogenic and adrenal tumors and gonadotropic pituitary tumors in gonadectomized rats, in: *Third Panamerican Congress of Endocrinology, Santiago de Chile*, p. 19.

HOUSSAY, B. A., HOUSSAY, A. B., CARDEZA, A. F., FOGLIA, V. G., AND PINTO, R. M., 1953, Adrenal tumors in gonadectomized rats, *Acta Physiol. Latinoam.* **3**:125.

HOUSSAY, B. A., HOUSSAY, A. B., CARDEZA, A. F., AND PINTO, R. M., 1955, Tumeurs surrénales oestrogéniques et tumeurs hypophysaires chez les animaux castrés, *Schweiz. Med. Wschr.* **85**:291.

HOWELL, J. S., MARCHANT, J., AND ORR, J. W., 1954, The induction of ovarian tumors in mice with 9:10-dimethyl-1:2-benzanthracene, *Brit. J. Cancer* **8**:635.

HUGGINS, C., 1967, Endocrine-induced regression of cancers, *Science* **156**:1050.

HUGGINS, C., AND MOULDER, P. V., 1945, Estrogen production by Sertoli cell tumors of the testis, *Cancer Res.* **5**:510.

HUGGINS, C., AND YANG, W. C., 1962, Induction and extinction of mammary cancer, *Science* **137**:257.

HUGGINS, C., BRIZIARELLI, G., AND SUTTON, H., 1959, Rapid induction of mammary carcinoma in the rat and the influence of hormones on the tumors, *J. Exp. Med.* **109**:25.

HUGGINS, C., GRAND, L. C., AND BRILLANTES, F. P., 1961, Mammary cancer induced by a single feeding of polynuclear hydrocarbon and its supression, *Nature* **189**:204.

HUSEBY, R. A., 1960, Studies of hormone dependency employing interstitial cell testicular tumors of mice, in: *Biological Activities of Steroids in Relation to Cancer* (G. Pincus, and E. P. Vollmer, eds.), pp. 211–223, Academic Press, New York.

HUSEBY, R. A., 1972, Hormonal factors in relation to cancer, in: *Environment and Cancer* (M. D. Anderson Hospital Symposium), pp. 372–393, Williams and Wilkins, Baltimore.

IGLESIAS, R., SALINAS, S., VUKUSIC, P., AND PANASEVICH, V., 1969, Transplantable gonadotrophic pituitary tumor of the AxC rat, *Proc. Am. Assoc. Cancer Res.* **10**:42.

IGLESIAS, R., SALINAS, S., VUKUSIC, P., GIRARDI, S., AND POLANCO, X., 1972, Functional transplantable ovarian tumors (OvT) developed in AxC rats grafted with the gonadotropic pituitary tumor (Gpic PT), *Proc. Am. Assoc. Cancer Res.* **13**:110.

ITO, A., MOY, P., KAUNITZ, H., KORTWRIGHT, K., CLARKE, S., FURTH, J., AND MEITES, J., 1972*a*, Incidence and character of the spontaneous pituitary tumors in strain CR and W/Fu male rats, *J. Natl. Cancer Inst.* **49**:701.

ITO, A., FURTH, J., AND MOY, P., 1972*b*, Growth hormone-secreting variants of a mammotropic tumor, *Cancer Res.* **32**:48.

IVERSEN, O. H., 1970, Some theoretical considerations on chalones and the treatment of cancer: A review, *Cancer Res.* **30**:1481.

JACOBS, B. B., AND HUSEBY, R. A., 1972, Brief communication: Hormone dependency of murine endocrine tumors *in vivo* and in organ culture: A correlative study, *J. Natl. Cancer Inst.* **49**:1205.

JENSEN, E. V., AND DESOMBRE, E. R., 1973, Estrogen–receptor interaction, *Science* **182**:126.

JENSEN, E. V., BLOCK, G. E., SMITH, S., KYSER, K., AND DESOMBRE, E. R., 1971, Estrogen receptors and breast cancer response to adrenalectomy, in: Prediction of Response in Cancer Therapy, *Natl. Cancer Inst. Monogr.* **34**:55.

JERNE, N. K., 1973, The immune system, *Sci. Am.* **229**:52.

JULL, J. W., AND PHILLIPS, A. J., 1969, The effects of 7,12-dimethylbenz(*a*)anthracene on the ovarian response of mice and rats to gonadotrophins, *Cancer Res.* **29**:1977.

KATO, J., 1970, *In vitro* uptake of tritiated oestradiol by the anterior hypothalamus and hypophysis of the rat, *Acta Endocrinol.* **64**:687.

KEEFER, D. A., STUMPF, W. E., AND SAR, M., 1973, Topographical localization of estrogen-concentrating cells in the rat spinal cord following $^3$H-estradiol administration, *Proc. Soc. Exp. Biol. Med.* **143**:414.

KIM, U., 1965, Pituitary function and hormonal therapy of experimental breast cancer, *Cancer Res.* **25**:1146.

KIM, U., AND FURTH, J., 1960*a*, Relation of mammary tumors to mammotropes. II. Hormone responsiveness of 3-methyl-cholanthrene-induced mammary carcinomas, *Proc. Soc. Exp. Biol. Med.* **103**:643.

KIM, U., AND FURTH, J., 1960*b*, Relation of mammotropes to mammary tumors. IV. Development of highly hormone-dependent mammary tumors, *Proc. Soc. Exp. Biol. Med.* **105**:490.

KIM, U., AND FURTH, J., 1960c, Relation of mammary tumors to mammotropes. I. Induction of mammary tumors in rats, *Proc. Soc. Exp. Biol. Med.* **103**:640.

KIM, U., FURTH, J., AND CLIFTON, K. H., 1960a, Relation of mammary tumors to mammotropes. III. Hormone responsiveness of transplanted mammary tumors, *Proc. Soc. Exp. Biol. Med.* **103**:646.

KIM, U., CLIFTON, K. H., AND FURTH, J., 1960b, A highly inbred line of Wistar rats yielding spontaneous mammo-somatotropic pituitary and other tumors, *J. Natl. Cancer Inst.* **24**:1031.

KIRKMAN, H., AND BACON, R. L., 1950, Malignant renal tumors in male hamsters (*Cricetus auratus*) treated with estrogen, *Cancer Res.* **10**:122.

KLEIN, G., 1973–1974, Immunological surveillance against neoplasia, *Harvey Lect.*, in press.

KNIGGE, K. M., SCOTT, D. E., AND WEINDL, A., eds., 1972, *Brain–Endocrine Interaction. Medium Eminence: Structure and Function*, Karger, Basel.

KRUSE, P. F., JR., AND PATTERSON, M. K., JR., 1973, *Tissue Culture: Methods and Applications*, Academic Press, New York.

KWA, H. G., 1961, *An Experimental Study of Pituitary Tumors*, Springer, Berlin.

LEFKOWITZ, R. J., ROTH, J., AND PASTAN, I., 1970a, Effects of calcium on ACTH stimulation of the adrenal: Separation of hormone binding from adenyl cyclase activation, *Nature (Lond.)* **228**:864.

LEFKOWITZ, R. J., ROTH, J., PRICER, W., AND PASTAN, I., 1970b, ACTH receptors in the adrenal: Specific binding of ACTH-$^{125}$I and its relation to adenyl cyclase, *Proc. Natl. Acad. Sci.* **65**:745.

LEWIS, A. A. M., AND DESHPANDE, N., 1973, The effect of hypophysectomy on the cortisol secretion in 4 patients with advanced metastatic breast cancer, *Brit. J. Surg.* **60**:493.

LEWIS, U. J., SINGH, R. N. P., AND SEAVEY, B. K., 1971, Human prolactin: Isolation and some properties, *Biochem. Biophys. Res. Commun.* **44**:1169.

LI, C. H., 1972, Hormones of the adenohypophysis, *Proc. Am. Phil. Soc.* **116**:365.

LI, C. H., 1973, Prolactin, *Calif. Med.* **118**:55.

LINDSAY, S., 1969, Ionizing radiation and experimental thyroid neoplasms: A review, in: *Thyroid Cancer* (C. Hedinger, ed.), pp. 161–171, Springer, Berlin.

LOCKE, W., AND SCHALLY, A. V., 1973, *The Hypothalamus and Pituitary in Health and Disease*, Thomas, Springfield, Ill.

LOEB, L., AND KIRTZ, M. M., 1939, The effect of transplants of anterior lobes of the hypophysis on the growth of the mammary gland and on the development of mammary gland carcinoma in various strains of mice, *Am. J. Cancer* **36**:56.

LOWENSTEIN, W. R., 1968, Communication through cell junctions: Implications in growth and differentiation, *Develop. Biol.* **19**:151 (Suppl. 2).

MACLEOD, R. M., SMITH, C., AND DEWITT, G. W., 1966, Hormonal properties of transplanted pituitary tumors and their relation to the pituitary gland, *Endocrinology* **79**:1149.

MACMAHON, B., COLE, P., AND BROWN, J., 1973, Etiology of human breast cancer: A review, *J. Natl. Cancer Inst.* **50**:21.

MARTIN, J. M., ÅKERBLOM, H. K., AND GARAY, G., 1968, Insulin secretion in rats with elevated levels of circulating growth hormone due to MtT-W15 tumor, *Diabetes* **17**:661.

MAZURKIEWICZ, J. E., AND NAKANE, P. K., 1972, Light and electron microscopic localization of antigens in tissues embedded in polyethylene glycol with a peroxidase-labeled antibody method, *J. Histochem. Cytochem.* **20**:969.

MCCORMICK, G. M., AND MOON, R. C., 1973, Effect of increasing doses of estrogen and progesterone on mammary carcinogenesis in the rat, *Europ. J. Cancer* **9**:483.

MCGUIRE, W. L., AND DELAGARZA, M., 1973a, Similarity of the estrogen receptor in human and rat mammary carcinoma, *J. Clin. Endocrinol. Metab.* **36**:548.

MCGUIRE, W. L., AND DELAGARZA, M., 1973b, Improved sensitivity in the measurement of estrogen receptor in human breast cancer, *J. Clin. Endocrinol. Metab.* **37**:986.

MCGUIRE, W. L., DELAGARZA, M., AND CHAMNESS, G. C., 1973, Estrogen receptor in a prolactin-secreting pituitary tumor (MtTW5), *Endocrinology* **93**:810.

MEITES, J., ed., 1970, *Hypophysiotropic Hormones of the Hypothalamus: Assay and Chemistry*, Williams and Wilkins, Baltimore.

MEITES, J., 1973, Control of prolactin secretion in animals, in: *Human Prolactin* (J. L. Pasteels and C. Robyn, eds.), pp. 105–118, Excerpta Medica, Amsterdam.

MESSIER, B., AND FURTH, J., 1962, A reversely responsive variant of a thyrotropic tumor with gonadotropic activity, *Cancer Res.* **22**:804.

MEŠTER, B., BRUNELLE, R., JUNG, I., AND SONNENSCHEIN, C., 1973, Estrogen-sensitive cells: Hormone receptors in tumors and cells in culture, *Exp. Cell Res.* **81**:447.

MINTON, J. P., AND DICKEY, R. P., 1973, Levodopa test to predict response of carcinoma of the breast to surgical ablation of endocrine glands, *Surg. Gynecol. Obstet.* **136:**971.

MOLTENI, A., NICKERSON, P. A., LATTA, J., AND BROWNIE, A. C., 1972, Hypertension in rats bearing an adrenocorticotropic hormone-, growth hormone-, and prolactin-secreting tumor (MtTF4), *Cancer Res.* **32:**114.

MOON, H. D., SIMPSON, M. E., LI, C. H., AND EVANS, H. M., 1950a, Neoplasms in rats treated with pituitary growth hormone. I. Pulmonary and lymphatic tissues, *Cancer Res.* **10:**297.

MOON, H. D., SIMPSON, M. E., LI, C. H., AND EVANS, H. M., 1950b, Neoplasms in rats treated with pituitary growth hormone. II. Adrenal glands, *Cancer Res.* **10:**364.

MOON, H. D., SIMPSON, M. E., LI, C. H., AND EVANS, H. M., 1950c, Neoplasms in rats treated with pituitary growth hormone. III. Reproductive organs, *Cancer Res.* **10:**549.

MOON, H. D., SIMPSON, M. E., LI, C. H., AND EVANS, H. M., 1951, Neoplasms in rats treated with pituitary growth hormone. V. Absence of neoplasms in hypophysectomized rats, *Cancer Res.* **11:**535.

MOORE, D. H., CHARNEY, J., KRAMARSKY, B., LASFARGUES, E. Y., SARKAR, N. H., BRENNAN, M. J., BURROWS, J. H., SIRSAT, S. M., PAYMASTER, J. C., AND VAIDYA, A. B., 1971, Search for a human breast cancer virus, *Nature (Lond.)* **229:**611.

MORIARTY, G. C., 1973, Adenohypophysis: Ultrastructural cytochemistry. A review, *J. Histochem. Cytochem.* **21:**855.

MORRIS, H. P., 1955, Experimental thyroid tumors, in: *The Thyroid* (Brookhaven Symposia in Biology No. 7), pp. 192–219, Associated Universities, Upton, N.Y.

MUNSON, P. L., HIRSCH, P. F., BREWER, H. B., REISFELD, R. A., COOPER, C. W., WÄSTHED, A. B., ORIMO, H., AND POTTS, J. T., JR., 1968, Thyrocalcitonin, *Rec. Prog. Horm. Res.* **24:**589.

NAGASAWA, H., AND YANAI, R., 1973, Effect of human placental lactogen on growth of carcinogen-induced mammary tumors in rats, *Int. J. Cancer* **11:**131.

NAGASAWA, H., CHEN, C.-L., AND MEITES, J., 1973, Relation between growth of carcinogen-induced mammary cancers and serum prolactin values in rats, *Proc. Soc. Exp. Biol. Med.* **142:**625.

NAKANE, P. K., 1970, Classifications of anterior pituitary cell types with immunoenzyme histochemistry, *J. Histochem, Cytochem.* **18:**9.

NOEL, G. L., SUH, H. K., AND FRANTZ, A. G., 1973, L-Dopa suppression of TRH-stimulated prolactin release in man, *J. Clin. Endocrinol. Metab.* **36:**1255.

OMENN, G. S., 1973, Pathobiology of ectopic hormone production by neoplasms in man, in: *Pathobiology Annual,* Vol. 3 (H. L. Ioachim, ed.), pp. 177–216, Appleton-Century-Crofts, New York.

ORR, J. W., 1962, Tumors of the ovary and the role of the ovary and its hormones in neoplasia, in: *The Ovary,* Vol. 2 (S. Zuckerman, ed.), pp. 533–561, Academic Press, New York.

PASTEELS, J. L., 1972, Tissue culture of human hypophyses: Evidence of a specific prolactin in man, in: *Lactogenic Hormones* (G. E. W. Wolstenholme and J. Knight, eds.), pp. 269–286, Churchill-Livingstone, Edinburgh.

PASTEELS, J. L., AND ROBYN, C., eds., 1973, *Human Prolactin,* Excerpta Medica, Amsterdam.

PHIFER, R. F., MIDGLEY, A. R., AND SPICER, S. S., 1972, Histology of the human hypophyseal gonadotropin secreting cells, in: *Gonadotropins* (B. B. Saxena, C. G. Beling, and H. M. Gandy, eds.), pp. 9–25, Wiley, New York.

PHIFER, R. F., MIDGLEY, A. R. AND SPICER, S. S., 1973, Immunohistologic and histologic evidence that follicle-stimulating hormone and luteinizing hormone are present in the same cell type in the human pars distalis, *J. Clin. Endocrinol. Metab.* **36:**125.

PIERCE, J. G., LIAO, T., HOWARD, S., SHOME, B., AND CORNELL, J., 1971, Studies on the structure of thyrotropin: Its relationship to luteinizing hormone, *Rec. Prog. Hor. Res.* **27:**165.

PLAPINGER, L., AND MCEWEN, B. S., 1973, Ontogeny of estradiol-binding sites in rat brain. I. Appearance of presumptive adult receptors in cytosol and nuclei, *Endocrinology* **93:**1119.

PLAPINGER, L., MCEWEN, B. S., AND CLEMENS, L. E., 1973, Ontogeny of estradiol-binding sites in rat brain. II. Characteristics of a neonatal binding macromolecule, *Endocrinology* **93:**1129.

POLLACK, R., AND SATO, G., eds., 1973, *Readings in Mammalian Cell Culture,* Cold Spring Harbor Laboratory, Cold Spring Harbor, N.Y.

PTASHNE, M., 1973–1974, Repressor, operators and promotors in bacteriophage λ, *Harvey Lect.,* in press.

RATHNAM, P., AND SAXENA, B. B., 1971, Subunits of luteinizing hormone from human pituitary glands, *J. Biol. Chem.* **246:**7087.

RILEY, P. A., LATTER, T., AND SUTTON, P. M., 1973, Hormone assays on breast-tumour cultures, *Lancet* **2:**818.

ROUS, P., 1943, The nearer causes of cancer, *J. Am. Med. Assoc.* **122:**573.

Rous, P., and Kidd, J. G., 1941, Conditional neoplasms and subthreshold neoplastic states, *J. Exp. Med.* **73**:365.

Russfield, A. B., 1966, *Tumors of Endocrine Glands and Secondary Sex Organs*, Public Health Service Publication No. 1332, Government Printing Office, Washington, D.C.

Schally, A. V., Arimura, A., and Kastin, A. J., 1973, Hypothalamic regulatory hormones, *Science* **179**:341.

Schlom, J., and Spiegelman, S., 1973, Evidence for viral involvement in murine and human mammary adenocarcinoma, *Am. J. Clin. Pathol.* **60**:44.

Shelesnyak, M. C., 1954, Ergotoxine inhibition of deciduoma formation and its reversal by progesterone, *Am. J. Physiol.* **179**:301.

Sinha, D., Pascal, R., and Furth, J., 1965, Transplantable thyroid carcinoma induced by thyrotropin, *Arch. Pathol.* **79**:192.

Smythe, G. A., and Lazarus, L., 1973, Blockade of the dopamine-inhibitory control of prolactin secretion in rats by 3,4-dimethoxyphenylethylamine (3,4-di-O-methyldopamine), *Endocrinology* **93**:147.

Spiegelman, S., and Schlom, J., 1972, Reverse transcriptase in oncogenic RNA viruses, in: *Virus–Cell Interactions and Viral Antimetabolites* (D. Sugar, ed.), pp. 115–133, Academic Press, London.

Steelman, S. W., Kelly, T. L., Norgello, H., and Weber, G. F., 1956, Occurrence of melanocyte stimulating hormone (MSH) in a transplantable pituitary tumor, *Proc. Soc. Exp. Biol. Med.* **92**:392.

Stein, G. S., Spelsberg, T. C., and Kleinsmith, L. J., 1974, Nonhistone chromosol proteins and gene regulation, *Science* **183**:817.

Steiner, A. L., Goodman, A. D., and Powers, S. R., 1968, Study of a kindred with pheochromocytoma, medullary thyroid carcinoma, hyperparathyroidism and Cushing's disease: Multiple endocrine neoplasia, type 2, *Medicine* **47**:371.

Sterental, A., Dominguez, J. M., Weissman, C., and Pearson, O. H., 1963, Pituitary role in the estrogen dependency of experimental cancer, *Cancer Res.* **23**:481.

Stoll, B. A., 1972, Brain catecholamines and breast cancer: A hypothesis, *Lancet* **1**:431.

Stoll, B. A., 1973, Hypothesis: Breast cancer regression under oestrogen therapy, *Brit. Med. J.* **3**:446.

Stumpf, W. E., 1969, Nuclear concentration of $^3$H-estradiol in tissues: Dry-mount autoradiography of vagina, oviduct, testis, mammary tumor, liver and adrenal, *Endocrinology* **85**:31.

Sunderman, F. W., and Sunderman, F. W., Jr., eds., 1971, *Laboratory Diagnosis of Endrocrine Diseases*, Green, St. Louis.

Sutherland, E. W., and Robison, G. A., 1966, The role of cyclic-3′,5′-AMP in responses to catecholamines and other hormones, *Pharmacol. Rev.* **18**:145.

Takizawa, S., Furth, J. J., and Furth, J., 1970, DNA synthesis in autonomous and hormone-responsive mammary tumors, *Cancer Res.* **30**:206.

Tashjian, A. H., Yasumura, Y., Levine, L., Sato, G. H., and Parker, M. L., 1968, Establishment of clonal strains of rat pituitary tumor cells that secrete growth hormone, *Endocrinology* **82**:342.

Taylor, S., and Foster, G., eds., 1970, *Calcitonin*, Springer, New York.

Temin, H. M., 1972, RNA-directed DNA synthesis, *Sci. Am.* **226**:24.

Thomas, J. A., and Mawhinney, M. G., 1973, *Synopsis of Endocrine Pharmacology*, University Park Press, Baltimore.

Turkington, R. W., 1971, Measurement of prolactin activity in human plasma by new biological and radioreceptor assays, *J. Clin. Invest.* **50**:94a.

Turkington, R. W., 1972, Secretion of prolactin by patients with pituitary and hypothalamic tumors. *J. Clin. Endocrinol. Metab.* **34**:159.

Ueda, G., and Furth, J., 1967, Sacromatoid transformation of transplanted thyroid carcinoma, *Arch. Pathol.* **83**:3.

Ueda, G., Hayakawa, K., Hamanaka, N., Yoshinare, S., Sato, Y., and Okudaira, Y., 1972, Enzyme histochemistry of experimental ovarian tumors in mice, *Acta Obstet. Gynecol. Jap.* **18**:16.

Ueda, G., Moy, P., and Furth, J., 1973, Multihormonal activities of normal and neoplastic pituitary cells as indicated by immunohistochemical staining, *Int. J. Cancer* **12**:100.

Vaitukaitis, J. L., and Ross, G. T., 1972, Antigenic similarities among the human glycoprotein hormones and their subunits, in: *Gonadotropins* (B. B. Saxena, C. G. Beling, and H. M. Gandy, eds.), pp. 435–443, Wiley, New York.

Vale, W., Grant, G., and Guillemin, R., 1973, Chemistry of the hypothalamic releasing factors—Studies on structure–function relationships, in: *Frontiers in Neuroendocrinology, 1973* (W. F. Ganong and L. Martini, eds.), pp. 375–413, Oxford University Press, New York.

WATANABE, H., ORTH, D. N., AND TOFT, D. O., 1973, Glucocorticoid receptors in pituitary tumor cells. I. Cytosol receptors, *J. Biol. Chem.* **248:**7625.

WEISZ, J., AND GUNSALUS, P., 1973, Estrogen levels in immature female rats: True or spurious—ovarian or adrenal? *Endocrinology* **93:**1057.

WELSCH, C. W., AND GRIBLER, C., 1973, Prophylaxis of spontaneously developing mammary carcinoma in C3H/HeJ female mice by suppression of prolactin, *Cancer Res.* **33:**2939.

WELSCH, C. W., ITURRI, G., AND MEITES, J., 1973, Comparative effects of hypophysectomy, ergocornine and ergocornine–reserpine treatments on rat mammary carcinoma, *Int. J. Cancer* **12:**206.

WIENER, N., 1948, *Cybernetics, or Control and Communication in the Animal and the Machine,* Technology Press, New York.

WILLIAMS, R. H., ed., 1968, *Textbook of Endocrinology,* Saunders, Philadelphia.

WILLIS, R. A., 1967, *Pathology of Tumours,* 4th ed., Butterworths, Washington, D.C.

WISH, L., FURTH, J., AND STOREY, R. H., 1950, Direct determinations of plasma, cell, and organ-blood volumes in normal and hypervolemic mice, *Proc. Soc. Exp. Biol. Med.* **74:**644.

WOLFSEN, A. R., MCINTYRE, H. B., AND ODELL, W. D., 1972, Adrenocorticotropin measurement by competitive binding receptor assay, *J. Clin. Endocrinol. Metab.* **34:**684.

WOLSTENHOLME, G. E. W., ed., 1966, *Histones—Their Role in the Transfer of Genetic Information* (Ciba Foundation Study Group 24), Little Brown, Boston.

WOLSTENHOLME, G. E. W., AND KNIGHT, J., eds., 1972, *Lactogenic Hormones,* Churchill-Livingstone, Edinburgh.

WOOLLEY, G. W., 1958, Tumors of the adrenal cortex, in: *Ciba Foundation Colloquia on Endocrinology,* Vol. 12 (G. E. W. Wolstenholme and M. O'Connor, eds.), pp. 122–136, Churchill, London.

WUTTKE, W., 1973, Dsicussion, in: *Human Prolactin* (J. L. Pasteels and C. Robyn, eds.), p. 143, Excerpta Medica, Amsterdam.

YALOW, R. S., Heterogeneity of peptide hormones, *Rec. Prog. Horm. Res.,* **30:**597.

YOKORO, K., AND FURTH, J., 1962, Determining the role of "mammotropins" in induction of mammary tumors in mice by virus, *J. Natl. Cancer Inst.* **29:**887.

YOKORO, K., FURTH, J., AND HARAN-GHERA, N., 1961, Induction of mammotropic pituitary tumors by X-rays in rats and mice: The role of mammotropes in development of mammary tumors, *Cancer Res.* **21:**178.

YOUNG, S., AND INMAN, R., eds., 1968, *Thyroid Neoplasia,* Academic Press, London.

ZUCKERMAN, S., ed., 1962, *The Ovary,* Vol. II, Academic Press, New York.

# 5

# Immunocompetence and Malignancy

CORNELIS J. M. MELIEF and ROBERT S. SCHWARTZ

> *The essential feature of a strategy of discovery lies in determining the sequence of choice of problems to solve. Now it is in fact very much more difficult to see a problem than to find a solution for it. The former requires imagination, the latter only ingenuity.*
>
> —J. D. BERNAL

## 1. Introduction*

In June of 1908, Paul Ehrlich, the founder of immunology, lectured at the University of Amsterdam on the subject of cancer. His remarks included the following: "the understanding of natural immunity really represents the key to carcinoma . . . . I have acquired the firm conviction that natural immunity does not depend on the presence of anti-microbial materials, but rather, it depends on purely cellular activities. I am certain that, in the enormously complicated course of fetal and post-fetal development, aberrant cells become unusually common. Fortunately, in the majority of people, they remain completely latent thanks to the organism's positive mechanisms. If such mechanisms did not exist, one might

---

* We assume that the reader has a working knowledge of the basic principles of immunology. Those who wish to brush up on recent advances may wish to consult either Roitt (1971) or Bach and Good (1972), both of which are excellent texts.

---

CORNELIS J. M. MELIEF and ROBERT S. SCHWARTZ ● Hematology Service, New England Medical Center Hospital, and the Department of Medicine, Tufts University School of Medicine, Boston, Massachusetts. Dr. Melief is the recipient of a fellowship from the Dutch Organization for the Advancement of Pure Research (ZWO). Supported by grants from USPHS (CA 10018) and the Damon Runyon Foundation.

121

expect carcinomas to have an enormous frequency. These cells may live in a latent state for 20, 30 or 40 years before changing to a significant tumor. This means, in light of my theory, that there has been a diminution of some vital cell activity [which] allows the rapid, parasitic growth of certain cells" (Ehrlich, 1957).*

Apparently, Ehrlich's amazing prescience was not appreciated, because, apart from a brief comment by Emery (1924), who expressed a similar notion, the idea that cellular immunity is important in the defense against neoplastic cells lay fallow for decades. However, the landmark experiments of Little (1941), Foley (1953), Prehn and Main (1957), and Klein (1966) revitalized immunological studies of cancer and set the stage for the development of one of the most powerful influences in the field. This is the theory of immunological surveillance.

There is general agreement that this concept in its modern form was formulated by Lewis Thomas, who, in 1959, proposed that "the phenomenon of homograft rejection will turn out to represent a primary mechanism for natural defense against neoplasia" (Thomas, 1959). This idea, which was offered extemporaneously in a discussion, fortunately recorded, of Medawar's experiments on transplantation immunity, was taken up by Burnet, who, besides expostulating on its profound biological and medical implications, first used the term *surveillance* as a coda for Thomas's concept (Burnet, 1963, 1970).

The theory that the immune system "represents a primary mechanism for natural defense against neoplasia" makes four predictions: (1) Neoplastic cells possess antigenic determinants that are absent from normal cells. (2) These antigens are immunogenic in the host of origin; i.e., they are autoantigens. (3) The immune response provoked by tumor-associated antigens protects the host by destroying neoplastic cells; i.e., the surveillance mechanism relies on an autoimmune reaction. (4) Tumor cells flourish in individuals with defective or suppressed immunity.

Abundant evidence supports the first three predictions, and we will not deal with them here because they have been thoroughly analyzed elsewhere (Hellström, 1969; Alexander, 1972; Klein, 1972). Instead, we will direct our attention to the theory's fourth prediction. This is its keystone. Moreover, the prediction that impaired immunity encourages the development and growth of cancer has important clinical implications. Investigations of the possibility of enhanced development of neoplasms during immunosuppressive therapy and renewed efforts toward the immunotherapy of cancer both originate from the notion that the immune system of the patient has failed to reject the neoplasm.

Before addressing ourselves to this problem, we should admit to the reader our skepticism. We feel that the theory of immunological surveillance has been overemphasized,† perhaps to the detriment of alternative views. We also believe that this theory has not been adequately challenged in the laboratory. Indeed, almost all experimental work stimulated by the theory seems to have been designed with the expressed or implied purpose of proving it. Yet a theory derives its strength from its ability to resist refutation (Popper, 1968). Left unchallenged,

---

* We are grateful to Dr. Barry Bloom for directing our attention to this article.
† Prehn (1970) has called it "overrated."

the theory of immunological surveillance is in danger of becoming a mere self-fulfilling prophecy. And when that stage in concept-making is reached, no further progress is possible. By writing this chapter, we hope to contribute toward breaking what we believe is a deadlock. By virtue of its extraordinary achievements, tumor immunology is becoming orthodox and predictable. Perhaps only the unorthodox and the unpredicted can advance it to the next major phase in its evolution.

## 2. Deliberate Immunosuppression and Malignancy in Experimental Animals

### 2.1. Immunosuppression and Infection with Oncogenic Viruses

#### 2.1.1. DNA Viruses

The polyoma virus,* which commonly infects both wild and laboratory mice (Gross, 1970), does not produce tumors under natural conditions even though it is potentially very oncogenic. Solid evidence indicates that this is so because thymus-dependent (T) lymphocytes efficiently eliminate any cell transformed to a malignant state by the virus.

Cells infected by the polyoma virus elaborate a new antigen, which, because it provokes the specific rejection of transplanted syngeneic polyoma tumors, is called a tumor-specific transplantation antigen (TSTA) (Koldovsky, 1969) or transplantation-resistance antigen (Law, 1969). Even transformed cells free of intact polyoma virus elaborate the TSTA (Ting and Law, 1965; Ting, 1966), so the relevant immunogenic determinant is not part of the virus itself but is made by the cell as a result of infection by the virus. Moreover, even high levels of antiviral antibody cannot protect mice against transplanted syngeneic polyoma tumors (Law, 1966).

Abundant evidence supports the view that the immunological response to TSTA induced by polyoma virus is mediated via thymus-dependent lymphocytes. Thymectomy or antilymphocyte serum (ALS)† treatment permits the appearance of tumors in mice and rats deliberately or naturally infected with polyoma virus (Vandeputte and De Somer, 1965; Allison and Taylor, 1967; Allison and Law, 1968; Chesterman et al., 1969; Vandeputte, 1969). In such immunological cripples, reconstitution with thymus, spleen, or lymph node cells prevents development of the neoplasms (Law and Ting, 1965; Allison and Taylor, 1967; Sjögren and Borum, 1971). Immunotherapy with lymphoid cells from sensitized donors is more effective in eliminating the neoplasms than is treatment with cells from normal donors (Law, 1969). This supports the argument that the neoplasms are rejected by immunologically specific mechanisms.

* Because the general principles derived from experiments with polyma are applicable to SV40 and oncògenic adenoviruses (Kirschstein et al., 1964; Allison et al., 1967; Allison and Taylor, 1967; Hoosier et al., 1968; Law, 1970b), these viruses will not be dealt with separately.

† ALS selectively depletes rodents of circulating T cells (Lance et al., 1973).

Recent evidence indicates that neither neonatal thymectomy nor treatment with ALS completely abolishes cellular immunity. Although the tissues of mice treated in either of these ways are severely depleted of lymphocytes, those few that do remain can exert specific killing effects on tumor cells *in vitro* (Sjögren and Borum, 1971). Therefore, impaired cellular immunity may not be the only reason for the progressive growth of polyoma-induced neoplasms. Another possibility is "blocking factor," which probably consists of a complex of tumor antigen and its corresponding antibody (Sjögren *et al.*, 1971). This factor prevents the killing of tumor cells by sensitized lymphocytes, probably by masking antigenic sites on the neoplastic cell. "Blocking factor" has been found in the serum of mice dying of progressively growing polyoma tumors (Sjögren and Borum, 1971). The story is further complicated by an "unblocking factor," which nullifies the effect of the "blocking factor." Infusion of serum containing "unblocking factor" into animals has caused regression of spreading polyoma tumors (Bansal and Sjögren, 1971, 1973). Neither thymectomy nor ALS treatment affects the production of "blocking factor," so an animal treated with, say, ALS, would be in double jeopardy if inoculated with a polyoma tumor: grossly impaired cellular immunity compounded by the biological effects of unimpaired production of "blocking factor."

Although the polyoma system seems to fulfill the four predictions of the theory of immunological surveillance, it is noteworthy that polyoma tumors are strongly antigenic and give rise to durable, high-grade immunity (Law, 1970*b*). By contrast, most naturally occurring neoplasms are only weakly antigenic (Klein, 1969). Therefore, the principles derived from the polyoma system may not apply directly to spontaneous neoplasms. We have also seen that even in mice with rapidly growing polyoma tumors there is an immune response: the production of "blocking factor." However, unlike cellular immunity, this response protects, not the host, but the tumor.

### 2.1.2. RNA Viruses

By contrast with the findings in the polyoma system, neonatal thymectomy *reduces* the incidence of leukemia in mice deliberately or naturally infected with Gross or Moloney leukemia virus (Gross, 1959; Moloney, 1962; Furth *et al.*, 1966; Law, 1966). However, in this instance the effects of thymectomy are related, not to immunosuppression, but to the removal of a microenvironment required for the development of leukemia. Hence, any tumor-promoting effect provided by immunosuppression after thymectomy will be obscured (Law, 1966).

Alternative immunosuppressive procedures are thus required to establish the relationship between immunocompetence and leukemogenesis due to oncornaviruses. The consensus is that treatment with ALS (Allison and Law, 1968; Hirsch and Murphy, 1968; Law, 1970*a*; Law and Chang, 1971; Varet *et al.*, 1971; Stutman and Dupuy, 1972; Zisblatt and Lilly, 1972), irradiation (Stutman and Dupuy, 1972), or cortisone (Shachat *et al.*, 1968) can increase susceptibility to tumors induced by a variety of C-type RNA viruses in mice and rats. Moreover, in those cases where oncogenesis by C-type RNA viruses does not require the thymic microenvironment (Rous sarcoma virus or murine sarcoma virus), thymectomy enhances rather than inhibits the development of neoplasms (Radzichovskaja, 1967; Ting, 1967; East and Harvey, 1968).

The effects of immunosuppression on oncogenesis by oncornaviruses include a reduction of the latency period, a decreased threshold dose of virus, an increase in tumor incidence, and, sometimes, alteration in the pathology of the disease. For example, Allison and Law (1968) observed a high incidence of subcutaneous reticulum cell sarcomas in ALS-treated mice given Moloney leukemia virus (MLV), an agent that usually causes a generalized leukemic process. Law (1970a) and Law and Chang (1971) found much higher levels of infective virus in spleen extracts of mice treated with both ALS and MLV as compared to mice given either ALS or MLV alone. In addition, antiviral antibody titers were reduced in mice treated with ALS and MLV. These findings contrast with the case of oncogenic DNA viruses, where titers of infectious virus and antiviral antibody are not altered by immunosuppression (Law and Ting, 1965; Vandeputte and De Somer, 1965; Law, 1966). Thus it remains to be determined whether immunosuppression facilitates tumor formation by oncornaviruses by suppressing antiviral immunity or, as in oncogenesis by DNA viruses, by suppressing the immune response against virus-induced antigens on tumor cells. This problem is of paramount importance for the development of an anticancer vaccine: what is the protective immunogen?

Stutman and Dupuy (1972) recently discovered several interesting relationships between the effect of ALS treatment on leukemogenesis by the Friend virus and two genes of the mouse, $Fv-1$ and $Fv-2$. Alleles at these loci determine resistance or susceptibility to the virus. ALS treatment could not overcome resistance to the virus in animals possessing "resistant" alleles at both $Fv-1$ and $Fv-2$. However, the effect of the allele for resistance ($r$) at $Fv-1$ was overcome by the ALS treatment provided that the animals had the allele for susceptibility ($s$) at $Fv-2$. In the reverse situation ($Fv-1^s$, $Fv-2^r$), ALS treatment also partially overcame the resistance. Thus ALS appears capable of modifying the effect of either $Fv-1^r$ or $Fv-2^r$, but not the combined effect of the two alleles. The effect of $Fv-1$ is especially noteworthy because it influences resistance to a wide range of murine leukemia viruses, including naturally occurring endogenous viruses (Pincus *et al.*, 1971). This study is of considerable importance to our understanding of the effects of immunosuppression on leukemogenesis because it demonstrates that unless a genetic factor permitting the action of an oncogenic agent is present, immunosuppression has no effect. The converse seems equally illuminating: in individuals "absolutely resistant" to an oncogenic virus, the immune mechanism is irrelevant.

## 2.2. Effects of Immunosuppression on Oncogenesis by Chemicals

Although the enhancing effect of immunosuppression, particularly by ALS, on oncogenesis following infection by oncogenic viruses is unquestionable, the evidence in the case of chemical carcinogens is less convincing.

In thymectomized animals, the incidence of lymphatic leukemia after carcinogen administration is as drastically reduced as it is in the case of oncornaviruses (Law and Miller, 1950; Cohen et al., 1973). Again, this observation is of no help in establishing the importance of cell-mediated immunity in the defense against neoplasia because thymectomy removes the microenvironment required for the generation of the neoplastic cells. More significant is the failure of thymectomy to influence the incidence of skin and mammary tumors induced in mice by methylcholanthrene (Law and Miller, 1950). There is no evidence that the thymus is required for the induction of these kinds of neoplasms. Cohen et al. (1973) observed a greatly increased incidence of papillomas of the forestomach in adult mice subjected to thymectomy and treated with the carcinogen N-[4-(5-nitro-2-furyl)-2-thiazolyl]acetamide. By contrast with neonatal thymectomy, it is doubtful that thymectomy of adult mice produces much immunosuppression (Miller, 1962). Nevertheless, it must be conceded that the effects of various immunosuppressants are greatly augmented by thymectomy (Schwartz, 1965); therefore, this result can be explained if the carcinogen is immunosuppressive. In the hands of several investigators, neonatal thymectomy followed by painting of the skin with a carcinogen shortened the latent period before the appearance of papillomas (Miller et al., 1963; Defendi and Roosa, 1964; Grant and Miller, 1965; Johnson, 1968). However, the final incidence of tumors in these studies was 100% in both the thymectomized and the control group, and no effects on the growth rate or conversion to carcinoma were noted. Several investigators not only failed to observe a shortening of the latent period before tumor appearance, but they also were unable to demonstrate any effect on the incidence, growth rate, and histological type of tumors in neonatally thymectomized mice treated with carcinogens (Balner and Dersjant, 1966; Law, 1966; Allison and Taylor, 1967).

Immunosuppression by ALS has resulted in either an increased incidence of tumors or a decreased latency period, or both, after treatment with chemical carcinogens (Balner and Dersjant, 1969; Cerelli and Treat, 1969; Friedrich-Freska and Hoffman, 1969; Woods, 1969; Rabbat and Jeejeebhoy, 1970). Others, however, have failed to uncover an enhancing effect of ALS treatment on chemical oncogenesis (Fisher et al., 1970; Wagner and Haughton, 1971). Grant and Roe (1969) found that ALS-treated germ-free mice did not develop tumors when given dimethylbenzanthracene, whereas about one-half of similarly treated, conventional mice did. The emergence of neoplasms in the latter group was perhaps due to the combined effects of immunosuppression and antigenic stimulation, a subject we shall return to later.

Denlinger et al. (1973) reported that the treatment of rats given N-methyl-N-nitrosourea (MNU), a potent neurological carcinogen, with ALS did not increase the incidence of tumors of the nervous system. The incidence of nonneural tumors was also unaffected, with the notable exception of bladder tumors, which developed in 25% of the rats given both MNU and ALS but in none of the animals given either one alone.

Results with ALS are often difficult to evaluate. For example, each batch of ALS must be calibrated in vivo for its immunosuppressive potency because in many cases "ALS" has little or no immunosuppressive action. Among the many reasons for this is the fact that, being a foreign protein, ALS elicits an antibody that sooner or later nullifies its effects. Rendering the experimental animal tolerant of the foreign protein (e.g., rabbit globulin) before treatment with ALS (e.g., rabbit anti–mouse lymphocyte globulin) can prevent this complication (Lance et al., 1973). Such considerations were taken into account by Stutman (1969), who rendered mice immunologically tolerant of the foreign protein and found that prolonged treatment with ALS failed to influence the incidence and latency period of tumors appearing after exposure to methylcholanthrene. Interestingly, the same treatment in mice not tolerant to rabbit globulin did shorten the latency period. However, the same effect was also produced by treatment with normal rabbit globulin! Such results indicate that prolonged antigenic stimulation—and not immunosuppression—was the accelerating factor. In other experiments with mice of the I strain, which are relatively resistant to the carcinogenic effects of methylcholanthrene, Stutman (1969) showed that prolonged treatment with ALS (after induction of immunological tolerance to rabbit globulin) did increase the incidence of methylcholanthrene-induced tumors from 14% to 37%. He commented that the results can be interpreted by "supporters of the immune surveillance theory . . . that, in the protracted presence of effective immunosuppression, the relative resistance of I mice to MCA oncogenesis is overcome. On the other hand, it is also clear that 60% of the similarly immunosuppressed animals . . . remained tumor-free during their lifespan, which suggests that other factors of a nonimmunologic type are operative."

The evidence that immunosuppression consistently augments the development of neoplasms by chemical carcinogens therefore seems unconvincing. We base our conclusion on two considerations: technical inadequacy of experimental design, which vitiates many of the data dealing with this subject, and, in those experiments that are based on sound immunological technique, the contribution of important nonimmunological mechanisms to resistance to carcinogenesis.

## 2.3. Effects of Immunosuppression on Development of Spontaneous Tumors

### 2.3.1. Natural Infection with Mammary Tumor Virus

Martinez 1964) was the first to observe that thymectomy at an early age greatly reduces the incidence of mammary tumors in strains of mice positive for mammary tumor virus (MTV).* Moreover, the latent period before tumor appearance was significantly longer in the thymectomized animals. Law (1966) made similar observations in MTV$^+$ female C3H/HeN mice. Extending these findings, Yunis et al. (1969) showed that reconstitution of thymectomized C3H MTV$^+$ female mice with syngeneic thymus tissue from either MTV$^+$ or MTV$^-$ animals abolished the inhibitory effect of thymectomy on mammary

---

* Natural carriers of this virus are termed MTV$^+$, whereas mice normally free of the agent are designated MTV$^-$.

carcinogenesis. Estrogen deficiency as a consequence of thymectomy cannot explain these findings, since the reduced tumor incidence was still observed after stimulation with exogenous hormone (Heppner *et al.*, 1968). Prehn's (1971) provocative explanation of these findings is that an immune response to mammary tumor–associated antigens actually stimulates growth of the neoplasm (see below).

In contrast to these results, Burstein and Law (1971) found an increased incidence of mammary tumors in neonatally thymectomized $F_1$ hybrids of C57BL and C3H mice (BC3HF$_1$), which are MTV$^-$. At 23 months of age, 40% of thymectomized animals had developed mammary carcinomas *vs.* only 4% of control animals. However, the thymectomized animals did not show an altered incidence of the two other commonly occurring spontaneous neoplasms of BC3HF$_1$ mice, hepatomas and reticulum cell sarcomas. The divergent effects of thymectomy on MTV- and non-MTV-induced mammary tumors remain unexplained; they are possibly related to a difference in antigenicity of the two types of tumor (Burstein and Law, 1971).

C3H mice in which the $H$-$2^k$ histocompatibility locus was replaced with $H$-$2^b$ by repeated backcrossing were much less susceptible to the development of mammary tumors by MTV (Mühlbock and Dux, 1971). Conceivably, the chromosomal region determining $H$-$2^b$ contains a gene coding for immunoresistance against either the MTV itself (Klein, 1973) or the tumor cell antigens it induces. However, this does not explain how thymectomy reduces the incidence of MTV-induced tumors, since most genes determining immunological responsiveness, such as the *Ir* gene, operate via the T-cell system (Katz and Benacerraf, 1972).

Like thymectomy, ALS was also shown to inhibit tumorigenesis by MTV (Lappé and Blair, 1970; Blair, 1971). Interestingly, a high proportion of animals had circulating antibodies against MTV after recovery from ALS-induced immunosuppression. This raises the possibility that thymectomy or ALS treatment in MTV$^+$ animals abrogates immunological tolerance to the virus or to virus-induced cellular antigens, as suggested by Yunis *et al.* (1969). Indeed, it is increasingly clear that thymus-derived lymphocytes consist of several subpopulations, which can either enhance or suppress immune responses (Katz and Benacerraf, 1972; Blair, 1972; Gershon *et al.*, 1972).

### 2.3.2. Murine Leukemia Viruses

Most, if not all, mice appear to carry the genetic information required for the assembly of murine leukemic viruses (MuLV) (Todaro and Huebner, 1972). Whether or not this information is actually expressed seems to depend on many other genes, an increasing number of which are being identified (Lilly, 1972; Lilly and Pincus, 1973). Some strains of mice, in which high levels of infectious virus are present very early in life, such as AKR, SJL, and NZB, have a high incidence of leukemia or lymphoma later in life. In the AKR mouse, the malignancy originates in the thymus or in the thymus-dependent lymphoid tissue (Siegler, 1968). It is thus not surprising that thymectomy early in life drastically reduces the incidence of leukemia in this animal (McEndy *et al.*, 1944; Allison, 1970).

In contrast to thymectomy, ALS treatment can shorten the latent period before
tumor development in natural carriers of infectious MuLV (Allison, 1970;
Burstein and Allison, 1970; Judd *et al.*, 1971; Hirsch *et al.*, 1973*a*). Vredevoe and
Hays (1969), however, observed a tendency toward prolongation of the latent
period of spontaneous leukemia in AKR mice treated with ALS; also, Nagaya and
Sieker (1969) failed to affect the incidence of leukemia after treatment of AKR
mice with ALS. Interpretation of these results is subject to the same pitfalls
mentioned in the case of ALS-treated mice given carcinogenic chemicals: unless
the immunosuppressive potency of the ALS employed by the investigator is
proven by bioassay, no conclusion can be drawn.

As mentioned previously, ALS, apart from its immunosuppressive properties,
also has certain actions not directly related to immunosuppression. One such
effect relevant to the preceding is its ability to lyse neoplastic lymphoid cells (Judd
*et al.*, 1971). Furthermore, it is not inconceivable that certain batches of
anti-mouse lymphocyte serum contain neutralizing antibodies against MuLV.
Considering the prevalence of MuLV virions or their antigens in mice (Todaro
and Huebner, 1972), this possibility deserves serious consideration. The presence
of such antibodies could, of course, offset any immunosuppressive effects of the
preparation. Because of the diverse effects of ALS, it is difficult to ascribe solely to
immunosuppression any influence of ALS on virus-induced lymphoid tumors.
Once again we are faced with the problem of interpreting results of what are most
likely inadequate experiments, experiments that have failed to take into account
the very complex nature of the system under analysis.

More decisive results have been obtained in mice that do not harbor infectious
virus early in life. Nehlsen (1971) studied the effect of long-term ALS treatment
on the incidence of tumors in 250 CBA mice. The ALS injections were started on
the day of birth and were continued every 4 days for 18 months. This treatment
caused a severe deficiency in cell-mediated immune capabilities, including inability to cause graft vs. host reactions, anergy to a chemical sensitizer (oxazolon),
impaired responses of lymphocytes to phytohemagglutinin, retention of skin
allografts for 6–18 months, and survival of skin xenografts for as long as 20–60
days. Nevertheless, the mice survived normally for 18 months, and, with the
exception of two lymphoblastic lymphomas in male mice 13 months of age, all
tumors that developed could be attributed to the polyoma virus. Sanford *et al.*
(1973) studied the incidence of spontaneous tumors in BALB/c mice. The life
spans of neonatally thymectomized and sham-thymectomized animals did not
differ (758 days and 796 days, respectively), nor did the overall incidence of
tumors (85% and 81%, respectively). However, the kinds of tumors as well as their
behavior were different in the two groups. In comparison to the control mice, the
incidence of lung and mammary tumors was lower in thymectomized animals,
whereas the incidence of hemangioendothelioma was slightly higher. Also, 10%
of the thymectomized mice developed tumors of a type not found in the control
mice, including two myoepitheliomas, one squamous cell carcinoma, and one
lipoma. Furthermore, multiple lung adenomas were seen in ten of 20 thymectomized mice, whereas only single adenomas occurred in control mice. Trainin and

Linker-Israeli (1971) similarly observed an increased incidence of presumably non-virus-induced lung adenomas in neonatally thymectomized SWR and Swiss mice. In addition to Nehlsen (1971) and Sanford *et al.* (1973), others have failed to note an increased incidence of neoplasms in virus-negative animals treated with ALS or thymectomy, or both (Law, 1970*a*; Denlinger *et al.*, 1973).

Thus present evidence concerning the development of spontaneous neoplasms in deliberately immunosuppressed mice is conflicting. On the one hand, some data indicate that treatment with ALS hastens the appearance of neoplasms in mice with a high spontaneous incidence of such tumors. On the other hand, there is evidence that documented, severe immunosuppression fails to influence the incidence of neoplasms in mice with a low rate of development of spontaneous tumors. On balance, the weight of the evidence favors the view that severe immunosuppression *by itself* does not influence the incidence of neoplasms in laboratory mice. Important evidence now emerging from studies of congenitally athymic mice, which are discussed next, supports this conclusion.

## 3. Spontaneous Immunosuppression and Malignancy in Experimental Animals

### 3.1. Congenitally Athymic (Nude) Mice

In "nude" mice, a single autosomal recessive mutant gene is responsible for both hairlessness and failure of thymic development (Flanagan, 1966; Pantelouris, 1968). The immunological deficiencies of nude mice are impressive and include inability to reject skin grafts from other mammals and even from birds, reptiles, or amphibians, as well as markedly impaired antibody production in response to thymus-dependent antigens* (Rygaard, 1969; Wortis, 1971; Reed and Jutila, 1972; Manning *et al.*, 1973). Wortis *et al.* (1971) showed that nude mice have a normal compartment of precursors for T cells and concluded that a defective thymic epithelium is responsible for their grossly impaired immunity. The B-cell system of these animals is intact, and immunological responses to so-called thymus-independent antigens,† such as lipopolysaccharide, are intact (Reed *et al.*, 1973).

There is every indication that these animals promise important information relevant to immunological surveillance. If cellular immunity is a principal defense against neoplastic cells, nude mice should have a very high incidence of spontaneous neoplasms. But as of this writing, there is no evidence from any group studying these mice that this prediction is upheld. In nude mice observed for as long as 7 months, no spontaneous tumors were found (in these studies the genetic background for the nude strain was BALB/c) (Reed and Jutila, unpublished observations).‡ One difficulty in evaluating these preliminary results is the

---

* Antigens requiring the presence of both T and B cells in order to stimulate the production of antibodies (Claman and Chaperon, 1969).
† Antigens requiring the presence only of B cells in order to stimulate the production of antibodies (Claman and Chaperon, 1969).
‡ A 6-month-old nude mouse that died of a reticulum cell sarcoma was recently reported (Custer *et al.*, 1973).

relatively early death of the nude mouse due to its extreme susceptibility to infection. Successful colonies require either specific pathogen-free or germ-free conditions. Conceivably, imposition of the germ-free environment could in itself lower the incidence of neoplasms, especially of the lymphoid type.

Nude mice were recently found to resist the carcinogenic effects of certain hydrocarbons such as 3,4-benzopyrene, methylcholanthrene, and dimethylbenzanthracene (DMBA) (Johnson *et al.*, 1974). In these experiments, 100% of the normal littermates of nudes developed tumors in response to skin painting with DMBA, but only one of 15 nude mice did so. The one nude animal developed a papilloma which spontaneously regressed after 1 month. Out of 12 nude mice grafted with thymic tissue (thus restoring their T-cell system) and treated with DMBA, all developed tumors. Hence skin abnormalities in nudes are unlikely to account for their unexpected resistance to chemical carcinogenesis. It should be mentioned here that mice carrying a hairless mutation not associated with congenital absence of the thymus (*hr/hr*) have also shown resistance to tumor formation after skin painting with chemical carcinogens (Giovanella *et al.*, 1970). The resistance in these mice has been ascribed to the skin abnormalities, although the evidence is circumstantial.

In addition to chemical oncogenesis, viral oncogenesis by Friend leukemia virus (FLV) was also found to be disturbed in nude mice. Kouttab *et al.* (1974) noted that although FLV administration shortened the life span of nude mice, they did not have evidence of leukemia at the time of death. Considerable evidence indicates that FLV suppresses B-lymphocyte function (Dent, 1972). More recently, T cells were also shown to be suppressed (see below), suggesting that both B and T cells or cooperative mechanisms between B and T cells are targets of FLV. Although it is not known to what extent interaction between B and T cells is required for the development of typical Friend disease, the evidence in nude mice indicates that T cells are involved.

It thus appears that nude mice fail to develop neoplasms spontaneously or when treated with either chemical carcinogens or oncogenic viruses, although the data are admittedly in a preliminary stage. The results are not inconsistent with the "immunostimulatory" theory—i.e., that immunity is *required* for the development of a neoplasm (Prehn, 1972). They are not consistent with the immunological surveillance theory, unless the notion that cellular immunity is a prime defense against neoplasms is abandoned.

### 3.2. Immunocompetence of Animals with a High Incidence of Tumors

Immunocompetence has been studied in three "high tumor" strains of mice, AKR, NZB, and SJL/J. Whereas most authors agree that leukemic AKR mice have decreased immunocompetence (Metcalf and Moulds, 1967), preleukemic AKR mice have been variously reported to have normal immune capabilities (Murphy and Syverton, 1961; Metcalf, 1963; Hechtel *et al.*, 1965; Metcalf and Moulds, 1967; Levine and Vas, 1970; Hargis and Malkiel, 1972) or decreased immunocompetence (Friedman, 1964; Doré *et al.*, 1969; Gottlieb *et al.*, 1972). These investigations were of both humoral and cell-mediated immunological functions, such as the capacity to produce antibody against sheep red blood cells, rejection of tumor transplants, capacity to mount graft vs. host reactions, production of IgG and reagin, and susceptibility to infection. Results of these studies lead us to conclude that if immunodeficiency exists in preleukemic AKR mice, its extent is certainly not impressive. The question of whether AKR mice are selectively hyporesponsive to the leukemia virus they harbor or to virus-induced cellular antigens remains largely unanswered (Hirsch et al., 1973a). In any case, AKR mice, like other MuLV-carrying mice, are not tolerant to their own virus, since both humoral and cell-mediated responses to viral antigens can be detected in vitro (Hirsch et al., 1969; Wahren and Metcalf, 1970; Oldstone et al., 1972; Profitt et al., 1973). Recently, evidence has been presented for the existence of two loci coding for virus expression in the genome of AKR mice (Rowe, 1972; Rowe and Hartley, 1972). Conceivably, the action of these genes can overcome the effects of antiviral immunity.

The immune status of SJL mice, which are genetically predisposed to the development of a "Hodgkin's-like" lymphoma, has been less extensively studied. In one experiment, antibody production to sheep red blood cells, rejection of skin allografts, delayed hypersensitivity, and capacity to cause graft vs. host reactions were determined (Haran-Ghera et al., 1973). No significant immune deficiencies were found in young SJL/J mice, but, as also noted in strains without a high incidence of spontaneous tumors (Makinodan and Peterson, 1964; Metcalf et al., 1966; Hanna et al., 1967; Legge and Austing, 1968), the immune reactions of SJL mice decreased with age. This occurred whether the animal was normal or had a tumor.

A third strain of mice in which tumors develop in an unusually high percentage and in which a diversity of immunological abnormalities occurs is the NZB line (East, 1970). Whereas young NZB mice produce unusually large amounts of antibodies (Playfair, 1968; Weir et al., 1968; Staples and Talal, 1969), old NZB mice have profoundly impaired cellular immunity (Stutman et al., 1968; Cantor et al., 1970; Leventhal and Talal, 1970; Teague et al., 1970; Gelfand and Steinberg, 1973). The deficiencies in cell-mediated immunity include retarded rejection of skin allografts, diminished capacity to mount graft vs. host reactions, and impaired in vitro responses of lymphocytes to phytohemagglutinin and allogeneic lymphocytes. A progressive loss of recirculating T cells was also demonstrated in NZB mice (Denman and Denman, 1970; Gelfand and Steinberg, 1973). It is not known to what extent the infection with oncornaviruses in NZB mice causes, results from, or is coincidental with the immunological abnormalities.

Recent developments in the genetics of leukemogenesis may shed new light on experiments of the type we have just described. There is clear evidence that viral oncogenesis in mice depends on multiple genes. For example, the combined action of several genes determines the ultimate balance between resistance and susceptibility to the induction of leukemia in mice by either endogenous or exogenous viruses (Lilly, 1972; Lilly and Pincus, 1973). Nonimmunological effects are exerted by some of these genes, the most notable being the Fv-1 and Fv-2 loci.

Another gene, *Rgv-1*, exerts its influences by immunological mechanisms.* *Rgv-1*
is located within the *H-2* complex of linkage group IX and its position coincides with the *Ir* region. The latter contains several genes determining the ability to respond immunologically to a variety of antigens (McDevitt and Benacerraf, 1969). In view of its chromosomal location, it is not surprising that all current evidence indicates that *Rgv-1* regulates the capacity to respond immunologically to MuLV and the cellular antigens it induces. For example, the antigenic system X.1 occurs on the surface of both the virions and the cells of a murine radiation-induced leukemia. Immunological responsiveness to this antigen has been traced to *Rgv-1*; alleles at this locus determine the animal's ability to produce antibody against X.1 and to reject X.1$^+$ leukemia cells (Sato *et al.*, 1973). In addition, *Rgv-1* may influence the expression of virus-induced cellular antigens: the antigen usually induced by Friend virus is not expressed in animals having the *Rgv-1* allele governing susceptibility to this agent (Lilly and Pincus, 1973).

Thus, at least in viral leukemogenesis in the mouse, there is strong circumstantial evidence that the genetic capacity to react immunologically to tumor-associated antigens influences the development of neoplasms. This may be of considerable importance in protection against neoplasia since mice prone to tumors induced by endogenous oncornaviruses, such as AKR, C58, SJL/J, NZB, and C3H, possess the *Rgv-1* allele for susceptibility. However, not all strains of mice with this allele have a high incidence of tumors. Clearly, leukemogenesis by endogenous oncornaviruses is a complex, multifactorial process involving not only several genes but also variations of the infectivity and oncogenicity of the virus itself (Rowe, 1972; Lilly and Pincus, 1973; Peters *et al.*, 1973).

In view of this, it seems an oversimplification to connect diminished immunological reactions against antigens such as foreign erythrocytes, skin grafts, and bacteria with the pathogenesis of neoplasms. Failure to respond to the etiological agent (virus) or to tumor-associated antigens of a spontaneous neoplasm seems more to the point. Recent findings on the genetic control of immunological responsiveness to oncornaviruses and the cellular antigens they induce bring these doubts into sharp focus and strongly imply that the demonstration of poor immunological responsiveness to a limited number of antigens does not necessarily imply poor responsiveness to tumor-associated antigens.

## 3.3. Immunosuppression by Oncogenic Viruses

Immunosuppression by oncogenic viruses has been reviewed by several authorities (Salaman, 1969; Notkins *et al.*, 1970; Dent, 1972; Friedman and Ceglowski, 1973). Nevertheless, a brief discussion of the major findings seems appropriate.

---

* The *Rgv-1* gene (resistance to Gross virus) was first identified in experiments concerning susceptibility to the Gross virus (Lilly *et al.*, 1964); subsequently it was also found to influence susceptibility to other leukemia viruses (Lilly, 1968; Tennant and Snell, 1968) as well as the mammary tumor virus (Nandi, 1967).

Almost all laboratory strains of leukemia-inducing RNA viruses have been found to suppress antibody formation. FLV has been most extensively studied in this regard. In general, the longer FLV is administered before antigen injection, the more profound the degree of immunosuppression. However, immunosuppression by FLV clearly precedes the onset of malignancy. Both IgM and IgG antibody responses to sheep red blood cells are affected after FLV infection, although the latter more than the former (Dent, 1972). Production of antibodies to "thymus-dependent" antigens such as sheep erythrocytes requires cooperation between T and B cells (Claman and Chaperon, 1969). Initially, FLV appeared to suppress preferentially the function of B lymphocytes (Bennett and Steeves, 1970). More recently, however, FLV was also shown to suppress T-cell-mediated immune functions, such as immunity to mycobacteria and rejection of skin allografts (Friedman and Ceglowski, 1971). Nevertheless, B-cell function is suppressed more rapidly and more profoundly than is T-cell function (Friedman *et al.*, 1973). In an earlier report, Gross passage A virus was also shown to prolong survival of skin allografts, in this instance across a non-*H-2* barrier (Dent *et al.*, 1965). In addition, a lymphatic leukemia-inducing virus isolated from irradiated SJL/J mice was found to depress the function of both T and B cells (Shearer *et al.*, 1973).

The general picture emerging from the literature is that laboratory strains of leukemogenic RNA viruses suppress both B- and T-cell functions. The suppression of T-cell function is especially intriguing, since immunosurveillance against cancer is thought to function via the T-cell system. Consequently, the important issue is raised here of whether or not suppression of T-cell function is a necessary prerequisite for tumor induction by these viruses. Although much can be said in favor of the notion that a causal relationship exists between immunosuppression by tumor viruses and oncogenesis (Dent, 1972), the evidence is entirely circumstantial. It is noteworthy that immunosuppression by naturally occurring leukemogenic viruses in their endogenous hosts has not been demonstrated. Moreover, in contrast to the lymphotropic RNA leukemia viruses, RNA sarcoma viruses and oncogenic DNA viruses have not generally been found to suppress immunological functions (Dent, 1972), although immunosuppressive procedures clearly enhance oncogenesis by these viruses. In addition, many nononcogenic viruses are known to be immunosuppressive (Salaman, 1969; Notkins *et al.*, 1970). Therefore, it seems that the true biological significance, if any, of immunosuppression by oncogenic viruses remains to be elucidated.

## 3.4. Immunosuppression by Carcinogenic Chemicals

Carcinogenic chemicals suppress both antibody production (Malmgren *et al.*, 1952; Stjernsward, 1965, 1966, 1967, 1969; Stutman, 1969; Ball, 1970; Szakal and Hanna, 1972) and cell-mediated immunity (Prehn, 1963; Stjernsward, 1965; Doell *et al.*, 1967; Ball, 1970; Lappé and Prehn, 1970; Szakal and Hanna, 1972). A number of observations sustain the hypothesis that carcinogenesis by these compounds is at least facilitated by, if not dependent on, their immunosuppressive properties. Thus carcinogenic hydrocarbons were found to be immunosuppressive, whereas noncarcinogenic hydrocarbons were not (Stjernsward, 1966). And mice resistant to carcinogenesis by 3-methylcholanthrene were also resistant to immunosuppression by this compound (Stutman, 1969). The duration of suppression of antibody production after carcinogen administration generally corresponds to the latency period before tumor appearance (Stjernsward, 1969; Szakal and Hanna, 1972). In one study (Szakal and Hanna, 1972), the suppression of both regional and systemic humoral immunity after treatment of Syrian hamsters with 7,12-dimethylbenzanthracene was transient, and maximal suppression coincided with the appearance of papillomas. Cell-mediated immunity was found to be depressed permanently, as measured by the survival of skin allografts, and this was considered to be essential for further development of the papillomas.

The evidence from these studies seems circumstantial and should be compared with contrasting observations. For example, additional immunosuppression by thymectomy or ALS treatment does not greatly increase the incidence of tumor after treatment with chemical carcinogens. Decisive evidence on this point was obtained by Andrews (1971), who placed methylcholanthrene-treated skin allografts on severely immunodepressed (thymectomy plus 450 r plus ALS) mice. Although the allografts were never rejected, 80% of the papillomas on the grafts regressed. Clearly, then, important nonimmunological mechanisms are responsible for the rejection of at least this kind of carcinogen-induced tumor. In other work, of three carcinogenic hydrocarbons (DMBA, benz[a]pyrene, and 3-methylcholanthrene) injected subcutaneously into newborn CFW/D mice, only one (DMBA) was found to suppress antibody production to sheep red blood cells, although all compounds induced tumors (Ball, 1970).

## 4. Immunosuppression and Malignancy in Human Beings

### 4.1. Immunodeficiency Diseases

Although it is widely held that neoplasms are common in patients with deficient immunity (Fraumeni, 1969; Kaplan, 1971; Good, 1972), their frequency is difficult to determine. The literature dealing with this topic consists largely of case reports, which give a distorted impression of the actual incidence. Thus far, a prospective study of large groups of patients with these diseases has not been undertaken for the purpose of determining the incidence of neoplasms. Table 1 provides data from several series of apparently unselected cases. Of the 678 patients (some of these may be duplicates), 33 had a neoplasm, for an incidence of about 5%. However, this figure is only an approximation and the true value could be substantially higher or lower. Note, for example, that in one series of patients with ataxia-telangiectasia, only 3 of 101 had a neoplasm (Boder and Sedgwick, 1963), whereas in a series of patients with Wiskott–Aldrich syndrome, 4 of 16 had a malignancy (Waldmann et al., 1972). Moreover, inclusion of 70 cases of

TABLE 1
*Tumors/Patients*

| Combined immunodeficiency | 0/70 | Hitzig (1968) |
|---|---|---|
| Wiskott–Aldrich syndrome | 1/18 | Cooper *et al.* (1968) |
| Wiskott–Aldrich syndrome | 4/16 | Waldmann *et al.* (1972) |
| Ataxia-telangiectasia | 1/20 | Waldmann *et al.* (1972) |
| Ataxia-telangiectasia | 3/101 | Boder and Sedgwick (1963) |
| Ataxia-telangiectasia | 8/125 | Peterson *et al.* (1964) |
| Hypogammaglobulinemia[a] | 8/176 | Editorial (1969) |
| Selective IgA deficiency | 5/102 | Ammann and Hong (1971) |
| Intestinal lymphangiectasia | 3/50 | Waldmann *et al.* (1972) |

[a] Common variable type.

combined immunodeficiency in this table may bias the result toward a lower than actual frequency, since patients with this condition usually die in infancy. If we accept 5% as tentative, the incidence of malignancy in the various immunodeficiency disorders is about 200 times the expected rate.

### 4.1.1. Classification of Immunodeficiency Diseases

Immunodeficiency diseases are a heterogeneous group, in which defects in T cells, B cells, or both predominate. The major forms these conditions take are as follows:

*a. Combined Immunodeficiency (Swiss-Type Agammaglobulinemia) (Hoyer et al., 1968).* Both humoral and cellular responses are lacking in combined immunodeficiency, probably because of the failure of precursors of T and B cells to develop. Death during infancy because of overwhelming infection is the rule.

*b. DiGeorge Syndrome (DiGeorge, 1968).* The thymus fails to develop in DiGeorge syndrome, whereas the B-cell population is normal in this very rare disorder. Cellular immunity is lacking and immunoglobulin synthesis is normal, although antibody production against thymus-dependent antigens is impaired.

*c. X-Linked Hypogammaglobulinemia (Bruton Type) (Gitlin and Janeway, 1956).* The converse of the DiGeorge syndrome, X-linked hypogammaglobulinemia, is characterized by a failure to produce antibodies and intact cellular immunity. Plasma cells are lacking, and the structure of the thymus is normal. If untreated, the disease is associated with an extraordinary susceptibility to infections by pyogenic bacteria.

*d. Common Variable Immunodeficiency (Douglas et al., 1970).* The onset of common variable immunodeficiency occurs in adults, and both men and women can be affected. The syndrome is heterogeneous, with hypogammaglobulinemia as the hallmark. Autoimmunity and gastrointestinal disorders are common. Defective cellular immunity is frequent, and, despite hypogammaglobulinemia, B

cells can be detected in the blood in some cases (Cooper *et al.*, 1971). The
fundamental defect may be an inability to "switch on" B cells.

*e. Dysgammaglobulinemia (Ammann and Hong, 1971).* Dysgammaglobulinemia is characterized by a selective deficiency of one or more classes of immunoglobulins. IgA deficiency is by far the commonest form of this group of disorders; its incidence may be as high as one in 600. Autoimmunity is common, but some persons with IgA deficiency are ostensibly normal.

*f. Ataxia-Telangiectasia (Waldmann, et al., 1972).* Ataxia-telangiectasia consists of a triad of cerebellar ataxia, telangiectasia of the skin and eyes, and immunodeficiency. The last is the basis of the frequent sinopulmonary infections in ataxia-telangiectasia. The immunodeficiency is complex; the usual findings are normal levels of IgG, deficiency of IgA and IgE, the presence of low molecular weight IgM, and diminished cellular immunity. The thymus is often absent or atrophic, and thymus-dependent areas of lymphoid tissue are depleted. The immunological disorder may result from the failure of thymus development.

*g. Wiskott–Aldrich Syndrome (Waldmann et al., 1972).* Wiskott–Aldrich syndrome consists of the triad of thrombocytopenia, eczema, and repeated infections and is inherited as an X-linked recessive. The immunodeficiency is severe and consists of defects in both cellular and humoral immunity. Immunoglubulin levels are normal or even increased (IgA and IgE). Both the synthetic and the catabolic rates of immunoglobulins G, A, and M are greatly increased. Despite this, antibody responses following immunization, especially with polysaccharide antigens, are depressed. The defect in cellular immunity is also paradoxical, because, although delayed hypersensitivity is absent, *in vitro* responses of lymphocytes to PHA are normal. The disease may represent an abnormality of the afferent limb of the immune response, perhaps in the recognition or processing of antigen.

### 4.1.2. Malignancy in Immunodeficiency Diseases

Table 2 lists 55 representative examples of patients with an immunodeficiency disease who developed a malignancy. These examples were culled from case reports and are not meant to provide epidemiological data, but rather to demonstrate the major features of the literature.

Several problems arise in coming to an understanding of the phenomena described in Table 2. First among these is whether the changes described in the lymphoid organs of these patients are truly neoplastic. Although no doubt exists in those examples where metastases revealed the malignant nature of the process (e.g., cases 8 and 20), in others the picture is not clear. This is especially so in combined immunodeficiency. The changes described in these cases are not, in our opinion, diagnostic of a lymphoreticular malignancy. Although Reed–Sternberg cells were noted in cases 3 and 4 (and therefore led to the diagnosis of Hodgkin's disease), this is not proof of malignancy since such cells have been found in

TABLE 2

*Fifty-Five Cases of Neoplasms in Patients with Immunodeficiency Diseases*

| Case | Immuno-deficiency | Age | Tumor | Comment | Reference |
|---|---|---|---|---|---|
| 1 | CID | 5 months | Lymphoreticular neoplasm | — | Jung et al. (1969) |
| 2 | CID | 3 months | "Histiocytosis" | GVHR? | Jung et al. (1969) |
| 3 | CID | 4 months | Reticulum cell hyperplasia | Reed–Sternberg cell | McKusick and Cross (1966) |
| 4 | CID | 5 months | Thymoma | Reed–Sternberg cell | Bermuth et al. (1970) |
| 5 | WAS | 3 yr | Acute myelogenous leukemia | Brother of case 6 | Ten Bensel et al. (1966) |
| 6 | WAS | 6 yr | Reticulum cell sarcoma | Metastases | Ten Bensel et al. (1966) |
| 7 | WAS | 13 yr | Reticulum cell sarcoma | Monoclonal gammopathy | Radl et al. (1967) |
| 8 | WAS | 2½ yr | Reticulum cell sarcoma | Metastases | Kildeberg (1961) |
| 9 | WAS | 2 yr | "Reticuloendotheliosis" | — | Coleman et al. (1961) |
| 10 | WAS | 9 yr | Thymoma | Lymphoepithelioma | Chaptal et al. (1966) |
| 11 | WAS | 3 yr | Reticulum cell sarcoma | Confined to brain | Brand and Marinkovich (1969) |
| 12 | WAS | 8 yr | Astrocytoma | Cerebellum | Amiet (1963) |
| 13 | WAS | 4½ yr | Histiocytosis (Letterer–Siwe) | Widespread tumors | Huber (1968) |
| 14 | WAS | 6½ yr | Malignant reticuloendotheliosis | Brother had WAS and acute leukemia | Taleb et al. (1969) |
| 15 | AT | 21 yr | Malignant lymphoma | — | Peterson et al. (1966) |
| 16 | AT | 10 yr | Reticulum cell sarcoma | — | Gotoff et al. (1967) |
| 17 | AT | 9 yr | Acute lymphocytic leukemia | — | Taleb et al. (1969) |
| 18 | AT | 18 yr | Glioma (frontal lobe) | — | Young et al. (1964) |
| 19 | AT | 13 yr | Cerebellar medulloblastoma | — | Shuster et al. (1966) |
| 20 | AT | 9 yr | Lymphosarcoma | Disseminated | Peterson et al. (1964) |
| 21 | AT | 5 yr | "Reticuloendotheliosis" | Histiocytosis X? | Peterson et al. (1964) |
| 22 | AT | 9 yr | Hodgkin's disease | Radiation reaction | Morgan et al. (1968) |
| 23 | AT | 15 yr | Reticulum cell sarcoma | — | Miller (1967) |
| 24 | AT | 14 yr | Acute lymphocytic leukemia | Brother of case 25 | Lampert (1969) |
| 25 | AT | 3 yr | Acute lymphocytic leukemia | — | Lampert (1969) |
| 26 | AT | 5 yr | Acute lymphocytic leukemia | Sister of case 27 | Hecht et al. (1966) |

| | | | | | |
|---|---|---|---|---|---|
| 27 | AT | 6 yr | Acute lymphocytic leukemia | | Hecht et al. (1966) |
| 28 | AT | 21 yr | Adenocarcinoma of stomach | Sister of case 29 | Haerer et al. (1969) |
| 29 | AT | 19 yr | Adenocarcinoma of stomach | — | Haerer et al. (1969) |
| 30 | AT | 10 yr | Lymphosarcoma | Radiation reaction | Gotoff et al. (1967) |
| 31 | AT | 30 months | Reticulum cell sarcoma | Thymus, mediastinum, lung | Feigin et al. (1970) |
| 32 | AT | 17 yr | Ovarian dysgerminoma | — | Dunn et al. (1964) |
| 33 | AT | 14 yr | Unspecified lymphoma | Stomach | Castaigne et al. (1969) |
| 34 | AT | — | Histiocytic lymphoma | Brother of case 13 | Castaigne et al. (1969) |
| 35 | AT | | Basal cell carcinoma | | |
| 36 | CVI | 12 yr | Lymphosarcoma | Localized to pharynx | Freeman et al. (1970) |
| 37 | CVI | 3¾ yr | Generalized lymphosarcoma | Sister of case 36 | Freeman et al. (1970) |
| 38 | CVI | 67 yr | Chronic lymphocytic leukemia | Sister of case 39 | Potolsky et al. (1971) |
| 39 | CVI | 45 yr | Lymphocytic lymphoma | | Potolsky et al. (1971) |
| 40 | CVI | 70 yr | Lymphosarcoma | | Potolsky et al. (1971) |
| 41 | CVI | 54 yr | Chronic lymphocytic leukemia | Sister of case 39 | Potolsky et al. (1971) |
| 42 | CVI | 50 yr | Reticulum cell sarcoma | Sister of case 39 | Potolsky et al. (1971) |
| 43 | CVI | 47 yr | Reticulum cell sarcoma | Brother of case 39 | Potolsky et al. (1971) |
| 44 | CVI | 50 yr | Lymphoblastic lymphoma | Hypo-γ 18 yr | Green et al. (1966) |
| 45 | CVI | 54 yr | Lymphosarcoma | — | Fudenberg and Solomon (1961) |
| 46 | CVI | 54 yr | Thymoma | | Douglas et al. (1970) |
| 47 | CVI | 28 yr | Lymphosarcoma | No tumor 16 yr later | Douglas et al. (1970) |
| 48 | CVI | 57 yr | Adenocarcinoma of stomach | Long history of infections | Hermans and Huizenga (1972) |
| 49 | CVI | 56 yr | Adenocarcinoma of stomach | Long history of infections | Hermans and Huizenga (1972) |
| 50 | CVI | 31 yr | Adenocarcinoma of stomach | Long history of infections | Hermans and Huizenga (1972) |
| 51 | CVI | 27 yr | Carcinoma of stomach | Long history of infections | Forssman and Herner (1964) |
| 52 | BA | | Malignant lymphoma | Dermatomyositis | Page et al. (1963) |
| 53 | BA | 5 yr | Acute lymphocytic leukemia | Brother of case 52 | Page et al. (1963) |
| 54 | BA | — | Hodgkin's disease | Identical twin | Pekonen et al. (1963) |
| 55 | BA | — | Monomyelocytic leukemia | — | Reisman et al. (1964) |

[a] CID, combined immunodeficiency disease; WAS, Wiskott–Aldrich syndrome; AT, ataxia-telangiectasia; CVI, common variable immunodeficiency; BA, Bruton's agammaglobulinemia.

benign, reactive disorders of lymphoid tissue (Strum *et al.*, 1970). Many of the pathological changes in combined immunodeficiency are entirely consistent with a graft vs. host reaction (GVHR). For example, case 2 was diagnosed as "histiocytosis," a characteristic finding in the acute GVHR, and the authors speculated on the possibility that instead of a neoplasm they were dealing with the end result of a GVHR (Jung *et al.*, 1969). Some cases of combined immunodeficiency may represent the result of a GVHR induced in the fetus by maternal lymphocytes that traversed the placenta (Kadowaki *et al.*, 1965).

Case 47 is of interest because she was diagnosed as having a "lymphosarcoma," yet 16 yr later there was no trace of the tumor. This extraordinary behavior of a "malignancy" in a patient with an immunodeficiency disease raises doubts about the validity of the diagnosis. If the lesion in this case and others is not neoplastic, what could it be? Perhaps we are dealing with unusual forms of lymphoid reactivity in patients with frequent infections (i.e., repeated antigenic stimuli) who lack normal immunoregulatory mechanisms. Experimentally, deregulated immune responses can lead to prolonged hyperplasia of lymphoid tissue (Sahiar and Schwartz, 1966). Relevant to this is the marked hyperplasia of lymphoid tissue without changes diagnostic of malignancy that can occur in patients with ataxia-telangiectasia (Peterson *et al.*, 1966; Ammann *et al.*, 1965). Conceivably, such hyperplastic changes could be misdiagnosed as neoplastic. In this connection, it is worth noting that many of the "tumors" in these cases were diagnosed only at autopsy because there were no clinical manifestations.

A second, related problem is the very high proportion of lymphoid tumors in these patients. Of the 55 malignancies in Table 2, 42 (80%) involved lymphoid tissue. Why should this be? One possibility has already been mentioned; i.e., that at least some of the "tumors" were not malignant, but either GVH reactions or highly abnormal kinds of reactive hyperplasia. Another possibility, which we shall discuss later, is that under conditions of combined immunosuppression and immunostimulation, lymphoid tissue is particularly susceptible to neoplastic transformation. We believe that if impaired immunological surveillance were the sole explanation for these cases, a much more representative variety of cancers should have been found. It seems more than coincidental that the very tissue which is abnormal in patients with immunodeficiency is the seat of the malignant change. Moreover, we would expect multiple neoplasms in the same immunodeficient patient if the immunological surveillance theory had a bearing on these cases. We have found no examples of this phenomenon in any of the 55 cases we studied.

We now come to the nonlymphoid tumors in immunodeficiency diseases. The development of brain tumors (cases 18 and 19) and an ovarian tumor (case 32) in ataxia-telangiectasia is interesting because in this condition it is these organs that undergo severe degenerative changes (McFarlin *et al.*, 1972). Is it conceivable that this is the basis of the tumors of these organs rather than some immunological dysfunction? Similarly, in the category of common variable immunodeficiency we see several cases of cancer of the stomach (cases 48, 49, 50, and 51). Two of these (cases 49 and 51) also had pernicious anemia, a disease known to predispose to this kind of cancer. Moreover, patients with common variable immunodeficiency are prone to achlorhydria and atrophic gastritis (Twomey *et al.*, 1970; Hermans and Huizenga, 1972), which are also associated with a high incidence of cancer of the stomach.

The case for an increased incidence of malignancy in X-linked hypogammaglobulinemia seems unsubstantiated. In two patients reported by Page *et al.* (1963), one also had dermatomyositis, which by itself can be associated with a high incidence of neoplasms, although in children the association is not as striking as it is in adults. One case associated with acute lymphocytic leukemia (Reisman *et al.*, 1964) and one with Hodgkin's disease (Pekonen *et al.*, 1963) are also recorded, but in view of the relatively high frequency of X-linked hypogammaglobulinemia we would expect many more such examples than the literature reports.

Intestinal lymphangiectasia is of considerable relevance to the problem of immunodeficiency diseases and malignancy. This disorder is characterized by losses of immunoglobulins and circulating lymphocytes through abnormal lymphoid channels in the gut. The result is hypogammaglobulinemia and lymphocytopenia, the latter leading to a profound depression in cellular immunity (Weiden *et al.*, 1972). These patients are thus analogous to animals undergoing thoracic duct drainage. Thus far, three of 50 patients with intestinal lymphangiectasia have developed neoplasms; all three were lymphomas, two of which involved primarily the gastrointestinal tract (Waldmann *et al.*, 1972).

A long-term study of ataxia-telangiectasia has revealed a new element of importance. Girls with the disease who pass through adolescence normally seem to avoid the development of severe pulmonary disease and neoplasia, whereas those who fail to develop secondary sexual characteristics or who do not menstruate regularly because of ovarian failure are predisposed to the infectious and malignant complications of ataxia-telangiectasia (Boder, 1973).

Immunodeficiency as an *effect* of the malignancy rather than its precursor needs to be excluded. This is well known to occur in Hodgkin's disease (Brown *et al.*, 1967). Immunodeficiency secondary to acute leukemia has also been described (Hersh *et al.*, 1971). This may have been the situation in case 55 (but no details are given). It is probably not applicable to those patients (e.g., cases 44 and 45) in whom a long history of hypogammaglobulinemia preceded development of leukemia.

Finally, the strong familial incidence of cancer in some of these patients is worth noting. This occurs particularly in ataxia-telangiectasia, where numerous family members without stigmata of ataxia-telangiectasia have cancer (Reed *et al.*, 1966). Is there, then, a genetic basis (excluding genes determining the immunodeficiency) for malignancy in some of these patients? In other words, the relationship between immunodeficiency and malignancy may not necessarily be cause and effect. Hecht *et al.* (1973) have provided an important clue to our understanding of this problem by their extraordinary study of a patient with ataxia-telangiectasia. Initially, they found in the blood a single lymphocyte that had a chromosomal translocation. During the next 52 months they scored 2676 metaphases of blood lymphocyte cultures and observed a progressive increase in the number of cells with the translocation. By the end of the study, about three-fourths of the lymphocytes had the abnormality. The chromosomal alterations occurred in the D group, where abnormalities are found in other cases of ataxia-telangiectasia, suggesting to the authors that "accidents" of a D chromosome could occur preferentially in this disease. The relationship between chromosomal abnormalities and the emergence of new clones of lymphocytes—as in Hecht's case—may be important in the development of lymphoid neoplasms in ataxia-telangiectasia.

The lack of evidence of an increased incidence of neoplasms in diseases with a secondary immunodeficiency, such as sarcoidosis (Hirschhorn et al., 1964) and leprosy (Waldorf et al., 1966; Bullock, 1968), compounds the difficulties in interpreting the significance of neoplasms in patients with a primary immunodeficiency. Although a systematic analysis of this question has not been carried out in sarcoidosis, the literature fails to reveal that malignancy is a feature of this condition (L. Siltzbach, personal communication, 1973). The incidence of neoplasms has been determined in 848 lepers; 19.7 cancer deaths were expected and 21 were observed (Oleinick, 1969). The defect in cellular immunity in lepromatous leprosy can be as severe as in any primary immunodeficiency disease, although anergy in patients with tuberculoid leprosy is less common (Turk and Bryceson, 1971), so we are left with the paradox of severe immunodeficiency without an increased incidence of malignancy.

If impaired immunological surveillance against malignant cells were the sole explanation for the development of tumors in patients with primary immunodeficiency diseases, we would anticipate (1) an incidence of neoplasms much higher than 5%, (2) a representative variety of cancers, and (3) multiple neoplasms in individual patients. By contrast, impaired immunological surveillance against microorganisms in these patients results in (1) an almost universal susceptibility to infections (2) infectious disorders mediated by mechanisms representative of the immunodeficiency and (3) simultaneous or repeated infection by multiple organisms. Thus everything known about the role of the immune system in infection is upheld by clinical evidence. But a Scotch verdict must be handed down in the case for immunological surveillance against neoplasms.

### 4.2. Neoplasms in Recipients of Organ Allografts

The dramatic announcement in 1969 by Penn and his colleagues of five cases of malignant lymphoma in recipients of kidney allografts* was soon followed by a series of similar observations. Penn has continued his observations, and many of these cases are described in detail in his monograph (Penn, 1970). A registry of 5170 recipients (including 5000 kidney and 170 heart allografts) was compiled (Schneck and Penn, 1971). Fifty-two (1%) of the patients had developed a

---

* These tumors arose *de vovo* and are to be distinguished from (1) the inadvertent transplantation of malignant cells contained in the kidney of a donor with a neoplasm or (2) the growth of residual tumor in a recipient who had cancer before the transplant operation (Starzl *et al.*, 1971).

neoplasm; 28 of the tumors were of epithelial origin (usually involving the skin, cervix, and tongue), 22 were lymphomas, and two were leiomyosarcomas. These cases were collected on an informal basis from transplantation centers around the world, and therefore the incidence of 1% may not be accurate. Penn and Starzl (1972) analyzed 366 of their own patients who were alive 6 months to 9½ years after receiving a kidney allograft. Tumors developed in 18 (4.9%). More recently, Penn (1974) reported 24 neoplasms in 347 (6.9%) recipients surviving at least 4 months after renal transplantation.

An analysis of 95 tumors arising in about 9000 transplant recipients revealed that the commonest type (30%) was a malignant lymphoma (Penn and Starzl, 1972). Other common neoplasms included skin cancer (21%), *in situ* carcinoma of the cervix (8%), and carcinoma of the lip (8%). Two patients had multiple neoplasms. Superficial epithelial cancers have been noted in other series of kidney allograft recipients; for example, 14% of 51 recipients developed malignant skin tumors (Walder *et al.*, 1971), and carcinoma of the cervix has been noted by others (Kay *et al.*, 1970). It is noteworthy that the high incidence of skin cancer in recipients of renal allografts has been reported from Australia, a sun-drenched continent known for the high incidence of skin cancer in its population.

Another analysis of recipients of renal allografts—this one involving 6297 persons—indicated that the risk of reticulum cell sarcoma in men was 350 times greater than expected. In women the figure was 700. But the incidence of the commonest neoplasm of women, breast cancer, was not increased. The excess risk appeared within a year of transplantation and remained at the same high level for at least 5 yr. Skin and lip cancers occurred up to 4 times more often than expected and other cancers were 2.5 times more common, in men only. The excess risk of other cancers appeared later than that for the lymphomas and became more pronounced as the interval since transplantation increased (Hoover and Fraumeni, 1973).

One puzzling feature of these patients is that the incidence of neoplasms at different institutions is highly variable. The development of tumors in 24 out of 347 of Penn's patients has already been mentioned. By contrast, neither Deodhar (1972) at the Cleveland Clinic nor R. Simmons (personal communication, 1973) at the University of Minneapolis has found such a high incidence. Only one of Deodhar's 330 patients had a tumor, and Simmons found as many neoplasms in transplant recipients as in patients maintained on hemodialysis. It seems important to determine the basis for this regional variation (Table 3).

In every case of the *de novo* appearance of a tumor, the transplant recipient was receiving immunosuppressive therapy. All of the 95 patients referred to previously (Penn and Starzl, 1972) were taking corticosteroids, and 92 of them were also taking azathioprine. Antilymphocyte globulin was given to 25 patients. The average time of appearance of the tumor was 30 months after initiation of the immunosuppressive therapy; 12% of the neoplasms appeared in less than 4 months after transplantation.

The overriding consideration in arriving at an explanation of how these neoplasms arose is the immunosuppressive therapy. Yet analysis of this obvious

TABLE 3

*Incidence of Tumors in Kidney Transplant Recipients from Three Different Medical Centers*

| Series | Number of patients | Post-transplant tumors | Pretransplant tumors |
|--------|--------------------|-----------------------|----------------------|
| Penn | 347 | 24 | — |
| Deodhar | 330 | 1 | — |
| Simmons | 480 | 9 | 11[a] |

[a] In two cases, nephrectomy was done because of renal tumor. In three other cases, the tumor was removed at least 10 yr before the transplantation procedure.

possibility raises some doubts. In the first place, the assumption that any patient taking an "immunosuppressive" drug is immunologically impaired is unwarranted. At least two studies have shown that patients treated either with azathioprine alone or with azathioprine plus prednisone can respond normally to conventional antigenic stimuli (Swanson and Schwartz, 1967; Lee *et al.*, 1971). Moreover, the observation that many of the transplant recipients who developed a tumor had suffered repeated rejection crises (McKhann, 1969) indicates a relatively intact immune system, at least with regard to the antigens of the graft. However, enhanced susceptibility to infection with organisms that are not pathogenic in nonimmunosuppressed individuals is common (Rifkind *et al.*, 1967). Studies of the immune status of these patients are clearly in order, and until an immunodeficient state is identified and related to those recipients who developed a neoplasm, the pathogenesis of the tumors remains an open question.

We deal next with the possibility that chronic uremia, which impairs cell-mediated immunity (Dammin *et al.*, 1957), is behind the development of the neoplasms. Virtually all the recipients were chronically uremic before the transplant operation, but no data state the duration of the pregrafting uremic state. We know of no demonstration that chronic uremia is associated with an increased incidence of cancer. Of 4600 patients treated with hemodialysis for chronic uremia, 1% died from malignancy (Burton *et al.*, 1971). But this figure cannot be evaluated because the ages of the patients are not given. Penn (1970), citing a personal communication from R. F. Barth, states that no case of antecedent chronic renal disease was found in a study of 500 patients with lymphoma. We therefore exclude uremia as a contributing factor in the transplant cases.*

The extraordinarily high incidence (at least 100 times the expected rate) of lymphomas (especially reticulum cell sarcomas) is as vexing in the transplant recipients as it is in the patients with immunodeficiency diseases. But a new element is added in the former instance: involvement primarily of the brain in the majority of cases. Involvement of the central nervous system is a remarkable and highly atypical feature of the lymphomas arising in recipients of organ allografts

* The immunological surveillance theory fails to explain why there is not an increased incidence of malignancy in chronic uremia in view of the profound suppression of cellular immunity associated with this condition.

(Schneck and Penn, 1970, 1971). Ordinarily, lymphomas involving primarily the brain are very rare (Rosenberg *et al.*, 1961). Yet of 22 tumors found in transplant recipients, the brain was the only site of neoplasm in eight cases. In three additional patients, the brain as well as other organs was involved (Schneck and Penn, 1971). Traditionally, the brain is thought of as immunologically "privileged" because it lacks a lymphatic system. In such a protected environment, antigenic neoplasms should flourish. But, if this were the case, why should lymphomas arise preferentially in the brain of an *already* immunosuppressed person? Why do the transplant recipients develop cerebral *lymphomas* and not gliomas? Why are central nervous system lymphomas rare in patients with immunodeficiency diseases?

If we assume that transplant recipients and patients with immunodeficiency diseases have comparable degrees of impaired immunosuppression (as mentioned above, this assumption may be false), then two outstanding differences between the two groups are apparent. The first is that the former group is treated with azathioprine and corticosteroids, which could alter the permeability of the blood–brain barrier to lymphoid cells. These agents might thus enhance the spread of neoplastic cells from microscopic extracerebral sites to the brain. The second difference between the two groups is, of course, the transplanted organ. It is known that a kidney graft contains large numbers of donor lymphocytes, presumably of the circulating type (Guttman and Lindquist, 1969). If only a few foreign lymphocytes gained entry into the brain, might this not provide a nidus for the development of a cerebral lymphoma?

This brings us to consider the more general relevance of the allograft in the development of neoplasms in transplant recipients. In order to analyze this question, the incidence of tumors in patients treated with immunosuppressive agents, but who are not allograft recipients, is required. Unfortunately, little is known about the incidence of cancer in these patients. Several case reports describe the development of tumors in patients receiving immunosuppressants for the treatment of systemic lupus erythematosus (Lipsmeyer, 1972; Manny *et al.*, 1972; Newman and Walter, 1973), nephrotic syndrome (Sharpstone *et al.*, 1969; Bashour *et al.*, 1973), and psoriasis (Rees *et al.*, 1964; Harris, 1971; Craig and Rosenbery, 1971). However, these are difficult to interpret because neoplasms may develop in some of these diseases even when no treatment is applied (Hoerni and Laporte, 1970). The most striking example of the complexities of this problem is the controlled trial of azathioprine in rheumatoid arthritis conducted by Harris *et al.* (1971). Of 54 patients, 27 received azathioprine and 27 a placebo. Three lymphomas developed, each in a patient treated with the placebo. The authors dryly noted, "it is interesting to speculate on the conclusions which might have been drawn had the (tumors) occurred in the azathioprine-treated group." McEwan and Petty (1972) state that they can find only three published cases of neoplasm in over 4000 cases of nontransplant patients treated with azathioprine. However, this figure cannot be accepted as the true incidence; only a prospective search for cancer in these patients (and appropriate controls) will provide the answer.

There is interesting new information concerning the occurrence of a *new* malignancy in patients treated for cancer with agents known to suppress immunity. Several cases of acute myelomonocytic leukemia have occurred in patients treated with melphalan for multiple myeloma (Kyle *et al.*, 1970). (It is our opinion that the leukemia is a natural evolution of multiple myeloma.) A greater than threefold risk of development of second neoplasms was found in 425 patients with Hodgkin's disease treated with intensive radiotherapy, with or without subsequent chemotherapy (Arseneau *et al.*, 1972). In light of the demonstration that the standard form of radiotherapy given following mastectomy depletes T cells from blood (Stjernsward *et al.*, 1972), it is of interest that irradiation to the mediastinum following removal of a seminoma may be associated with an increased risk of a second neoplasm (Ytredal and Bradfield, 1972).

## 5. Conclusions

According to Burnet (1970), "when aberrant cells with proliferative potential arise in the body, they will carry new antigenic determinants on their cell surface. When a significant amount of new antigen has developed, a thymus-dependent immunological response will be initiated which eventually eliminates the aberrant cells in essentially the same way as a homograft is destroyed." We fully agree that all the criteria of a surveillance mechanism have been met in certain instances, such as polyma virus-induced tumors. However, we remain doubtful of the *general* applicability of the theory to the pathogenesis of cancer. Some of our doubt springs from semantic and technical problems:

1. Proponents of the theory of immunological surveillance have stressed repeatedly that "adaptive immunity evolved to minimize the dangers of malignant disease." This kind of statement, we feel, puts the idea beyond the reach of orderly discussion. Such teleological reasoning fails to acknowledge the existence of a parallel system of adaptive immunity—blocking antibody—which, according to all present evidence, protects the tumor against the cell-mediated immunity of the host. We feel it is time to abandon this kind of argument, which is of no value in coming to grips with the substantive issues.

2. Let us admit that, apart from a few exceptions, the cause of spontaneous cancer is unknown. It seems highly unlikely, for example, that the virulent strains of Friend, Moloney, and Rauscher viruses that are used to demonstrate immunosuppression by oncogenic viruses have any relevance to malignancies as they develop naturally. The same comment applies to the administration of large doses of carcinogenic chemicals to newborn animals, to the study of immunity in strains of mice with a 100% incidence of neoplasms, to the use of viruses which are not oncogenic in the strain of origin, and to all other systems that skirt the fundamental problem of spontaneous malignancy in genetically heterogeneous populations.

3. Assuming that at least some human neoplasms are induced by viruses (and this to us seems reasonable), the issue of defense mechanisms against oncogenic

viruses *qua* infectious agents must be separated from that of the defense against the cells they have transformed to a malignant state.* Very important conceptual and practical implications flow from these different phenomena. Earlier, we pointed out that several genes determine susceptibility or resistance to certain oncogenic viruses; some of these genes operate via nonimmunological mechanisms and they can be of overriding importance in determining the development of malignancy, even in severely immunosuppressed individuals. We feel that, in most experiments designed to examine immunological surveillance against neoplasms, this fundamental problem has been neglected. The most glaring example is the deliberate superinfection of mice with highly virulent oncogenic viruses combined with profound immunosuppression. In our opinion, all experiments of this type are useless because they fail to mirror spontaneous neoplasia. Quite simply, they are artifacts.

4. Although "immunosuppression" is a key notion in the concept of immunological surveillance, it is nowhere defined satisfactorily. The result is that virtually all experimental models have relied on techniques that yield profound degrees of immunosuppression, such as neonatal thymectomy, ALS treatment, or thymectomy combined with ALS. Apart from those patients with certain immunodeficiency diseases, there is no evidence that individuals with early neoplasms or with premalignant lesions have comparable defects in immunity. Indeed, there is little evidence that they have *any* immunodeficiency. We therefore conclude that the relevance of all such data to spontaneous neoplasms is highly doubtful except in one respect: the *failure* of profoundly immunosuppressed experimental animals to develop neoplasms sharply diminishes the force of the surveillance theory.

Possibly, the search for immunodeficiency has been misguided. Instead of cataloging responses to antigens with no conceivable relationship to the neoplasm, investigators of this problem may be better advised to determine the subject's ability to respond to antigens of his own neoplasm. This has already begun, and the results thus far are startling: in virtually every case of cancer studied in human beings, evidence for cell-mediated immunity against antigens of the tumor (either from the patient or from a histologically similar allogeneic tumor) has been found. This has been reported in sarcoma (Cohen *et al.*, 1973), neuroblastoma (Hellström *et al.*, 1970*b*), melanoma (Hellström and Hellström, 1973), carcinoma of the colon (Hellström *et al.*, 1970*a*) and bladder (Bubenik *et al.*, 1970), Burkitt's lymphoma (Fass *et al.*, 1970), and several other malignancies (Chu *et al.*, 1967; Oren and Herberman, 1971; Herberman, 1973). In many instances, notably in patients with rapidly advancing tumors, a blocking factor that specifically inhibits the cytotoxic effect of sensitized cells is also present (Hellström *et al.*, 1969, 1971). Therefore, the immunological defect in these cases is not due to immunosuppression, but to an immune response that protects the tumor instead

---

* The role of antiviral immunity in protection against neoplasms is nicely illustrated by the case of herpes virus saimiri, which causes no disease in its natural host, the squirrel monkey. However, when it is injected into marmosets and owl monkeys, which are normally free of this virus, a malignant lymphoma develops. The squirrel monkey—the natural host of this agent—produces antibody to this virus more regularly than marmosets and owl monkeys do (Falk *et al.*, 1973).

of the patient. It could be argued that such data detract nothing from the central theme of the surveillance theory: after all, in the final analysis cellular immunity failed to eliminate the tumor. However, the practical implications of these results are vastly different from the proposal that immunodeficiency is a major element in the development of cancer. It is one thing to deal therapeutically with the problem of blocking factor and quite another to devise methods of augmenting the immune response.

Conceivably, the theory of immunological surveillance can surmount these difficulties—or its proponents may have immediate answers—but even so, there remains an issue which to us seems of great importance. This is the extraordinary susceptibility of immunologically impaired individuals to develop malignant lymphoproliferative diseases. The reader is reminded that over 80% of the neoplasms in patients with spontaneous immunodeficiency and about 60% of those in recipients of organ transplants are lymphomas. Put another way, in a woman who receives a kidney transplant the risk of developing a reticulum cell sarcoma is about 700 times the risk of her developing cancer of the breast (Hoover and Fraumeni, 1973). If these figures are sustained by further experience, the theory of immunological surveillance cannot have general validity.

Can we explain these events without invoking a surveillance mechanism? At least two alternatives occur to us. In the first place, impaired defense mechanisms against oncogenic viruses have not been excluded. The marked susceptibility of heavily immunosuppressed recipients of renal allografts to viral infections is well documented. The common kinds of malignancy that do occur in immunosuppressed persons—lymphomas and superficial epithelial cancers of the lip, skin, and cervix—are precisely those in which oncogenic viruses are suspected to be etiological. This is what we referred to earlier as immunity against an infectious agent—and not immunity against a neoplasm.

Another possibility is that the development of lymphoid tumors in immunodeficiency states results from impaired regulation of lymphoid tissue. In other words, defective negative feedback loops permit unchecked proliferative activity in lymphoid tissue (Schwartz, 1972).

Several important feedback loops control the activity of antibody-forming tissue (Schwartz, 1971). Apart from the amount of antigen available to lymphocytes, the most important among these is the control of antibody synthesis by antibody. The feedback control of the synthesis of IgM antibodies by IgG antibodies is a typical example. This mechanism is highly specific and presumably acts by neutralization of the antigen. When IgG antibodies are not made (as, for example, in a partially immunosuppressed individual), IgM synthesis and hyperplasia of lymphoid tissue continue for a long time. Infusion of antigen-specific IgG antibodies immediately stops the abnormalities (Sahiar and Schwartz, 1966). Recently, considerable interest has focused on cellular feedback mechanisms. Regulation of thymus-independent (B) lymphocytes by T lymphocytes has been clearly demonstrated in several systems (Katz and Benacerraf, 1972). Interestingly enough, certain schedules of ALS—and perhaps other immunosuppressants—eliminate "suppressor" T cells with a sharp *increase* in antibody formation (Baker *et al.*, 1970).

Two experimental models are consistent with the notion that unrestrained proliferative activity of lymphoid tissue can culminate in neoplasia: persistent antigenic stimulation combined with partial immunosuppression (Krueger, 1972), and chronic graft vs. host reactions (Armstrong *et al.*, 1970). We believe that the following clinical events are representative of similar phenomena: antigenic stimulation by organ allografts in partially immunosuppressed recipients; uncontrolled lymphoid hyperplasia in patients with spontaneous and partial immunodeficiency; development of Burkitt's lymphoma in individuals who are partially immunosuppressed as a result of infestation by malaria parasites (Greenwood *et al.*, 1972; O'Conor, 1970); appearance of malignant lymphoproliferative diseases in association with certain autoimmune disorders (Talal and Bunim, 1964; Hoerni and Laporte, 1970).

Recent work has added a new dimension to the implications of immunoregulation in the pathogenesis of certain malignancies. This is the finding that antigenic stimuli can activate latent endogenous oncornaviruses (Hirsch *et al.*, 1970). Indeed, a reaction as seemingly innocuous as the rejection of a skin allograft can lead to the appearance of infectious oncornaviruses in the spleens of mice (Hirsch *et al.*, 1973*b*). Such immunologically activated viruses can be oncogenic (Armstrong *et al.*, 1973). Evidence is now accumulating that C-type RNA viruses replicate preferentially in transformed lymphocytes; this means that a deregulated immune response—one in which recruitment of newly transformed lymphocytes is unimpeded—can provide the ideal environment favoring the activation and replication of oncornaviruses (Schwartz, 1971).

The theory of immunological surveillance has held centerstage for a dozen years. Its usefulness in provoking experiments and, more important, in bringing a sense of definition and purpose to tumor immunology cannot be overestimated. However, alternative ideas are now possible because of the incredibly rich body of data that has emerged since the theory was first advanced. Indeed, recent experimental results now permit a serious examination of the notion that the immune reaction *stimulates* the growth of tumors (Prehn, 1971).

We end this chapter as we began, with a quotation from Ehrlich's address to the University of Amsterdam: "The deeper one explores these mechanisms in the experimental animal, the greater are the chances of offering treatment in human disease. Indeed, this was the reason I have brought to your attention the purely theoretical interpretation of current advances in experimental cancer research—it is especially true for the art of medicine that *Natura artis magistra*" (Ehrlich, 1957).

## 6. References

ALEXANDER, P., 1972, Foetal "antigens" in cancer, *Nature (Lond.)* **235**:137.
ALLISON, A. C., 1970, Tumour development following immunosuppression, *Proc. Roy. Soc. Med.* **63**:1077.
ALLISON, A. C., AND LAW, L. W., 1968, Effects of antilymphocyte serum on virus oncogenesis, *Proc. Soc. Exp. Biol. Med.* **127**:207.

ALLISON, A. C., AND TAYLOR, R. B., 1967, Observations on thymectomy and carcinogenesis, *Cancer Res.* **27**:703.

ALLISON, A. C., BERMAN, L. D., AND LEVEY, R. H., 1967, Increased tumour induction by adenovirus type 12 in thymectomized mice and mice treated with antilymphocyte serum, *Nature (Lond.)* **215**:185.

AMIET, A., 1963, Aldrich's syndrome: A report of two cases, *Ann. Paediat.* **201**:515.

AMMANN, A. J., AND HONG, R., 1971, Selective IgA deficiency: Presentation of 30 cases and a review of the literature, *Medicine* **50**:223.

AMMANN, P., LOPEZ, R., AND BUTLER, R., 1965, Das Ataxia-telangiecktasie-syndrom (Louis-Bar syndrom) aus immunologischer Sicht, *Helv. Paediat. Acta* **20**:137.

ANDREWS, E. J., 1971, Evidence of the nonimmune regression of chemically induced papillomas in mouse skin, *J. Natl. Cancer Inst.* **47**:653.

ARMSTRONG, M. Y. K., GLEICHMANN, E., GLEICHMANN, H., BELDOTTI, L., AND ANDRE-SCHWARTZ, R. S., 1970, Chronic allogeneic disease. II. Development of lymphomas, *J. Exp. Med.* **132**:417.

ARMSTRONG, M. Y. K., RUDDLE, N. H., LIPMAN, M. B., AND RICHARDS, F. F., 1973, Tumor induction by immunologically activated murine leukemia virus, *J. Exp. Med.* **137**:1163.

ARSENEAU, J. C., SPONZO, R. W., LEVIN, D. L., SCHNIPPER, L. E., BONNER, H., YOUNG, R. C., CANELLOS, G. P., JOHNSON, R. E., AND DEVITA, V. T., 1972, Nonlymphomatous malignant tumors complicating Hodgkin's disease, *New Engl. J. Med.* **287**:1119.

BACH, F. H., AND GOOD, R. A., 1972, *Clinical Immunobiology*, Vol. 1, Academic Press, New York.

BAKER, P. J., BARTH, R. F., STASHOK, P. W., AND AMSBAUGH, D. F., 1970, Enhancement of the antibody response to type III pneumococcal polysaccharide in mice treated with antilymphocyte serum, *J. Immunol.* **104**:1313.

BALL, J. K., 1970, Immunosuppression and carcinogenesis: Contrasting effects with 7,12-dimethylbenz (a) anthracene benz (a) pyrene and 3-methylcholanthrene, *J. Natl. Cancer Inst.* **44**:1.

BALNER, H., AND DERSJANT, H., 1966, Neonatal thymectomy and tumor induction with methylcholanthrene in mice, *J. Natl. Cancer Inst.* **36**:513.

BALNER, H., AND DERSJANT, H., 1969, Increased oncogenic effect of methylcholanthrene after treatment with antilymphocyte serum, *Nature (Lond.)* **224**:376.

BANSAL, S. C., AND SJÖGREN, H. O., 1971, "Unblocking" serum activity *in vitro* in the polyoma system may correlate with antitumour effect of antiserum *in vivo*, *Nature New Biol.* **233**:76.

BANSAL, S. C., AND SJÖGREN, H. O., 1973, Regression of polyoma tumor metastasis by combined unblocking and BCG treatment: Correlation with induced alterations in tumor immunity status, *Int. J. Cancer* **12**:179.

BASHOUR, B. N., MANCER, K., AND RANCE, C. P., 1973, Malignant mixed mullerian tumor of the cervix following cyclophosphamide therapy for nephrotic syndrome, *J. Pediat.* **82**:292.

BENNETT, M., AND STEEVES, R. A., 1970, Immunocompetent cell functions in mice infected with Friend leukemia virus, *J. Natl. Cancer Inst.* **44**:1107.

BERMUTH, G. V., MINIELLY, J. A., LOGAN, G. B., AND GLEICH, G. J., 1970, Hodgkin's disease and thymic alymphoplasia in a 5 month old infant, *Pediatrics* **45**:792.

BLAIR, P. B., 1971, Immunological aspects of the relationship between host and oncogenic virus in the mouse mammary tumor system, *Israel J. Med. Sci.* **7**:161.

BLAIR, P. B., 1972, Effect of transient immunosuppression on host response to neonatally introduced oncogenic virus, *Cancer Res.* **32**:356.

BODER, E., 1973, Ataxia-telangiectasia: Recent clinical and pathological observations, in: *Proceedings of the Second International Workshop on Immunodeficiency Diseases in Man* (D. Bergsma and R. A. Good, eds.), The National Foundation, New York.

BODER, E., AND SEDGWICK, R. P., 1963, Ataxia telangiectasia: A review of 101 cases, in: *Cerebellum, Posture and Cerebral Palsy* Little Club Clinics in Developmental Medicine No. 8, (G. E. Walsh, ed.), pp. 110–118, J. B. Lippincott, Philadelphia.

BRAND, M. M., AND MARINKOVICH, V. A., 1969, Primary malignant reticulosis of the brain in Wiskott–Aldrich syndrome: Report of a case, *Arch. Dis. Child.* **44**:536.

BROWN, R. S., HAYNES, H. A., FOLEY, H. T., GODWIN, H. A., BERARD, C. W., AND CARBONE, P. P., 1967, Hodgkin's disease: Immunologic, clinical and histologic features of 50 untreated patients, *Ann. Int. Med.* **67**:291.

BUBENIK, J., PERLMANN, P., HELMSTEIN, K., AND MOBERGER, G., 1970, Cellular and humoral immune responses to human urinary bladder carcinomas, *Int. J. Cancer* **5**:310.

BULLOCK, W. E., 1968, Studies of immune mechanisms in leprosy. I. Depression of delayed allergic responses to skin test antigens, *New Engl. J. Med.* **278**:298.

BURNET, F. M., 1963, The evolution of bodily defense, *Med. J. Austral.* **2**:817.

BURNET, F. M., 1970, The concept of immunological surveillance, *Prog. Exp. Tumor Res.* **13**:1.

BURSTEIN, N. A., AND ALLISON, A. C., 1970, Effect of antilymphocyte serum on the appearance of reticular neoplasms in SJL/J mice, *Nature (Lond.)* **225**:1139.

BURSTEIN, N. A., AND LAW, L. W., 1971, Neonatal thymectomy and nonviral mammary tumors in mice, *Nature (Lond.)* **231**:450.

BURTON, B. T., KRUEGER, K. K., AND BRYAN, F. A., 1971, National Registry of Long-Term Dialysis Patients, *J. Am. Med. Assoc.* **218**:718.

CANTOR, H., ASOFSKY, R., AND TALAL, N., 1970, Synergy among lymphoid cells mediating the graft versus host response. I. Synergy in graft versus host reactions produced by cells from NZB/Bl mice, *J. Exp. Med.* **131**:223.

CASTAIGNE, P., CAMBIER, J., AND BRUNET, P., 1969, Ataxie-telangiectasies, desordres immunitaires, lymphosarcomatose terminale chez deux frères, *Presse Med.* **77**:347.

CERELLI, G. J., AND TREAT, R. C., 1969, The effect of antilymphocyte serum on the induction and growth of tumor in the adult mouse, *Transplantation* **8**:774.

CHAPTAL, J., ROYER, P., JEAN, R., ALAGILLE, D., BONNET, H., LAGARDE, E., ROBINET, M., AND RIEU, D., 1966, Syndrome de Wiskott–Aldrich avec survie prolongée (gans) évolution mortelle par thymosarcome, *Arch. Franc. Pediat* **23**:907.

CHESTERMAN, F. C., GAUGAS, J. M., HIRSCH, M. S., REES, R. J. W., HARVEY, J. F., AND GILCHRIST, C., 1969, Unexpected high incidence of tumours in thymectomized mice treated with anti-lymphocyte globulin and *Mycobacterium leprae*, *Nature (Lond.)* **221**:1033.

CHU, E. H. Y., STJERNSWARD, J., CLIFFORD, P., AND KLEIN, G., 1967, Reactivity of human lymphocytes against autochthonous and allogeneic normal and tumor cells *in vitro*, *J. Natl. Cancer Inst.* **39**:595.

CLAMAN, H. N., AND CHAPERON, E. A., 1969, Immunologic complementation between thymus and marrow cells—A model for the two-cell theory of immunocompetence, *Transpl. Rev.* **1**:92.

COHEN, A. M., KETCHAM, A. S., AND MORTON, D. L., 1973, Tumor-specific cellular cytotoxicity to human sarcomas: Evidence for a cell-mediated host immune response to a common sarcoma cell-surface antigen, *J. Natl. Cancer Inst.* **50**:585.

COHEN, S. M., HEADLEY, D. B., AND BRYAN, G. T., 1973, The effect of adult thymectomy and adult splenectomy on the production of leukemia and stomach neoplasms in mice by *N*-(4-(5-nitro-2-furyl)-2-thiazolyl) acetamide, *Cancer Res.* **33**:637.

COLEMAN, A., LEIKIN, S., AND GUIN, G. H., 1961, Aldrich's syndrome, *Clin. Proc. Child. Hosp. (Wash.)* **17**:22.

COOPER, M. D., CHASE, H. P., LOWMAN, J. T., KRURT, W., AND GOOD, R. A., 1968, Wiskott–Aldrich syndrome, *Am. J. Med.* **44**:499.

COOPER, M. D., LAWTON, A. R., AND BOCKMAN, D. E., 1971, Agammaglobulinemia with B lymphocytes: Specific defect of plasma-cell differentiation, *Lancet* **2**:791.

CRAIG, S. R., AND ROSENBERY, E. W., 1971, Methotrexate-induced carcinoma? *Arch. Dermatol.* **103**:505.

CUSTER, R. P., OUTZEN, H. C., EATON, G. J., AND PREHN, R. J., 1973, Does the absence of immunologic surveillance affect the tumor incidence in "nude" mice? First recorded spontaneous lymphoma in a "nude" mouse, *J. Natl. Cancer Inst.* **51**:707.

DAMMIN, G. J., COUCH, N. P., AND MURRAY, J. E., 1957, Prolonged survival of skin homografts in uremic patients, *Ann. N.Y. Acad. Sci.* **64**:967.

DEFENDI, V., AND ROOSA, R. A., 1964, The role of the thymus in carcinogenesis, in: *The Thymus* (V. Defendi and D. Metcalf, eds.), p. 121, Wistar Institute Press, Philadelphia.

DENLINGER, R. H., SWENBERG, J. A., KOESTNER, A., AND WECHSLER, W., 1973, Differential effect of immunosuppression on the induction of nervous system and bladder tumors by *N*-methyl *N*-nitrosurea, *J. Natl. Cancer Inst.* **50**:87.

DENMAN, A. M., AND DENMAN, E. J., 1970, Depletion of long-lived lymphocytes in old New Zealand Black mice, *Clin. Exp. Immunol.* **6**:457.

DENT, P., 1972, Immunosuppression by oncogenic viruses, *Prog. Med. Virol.* **14**:1.

DENT, P. B., PETERSON, R. D. A., AND GOOD, R. A., 1965, A defect in cellular immunity during the incubation period of passage A leukemia in C3H mice, *Proc. Soc. Exp. Biol. Med.* **119**:869.

DEODHAR, S., 1972, Discussion, in: *Conference on Immunology of Carcinogenesis*, p. 217, National Cancer Institute Monograph 35, National Cancer Institute, Bethesda, Md.

DIGEORGE, A. M., 1968, Congenital absence of the thymus and its immunologic consequences: Concurrence with congenital hypoparathyroidism, in: *Immunologic Deficiency Diseases of Man* (R. A. Good and D. Bergsma, eds.), pp. 116–123, The National Foundation, New York.

DOELL, R. G., DeVAUX ST. CYR, C., AND GRABAR, P., 1967, Immune reactivity prior to development of thymic lymphoma in C57Bl mice, *Int. J. Cancer* **2**:103.

DORÉ, J. F., SCHNEIDER, M., AND MATHÉ, G., 1969, Réactions immunitaires chez les souris AKR leucemiques ou preleucemiques, *Rev. Franc. Etudes Clin. Biol.* **14**:1003.

DOUGLAS, S. D., GOLDBERG, L. S., AND FUDENBERG, H. H., 1970, Clinical, serologic and leukocyte function studies on patients with idiopathic "acquired" agammaglobulinemia and their families, *Am. J. Med.* **48**:48.

DUNN, H. G., MEUWISSEN, H., LIVINGSTON, C. S., AND PUMP, K. K., 1964, Ataxia telangiectasia, *Canad. Med. Assoc. J.* **91**:1106.

EAST, J., 1970, Immunopathology and neoplasms in NZB and SJL/J mice, *Prog. Exp. Tumor Res.* **13**:88.

EAST, J., AND HARVEY, J. J., 1968, The differential action of neoatal thymectomy in mice infected with murine sarcoma virus-Harvey (MSV-H), *Int. J. Cancer* **3**:614.

EDITORIAL, 1969, Hypogammaglobulinemia in the United Kingdom, *Lancet* **1**:163.

EHRLICH, P., 1957, Uber den jetzigen Stand der Karzinomforschung, in: *The Collected Papers of Paul Ehrlich*, Vol. II, p. 550, Pergamon Press, London.

EMERY, C. W. A., 1924, Early pregnancy and epitheliomata, *Brit. Med. J.* **2**:1149.

FALK, L. A., WOLFE, L. G., AND DEINHARDT, F., 1973, Herpesvirus saimiri: Experimental infection of squirrel monkeys (*Saimiri sciureus*), *J. Natl. Cancer Inst.* **51**:165.

FASS, L., HERBERMAN, R. B., AND ZIEGLER, J. L., 1970, Cutaneous hypersensitivity reactions to autologous extracts of Burkitt's lymphoma cells, *New Engl. J. Med.* **282**:776.

FEIGIN, R. D., VIETTI, T. J., WYATT, R. G., KAUFMAN, D. G., AND SMITH, C. H., 1970, Ataxia telangiectasia with granulocytopenia, *J. Pediat.* **77**:431.

FISHER, J. C., DAVIS, R. C., AND MANNICK, J. A., 1970, The effects of immunosuppression on the induction and immunogenicity of chemically induced sarcomas, *Surgery* **68**:150.

FLANAGAN, S. P., 1966, "Nude," a new hairless gene with pleiotropic effects, *Genet. Res. (Camb.)* **8**:295.

FOLEY, E. J., 1953, Antigenic properties of methylcholanthrene-induced tumors in mice of the strain of origin, *Cancer Res.* **13**:835.

FORSSMAN, O., AND HERNER, B., 1964, Acquired agammaglobulinaemia and malansorption, *Acta Med. Scand.* **176**:779.

FRAUMENI, J. F., 1969, *Constitutional disorders of Man Predisposing to Leukemia and Lymphoma*, p. 221, National Cancer Institute Monograph 32, National Cancer Institute, Bethesda, Md.

FREEMAN, A. I., SINKS, L. F., AND COHEN, M. M., 1970, Lymphosarcoma in siblings associated with cytogenetic abnormalities, immune deficiency and abnormal erythropoiesis, *J. Pediat.* **77**:996.

FRIEDMAN, H., 1964, Distribution of antibody plaque forming cells in various tissues of several strains of mice injected with sheep erythrocytes, *Proc. Soc. Exp. Biol. Med.* **117**:526.

FRIEDMAN, H., AND CEGLOWSKI, W. S., 1971, Defect in cellular immunity of leukemia virus–infected mice assessed by macrophage migration-inhibition assay, *Proc. Soc. Exp. Biol. Med.* **136**:154.

FRIEDMAN, H., AND CEGLOWSKI, W. S., 1973, Cellular immunity and leukemia virus infection, in: *Virus Tumorigenesis and Immunogenesis* (W. S. Ceglowski and H. Friedman, eds.), p. 299, Academic Press, New York and London..

FRIEDMAN, H., MELNICK, H., MILLS, L., AND CEGLOWSKI, W. S., 1973, Depressed allograft immunity in leukemia virus infected mice, *Transpl. Proc.* **5**:981.

FRIEDRICH-FRESKA, H., AND HOFFMAN, M., 1969, Immunological defense against preneoplastic stages of diethyl-nitrosamine-induced carcinomas in rat liver, *Nature (Lond.)* **223**:1162.

FUDENBERG, H., AND SOLOMON, A., 1961, "Acquired agammaglobulinemia" with auto-immune hemolytic disease: Graft versus host reaction? *Vox Sang.* **6**:68.

FURTH, J., KUNII, A., IOACHIM, H., SANEL, F. T., AND MOY, P., 1966, Parallel observations on the role of the thymus in leukaemogenesis, immunocompetence and lymphopoiesis, in: *The Thymus: Experimental and Clinical Studies* (G. E. W. Wolstenholme and R. Potter, eds.), p. 288, Little, Brown, Boston.

GELFAND, M. E., AND STEINBERG, A. D., 1973, Mechanism of allograft rejection in New Zealand mice. I. Cell synergy and its age-dependent loss, *J. Immunol.* **110**:1652.

GERSHON, R. K., COHEN, P., HENCIN, R., AND LIEBHABER, S. A., 1972, Suppressor T cells, *J. Immunol.* **108**:586.

GIOVANELLA, B. C., LIEGEL, J., AND HEIDELBERGER, C., 1970, The refractoriness of the skin of hairless mice to chemical carcinogenesis, *Cancer Res.* **30**:2590.

GITLIN, D., AND JANEWAY, C. A., 1956, Agammaglobulinemia, congenital, acquired and transient forms, *Prog. Hematol.* **1**:318.

GOOD, R. A., 1972, Relations between immunity and malignancy, *Proc. Natl. Acad. Sci.* **69**:1026.

GOTOFF, S. P., AMIRMOKRI, E., AND LIEBNER, E. J., 1967, Ataxia telangiectasia: Neoplasia, untoward response to x-irradiation and tuberous sclerosis, *Am. J. Dis. Child.* **114:**617.

GOTTLIEB, C. F., PERKINS, E. H., AND MAKINODAN, T., 1972, Genetic regulation of the thymus dependent humoral immune response in leukemia prone AKR (*H-2^k*) and nonleukemic C3H (*H-2^k*) mice, *J. Immunol.* **109:**974.

GRANT, G. A., AND MILLER, J. F. A. P., 1965, Effect of neonatal thymectomy on the induction of sarcomata in C57BL mice, *Nature (Lond.)* **205:**1124.

GRANT, G. A., AND ROE, F. J. C., 1969, Effect of germ free status and antilymphocyte serum on induction of various tumors in mice by a chemical carcinogen given at birth, *Nature (Lond.)* **223:**1060.

GREEN, T., LITURN, S., ADLERSBERG, R., AND RUBIN, I., 1966, Hypogammaglobulinemia with late development of a lymphosarcoma: A case report, *Arch. Int. Med.* **118:**592.

GREENWOOD, B. M., BRADLEY-MOORE, A. M., PALIT, A., AND BRIJCESON, A. D. M., 1972, Immunosuppression in children with malaria, *Lancet* **1:**1969.

GROSS, L., 1959, Effect of thymectomy on development of leukemia in C3H mice inoculated with leukemic "passage" virus, *Proc. Soc. Exp. Biol. Med.* **100:**325.

GROSS, L., 1970, *Oncogenic Viruses*, Pergamon Press, New York.

GUTTMAN, R. D., AND LINDQUIST, P. R., 1969, Renal transplantation in inbred rats: Reduction of allograft immunogenicity by cytotoxic drug pretreatment of donors, *Transplantation* **8:**490.

HAERER, A. F., JACKSON, J. F., AND EVERS, C. G., 1969, Ataxia telangiectasia with gastric carcinoma, *J. Am. Med. Assoc.* **210:**1884.

HANNA, M. G., NETTESHEIM, P., AND OGDEN, L., 1967, Reduced immune potential of aged mice: Significance of morphologic changes in lymphatic tissue, *Proc. Soc. Exp. Biol. Med.* **125:**882.

HARAN-GHERA, N., BEN YAAKOV, M., PELED, A., AND BENTWICH, Z., 1973, Immune status of SJL/J mice in relation to age and spontaneous tumor development, *J. Natl. Cancer Inst.* **50:**1227.

HARGIS, B. J., AND MALKIEL, S., 1972, The immunocapacity of the AKR mouse, *Cancer Res.* **32:**291.

HARRIS, C. C., 1971, Malignancy during methotrexate and steroid therapy for psoriasis, *Arch. Dermatol.* **103:**501.

HARRIS, J., JESSOP, J. D., AND DE SAINTONGE, D. M. C., 1971, Further experience with azathioprine in rheumatoid arthritis, *Brit. Med. J.* **4:**463.

HECHT, F., KOLER, R. D., RIGAS, D. A., DAHNKE, G. S., CASE, M. P., TISDALE, V., AND MILLER, R. W., 1966, Leukemia and lymphocytes in ataxia telangiectasia, *Lancet* **2:**1193.

HECHT, F., MCCAW, B. K., AND KOLER, R. D., 1973, Ataxia-telangiectasia—Clonal growth of translocation lymphocytes, *New Engl. J. Med.* **289:**286.

HECHTEL, M., DISHON, T., AND BRAUN, W., 1965, Hemolysin formation in newborn mice of different strains, *Proc. Soc. Exp. Biol. Med.* **120:**728.

HELLSTRÖM, I., AND HELLSTRÖM, K. E., 1973, Some recent studies on cellular immunity to human melanomas, *Fed. Proc.* **32:**156.

HELLSTRÖM, I., HELLSTRÖM, K. E., EVANS, C. A., HEPPNER, G. H., PIERCE, G. E., AND YANG, J. P. S., 1969, Serum-mediated protection of neoplastic cells from inhibition by lymphocytes immune to their tumor-specific antigens, *Proc. Natl. Acad. Sci.* **62:**362.

HELLSTRÖM, I., HELLSTRÖM, K. E., AND SHEPARD, T. H., 1970a, Cell-mediated immunity against antigens common to human colonic carcinomas and fetal gut epithelium, *Int. J. Cancer* **6:**346.

HELLSTRÖM, I., HELLSTRÖM, K. E., BILL, A. H., PIERCE, G. E., AND YANG, J. P. S., 1970b, Studies on cellular immunity to human neuroblastoma cells, *Int. J. Cancer* **6:**172.

HELLSTRÖM, I., HELLSTRÖM, K. E., SJÖGREN, H. O., AND WARNER, G. A., 1971, Serum factors in tumor-free patients cancelling the blocking of cell-mediated immunity, *Int. J. Cancer* **8:**185.

HELLSTRÖM, K. E., AND HELLSTRÖM, I., 1969, Cellular immunity against tumor antigens, *Advan. Cancer Res.* **12:**167.

HEPPNER, G. H., WOOD, P. C., AND WEISS, D. W., 1968, Studies on the role of the thymus in viral tumorigenesis. I. Effect of thymectomy on induction of hyperplastic alveolar nodules and mammary tumors in BALB/c and C3H mice, *Israel J. Med. Sci.* **4:**1195.

HERBERMAN, R. B., 1973, *In vivo* and *in vitro* assays of cellular immunity to human tumor antigens, *Fed. Proc.* **32:**160.

HERMANS, P. C., AND HUIZENGA, K. A., 1972, Association of gastric carcinoma with idiopathic late-onset immunoglobulin deficiency, *Ann. Int. Med.* **76:**605.

HERSH, E. M., WHITECAR, J. P., MCCREDIE, K. B., BODEY, G. P., AND FREIREICH, E. J., 1971, Chemotherapy, immunocompetence, immunosuppression and prognosis in acute leukemia, *New Engl. J. Med.* **285:**1211.

HIRSCH, M. S., AND MURPHY, F. A., 1968, Effects of antithymocyte serum on Rauscher virus infection of mice, *Nature (Lond.)* **218**:478.

HIRSCH, M. S., ALLISON, A. C., AND HARVEY, J. J., 1969, Immune complexes in mice infected neonatally with Moloney leukemogenic and murine sarcoma viruses, *Nature (Lond.)* **223**:739.

HIRSCH, M. S., BLACK, P. H., TRACY, G. S., LEIBOWITZ, S., AND SWARTZ, R. S., 1970, Leukemia virus activation in chronic allogeneic disease, *Proc. Natl. Acad. Sci.* **67**:1914.

HIRSCH, M. S., BLACK, P. H., WOOD, M. L., AND MONACO, A. P., 1973a, Effects of pyran copolymer on leukemogenesis in immunosuppressed AKR mice, *J. Immunol.* **111**:91.

HIRSCH, M. S., ELLIS, D. A., BLACK, P. H., MONACO, A. P., AND WOOD, M. L., 1973b, Leukemia virus activation during homograft rejection, *Science* **180**:500.

HIRSCHHORN, K.,SCHREIBMAN, R. R., BACH, F. H., AND SILTZBACH, L. E., 1964, *In vitro* studies of lymphocytes from patients with sarcoidosis and lymphoproliferative diseases, *Lancet* **2**:842.

HITZIG, W. G., 1968, The Swiss type of agammaglobulinemia, in: *Immunologic Deficiency Diseases in Man* (R. A. Good and D. Bergsma, eds.), p. 53, The National Foundation, New York.

HOERNI, B., AND LAPORTE, G., 1970, Immunological disorders in the aetiology of lymphoreticular neoplasms, *Rev. Europ. Etud. Clin. Biol.* **15**:841.

HOOVER, R., AND FRAUMENI, J. F., JR., 1973, Risk of cancer in renal-transplant recipients, *Lancet* **2**:55.

HOYER, J. R., COOPER, M. C., GABRIELSON, A. E., AND R. A., 1968, Lymphopenic forms of congenital immunologic deficiency diseases, *Medicine* **47**:201.

HUBER, F., 1968, Experience with various immunologic deficiencies in Holland, in: *Immunologic Deficiency Diseases in Man* (R. A. Good and D. Bergsma, eds.), p. 53, The National Foundation, New York.

JOHNSON, E. A., REED, N. D., JUTILA, J. W., AND HILL, W. D., 1974, Submitted for publication.

JOHNSON, S., 1968, Effect of thymectomy on the induction of skin tumors by dibenzanthracene and of breast tumors by dimethylbenzanthracene in mice of the IF strain, *Brit. J. Cancer* **22**:755.

JUDD, K. P., STEPHENS, K., AND TRENTIN, J. J., 1971, Effects of heterologous antilymphocyte antibody on the development of spontaneous and transplanted lymphoma in AKR mice, *Cancer* **27**:1161.

JUNG, K. S. K., HOFFMAN, G. C., AND LONSDALE, D., 1969, Lymphoproliferative lesion in congenital thymic aplasia associated with agammaglobulinemia, *Am. J. Clin. Pathol.* **52**:726.

KADOWAKI, J. I., THOMPSON, R. I., ZUELZER, W. W., WOOLEY, P. V., BROUGH, A. J., AND GRUBER, D., 1965, XX/XY lymphoid chimaerism in congenital immunological deficiency syndrome with thymic alymphoplasia, *Lancet* **2**:1152.

KAPLAN, H. S., 1971, Role of immunologic disturbance in human oncogenesis: Some facts and fancies, *Brit. J. Cancer* **25**:620.

KATZ, D. H., AND BENACERRAF, B., 1972, The regulatory influence of activated T cells on B cell responses to antigen, *Advan. Immunol.* **15**:1.

KAY, S., FRABLE, W. J., AND HUME, D. M., 1970, Cervical dysplasia and cancer developing in women on immunosuppression therapy for renal homotransplantation, *Cancer* **26**:1048.

KILDEBERG, P., 1961, The Aldrich syndrome: Report of a case and discussion of pathogenesis, *Prediatrics* **27**:362.

KIRSCHSTEIN, R., RABSON, A. S., AND PETERS, E. A., 1964, Oncogenic activity of adenovirus 12 in thymectomized BALB/c and C3H/HeN mice, *Proc. Soc. Exp. Biol. Med.* **117**:198.

KLEIN, G., 1972, Tumor immunology, escape mechanisms, *Ann. Inst. Pasteur* **122**:593.

KLEIN, G., 1966, Tumor antigens. *Ann. Rev. Microbiol.* **20**:223.

KLEIN, G., 1969, Experimental studies in tumor immunology, *Fed. Proc.* **28**:1739.

KLEIN, G., 1973, Tumor immunology, *Transpl. Proc.* **5**:31.

KOLDOVSKY, P., 1969, *Tumor Specific Transplantation Antigen*, Springer, New York.

KOUTTAB, N. M., JUTILA, J. W., AND REED, N. D., Submitted for publication.

KRUEGER, G. R. F., 1972, Chronic immunosuppression and lymphomagenesis in man and mice, in: *Conference on Immunology of Carcinogenesis*, p. 138, National Cancer Institute Monograph 35, National Cancer Institute, Bethesda, Md.

KYLE, R. A., PIERRE, R. V., AND BAYRD, E. D., 1970, Multiple myeloma and acute myelomonocytic leukemia, *New Engl. J. Med.* **283**:1121.

LAMPERT, F., 1969, Akute lymphoblastische Leukämie bei Geschwistern mit progressiver Kleinhernataxie (Louis-Bar syndrom), *Deutsch. Med. Wschr.* **94**:217.

LANCE, E. M., MEDAWAR, P. B., AND TAUT, R. N., 1973, Antilymphocyte serum, *Advan. Immunol.* **17**:2.

LAPPE, M. A., AND BLAIR, P. B., 1970, Interference with mammary tumorigenesis by antilymphocyte serum, *Proc. Am. Assoc. Cancer Res.* **11**:47.

LAPPE, M. A., AND PREHN, R. J., 1970, The predictive value of skin allograft survival times during the development of urethan-induced lung adenomas in BALB/c mice, *Cancer Res.* **30**:1357.

LAW, L. W., 1966, Studies of thymic function with emphasis on the role of the thymus in oncogenesis, *Cancer Res.* **26**:551.

LAW, L., 1969, Studies of the significance of tumor antigens in induction and repression of neoplastic disease, *Cancer Res.* **29**:1.

LAW, L. W., 1970a, Effects of antilymphocyte serum on the induction of neoplasms of lymphoreticular tissues, *Fed. Proc.* **29**:171.

LAW, L. W., 1970b, Studies of tumor antigens and tumor specific immune mechanisms in experimental systems, *Transpl. Proc.* **2**:117.

LAW, L. W., AND CHANG, S. S., 1971, Effects of antilymphocyte serum (ALS) on the induction of lymphocytic leukemia in mice, *Proc. Soc. Exp. Biol. Med.* **136**:420.

LAW, L. W., AND MILLER, J. H., 1950, The influence of thymectomy on the incidence of carcinogen-induced leukemia in strain DBA mice, *J. Natl. Cancer Inst.* **11**:425.

LAW, L. W., AND TING, R. C., 1965, Immunologic competence and induction of neoplasms by polyoma virus, *Proc. Soc. Exp. Biol. Med.* **119**:823.

LEE, A. K. Y., MACKAY, I. R., ROWLEY, M. J., AND YAP, C. Y., 1971, Measurement of antibody-producing capacity to flagellin in man. IV. Studies in autoimmune disease, allergy and after azathioprine treatment, *Clin. Exp. Immunol.* **9**:507.

LEGGE, J. S., AND AUSTING, C. M., 1968, Antigen localization and the immune response as a function of age, *Austral. J. Exp. Biol. Med. Sci.* **46**:361.

LEVENTHAL, B. G., AND TALAL, N., 1970, Response of NZB and NZB/NZW spleen cells to mitogenic agents, *J. Immunol.* **104**:918.

LEVINE, B. B., AND VAS, N. M., 1970, Effect of combinations of inbred strain, antigen, and antigen dose on immune responsiveness and reagin production in the mouse, *Int. Arch. Allergy Appl.* **39**:156.

LILLY, F., 1968, The effect of histocompatibility-2 type on response to Friend leukemia virus in mice, *J. Exp. Med.* **127**:465.

LILLY, F., 1972, Mouse leukemia: A model of a multiple gene disease, *J. Natl. Cancer Inst.* **49**:927.

LILLY, F., AND PINCUS, T., 1973, Genetic control of murine viral leukemogenesis, *Advan. Cancer Res.* **17**:231.

LILLY, F., BOYSE, E. A., AND OLD, L. J., 1964, Genetic basis of susceptibility to viral leukemogenesis, *Lancet* **2**:1207.

LIPSMEYER, E. A., 1972, Development of malignant cerebral lymphoma in a patient with systemic lupus erythematosus treated with immunosuppression, *Arthritis. Rheum.* **15**:183.

LITTLE, C. C., 1941, The genetics of tumor transplantation, in: *Biology of the Laboratory Mouse* (G. D. Snell, ed.), pp. 279–309, Blakiston, Philadelphia.

MAKINODAN, T., AND PETERSON, W. J., 1964, Growth and senescence of the primary antibody-forming potential of the spleen, *J. Immunol.* **93**:886.

MALMGREN, R. A., BENNISON, B. E., AND MCKINLEY, T. W., 1952, Reduced antibody titers in mice treated with carcinogenic and cancer chemotherapeutic agents, *Proc. Soc. Exp. Biol. Med.* **79**:484.

MANNING, D. D., REED, N. D., AND SHAFFER, C. F., 1973, Maintenance of skin xenografts of widely divergent phylogenetic origin on congenitally athymic (nude) mice, *J. Exp. Med.* **138**:488.

MANNY, N., ROSENMAN, E., AND BENBASSAT, J., 1972, Hazard of immunosuppressive therapy, *Brit. Med. J.* **2**:291.

MARTINEZ, C., 1964, Effect of early thymectomy on development of mammary tumours in mice, *Nature (Lond.)* **203**:1188.

MCDEVITT, H. O., AND BENACERRAF, B., 1969, Genetic control of specific immune responses, *Advan. Immunol.* **11**:31.

MCENDY, D. P., BOON, M. C., AND FURTH, J., 1944, On the role of thymus, spleen and gonads in the development of leukemia in a high leukemia stock of mice, *Cancer Res.* **4**:377.

MCEWAN, A., AND PETTY, L. G., 1972, Oncogenicity of immunosuppressive drugs, *Lancet* **1**:326.

MCFARLIN, D. E., STROBER, W., AND WALDMANN, T. A., 1972, Ataxia telangiectasia, *Medicine* **51**:281.

MCKHANN, C. F., 1969, Primary malignancy in patients undergoing immunosuppression for renal transplantation, *Transplantation* **8**:209.

MCKUSICK, V. A., AND CROSS, H. E., 1966, Ataxia telangiectasia and Swiss-type agammaglobulinemia, *J. Am. Med. Assoc.* **195**:119.

METCALF, D., 1963, The fate of parental preleukemic cells in leukemia susceptible and leukemia resistant $F_1$ hybrid mice, *Cancer Res.* **23**:1774.

METCALF, D., AND MOULDS, R., 1967, Immune responses in preleukemic and leukemic AKR mice, *Int. J. Cancer* **2**:53.

METCALF, D., MOULDS, R., AND PIKE, B., 1966, Influence of the spleen and thymus on immune responses in aging mice, *Clin. Exp. Immunol.* **2**:109.

MILLER, D. G., 1967, The association of immune disease and malignant lymphoma, *Ann. Int. Med.* **66**:511.

MILLER, J. F. A. P., 1962, Role of the thymus in transplantation, *Ann. N.Y. Acad. Sci.* **99**:340.

MILLER, J. F. A. P., GRANT, G. A., AND ROE, F. J. C., 1963, Effect of thymectomy on the induction of skin tumors by 3,4-benzopyrene, *Nature (Lond.)* **199**:920.

MOLONEY, J. B., 1962, The murine leukemias, *Fed. Proc.* **21**:19.

MORGAN, J. L., HOLCOMB, T. M., AND MORRISSEY, R. W., 1968, Radiation reaction in ataxia telangiectasia, *Am. J. Dis. Child.* **116**:557.

MÜHLBOCK, O., AND DUX, A., 1971, Histocompatibility genes and susceptibility to mammary tumor virus in mice, *Transpl. Proc.* **3**:1247.

MURPHY, W. H., AND SYVERTON, J. T., 1961, Relative immunologic capacity of leukemic and low-leukemic strains of mice to resist infection, *Cancer Res.* **21**:921.

NAGAYA, H., AND SIEKER, H. O., 1969, Effects of antithymus serum and antilymphocyte serum on the incidence of lymphoid leukemia, *Proc. Soc. Exp. Biol. Med.* **131**:891.

NANDI, S., 1967, The histocompatibility-2 locus and susceptibility to Bittner virus borne by red blood cells in mice, *Proc. Natl. Acad. Sci.* **58**:485.

NEHLSEN, S. L., 1971, Immunosuppression, virus and oncogenesis in mice, *Transpl. Proc.* **3**:811.

NEWMAN, D. M., AND WALTER, J. B., 1973, Multiple dermatofibromas in patients with systemic lupus erythematosus on immunosuppressive therapy, *New Engl. J. Med.* **289**:842.

NOTKINS, A. L., MERGENHAGEN, S. E., AND HOWARD, R. J., 1970, Effect of virus infections on the function of the immune system, *Ann. Rev. Microbiol.* **24**:525.

O'CONOR, G. T., 1970, Persistent immunologic stimulation as a factor in oncogenesis, with special reference to Burkitt's tumor, *Am. J. Med.* **48**:279.

OLDSTONE, M. B. A., AOKI, T., AND DIXON, F. J., 1972, The antibody response to murine leukemia virus: Absence of classical immunologic tolerance, *Proc. Natl. Acad. Sci.* **69**:134.

OLEINICK, A., 1969, Altered immunity and cancer risk: A review of the problem and analysis of the cancer mortality experience in leprosy patients, *J. Natl. Cancer Inst.* **43**:775.

OREN, M. E., AND HERBERMAN, R. B., 1971, Delayed cutaneous hypersensitivity reactions to membrane extracts of human tumor cells, *Clin. Exp. Immunol.* **9**:45.

PAGE, A. R., HANSEN, A. E., AND GOOD, R. A., 1963, Occurrence of leukemia and lymphoma in patients with agammaglobulinemia, *Blood* **21**:197.

PANTELOURIS, F. M., 1968, Absence of thymus in a mouse mutant, *Nature (Lond.)* **217**:370.

PEKONEN, R., SIURALA, M., AND VUOPIO, P., 1963, Inherited agammaglobulinemia with malabsorption and marked alterations in the gastrointestinal mucosa, *Acta Med. Scand.* **173**:549.

PENN, I., 1970, *Malignant Tumors in Organ Transplant Recipients*, Springer, New York.

PENN, I., 1974, Malignancies in renal transplant recipients, in: *Seventh Miles International Symposium*, in press.

PENN, I., AND STARZL, T. E., 1972, Malignant tumors arising *de novo* in immunosuppressed organ transplant recipients, *Transplantation* **14**:407.

PENN, I., HAMMOND, W., BRETTSCHNEIDER, L., AND STARZL, T. E., 1969, Malignant lymphomas in transplantation patients, *Transpl. Proc.* **1**:106.

PETERS, R. L., SPAHN, G. J., RABSTEIN, L. S., KELLOFF, G. J., AND HUEBNER, R. J., 1973, Neoplasm induction by murine type-C viruses passaged directly from spontaneous non-lymphorecticular tumours, *Nature New Biol.* **244**:103.

PETERSON, R. D. A., KELLY, W. D., AND GOOD, R. A., 1964, Ataxia telangiectasia: Its association with a defective thymus, immunological deficiency disease, and malignancy, *Lancet* **1**:1189.

PETERSON, R. D. A., COOPER, M. D., AND GOOD, R. A., 1966, Lymphoid tissue abnormalities associated with ataxia-telangiectasia, *Am. J. Med.* **41**:342.

PINCUS, T., ROWE, W. P., AND LILLY, F., 1971, A major genetic locus affecting resistance to infection with murine leukemia viruses. II. Apparent identity to a major locus described for resistance to Friend murine leukemia virus, *J. Exp. Med.* **133**:1234.

PLAYFAIR, J. H. L., 1968, Strain differences in the murine response of mice. I. The neonatal response to sheep red cells, *Immunology* **15**:35.

POPPER, K., 1968, *The Logic of Scientific Discovery*, Harper and Row, New York.

POTOLSKY, A. I., HEATH, C. W., BUCKLEY, C. E., AND ROWLANDS, D. T., 1971, Lymphoreticular malignancies and immunologic abnormalities in a sibship, *Am. J. Med.* **50**:42.

PREHN, R. T., 1963, Function of depressed immunological reactivity during carcinogenesis, *J. Natl. Cancer Inst.* **31**:791.

PREHN, R. T., 1970, Critique of surveillance hypothesis, in: *Immune Surveillance* (R. T. Smith and M. Landy, eds.), p. 460, Academic Press, New York.

PREHN, R. T., 1971, Perspectives in oncogenesis: Does immunity stimulate or inhibit neoplasia? *J. Reticuloendothel. Soc.* **10**:1.

PREHN, R. T., 1972, The immune reaction as a stimulator of tumor growth, *Science* **176**:170.

PREHN, R. T., AND MAIN, J. M., 1957, Immunity to methylcholanthrene-induced sarcomas, *J. Natl. Cancer Inst.* **18**:769.

PROFITT, M. R., HIRSCH, M. S., AND BLACK, P. H., 1973, Absence of cell-mediated immunologic tolerance to leukemia virus in carrier mice, *J. Immunol.* **110**:1183.

RABBAT, A. G., AND JEEJEEBHOY, H. F., 1970, Heterologous antilymphocyte serum (ALS) hastens the appearance of methylcholanthrene-induced tumours in mice, *Transplantation* **9**:164.

RADL, MASOPUST, J., HOUSTEK, J., AND HRODEK, O., 1967, Paraproteinaemia and unusual dysgammaglobulinemia in a case of Wiskott–Aldrich syndrome: An immunochemical study, *Arch. Dis. Child.* **42**:608.

RADZICHOVSKAJA, R., 1967, Effect of thymectomy on Rous virus tumor growth induced in chickens, *Proc. Soc. Exp. Biol. Med.* **126**:13.

REED, N. D., AND JUTILA, J. W., 1972, Immune response of congenitally thymusless mice to heterologous erythrocytes, *Proc. Soc. Exp. Biol. Med.* **139**:1234.

REED, N. D., MANNING, J. K., AND RUDBACH, J. A., 1973, Immunological responsiveness of mice to LPS from *Escherichia coli*, *J. Infect. Diseases* (Endotoxin Suppl.).

REED, W. B., EPSTEIN, W. L., BODER, E., AND SEDGWICK, R., 1966, Cutaneous manifestations of ataxia telangiectasia, *J. Am. Med. Assoc.* **195**:746.

REES, R. B., BENNETT, J. H., HAMLIN, E. M., AND MAIBACH, H. I., 1964, Aminopterin for psoriasis, *Arch. Dermatol.* **90**:544.

REISMAN, L. E., MITANI, M., AND ZUELZER, W. W., 1964, Chromosome studies in leukemia. I. Evidence for the origin of leukemic stem lines from aneuploid mutants, *New Engl. J. Med.* **270**:591.

RIFKIND, D., MARCHIORO, T. L., AND SCHNECK, S. A., 1967, Systemic fungal infections complicating renal transplantation, *Am. J. Med.* **43**:28.

ROITT, I., 1971, *Essential Immunology*, Davis, London.

ROSENBERG, S. A., DIAMOND, H. D., JASLOWITZ, B., AND CRAVER, L. F., 1961, *Medicine* **40**:31.

ROWE, W. P., 1972, Studies of genetic transmission of murine leukemia virus by AKR mice. I. Crosses with $Fv-1^n$ strains of mice, *J. Exp. Med.* **136**:1272.

ROWE, W. P., AND HARTLEY, J. W., 1972, Studies of genetic transmission of murine leukemia virus by AKR mice. II. Crosses with $Fv-1^b$ strains of mice, *J. Exp. Med.* **136**:1286.

RYGAARD, J., 1969, Immunobiology of the mouse mutant "nude": Preliminary investigations, *Acta Pathol. Microbiol. Scand.* **77**:761.

SAHIAR, K., AND SCHWARTZ, R. S., 1966, The immunoglobulin sequence. II. Histological effects of the suppression of $\gamma$M and $\gamma$G antibody synthesis, *Int. Arch. Allergy* **29**:52.

SAINT GEME, J. W., JR., PRINCE, J. T., BURKE, B. A., GOOD, R. A., AND KRIVITT, W., 1966, Impaired cellular resistance to herpes-simplex virus in Wiskott–Aldrich syndrome, *New Engl. J. Med.* **273**:229.

SALAMAN, M. H., 1969, Immunosuppression by oncogenic viruses, *Antibiot. Chemother.* **15**:393.

SANFORD, B. H., KOHN, H. J., DALY, J. J., AND SOO, S. F., 1973, Longterm spontaneous tumor incidence in neonatally thymectomized mice, *J. Immunol.* **110**:1437.

SATO, H., BOYSE, E. A., AOKI, T., IRITANI, C., AND OLD, L. J., 1973, Leukemia associated transplantation antigens related to murine leukemia virus. The X.1 system: immune response controlled by a locus linked to *H-2*, *J. Exp. Med.* **138**:593.

SCHNECK, S. A., AND PENN, I., 1970, Cerebral neoplasms associated with renal transplantation, *Arch. Neurol.* **22**:226.

SCHNECK, S. A., AND PENN, I., 1971, *De-novo* brain tumors in renal-transplant recipients, *Lancet* **1**:983.

SCHWARTZ, R. S., 1965, Immunosuppressive drugs, *Prog. Allergy* **9**:246.

SCHWARTZ, R. S., 1971, Immunoregulation by antibody, *Prog. Immunol.* **1**:1081.

SCHWARTZ, R. S., 1972, Immunoregulation, oncogenic viruses and malignant lymphomas, *Lancet* **1**:1266.

SHACHAT, D. A., FEFER, A., AND MOLONEY, J. B., 1968, Effect of cortisone on oncogenesis by murine sarcoma virus (Moloney), *Cancer Res.* **28**:517.

SHARPSTONE, P., OGG, C. S., AND CAMERON, J. S., 1969, Nephrotic syndrome due to primary renal disease in adults. II. A controlled trial of prednisone and azathioprine, *Brit. Med. J.* **2**:535.

SHEARER, G, M., MOZES, E., HARAN-GHERA, N., AND BENTWICH, Z., 1973, Cellular analysis of immunosuppression to synthetic polypeptide immunogens induced by a murine leukemia virus, *J. Immunol.* **110**:736.

SHUSTER, J., HART, Z., STIMSON, C. W., BROUGH, A. J., AND POULIK, M. D., 1966, Ataxia telangiectasia with cerebellar tumor, *Pediatrics* **37**:776.

SIEGLER, R., 1968, Pathology of murine leukemias, in: *Experimental Leukemia* (M. A. Rich, ed. ), p. 51, Appleton-Century-Crofts, New York.

SJÖGREN, H. O., AND BORUM, K., 1971, Tumor-specific immunity in the course of primary polyoma and Rous tumor development in intact and immunosuppressed rats, *Cancer Res.* **31**:890.

SJÖGREN, H. O., HELLSTRÖM, I., BANSAL, S. C., AND HELLSTRÖM, K. E., 1971, Suggestive evidence that the "blocking antibodies" of tumor-bearing individuals may be antigen–antibody complexes, *Proc. Natl. Acad. Sci.* **68**:1372.

STAPLES, P. J., AND TALAL, N., 1969, Relative inability to induce tolerance in adult NZB and NZB/NZW $F_1$ mice, *J. Exp. Med.* **129**:123.

STARZL, T. E., PENN, I., PUTNUM, C. W., GROTH, C. G., AND HALGRIMSON, C. G., 1971, Iatrogenic alterations of immunologic surveillance in man and their influence on malignancy, *Transpl. Rev.* **7**:112.

STJERNSWARD, J., 1965, Immunodepressive effect of 3-methylcholanthrene: Antibody formation at cellular level and reaction against weakly antigenic homografts, *J. Natl. Cancer Inst.* **35**:885.

STJERNSWARD, J., 1966, Effect of non-carcinogenic and carcinogenic hydrocarbons on antibody forming cells measured at cellular level *in vitro*, *J. Natl. Cancer Inst.* **36**:1189.

STJERNSWARD, J., 1967, Further immunological studies of chemical carcinogenesis, *J. Natl. Cancer Inst.* **38**:515.

STJERNSWARD, J., 1969, Immunosuppression by carcinogens, *Antibiot. Chemother.* **15**:213.

STJERNSWARD, J., JONDAL, M., VANKY, F., WIGZELL, H., AND SEALY, R., 1972, Lymphopenia and change in distribution of human B and T lymphocytes in peripheral blood induced by irradiation for mammary carcinoma, *Lancet* **1**:1352.

STRUM, S. B., PARK, J. K., AND RAPPAPORT, H., 1970, Observation of cells resembling Sternberg–Reed cells in conditions other than Hodgkin's disease, *Cancer* **26**:176.

STUTMAN, O., 1969, Carcinogen-induced immune depression: Absence in mice resistant to chemical oncogenesis, *Science* **166**:620.

STUTMAN, O., AND DUPUY, J. M., 1972, Resistance to Friend leukemia virus in mice: Effect of immunosuppression, *J. Natl. Cancer Inst.* **49**:1283.

STUTMAN, O., YUNIS, E. J., AND GOOD, R. A., 1968, Deficient immunologic functions of NZB mice, *Proc. Soc. Exp. Biol. Med.* **127**:1204.

SWANSON, M., AND SCHWARTZ, R. S., 1967, Immunosuppressive therapy: The relation between clinical response and immunologic competence, *New Engl. J. Med.* **277**:163.

SZAKAL, A. K., AND HANNA, M. G., 1972, Immune suppression and carcinogenesis in hamsters during topical application of 7,12-dimethylbenz(a)anthracene, in: *Conference on Immunology of Carcinogenesis*, p. 173, National Cancer Institute Monograph 35, National Cancer Instute, Bethesda, Md.

TALAL, N., AND BUNIM, J. J., 1964, The development of malignant lymphoma in the course of Sjögren's syndrome, *Am. J. Med.* **36**:529.

TALEB, N., TOHME, S., GHOSTINE, S., BARMADA, B., AND NAHAS, S., 1969, Association d'une ataxie telangiectasie avec une leucemie aigue lymphoblastique, *Presse Med.* **77**:345.

TEAGUE, P. O., YUNIS, E. J., RODEY, G., FISH, A. J., STUTMAN, O., AND GOOD, R. A., 1970, Autoimmune phenomena and renal disease in mice: Role of thymectomy, aging and involution of immunologic capacity, *Lab. Invest.* **22**:121.

TEN BENSEL, R. W., STADLAN, E. M., AND KRIVIT, W., 1966, The development of malignancy in the course of the Aldrich syndrome, *J. Pediat.* **68**:761.

TENNANT, J. R., AND SNELL, G. D., 1968, The *H-2* locus and viral leukemogenesis as studied in congenic strains of mice, *J. Natl. Cancer Inst.* **41**:597.

THOMAS, L., 1959, Discussion, in: *Cellular and Humoral Aspects of the Hypersensitive States* (H. S. Lawrence, ed.), pp. 529–532, Hoeber-Harper, New York.

TING, R. C., 1966, Effect of thymectomy on transplantation resistance induced by polyoma tumor homografts, *Nature (Lond.)* **211**:1000.

TING, R. C., 1967, Tumor induction in thymectomized rats by murine sarcoma virus (Moloney) and properties of the induced virus-free tumor cells, *Proc. Soc. Exp. Biol. Med.* **126**:778.

TING, R. C., AND LAW, L. W., 1965, The role of thymus in transplantation resistance induced by polyoma virus, *J. Natl. Cancer Inst.* **34**:521.

TODARO, G. J., AND HUEBNER, R. J., 1972, The viral oncogene hypothesis: New evidence, *Proc. Natl. Acad. Sci.* **69**:1009.

TRAININ, N., AND LINKER-ISRAELI, M., 1971, Increased incidence of spontaneous lung adenomas in mice following neonatal thymectomy, *Israel J. Med. Sci.* **7**:36.

TURK, J. L., AND BRYCESON, D. M., 1971, Immunological phenomena in leprosy and related diseases, *Advan. Immunol.* **13**:209.

TWOMEY, J. J., JORDAN, P. H., LAUGHTER, A. H., MEUWISSEN, H. J., AND GOOD, R. A., 1970, The gastric disorder in immunoglobulin-deficient patients, *Ann. Int. Med.* **72**:499.

VANDEPUTTE, M., 1969, Antilymphocyte serum and polyoma oncogenesis in rats, *Transpl. Proc.* **1**:100.

VANDEPUTTE, M., AND DE SOMER, P., 1965, Influence of thymectomy on viral oncogenesis in rats, *Nature (Lond.)* **206**:520.

VAN HOOSIER, G. L., GIST, C., AND TRENTIN, J. J., 1968, Enhancement by thymectomy of tumor formation by oncogenic adenoviruses, *Proc. Soc. Exp. Biol. Med.* **128**:467.

VARET, B., LEVY, J. P., LECLERC, J. C., AND KOURILSKY, F. M., 1971, Effect of antithymocytic serum on viral leukemia, erythroblastosis, and sarcoma in mice, *Int. J. Cancer* **7**:313.

VREDEVOE, D. L., AND HAYS, E. F., 1969, Effect of antilymphocytic and antithymocytic sera on the development of mouse lymphoma, *Cancer Res.* **29**:1685.

WAGNER, J. L., AND HAUGHTON, G., 1971, Immunosuppression by antilymphocyte serum and its effects on tumors induced by 2-methylcholanthrene in mice, *J. Natl. Cancer Inst.* **46**:1.

WAHREN, B., AND METCALF, D., 1970, Cytotoxicity *in vitro* of preleukaemic lymphoid cells on syngeneic monolayers of embryo or thymus cells, *Clin. Exp. Immunol.* **7**:373.

WALDER, B. K., ROBERTSON, M. R., AND JEREMY, D., 1971, Skin cancer and immunosuppression, *Lancet* **2**:1282.

WALDMANN, T. A., STROBER, W., AND BLAESE, R. M., 1972, Immunodeficiency disease and malignancy, *Ann. Int. Med.* **77**:605.

WALDORF, D. S., SHEAGREN, J. N., TRAUTMAN, J. R., AND BLOCK, J. B., 1966, Impaired delayed hypersensitivity in patients with lepromatous leprosy, *Lancet* **2**:773.

WEIDEN, P. L., BLAESE, R. M., STROBER, W., BLOCK, J. B., AND WALDMANN, T. A., 1972, Impaired lymphocyte transformation in intestinal lymphangiectasia: Evidence for at least two functionally distinct lymphocyte populations in man, *J. Clin. Invest.* **51**:1319.

WEIR, D. M., MCBRIDE, W., AND NAYSMITH, J. D., 1968, Immune response to a soluble protein antigen in NZB mice, *Nature (Lond.)* **219**:1276.

WOODS, D. A., 1969, Influence of antilymphocyte serum on DMBA induction of oral carcinomas, *Nature (Lond.)* **224**:276.

WORTIS, H. H., 1971, Immunological responses of "nude" mice, *Clin. Exo. Immunol.* **8**:305.

WORTIS, H. H., NEHLSEN, S., AND OWEN, J. J., 1971, Abnormal development of the thymus in "nude" mice, *J. Exp. Med.* **134**:681.

YOUNG, R. R., AUSTEN, K. F., AND MOSER, H. W., 1964, Abnormalities of serum gamma-1-A globulin and ataxia telangiectasia, *Medicine* **43**:423.

YTREDAL, D. O., AND BRADFIELD, J. S., 1972, Seminoma of the testicle: Prophylactic mediastinal irradiation versus periaortic and pelvic irradiation alone, *Cancer* **30**:628.

YUNIS, E. J., MARTINEZ, C., SMITH, J., STUTMAN, O., AND GOOD, R. A., 1969, Spontaneous mammary adenocarcinoma in mice: Influence of thymectomy and reconstitution with thymus grafts or spleen cells, *Cancer Res.* **29**:174.

ZATZ, M. M., MELLORS, R. C., AND LANCE, E. M., 1971, Changes in lymphoid populations of aging CBA and NZB mice, *Clin. Exp. Immunol.* **8**:491.

ZISBLATT, M., AND LILLY, F., 1972, The effect of immunosuppression on oncogenesis by murine sarcoma virus, *Proc. Soc. Exp. Biol. Med.* **141**:1036.

# 6

# Pathogenesis of Plasmacytomas in Mice

MICHAEL POTTER

## 1. Introduction

The malignant plasmacytoma is a rare tumor type that occurs naturally in several mammals—the dog (Osborne *et al.*, 1968), the cat (Farrow and Penny, 1971), the hamster (Cotran and Fortner, 1962), the rat (Bazin *et al.*, 1972), the mouse (Dunn, 1954, 1957), and man (Azar, 1973). Because plasmacytomas occur infrequently, it is difficult to study their pathogenesis. It is possible, however, to induce plasmacytomas in high frequency in a few uniquely susceptible inbred strains of mice by the intraperitoneal implantation of solid plastic materials (Merwin and Algire, 1959; Merwin and Redmon, 1963) or the intraperitoneal injection of mineral oils and related substance (Potter and Robertson, 1960; Potter and Boyce, 1962; Anderson and Potter, 1969). While this unusual method of induction is a laboratory method and has no apparent relationship to any known natural form of plasmacytoma development, it provides a means for studying the pathogenesis of plasmacytomas. In many forms of carcinogenesis, a specific differentiated cell type is the selective target. The reasons for cytotropism in the carcinogenic process are an intriguing problem. In plasma cell tumor formation in mice, the problem is even more complex because a segment of the plasma cell population appears particularly vulnerable. At present, immunology is an area of biology that has captured broad interest, and from many investigations have come a wealth of data on the differentiation, development, physiology, and proliferation of plasma cells. These data provide the background for understanding the normal plasma cell and the process of plasmacytoma formation. In this chapter, the pathogenesis of the induction of peritoneal plasmacytomas will be the main topic. The

MICHAEL POTTER • National Cancer Institute, Laboratory of Cell Biology, Bethesda, Maryland.

underlying mechanisms of peritoneal plasmacytoma formation in the mouse are not yet established, but it is hoped that insight gained from this study will provide a basis for understanding how plasmacytomas may develop "spontaneously" in the mouse and in other species, including man.

## 2. "Spontaneous" Plasmacytomas

### 2.1. Ileocecal Plasmacytomas in Mice

Dunn (1954, 1957) described "spontaneous" plasmacytomas that appeared to develop in the ileocecum of old mice. The smallest lesions detected on routine autopsy were areas of inflammation in the wall of the ileocecum (approximately 5 mm in diameter). The mucosa overlying the area was ulcerated. Within the lesions in the ileocecum, inflammatory reactive tissues containing well-differentiated plasma cells as well as plasma cells with distorted morphology were seen infiltrating the wall of the intestine, the lymphatics, and the regional mesenteric lymph node. Dunn noted that these rare tumors were most commonly seen in C3H mice; however, one case occurred in a Carworth Farms No. 1 mouse, and subsequently Yancey (1964) described a case in a (BALB/c × A/He)F₁ hybrid mouse. Dunn had no difficulty in classifying the large ileocecal tumors as plasmacytomas.

Pilgrim established two C3H plasmacytomas (X5563, X5647) in transplant and sent them to Dunn, who in turn gave them to the author for serological study (Potter *et al.*, 1957). Both tumors were shown to produce immunoglobulin (Potter *et al.*, 1957; Fahey *et al.*, 1960): X5563 produced an IgG ($\gamma_{2a}$ type) M component and X5647 produced an IgA M component. Since the successful transplantation of these two tumors, only three more ileocecal tumors have been transplanted in the mouse (Potter and Fahey, 1960). Yancey (1964) described one of these, YPC-1, an ileocecal plasmacytoma associated with ascites formation that developed in a (BALB/c × A/He)F₁ mouse; this ileocecal tumor was also associated with a small adenocarcinoma of cecum. Three of the transplanted plasmacytomas of ileocecal origin produced IgA myeloma proteins and one an IgG ($\gamma_{2a}$) immunoglobulin.

Pilgrim (1965) made a detailed study of the ileocecal region in old C3H mice and found that over 90% of them had mucosal ulcers in the ileoceum. The small ulcerations in the ileoceum suggest an important pathogenetic sequence, mainly that the ulceration of the mucosa is the primary event which permits the development of infection and a chronically inflamed tissue. Among 125 ileocecums examined by Pilgrim, 28 plasmacytomas were found microscopically; however, none of these was successfully established in transplant.

### 2.2. Ileocecal Immunocytomas in Rats

Bazin *et al.* (1972) identified monoclonal immunoglobulinsecreting tumors in rats and named these tumors "immunocytomas." Immunocytomas are closely related, if not actually homologous, to the ileocecal plasmacytomas in mice. In contrast to the single mesenteric node in mice, the rat has a chain of mesenteric lymph nodes; the cecum is drained by one located near the ileocecal junction, the ileocecal lymph node, and this is where immunocytomas appear to develop.

A review of the literature by Bazin *et al.* (1972) indicated that ileocecal lymph node tumors in the rat have been known for many years, the first description dating back to 1911. The pathological classification of the tumors varied—"malignant lymphoma," "polymorphous cell sarcoma," "lymphoblastic lymphosarcoma," "reticulum cell sarcoma," "lymphosarcoma," and "lymphoblastic reticulosarcoma" having been employed by various authors. The first clue that these tumors were derived from immunoglobulin-secreting cell types was found by Deckers (1963), who demonstrated M components associated with four of these tumors. Immunocytomas in rats are readily transplantable. According to Bazin *et al* (1972), histological and cytological studies show that cell types predominant in immunocytomas are poorly differentiated and cannot be readily classified as in plasmacytomas. However, the imprints and electron micrographs of the tumors are not unlike those of plasmacytomas in mice. Further detailed study is needed.

The histogenesis of these tumors has not been examined, chiefly because of the rarity of primary tumors. Bazin *et al.* (1973) have been able by selective breeding to obtain in strain LOU/Wsl rats a 23% incidence of immunocytomas. The mean age at appearance of immunocytomas is about 12–14 months. The possibility that these tumors originate in the wall of the cecum, as they all appear to do in the mouse, is not at all clear at present. In some earlier studies, ulceration of the ileocecum was described; However, the subsequent descriptions by Bazin's group suggest that the tumors involve the gut wall secondarily.

Roughly 73% of transplantable immunocytomas (Bazin *et al.*, 1973) have been shown to secrete immunoglobulin: of 184 examined, 23 or 3.3% produced IgM, 0.6% IgA, 35.9% $IgG_1$, 6% $IgG_{2a}$, 0.6% $IgG_{2b}$, 6.0% $IgG_{2c}$, and 34.2% IgE. The unusual and exciting finding of Bazin's group has been the existence of a large number of IgE myeloma proteins (this is the immunoglobulin class associated with reaginic antibody and with helminth infestations). IgE is a rare myeloma type in man and has not been seen in the mouse. The immunocytomas in rats offer an unusual new model system involving a very specialized component of the immune system.

## 2.3. Comment

The association of immunoglobulin-producing tumors in mice and rats with the gastrointestinal tract suggests that a regional disease in the gastrointestinal tract is a pathogenetic factor. The infestation of rats and mice with helminths and protozoans coupled with the normal flora could provide the specific agent that invades and damages the mucosa, thus beginning a chain of events from chronic inflammation to plasmacytoma development.

## 3.1. *Plasmacytomagenic Peritoneal Granuloma Inducing Agents*

Merwin and Algire (1959) first found peritoneal plasmacytomas in BALB/c mice that had been implanted with Millipore diffusion chambers (MDC) containing allogeneic tissue. In later experiments, Merwin and Redmon (1963) placed MDC of different sizes, with and without tissue, as well as components of the chambers and related materials, intraperitoneally in BALB/c mice to determine the nature of the plasmacytomagenic material (Table 1). Fifty-four percent of mice implanted with large empty MDC, 21 mm in diameter, developed plasmacytomas. A much lower incidence was observed with empty 17.5 mm MD6 and no plasmacytomas were obtained with MDC of 14 mm diameter. Tissue-containing 17.5 mm MDC induced a greater incidence of plasmacytomas than empty chambers, suggesting an additive effect of the tissue. Discs of only Millipore membrane or Lucite induced 10% and 18.5% plasmacytomas, respectively. Sharp-edged borings from Lucite blocks 1 mm in diameter were placed intraperitoneally and found to be highly effective materials; 50% of the mice

TABLE 1

*Materials That Evoke a Chronic Peritoneal Granuloma and Plasmacytomas in BALB/c Mice*

| Material | Number of plasmacytomas total (%) | Reference |
|---|---|---|
| 21.0-mm Millipore chamber, empty | 14/26 (54) | Merwin and Redmon (1963) |
| 17.5-mm Millipore chamber, empty | 2/27 (7.3) | Merwin and Redmon (1963) |
| 17.5-mm Millipore chamber + tumor tissue | 21/96 (22) | Merwin and Redmon (1963) |
| 14.0-mm Millipore chamber, empty | 0/25 (0) | Merwin and Redmon (1963) |
| 14.0-mm Millipore chamber + tumor tissue | 7/177 (3.99) | Merwin and Redmon (1963) |
| 14- or 17.5-mm Millipore discs | 3/30 (10) | Merwin and Redmon (1963) |
| 14- or 15.5-mm Lucite discs | 2/11 (18.5) | Merwin and Redmon (1963) |
| Lucite borings | 11/20 (56) | Merwin and Redmon (1963) |
| Freund's adjuvant, 0.5 ml ×1 | 37/64 (57.8) | Potter (1967) |
| Lieberman's staphylococcal adjuvant | | Potter (1967) |
| Primol D, 0.5 ml ×1 | 27/56 (39.2) | Potter (1967) |
| Bayol F, 0.5 ml ×3, bimonthly intervals | 78/128 (61.0) | Potter and Boyce (1962) |
| Bayol F, 0.5 ml ×1 | 14/119 (11.7) | Potter Boyce (1962) |
| Drakeol 6VR, 0.5 ml ×3 | 15/32 (47.0) | Potter (1967) |
| Drakeol 6VR, 0.5 ml ×1 | 3/32 (9.4) | Potter (1967) |
| Pristane (2,6,10,14-tetramethyl-pentadecane), 0.5 ml ×3 | 73/120[a] (61) | Anderson and Potter (1969) |
| Pristane, 0.5 ml ×1 | 8/55[a] (14.3) | this chapter |
| Squalane | — (23) | Anderson (1970) |
| 7n-Hexyloctadecane | — (60) | Anderson (1970) |

[a] Based on incidence at 300 days, see Fig. 1.

developed plasmacytomas. Discs and chambers caused the formation of both fibrosarcomas and plasmacytomas. The fibrosarcomas arose in the capsules surrounding the discs or chambers, and the plasmacytomas were found elsewhere on the peritoneal surfaces.

The induction in 1959 of plasmacytomas by MDC containing allogeneic tissue suggested that some component of the chambers, in particular the allogeneic tissue, was producing a sustained immune response. Other agents that stimulated immune responses over extensive periods of time were tested for plasmacytomagenic activity in the BALB/c peritoneum. At that time, Lieberman *et al.* (1960) had shown the effectiveness of a staphylococcal adjuvant mixture for inducing ascites fluid containing antibody in mice. This mixture contained 1 part incomplete Freund's adjuvant (8.5 parts Bayol F, 1.5 parts mannide monooleate) and 1 part heat-killed staphylococci. An intraperitoneal injection of 0.5 ml of this mixture induced plasmacytomas in BALB/c mice (Potter and Robertson, 1960), but multiple injections were more effective (Potter and Boyce, 1962). Since this adjuvant mixture contained several different materials, tests were made on individual components to determine whether any alone was plasmacytomagenic. It was found that the mineral oil component Bayol F actively induced plasmacytomas (Potter and Boyce, 1962). A systematic dose study was not made, but it was found that three 0.5-ml injections of the oil spaced 2 months apart were more effective than a single injection (Potter and Boyce, 1962; Potter, 1967). A variety of light and heavy white mineral oils including oils of USP grade that contain no fluorescent materials, e.g., Primol D, Drakeol 6VR, and Ervol, have been shown to induce plasmacytomas in BALB/c mice (Potter, 1967; Anderson, 1970). Mineral oils are chemically heterogeneous, and only a few chemically defined light oily substances are available. The straight-chain alkane *n*-hexadecane proved to be highly toxic (Potter, unpublished observations that could not be evaluated); however, a branched-chain, low viscosity oily substance, pristane (2,6,10,14-tetramethylpentadecane), was very plasmacytomagenic (Anderson and Potter, 1969). Pristane is well tolerated by mice, and when intraperitoneally given to BALB/c mice in three 0.5-ml doses spaced 2 months apart induced a high incidence (60–70%) of plasmacytomas (Fig. 1) (Anderson and Potter, 1969). In subsequent studies, Anderson (1970) has shown that squalane and the synthetically prepared 7*n*-hexyloctadecane are plasmacytomagenic. These compounds, however, are available only in limited quantities.

Crude petroleum from various geographic sources contains from 0.03 to 0.5% pristane (Bendoraitis *et al.*, 1962). Commercially, pristane is obtained from the livers of plankton-feeding vertebrates taken from the general vicinity of the Gulf of Maine (Blumer *et al.*, 1969). Blumer and his associates have outlined the migration of pristane in the food chain of marine animals (Fig. 2) (Blumer, 1965; Blumer and Thomas, 1965; Blumer *et al.*, 1969). Pristane is derived from phytol produced by phytoplankton. Phytol is converted to pristane and other intermediates by zooplankton and then consumed by plankton-feeding vertebrates such as the basking shark, sperm whale, alewife, and herring, where it is stored in the body fat and liver. The proportion of intermediates and other derivatives (Fig.

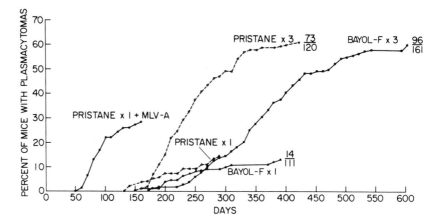

FIGURE 1. Induction of plasmacytomas. The percentage of plasmacytomas is the total number of plasmacytomas over the total number of mice at the start of the experiment and represents the total yield. Each curve represents the average of several experiments. "Pristane ×1" and "Pristane ×1 + MLV-A" are the data from three experiments (Potter *et al.*, 1973) in Table 4. The "Pristane ×1" group has been updated. "Pristane ×3" represents two experiments run in 1969 and 1971. "Bayol-F ×3" represents three experiments run in 1960, 1962, and 1970. "Bayol-F ×1" represents three experiments run in 1960 and 1961 (Potter, 1967; Potter and Boyce, 1962).

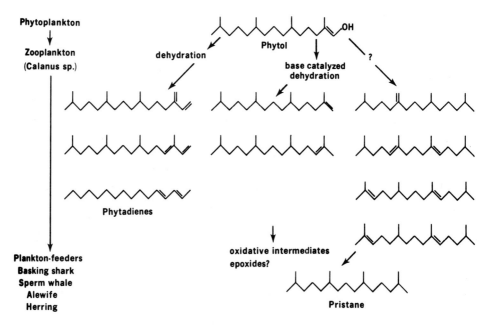

FIGURE 2. Isoprenoid hydrocarbons in the marine food chain. The data in this chart were derived from the publications of Dr. Max Blumer and associates of the Woods Hole Oceanographic Institute (Blumer, 1965; Blumer and Thomas, 1965; Blumer *et al.*, 1969).

2) found in the body fat of zooplankton remains much the same in the vertebrate tissues, as these compounds are not further metabolized. From 1 to 3% of commercially pure pristane may contain mono- and diolefins described and identified by Blumer and colleagues (Blumer, 1965; Blumer and Thomas, 1965; Blumer *et al.*, 1969) as well as traces of squalene. The oxidation of olefins could give rise to epoxide derivatives. It is of interest, then, that Van Duuren *et al.* (1963, 1967) have shown that compounds such as 1,2-epoxyhexadecane and hexaepoxy-squalene are weakly carcinogenic for the mouse epidermis. The possibility that pristane contains potential carcinogenic materials is being investigated currently in our laboratory.*

The earliest plasmacytomas are detected between 138 and 180 days after the first injection of oil and continue thereafter to develop until the mice are 2 yr old. The rate at which plasmacytomas develop varies with the type of oil used. With three injections of heterogeneous light oil such as Bayol F, plasmacytomas develop slowly over a prolonged period (Fig. 1) (180–600 days); by contrast, with three injections of pristane the tumors develop precipitously between 150 and 300 days after the first injection of oil.

The more rapid formation of tumors with pristane is as yet unexplained but suggests that pristane itself has a special property which accelerates plasmacytoma development or that it contains a cocarcinogenic substance as described above.

As may be seen from Fig. 1 three injections of oil given over a 4-month period are much more effective than a single injection.

### 3.2. Genetic Basis of Susceptibility

There have been several attempts to induce plasmacytomas in other strains of mice by both the implantation of plastic discs and the injection of mineral oils (Merwin and Redmon, 1963; Potter, 1967; Yamada *et al.*, 1969). A summary of the existing data is given in Table 2. As may be seen, most other inbred strains tried have been found to be resistant. An occasional plasmacytoma has been observed, but in all cases except NZB the incidence is far below that observed in the BALB/c. Several types of first-generation hybrids of BALB/c and other strains have also been tested. (BALB/c × C57BL)F₁ and (BALB/c × A/He)F₁ have a low incidence. An exceptional hybrid is the (NZB × BALB/c)F₁, in which an unusually high incidence approaching that in BALB/c was induced (Goldstein *et al.*, 1966). This observation prompted Noel Warner of the Hall Institute in Melbourne to investigate NZB itself. Warner (personal communication) has obtained an incidence of plasmacytomas in NZB of approximately 40%, clearly indicating that this strain of mouse is highly susceptible. The development of autoimmune disease and its complications in NZB mice decreases the yield of plasmacytomas.

*The author wishes to thank Dr. Max Blumer of the Oceanographic Institute at Woods Hole for pointing out this interesting possibility.

TABLE 2

*Effect of Intraperitoneal Implantation of Plastics or Injection of Mineral Oil in Strains of Mice Other Than BALB/c*

| | Number of plasmacytomas/total | |
|---|---|---|
| | Plastic | Oil |
| Inbred strain | | |
| C3H, C3Hf | 4/224[a] | 1/55[b] |
| DBA/2 | 0/63[a] | 0/36[b] |
| C57BL/6 | 0/28[a] | |
| C57BL/Ka | — | 0/52[b] |
| SWR | 1/25[a] | 0/30[b] |
| A/He | — | 0/26[b] |
| AL/N | — | 1/59[b] |
| Hybrids | | |
| (NZB × BALB/c)F₁ | | 7/31[c] |
| (BALB/c × A/He)F₁ | 3/40[a] | |
| (BALB/c × DBA/2)F₁ | 0/14[a] | 0/82[b] |
| (BALB/c × AL/N)F₁ | | 4/32[b] |
| (BALB/c × C57BL/Ka)F₁ | | 5/25[b] |
| (BALB/c × NH)F₁ | | 2/40[b] |

[a] Adapted from Merwin and Redmon (1963).
[b] Potter (1967).
[c] Goldstein *et al.* (1966).

## 3.3. The Peritoneal Site

Thus far, plasmacytomas have been induced only in the peritoneal cavity. Injection of oils or adjuvants subcutaneously results in the formation of large cysts. Fibrosarcomas develop in the cyst capsules surrounding adjuvants but have not been observed thus far around loculated subcutaneous mineral oils (Potter, unpublished observations). No subcutaneous plasmacytomas have been found in the mouse; however, Oppenheimer *et al.*, (1955) reported one in a rat that had received a cellophane implant into the subcutaneous tissues. The peritoneal site as compared to other sites provides (1) a large area over which oil or plastic material may be distributed and (2) a potential space in which cells may enter. The peritoneum contains a population of free cells, the peritoneal exudate cells, that probably provide the precursors of plasmacytoma cells. The physiological function of these cells is to police the peritoneal space. The peritoneum of the mouse is very resistant to infection with most common bacteria, and this reflects in part the effectiveness of the local cellular defense system. Peritoneal exudate cells are macrophages, small and large lymphocytes, mast cells, and mesothelial cells (Carr, 1967). Peritoneal exudate cells originate from circulating cells (Volkman, 1966; Koster and McGregor, 1971) and from the small patches of lymphoreticular tissue in the omentum, the "tâches laiteuses" of Ranvier or milk spots (Carr, 1967). The precursors of peritoneal macrophages are found chiefly in the bone marrow and blood (Volkman, 1966), while the precursors of the small and large lymphocytes are in the thoracic duct fluid (Koster and McGregor, 1971). In rats presensitized to *Listeria monocytogenes* antigen and then challenged intraperitoneally with *Listeria* organisms, the influx of short-lived, large and medium lymphocytes was particularly vigorous (Koster and McGregor, 1971). Evidence that long-lived small lymphocytes also enter the peritoneum could not be found in this study.

Inflammation is an important feature of plasmacytoma formation in the mouse. The only studies dealing directly with this problem (Takakura *et al.*, 1966; Hollander *et al.*, 1968) demonstrated that the subcutaneous administration of 0.1 or 0.5 mg cortisol five times per week to BALB/c mice continuously during and after the three intraperitoneal injections of mineral oil entirely prevented or vastly reduced the incidence of plasmacytomas. The total number of peritoneal exudate cells was $29.4 \times 10^4/\text{mm}^3$ in mineral oil treated mice and $1.4 \times 10^3/\text{mm}^3$ in those treated with cortisol plus mineral oil. Histologically the granulomatous tissue was reduced to only small pinpoint lesions on the omentum, and most of the mineral oil apparently remained in the peritoneal space.

Antigenic stimulation from the normal microbial flora is known to play an important role in plasmacytoma formation. McIntire and Princler (1969) found a greatly reduced incidence of plasmacytomas in germ-free mice injected with mineral oil, and we (Asofsky and Potter, unpublished observations) have confirmed this. A relatively large number of myeloma proteins (about 5%) induced in BALB/c mice have been found to bind antigens of bacterial origin (Potter, 1970, 1971); many of these antigens are produced by microorganisms isolated from our BALB/c mouse colony. These observations suggest that cells sensitized by the normal microbial flora are potential precursors of some plasmacytomas. The migration of these cells into the peritoneum where plasmacytomas develop may require antigen to be present in the peritoneum, or possibly the sustained inflammation in the peritoneum may simply increase the entry of all circulating cells.

A characteristic of peritoneal plasmacytomas in the mouse is the relatively high frequency (66%) of tumors differentiated to make IgA-class myeloma proteins (see Potter, 1972). In multiple myeloma in man, the preponderant class is IgG (Zawadzki *et al.* 1967). IgA-producing cells are found normally in great abundance in the lamina propria of the gastrointestinal tract, where they represent over 80% of all immunoglobulin-producing cells (Crabbé *et al.*, 1970). The bulk of IgA produced by lamina propria plasma cells is secreted across the mucosal epithelium into the lumen of the gut (Tomasi and Bienenstock, 1968). Comoglio and Guglielmone (1973) have demonstrated that IgA produced by subcutaneously transplanted plasmacytomas can be actively secreted across the gastointestinal epithelium or into the saliva. This suggests that the proximity of plasma cells to the mucosal epithelium is not a necessary prerequisite for secretion. Secretory IgA is thought to interact with antigen in the lumen of the gastrointestinal tract and with other secretions and thereby form a first line of defense for the organism. The peritoneum has not yet been implicated in the formation of secretory immunoglobulin, and thus the location of IgA-producing plasmacytomas here may reflect an unnatural location. This question cannot be settled, however, until the predominant class of immunoglobulins formed in omental tissues and milk spots is determined.

IgA cells in the lamina propria of the intestine apparently turn over rapidly. Mattioli and Tomasi (1973) have estimated the half-life of the major population of IgA-producing cells in this tissue to be 4.7 days. Presumably the bulk of the new cells arrive from the circulation and constitute a potential source of precursors for plasmacytomas.

### 3.4. Role of the Oil Granuloma

Because of the ease of injecting oily liquid substances intraperitoneally, the oil granuloma has been the most extensively studied peritoneal granulomatous tissue. This tissue begins to form almost immediately after the injection of oil. The oil first causes an inflammatory reaction characterized by the presence of lymphocytes, granulocytes, and plasma cells in the mesentery; furthermore, macrophages become very active and begin phagocytizing oil droplets. In the process the oil-laden macrophages adhere to the peritoneal surfaces and begin the buildup of oil granuloma tissue. This consists primarily of oil-laden macrophages or large drops of oil surrounded by many macrophages. Eventually these oil-containing cells become organized on the peritoneal surfaces and form a very extensive new tissue that is vascularized and covered with mesothelium (Potter and MacCardle, 1964).

#### 3.4.1. Growth Factors

Some insight into the mechanism of action of the oil granuloma in plasmacytoma development has been derived from studies on the transplantation of relatively low numbers of primary plasmacytoma cells (Potter *et al.*, 1972). It was found that when doses of $10^5$ or fewer cells obtained from the peritoneal fluid of a mouse with a primary plasmacytoma were transplanted intraperitoneally in normal BALB/c mice only three of 15 tumors grew progressively. By contrast, $10^5$ or fewer cells from all of these same tumors grew in mice previously conditioned with a single intraperitoneal injection of pristane. The tumors developed within several weeks, and in all the cases studied the immunoglobulins produced by the tumors were the same as in the original primary tumor. In cases where the primary host lacked a demonstrable M component, the M components in all the recipients had the same electrophoretic mobility. In some of the cases investigated, as few as $10^3$ primary plasmacytoma cells were successfully transplanted. In subsequent unpublished studies, it has been found that the conditioning injection of pristane can be given either simultaneously with the cells or within seven days. These results indicate that the injection of pristane either directly or indirectly provides factors that favor the progressive proliferation on neoplastic plasma cells. Hypothetically these same factors may play a role in the development of the primary neoplasmas. There is some indirect but suggestive evidence from *in vitro* studies of plasmacytoma growth that special factors may be required for the growth of plasmacytoma cells. Namba and Hanaoka (1972), in attempting to adapt the MOPC104E plasmacytoma to tissue culture, noted that their plasmacytoma cells grew initially in culture for a period of about 30 days and then began declining in numbers; simultaneously, the macrophages disappeared from the culture flask. Namba and Hanaoka (1972) were able to rescue cultures of MOPC104E cells by transfer of the declining cell cultures to dishes containing proliferating phagocytic cells, or by culturing the cells with conditioned medium from various types of cultures of phagocytic cells, including adherent cells obtained from the tumor itself, spleen, or peritoneum. Conditioned medium obtained from fibroblasts did not contain the factor. Normal mouse serum also contained a factor that stimulated growth. The potency of mouse serum could be increased over eighteenfold that of normal serum if the mice were previously injected intraperitoneally with 0.2 ml complete Freund's adjuvant. The peak activity was observed on the sixteenth day after injection but remained high for over 30 days. These workers also found that mitotic activity of MOPC104E cells could be stimulated by the addition of $3',5'$-cyclic AMP $(0.5 \, \mu/\text{ml})$ to the cultures.

In an independent study, Metcalf (1973) has been able to obtain microcolonies of plasmacytoma cells in agar. In this study, 25 different plasmacytomas were tested directly from *in vivo* transplant lines. Nineteen produced colonies in agar when a factor from whole mouse blood or from washed red blood cells of mouse or other mammals was added. Cloning efficiencies from 0.01 to 21.6% were obtained. The colony-enhancing factor was not present in normal serum but could be obtained from the serum of endotoxin-infected mice.

These *in vitro* studies of plasmacytoma growth indicate that special factors are required for growth and that they can be supplied from various sources. The Namba and Hanaoka (1972) serum factor appearing after intraperitoneal injection of Freund's adjuvant, which is also obtained from cultures of phagocytic cells, may possibly be produced by the large population of phagocytic cells in the oil granuloma. The serum factor described by Metcalf (1973) appearing after the injection of endotoxin may be similar to or even different from the factor described by Namba and Hanaoka. Other nutritional factors have been described by Park *et al.* (1971).

### 3.4.2. Local Immunosuppression

A second biological action of the oil granuloma on plasmacytoma formation may be in the form of a protective effect on tumor cell growth. It is known that transplantable plasmacytoma cells have several types of potential cell surface antigens, e.g., PC1 and XVEA (Aoki and Takahashi, 1972; Herberman and Aoki, 1972), tumor-specific transplantation antigens (Lespinats, 1969; Röllinghoff *et al.*, 1973; Williams and Krueger, 1972), and immunoglobulin idiotypic determinants (Lynch *et al.*, 1972). Since these may also be found on developing primary tumor cells, the question of how the tumor escapes from some form of immune elimination arises. Possibly the oil granuloma has an immunosuppressive action.

Kripke and Weiss (1970) postulated that the mineral oil might be immunosuppressive, but in their studies they looked for a general immunosuppressive effect and were able to obtain minimal evidence. We have observed that an established immunity to a transplantable plasmacytoma (Adj PC5) can be abrogated in mice that have been previously conditioned with an intraperitoneal injection of pristane (Potter and Walters, 1973). The effect is local, however, and occurs only when tumor cell challenges are introduced intraperitoneally into mice that have received a prior intraperitoneal injection of pristane. Similar challenge doses of tumor cells given subcutaneously to immune intraperitoneal pristane–treated mice were rejected as efficiently as in normal mice.

Several intriguing actions of macrophages on tumor immunity have been demonstrated in other systems that might be related to local abrogation of immunity in intraperitoneal pristane–conditioned mice. Hersey and MacLennan (1973) observed, for example, that macrophages can protect lymphoma tumor cells from cell-mediated and humoral immune cytolysis. In this system, they postulate that macrophages can actually phagocytize tumor cells, or provide protection by coming in close contact with them. They envisage that the macrophages in some way facilitate in clearing the antigenic materials from the fluid mosaic cell surface, thereby protecting against cytotoxic effects.

### 3.5. Role of Viruses in Plasmacytoma Development

Viruses have been strongly implicated in peritoneal plasmacytomagenesis in mice, but their precise mode of action has not yet been defined. Two general ways in which viruses may be involved in plasmacytoma formation are (1) activation of endogenous viruses and (2) infection with a plasmacytomagenic virus. There is evidence to support both modes of action. First, there is substantial evidence that C-type RNA viruses of the murine leukemia virus (MuLV) complex are activated in plasmacytoma cells, and, second, a defective C-type RNA virus (Abelson virus or MLV-A) has been shown to induce plasmacytomas rapidly in pristane-primed mice (Potter et al., 1973).

#### 3.5.1. Endogenous Viruses

In a number of studies, C-type RNA viral particles (Watson et al., 1970; Volkman and Krueger, 1973), or viral-associated antigens (Stockert et al., 1971; Hyman et al., 1972; Takahashi et al., 1970, 1971a,b; Aoki and Takahashi, 1972; Herberman and Aoki, 1972) have been demonstrated in transplantable plasmacytomas. The etiological significance of these findings is clouded by the fact that C-type RNA viruses of the MuLV system have been implicated in most neoplasms of the lymphoreticular tissues in mice and by the fact that the BALB/c strain of mouse in which these tumors developed is known to carry several different forms of C-type RNA viruses. Furthermore, many of these studies have been done with tissue culture lines of plasmacytomas, and in vitro cultivation alone is known to activate latent C-type RNA viruses (Aaronson et al., 1969). Aoki et al. (1973) have more

closely implicated the activation of C-type RNA viruses in plasmacytoma formation by demonstrating virus particles in primary plasmacytomas.

By use of the technique of immunoelectromicroscopy, at least three different
serological kinds of C-type particles have been demonstrated in primary BALB/c
plasmacytomas. One of these carries the viral envelope antigens (VEA) of
Gross-type leukemia virus; a second type of particle, MuMAV (murine
myeloma–associated virus), has the XVEA envelope virion antigen; and a third
lacks either of these. Evidence that transplantable plasmacytomas carry these
same types of viral particles has been available for some time (Aoki and Takahashi,
1972; Herberman and Aoki, 1972). The findings of Aoki *et al.* (1973) suggest that
these C-type RNA viruses become activated during plasmacytoma development,
but do not prove that virus activation itself is a plasmacytomagenic event. The fact
that three different serological types of viruses were found indicates that the viral
activation event also involved several types of viruses. All three types may be
equally capable of transforming cells on activation, or possibly only one has
plasmacytomagenic properties. Therefore, much remains to be learned about the
endogenous C-type RNA viruses in the BALB/c mouse.

There have been several studies of endogenous viruses in the BALB/c mouse.
Peters *et al.* (1972*b,c*) have studied the appearance of the group-specific gs antigen
and the infectious viruses in normal and tumor-bearing BALB/c mice during the
entire life span. To study infectious C-type viruses, Peters *et al.* (1972*a,b,c*) added
10% spleen extracts from BALB/c mice of various ages with and without tumors to
BALB/c and NIH embryo cells and cocultivated the cells for 19–20 days, at which
time the cultures were assayed for viral antigens with a complement fixation test
using antiserum from rats immunized with tumors induced by the Moloney strain
of murine sarcoma virus (M-MSV). They found that infectious virus, i.e., virus
that propagated in embryo cells following infection with spleen extracts, was
present in only 10% of BALB/c mice under 6 months of age, but thereafter
46–62% of the mice produced infectious virus. Isolations of viruses occurred on
both Fv–1$^n$ and Fv–1$^b$ indicator cell types.

Isolations of infectious viruses on BALB/c cells were relatively infrequent (less
than 6%) before 12 months of age but thereafter increased in frequency and
exceeded isolations on NIH cells. These results suggested the existence of at least
two viruses in the MuLV complex with different tropisms, an N-tropic virus that
occurred at 6 months and afterward and a B-tropic virus that appeared usually
after 2 years of age.

These interesting findings may be related to the long latent period for the
development of plasmacytomas after the injection of mineral oils such as Bayol F
(Fig. 1). It has been noted many times that heterogeneous oils such as Bayol F
evoke plasmacytomas with a much longer latent period than that of pristane-
induced ones. The latent period with the oils coincides with the time at which
spontaneous activation of endogenous C-type viruses was found in the study of
Peters *et al.* (1972*a,b,c*).

The infectivity of extracts of reticulum cell and other neoplasms of BALB/c
mice has been examined in a variety of studies (Table 3), beginning with the

TABLE 3

Effect of Injection of Extracts of Tumor or Other Tissues from BALB/c Mice into 0- to 7-Day-Old BALB/c on the Incidence of Lymphoreticular Neoplasms

| Tissue source | Properties of virus | | Lymphoreticular neoplasms | | | | | | | | | References |
|---|---|---|---|---|---|---|---|---|---|---|---|---|
| | XC test | N-or-tropism | Untreated control | | | Tissue control | | | Injected extract | | | |
| | | | Number of mice | Percent tumors | LP[a] | Number of mice | Percent tumors | LP[a] | Number of mice | Percent tumors | LP[a] | |
| MCA sarcoma | + | B | 32 | 16 | 22–24 | 42 | 13 | 18–24 | 20 | 45 | <12 | Bassombrio (1973) |
| MCA carcinoma | + | — | — | — | — | — | — | — | 43 | 44 | 18–24 | Peters et al. (1973) |
| Lymphoma | + | B | — | — | — | 904[b] | 12.5 | 48–49 | 470 | 32 | — | |
| | | non-B | — | — | — | — | — | — | 990 | 13 | — | |
| Reticulosarcoma | + | B | — | — | — | 85[c] | 15 | — | 68[c] | 59 | — | Ebbesen et al. (1973) |
| | + | N | — | — | — | — | — | — | 30[c] | 40 | — | |
| Reticulum cell sarcoma | ND | — | 70 | 23 | — | — | — | — | 66 | 60 | — | Ebbesen et al. (1968) |
| | ND | ND | 183 | 1 | — | — | — | — | 150 | 47.5[d] | 2–10 | Stansly and Soulé (1962) |

[a] LP, Average latent period in months.
[b] CoMul-negative mice injected with tumor or with spleen of tumor-bearing mouse.
[c] Pathogen-free BALB/c.
[d] Neoplasms only; hyperplasms were excluded.

observations of Stansly and Soulé (1962), who first noted the lymphoma-inducing properties of extracts of a reticulum cell sarcoma from a BALB/c mouse. They injected the Ehrlich ascites tumor into 15 newborn BALB/c mice, two of which developed reticulum cell sarcomas between 330 and 354 days later. Cell-free extracts of these tumors induced lymphomas (reticulum cell neoplasms and lymphosarcomas) in 47.5% of BALB/c mice. Ebbesen *et al* (1968) observed that conventional BALB/c female mice inoculated with extracts of tissues from mice with reticulosarcomas developed an increased incidence of reticulum cell sarcomas at about 19 months of age. In conventional mice, many of these tumors were shown to be associated with immunoglobulin production (paraproteinemia) and plasma cell morphology (Rask-Nielsen *et al.* 1968). Peters *et al.* (1973), Basombrio (1973), and Ebbesen *et al.* (1973) have investigated the ability of tissue extracts of BALB/c origin known to contain C-type RNA viruses to increase lymphoma development in BALB/c mice. In general, extracts containing B-tropic C-type RNA viruses were more effective than extracts containing N-tropic C-type RNA viruses. In the experiments of Ebbesen *et al.* (1973), pathogen-free BALB/c recipients were used, and only a few of the neoplasms were associated with paraproteinemia.

Aaronson and Stephenson (1973) have also found evidence of at least two types of endogenous C-type viruses in BALB/c, which they named BALB:virus-1 and BALB:virus-2. These viruses were isolated from BALB/c cells by *in vitro* exposure of cells to 20 $\mu$g/ml of IDU (iododeoxyuridine) and then cocultivation of these cells with NIH-3T3 cells or with NRK (normal rat kidney) cells. The two viruses were separated by their respective tropisms in NIH $\times$ (NIH $\times$ BALB/c)$F_1$ cells. The activation of the respective viruses is apparently controlled by separate genetic loci which segregate in appropriate backcrosses. The BALB:viruses-1 grows in both NIH and NRK cells, and the BALB:virus-2 grows only in NRK cells. Serologically both viruses can be neutralized by antisera that are specific for Gross-type MuLV (rat anti–AKR lymphoma); in addition, BALB:virus-2 is neutralized by an antiserum to an MuLV isolated from NZB mice.

It has been known for some time that strain NZB tissues have many C-type virus particles belonging to the MuLV complex, but these are not infectious for any of the standard types of indicator cells. Most viruses of the MuLV system can rescue murine sarcoma virus from nonproducer transformed cells.

Levy and Pincus (1970) cocultivated NZB cells with a hamster cell line that had been transformed with Moloney murine sarcoma virus and rescued a pseudotype virus, M-MSV(NZB), that was infectious for (NRK) cells but not for BALB/c or NIH mouse cells.

### 3.5.2. Intracisternal A Particles

Intracisternal A particles (double-membrane particles that bud from the rough endoplasmic reticulum) have been found by electron microscopy in every plasmacytoma of BALB/c origin thus far examined (Dalton *et al.*, 1961; Dalton and Potter, 1968). In transplantable tumors, large numbers of particles are often seen. Relatively pure preparations of the particles have been isolated from plasmacytomas and found to contain a small amount of RNA (Kuff *et al.*, 1968, 1972), a DNA polymerase enzyme with somewhat unusual substrate requirements (Wilson and Kuff, 1972), and a structural protein that differs from gs antigen (Kuff *et al.*, 1972) of the MuLV system. Furthermore, intracisternal A particles do not have the MuLV associated gs antigens.

Intracisternal A particles, have not yet been shown to be infective for any other cell type as yet, and thus it has not been possible to demonstrate that they play a role in plasmacytoma formation. A number of other neoplastic and normal cell types have also been shown to have these particles (Wivel and Smith, 1971). In most studies of normal plasma cells, intracisternal A particles have not been found. If these particles represent a defective virus, it is possible that their activation may play a role in plasmacytoma development. Thus far, however, intracisternal A particles have been found to have an intracytoplasmic location, and they probably do not affect the cell membrane.

### 3.5.3. Comment

The presence of endogenous C-type RNA viruses in plasmacytomas presents several questions. For example (1) Can any or all of the endogenous C-type viruses or the intracisternal A particles transform plasma cells, or is this restricted to viruses with special plasmacytotropic properties? (2) Is the restricted strain susceptibility of BALB/c and NZB related to a specific virus? None of these questions can be conclusively answered with existing data. There is, however, some suggestive evidence that specific forms of C-type RNA viruses may be involved. First, a B-tropic virus of BALB/c origin has been associated with the production of reticulum cell neoplasms in BALB/c mice (Table 3). Some of these tumors have morphological characteristics of plasma cells, i.e., the plasma cell leukemias of Rask-Nielsen (Ebbesen *et al.*, 1968) and paraproteinemia (Rask-Nielsen *et al.*, 1968). These reticular neoplasms may be the type produced by an immunocytotropic or plasmacytotropic virus in the *intact* mouse. The intraperitoneal injection of mineral oil may reveal other actions of these endogenous viruses, and for a variety of reasons they may now be able to transform some types of fully differentiated plasma cells. In the BALB/c mouse, the IgA-forming plasma cells appear to be a particularly vulnerable population of immunocytes.

The striking association of plasmacytoma development with specific inbred strains BALB/c and NZB could be related to a special virus. A possible example might be a rat-cell tropic virus found in NZB (Levy and Pincus, 1970) and BALB/c (Aaronson and Stephenson, 1973).

### 3.5.4. *Rapid Induction of Plasmacytomas in Pristane-Primed Mice by Abelson Virus*

A method for rapidly inducing plasmacytomas in BALB/c mice has been developed using pristane and Abelson virus (MLV-A) (Potter *et al.*, 1973). Adult mice are given a single 0.5-ml injection of pristane and 39–57 days later an injection of MLV-A. Plasmacytomas and lymphosarcomas begin to develop within 21 days after the injection of the virus, and 43–60% of the mice ultimately develop lymphosarcomas and 25–36% plasmacytomas (Table 4 and Fig. 1). The plasmacytomas develop long before the appearance of plasmacytomas in mice that receive only a single injection of pristane (Table 4 and Fig. 1). The rapidity with which these plasmacytomas develop indicates that they are derived from cells that have been transformed by MLV-A. The predominant form of immunoglobulin is IgA.

MLV-A was originally isolated by Abelson and Rabstein (1970a,b) from a BALB/c mouse that had received prednisolone continuously from birth and an intraperitoneal injection of Moloney leukemia virus (MolLV) (Pfizer lot 3042–278) at 28 days of age. The purpose of the prednisolone was to maintain a steroid-induced atrophy of the thymus. It had been previously reported (Moloney, 1962; Dunn and Deringer, 1968) that MolLV produced different types of reticular neoplasms in surgically thymectomized mice than in intact hosts. In the intact host, the tropism of the virus was for thymic cells (Dunn et al., 1961). In thymectomized hosts, myeloid leukemias and reticulum cell neoplasms developed. In the Abelson and Rabstein study (1970a), of 85 mice that were maintained on high doses of prednisolone and injected with MolLV, 50 developed lymphocytic leukemia, seven granulocytic neoplasms, one a stem cell leukemia, and six lymphosarcoma. One mouse that developed a lymphosarcoma at 93 days of age was the source of MLV-A. The lymphosarcoma in the original mouse involved the peripheral lymph nodes as well as tumors extending from the right hip region and others from the thoracic, lumbar, and sacral vertebrae and from the parietal bones of the skull. There were large tumor follicles in the spleen, but the viscera were not infiltrated. The thymus was normal. Microscopically the tumor consisted of large immature lymphocytes, many of which had an indented nucleus. This same type of nonthymic lymphoma of bone marrow and lymph nodes was transmitted by cellular transfer or by inoculation of either newborn or adult noncortisonized mice with cell-free filtrates. Attempts to isolate a similar virus from the other five lymphosarcomas in the study were unsuccessful (Abelson and Rabstein, 1970b).

MLV-A is currently thought to be a C-type RNA virus that has an MolLV helper component and a defective MLV-A component. The defective MLV-A component is possibly responsible for the plasmacytomagenic properties of the virus. It has been assumed, although not yet proved, that MLV-A has a general tropism for B lymphocytes. This is supported by the nonthymic origin of the lymphosarcomas. It is tempting to speculate that when a mouse is given an intraperitoneal injection of pristane B lymphocytes are stimulated to develop into plasma cells. MLV-A infection then transforms B lymphocytes in various stages of development, including some cells that have differentiated to the plasma cell stage. It must be assumed here that priming with pristane increases the target cell population. One extremely interesting question will be whether plasmacytoma formation by pristane and MLV-A will occur only in BALB/c mice or whether this will be a general mechanism for plasmacytoma induction.

TABLE 4

Induction of Plasmacytomas (PCT) and Lymphosarcomas (LS) by MLV-A in Pristane-Treated BALB/c Mice

| Experiment No. | Group | Pristane[a] (0.5 ml) | MLV-A on day[b] | Virus pool[c] | Total number of mice | Number of mice with | | Average latent period (range)[d] | |
|---|---|---|---|---|---|---|---|---|---|
| | | | | | | LS (%) | PCT (%) | LS | PCT |
| I | A | — | 39 | 1 | 14 | 2 (14) | 0 (0) | 73 (58–89) | — |
| | B | + | — | — | 16 | 0 (0) | 1 (6) | — | (285) |
| | C | + | 39 | 1 | 16 | 10 (62) | 4 (24) | 70 (40–129) | 59 (46–73) |
| II | A1 | — | 57 | 2 | 16 | 10 (60) | 0 (0) | 44 (36–55) | — |
| | A2 | — | 57 | 2F | 8 | 4 (50) | 0 (0) | 42 (32–47) | — |
| | B | + | — | — | 24 | 0 (0) | 6 | — | 217 (138–290) |
| | C1 | + | 57 | 2 | 32 | 20 (62) | 8 (25) | 55 (30–120) | 49 (21–93) |
| | C2 | + | 57 | 2F | 14 | 6 (43) | 5 (36) | 40 (30–48) | 46 (20–82) |
| III | B | + | — | — | 16 | 0 (0) | 1 (6) | — | (189) |
| | C | + | 39 | 3 | 30 | 18 (60) | 9 (30) | 37 (26–67) | 47 (28–58) |

[a] Pristane was injected intraperitoneally when the mice were approximately 2 months of age.

[b] Days after pristane.

[c] MLV-A pools 1 and 2 were 1.7% and 10% extracts of primary lymphosarcomas, respectively. Pool 2F was a 0.45-m$\mu$m Millipore filtrate of pool 2. Pool 3 was a 10% extract of a transplanted lymphosarcoma. Infectivity titers (per 0.1 ml) were as follows: pool 1, $10^{4.9}$ plaque-forming units (pfu) and $10^{1.8}$ tumor (lymphosarcoma) producing units 50 (TPD$_{50}$); Pool 2, $10^{5.7}$ pfu and $10^{2.6}$ TPD$_{50}$; pool 2F, $10^{5.2}$ pfu; pool 3, $1.6 \times 10^5$ pfu and $10^2$ TPD$_{50}$.

[d] Average latent period was determined as the number of days after the injection of MLV-A, except for mice in group B, for which it was determined as the number of days after pristane.

## 4. Summary

Circumstantial evidence suggests that ileocecal plasmacytomas in mice and immunocytomas in rats may originate in chronically inflamed tissues in the lamina propria of the gut. Because these neoplasms occur rarely, the pathogenesis has not yet been worked out.

Induction of plasmacytomas in mice has a number of different requirements. Plasmacytoma development

1. Depends on the formation of an abnormal granulomatous tissue in the peritoneum. This tissue probably plays an indirect role in plasmacytomagenesis by supplying growth factors for plasma cells, by being a locally immunosuppressed environment, and by providing a source of precursor cells.
2. Involves predominantly a specific segment of the immunocyte population—the IgA differentiated cells.
3. Occurs only in certain inbred strains, BALB/c and NZB, and hence is not a general susceptibility of all strains of mice.
4. May require the activation of endogenous C-type RNA viruses or intracisternal A particles to induce transformation.

A new, rapid method for inducing plasmacytomas in BALB/c mice with Abelson virus (MLV-A) and pristane in as short a period as 80 days has been developed.

## 5. References

AARONSON, S. A., AND STEPHENSON, J. R., 1973, Independent segregation of loci for activation of biologically distinguishable RNA C-type viruses in mouse cells, *Proc. Natl. Acad. Sci.* **70:**2055–2058.

AARONSON, S. A., HARTLEY, J. W., AND TODARO, G. J., 1969, Mouse leukemia virus "spontaneous" release by mouse embryo cells after long term *in vitro* cultivation, *Proc. Natl. Acad. Sci.* **64:**87.

ABELSON, H. T., AND RABSTEIN, L. S., 1970a, Influence of prednisolone on Moloney leukemogenic virus in BALB/c mice, *Cancer Res.* **30:**2208-2212.

ABELSON, H. T., AND RABSTEIN, L. S., 1970b, Lymphosarcoma: Virus-induced thymic-independent disease in mice, *Cancer Res.* **30:**2213–2222.

ANDERSON, P. N., 1970, Plasma cell tumor induction in BALB/c mice, *Proc. Am. Assoc. Cancer Res.* **11:**3 (abst.).

ANDERSON, P. N., AND POTTER, M., 1969, Induction of plasma cell tumors in BALB/c mice with 2,6,10,14-tetramethylpentadecane (pristane), *Nature (Lond.)* **222:**994–995.

AOKI, T., POTTER, M., AND STURM, M. M., 1973, Analysis by immunoelectron microscopy of type-C viruses associated with primary and short-term transplanted mouse plasma (H) tumors *J. Natl. Cancer Inst.* **51:**1609–1617.

AOKI, T., AND TAKAHASHI, T. L., 1972, Viral and cellular surface antigens of murine leukemias and myelomas, *J. Exp. Med.* **135:**443–457.

AZAR, H. A., 1973, Pathology of multiple myeloma and related growths, in: *Multiple Myeloma and Related Disorders* (H. A. Azar and M. Potter, eds.), pp. 1–85, Harper and Row, Hagerstown.

BASOMBRIO, M. A., 1973, Lymphomas in BALB/c mice inoculated with supernatants from chemically induced sarcomas, *J. Natl. Cancer Inst.* **51:**1157-1162.

BAZIN H., DECKERS, C., BECKERS, A., AND HEREMANS, J. F., 1972, Transplantable immunoglobulin secreting tumours in rats. I. General features of Lou/Wsl strain rat immunocytomas and their monoclonal proteins, *Int. J. Cancer* **10:**568–580.

BAZIN, H., BECKERS, A., DECKERS, C., AND MORIAME, M., 1973, Transplantable immunoglobulin-secreting tumors in rats. V. Monoclonal immunoglobulins secreted by 250 ileocecal immunocytomas in Lou/Wsl rats, *J. Natl. Cancer Inst.* **51:**1359–1362.

BENDORAITIS, J. G., BROWN, B. L., AND HEPNER, L. S., 1962, Isoprenoid hydrocarbons in petroleum isolation of 2,6,10,14-tetramethylpentadecane by high temperature gas–liquid chromatography, *Anal. Chem.* **34:**49–53.

BLUMER, M., 1965, "Zamene," isomeric $C_{19}$ mono-olefins from marine zooplankton, fishes, and mammals, *Science* **148:**370–371.

BLUMER, M., AND THOMAS, D., 1965, Phytadienes in zooplankton, *Science* **147:**1148–1149.

BLUMER, M., MULLIN, M. M., AND THOMAS, D. W. 1963, Pristane in zooplankton, *Science* **140:**974.

BLUMER, M., ROBERTSON, J. C., GORDON, J. E., AND SASS, J., 1969, Phytol derived $C_{19}$ di- and triolefinic hydrocarbons in marine zooplankton and fishes, *Biochemistry* **8:**4067–4074.

CARR, I., 1967, The fine structure of cells of the mouse peritoneum, *Z. Zellforsch.* **80:**534–555.

COMOGLIO, P. M., AND GUGLIELMONE, R., 1973, Immunohistochemical study of IgA transepithelial transfer into digestive tract secretions in the mouse, *Immunology* **25:**71–80.

COTRAN, R. S., AND FORTNER, J. B., 1962, Serum protein abnormality in a transplantable plasmacytoma of the Syrian hamster, *J. Natl. Cancer Inst.* **28:**1193–1205.

CRABBÉ, P. A., NASH, D. R., BAXIN, H., EYSSEN, H., AND HEREMANS, J. F., 1970, Immunochemical observations on lymphoid tissues from conventional and germ free mice, *Lab. Invest.* **22:**448–457.

DALTON, A. J., AND POTTER, M., 1968, Electronmicroscope study of the mammary tumor agent in plasma cell tumors, *J. Natl. Cancer Inst.* **40:**1375–1385.

DALTON, A. J., POTTER, M,, AND MERWIN, R. M., 1961, Some ultrastructural characteristics of a series of primary and transplanted plasma cell tumors of the mouse, *J. Natl. Cancer Inst.* **26:**1221–1267.

DECKERS, C., 1963, Etude electrophoretique et immunoelectrophoretique des proteines du rat atteint de leucosarcome, *Protides Biol. Fluids* **11:**105–108.

DUNN, T. B., 1954, Normal and pathologic anatomy of the reticular tissue in laboratory mice with a classification and discussion of neoplams, *J. Natl. Cancer Inst.* **14:**1281–1433.

DUNN, T. B., 1957, Plasma-cell neoplasms beginning in the ileocecal area in strain C3H mice, *J. Natl. Cancer Inst.* **19:**371–391.

DUNN, T. B., AND DERINGER, M. K., 1968, Reticulum cell neoplasm, type B or the "Hodgkin's-like lesion" of the mouse, *J. Natl. Cancer Inst.* **40:**771–821.

DUNN, T. B., MOLONEY, J. B., GREEN, A. W., AND ARNOLD, B., 1961, Pathogenesis of a virus induced leukemia in mice, *J. Natl. Cancer Inst.* **26:**189–221.

EBBESEN, P., RASK-NIELSEN, R., AND McINTIRE, K. R., 1968, Plasmacell leukemia in BALB/c mice inoculated with subcellular material. I Incidence and morphology, *J. Natl. Cancer Inst.* **41:**473–493.

EBBESEN, P., RASK-NIELSEN, R., HARTLEY, J. W., AND ROWE, W. P., 1973, Murine reticulum cell neoplasms (Hodgkin's-like lesions) induced in BALB/c mice with field isolates of murine leukemia virus, *Europ. J. Cancer* **9:**173–179.

FAHEY, J. L., POTTER, M., GUTTER, F. J., AND DUNN, T. B., 1960, Distinctive myeloma globulins associated with a new plasma cell neoplasm of strain C3H mice, *Blood* **15:**103–113.

FARROW, B. R. H., AND PENNY, R., 1971, Multiple myeloma in a cat, *J. Am. Vet. Med. Assoc.* **158:**606–611.

GOLDSTEIN, G. L., WARNER, N. L., AND HOLMES, M. C., 1966, Plasma cell tumor induction in (NZB × BALB/c)f1 hybrid mice, *J. Natl. Cancer Inst.* **37:**135–143.

HERBERMAN, R. B., AND AOKI, T., 1972, Immune and natural antibodies to syngeneic murine plasma cell tumors, *J. Exp. Med.* **136:**94–111.

HERSEY, P., AND MacLENNAN, I. C. M., 1973, Macrophage dependent protection of tumor cells, *Immunology* **24:**385–393.

HOLLANDER, W. P., TAKAKURA, K., AND YAMADA, H., 1968, Endocrine factors in the pathogenesis of plasma cell tumors, *Rec. Prog. Horm. Res.* **24:**81–137.

IIYMAN, R., RALPH, P., AND SARKAR, S., 1972, Cell-specific antigens and immunoglobulin synthesis of murine myeloma cells and their variants, *J. Natl. Cancer Inst.* **48:**173–184.

KOSTER, F. T., AND McGREGOR, D. C., 1971, The mediator of cellular immunity. III. Lymphocyte traffic from the blood into the inflamed peritoneal cavity, *J. Exp. Med.* **133:**864–876.

KRIPKE, M. L., AND WEISS, D. W., 1970, Studies on the immune responses of BALB/c mice during tumor induction by mineral oil, *Int. J. Cancer* **6:**422–430.

KUFF, E. L., WIVEL, N. A., AND LUEDERS, K. R., 1968, The extraction of intracisternal A particles from a mouse plasma cell tumor, *Cancer Res.* **28:**2137–2148.

KUFF, E. L., LUEDERS, K. K., OZER, H. L., AND WIVEL, N. A., 1972, Some structural and antigenic properties of intracisternal A particles occurring in mouse tumors, *Proc. Natl. Acad. Sci.* **69:**218.

LESPINATS, G., 1969, Induction d'une immunite vis-à-vis de la greffe de plasmacytosarcomes chez la souris BALB/c, *Europ. J. Cancer* **5:**421–426.

LEVY, J. A., AND PINCUS, T., 1970, Demonstration of biological activity of a murine leukemia virus of New Zealand black mice, *Science* **170:**326–327.

LIEBERMAN, R., DOUGLAS, J. O., AND MANTEL, N., 1960, Production in mice of ascitic fluid containing antibodies induced by *Staphylococcus*– or *Salmonella*–adjuvant mixtures, *J. Immunol.* **84:**514–529.

LYNCH, R. G., GRAFF, R. J., SIRISINHA, S., SIMMS, E. S., AND EISEN, H. N., Myeloma proteins as tumor-specific transplantation antigens, *Proc. Natl. Acad. Sci.* **69:**1540–1544.

MATTIOLI, C. A., AND TOMASI, T. B., JR., 1973, The life span of IgA plasma cells from mouse intestine, *J. Exp. Med.* **138:**452–460.

MCINTIRE, K. R., AND PRINCLER, G. L., 1969, Prolonged adjuvant stimulation in germ-free BALB/c mice: Development of plasma cell neoplasia, *Immunology* **17:**481–487.

MERWIN, R. M., AND ALGIRE, G. H., 1959, Induction of plasma cell neoplasms and fibrosarcomas in BALB/c mice carrying diffusion chambers, *Proc. Soc. Exp. Biol. Med.* **101:**437-439.

MERWIN, R. M., AND REDMON, L. W., 1963, Induction of plasma cell tumors and sarcomas in mice by diffusion chambers placed in the peritoneal cavity, *J. Natl. Cancer Inst.* **31:**998–1007.

METCALF, D., 1973, Colony formation in agar by murine plasmacytoma cells: Potentiation by hematopoietic cells and serum, *J. Cell. Physiol.* **81:**397–410.

MOLONEY, J. B., 1962, The murine leukemias, *Fed. Proc.* **21:**19–31.

NAMBA, Y., AND HANAOKA, M., 1972, Immunocytology of cultured IgM-forming cells of mouse, I. Requirement of phagocytic cell factor for the growth of IgM-forming tumor cells in tissue culture, *J. Immunol.* **109:**1193–1200.

OPPENHEIMER, B. S., OPPENHEIMER, E. T., DANISHETSKY, I., STOUT, A. P., AND ELRICH, F. R., 1955, Further studies of polymers as carcinogenic agents in animals, *Cancer Res.* **15:**333–340.

OSBORNE, C. A., PERMAN, V., SAUTTER, J. H., STEVENS, J. B., AND HANLON, G. F., 1968, Multiple myeloma in the dog, *J. Am. Vet. Med. Assoc.* **153:**1300–1319.

PARK, C. H., BERGSAGEL, D. E., AND MCCULLOCH, E. A., 1971, Mouse myeloma tumor stem cells a primary culture assay, *J. Natl. Cancer Inst.* **46:**411–422.

PETERS, R. L., RABSTEIN, L. S., SPAHN, G.-J., MADISON, R. M., AND HUEBNER, R. J., 1972a, Incidence of spontaneous neoplasms in breeding and retired breeder BALB/c Cr mice throughout the natural life span, *Int. J. Cancer* **10:**273–282

PETERS, R. L., HARTLEY, J. W., SPAHN, G. J., RABSTEIN, L. S., WHITMORE, L. S., TURNER, H. C., AND HUEBNER, R. J., 1972b, Prevalence of the group-specific (gs) antigen and infectious virus expressions of the murine C-type RNA viruses during the life span of BALB/c Cr mice, *Int. J. Cancer* **10:**283–289.

PETERS, R. L., RABSTEIN, L. S.; SPAHN, G. J., TURNER, H. C., AND HUEBNER, R. J., 1972c, Incidence of group-specific (gs) antigens of type C RNA tumor viruses in spontaneous neoplasms of BALB/cCr mice, *Int. J. Cancer* **10:**290–295.

PETERS, R. L., SPAHN, G. J., RABST3EIN, L. S., KELLOFF, G. J., AND HUEBNER, R. J., 1973, Neoplasm induction by murine type C viruses passaged directly from spontaneous nonlymphoreticular tumors, *Nature New Biol.* **244:**103–105.

PILGRIM, H. I., 1965, The relationship of chronic ulceration of the ileocecal junction to the development of reticuloendothelial tumors in C3H mice, *Cancer Res.* **25:**53–65.

POTTER, M., 1967, The plasma cell tumors and myeloma proteins of mice, in: *Methods in Cancer Research, Vol. II* (H. Busch, ed.), pp. 105–157, Academic Press, New York.

POTTER, M., 1970, Mouse IgA myeloma proteins that bind polysaccharide antigens of enterobacterial origin, *Fed Proc.* **29:**85–91.

POTTER, M., 1971, Antigen binding myeloma proteins in mice, *Ann N.Y. Acad Sci.* **190:**306–321.

POTTER, M., 1972, Immunoglobulin producing tumors and myeloma proteins in mice, *Physiol. Rev.* **52:**631–719.

POTTER, M., AND BOYCE, C., 1962, Induction of plasma cell neoplasms in strain BALB/c mice with mineral oil and mineral oil adjuvants, *Nature (Lond.)* **193:**1086–1087.

POTTER, M., AND FAHEY, J. L., 1960, Studies on eight transplantable plasma cell neoplasms in mice, *J. Natl. Cancer Inst.* **24:**1153–1165.

POTTER, M., AND MACCARDLE, R. C., 1964, Histology of developing plasma cell neoplasia induced by mineral oil in BALB/c mice, *J. Natl. Cancer Inst.* **33:**497–515.

POTTER, M., AND ROBERTSON, C. L., 1960. Development of plasma cell neoplasms in BALB/c mice after intraperitoneal injection of paraffin oil adjuvant–heat killed staphylococcus mixtures, *J. Natl. Cancer Inst.* **25**:847–861.

POTTER, M., AND WALTERS, J. L., 1973, Effects of intraperitoneal pristane on established immunity to the Adj-PC-5 plasmacytoma, *J. Natl. Cancer Inst.* **51**:875–881.

POTTER, M., FAHEY, J. L., AND PILGRIM, H. I., 1957, Abnormal serum protein and bone destruction in transmissible mouse plasma cell neoplasm (multiple myeloma), *Proc. Soc. Exp. Biol. Med.* **94**:327–333.

POTTER, M., PUMPHREY, J. G., AND WALTERS, J. L., 1972, Growth of primary plasmacytomas in the mineral oil–conditioned peritoneal environment, *J. Natl. Cancer Inst.* **49**:305–308.

POTTER, M., SKLAR, M. D., AND ROWE, W. P., 1973, Rapid viral induction of plasmacytomas in pristane primed BALB/c mice, *Science* **182**:592–594.

RASK-NIELSEN, R., MCINTIRE, K. R., AND EBBESEN, P., 1968, Plasma-cell leukemia in BALB/c mice inoculated with subcellular material. II. Serological changes, *J. Natl. Cancer Inst.* **41**:495–504.

RÖLLINGHOFF, M., ROUSE, B. T., AND WARNER, N. L., 1973, Tumor immunity to murine plasma cell tumors. I. Tumor–associated transplantation antigens of NZB and BALB/c plasma cell tumors, *J. Natl. Cancer Inst.* **50**:159–172.

STANSLY, P. G., AND SOULÉ, H. D., 1962, Transplantation and cell-free transmission of a reticulum-cell sarcoma in BALB/c mice, *J. Natl. Cancer Inst.* **29**:1083–1105.

STOCKERT, E., OLD, L. J., AND BOYSE, E. A., 1971, The $G_{ix}$ system: A cell surface antigen associated with murine leukemia virus; implications regarding chromosomal integration of the viral genome. *J. Exp. Med.* **133**:1334–1355.

TAKAHASHI, T., OLD, L. J., AND BOYSE, E. A., 1970, Surface allo antigens of plasma cells, *J. Exp. Med.* **131**:1325–1341.

TAKAHASHI, T., OLD, L. J., HSU, C. J., AND BOYSE, E. A., 1971*a*, A new differentiation antigen of plasma cells, *Europ. J. Immunol.* **1**:478.

TAKAHASHI, T., OLD, L. J., MCINTIRE, K. R., AND BOYSE, E. A., 1971*b*, Immunoglobulin and other surface antigens of cells of the immune system, *J. Exp. Med.* **134**:815–832.

TAKAKURA, K., MASON, W. B., AND HOLLANDER, W. P., 1966, Studies on the pathogenesis of plasma cell tumors. I. Effect of cortison on development of plasma cell tumors, *Cancer Res.* **26**:596–599.

TOMASI, T. B. JR., AND BIENENSTOCK, J., 1968, Secretory immunoglobulins, *Advan. Immunol.* **9**:1–96.

VAN DUUREN, B. L., NELSON, N., ORRIS, L., PALMES, E. D., AND SCHMITT, F. L., 1963, Carcinogenicity of epoxides, lactones, and peroxy compounds, *J. Natl. Cancer Inst.* **31**:41–55.

VAN DUUREN, B. L., LANGSETH, L., GOLDSCHMIDT, B. M., AND ORRIS, L., 1967, Carcinogenicity of epoxides, lactones and peroxy compounds. VI. Structure and carcinogenic activity, *J. Natl. Cancer Inst.* **39**:1217–1228.

VOLKMAN, A., 1966, The origin and turnover of mononuclear cells in peritoneal exudates in rats, *J. Exp. Med.* **124**:241–253.

VOLKMAN, L. E., AND KRUEGER, R. G., 1973, XC cell cytopathogenicity as an assay for murine myeloma C-type virus, *J. Natl. Cancer Inst.* **51**:1205–1210.

WATSON, J., RALPH, P., AND SARKAR, S., 1970, Leukemia viruses associated with mouse myeloma cells, *Proc. Natl. Acad. Sci.* **66**:344–351.

WILLIAMS, W. H., AND KRUEGER, R. G., 1972, Tumor-associated transplantation antigens of myelomas induced in BALB/c mice, *J. Natl. Cancer Inst.* **49**:1613–1620.

WILSON, S. H., AND KUFF, E. L., 1972, A novel DNA polymerase activity found in association with intracisternal-A particles, *Proc. Natl. Acad. Sci.* **69**:-531.

WIVEL, N. A., AND SMITH, G. H., 1971, Distribution of intracisternal A particles in a variety of normal and neoplastic mouse tissues, *Int. J. Cancer* **7**:167–175.

YAMADA, H., MASHBURN, L. T., TAKAKURA, K., AND HOLLANDER, V. P., 1969, The correlation between plasma cell tumor development and antibody response in inbred strains of mice, *Proc. Soc. Exp. Biol. Med.* **131**:947–850.

YANCEY, S. T., 1964, Plasma cell neoplasm arising in a CAF$_1$ mouse: Characteristics and response to certain chemotherapeutic agents, *J. Natl. Cancer Inst.* **33**:373–382.

ZAWADZKI, Z. A., EDWARDS, G. A., AND ADAMS, R. V., 1967, M-components in immunoproliferative disorders. Electrophoretic and immunological analysis of 200 cases. *Am. J. Clin. Path.* **48**:418–430.

# Chemical Carcinogenesis

# 7

# Metabolism of Chemical Carcinogens

## J. H. WEISBURGER and G. M. WILLIAMS

### 1. Cancer, a Class of Diseases Due Mainly to Environmental Factors: Synthetic or Naturally Occurring

In the mind of the lay and even professional public, cancer of various types has been considered to be a "spontaneous" condition (Weisburger, 1973a). The concept that some types of cancer might, however, be caused by environmental factors traces back to the observation of Pott in the late eighteenth century that human scrotal cancer in Great Britain was associated with the occupation of his patients, namely sweeping chimneys. Since that time, people in other occupations have been demonstrated to have certain risks of developing cancer at some sites. Overall, however, occupational cancers are relatively rare events which affect only limited numbers of individuals. The bulk of human cancers were until recently considered to stem from unknown elements. It was a consideration of international incidence rates of various types of cancer, and the fact that the incidence depends in part on the site of residence, which underwrote the concept that many types of human cancer are caused, mediated, or modified by environmental factors (Wynder and Mabuchi, 1972; Higginson and Muir, 1973). Thus examination of the incidence of two types of cancer of the digestive tract, namely stomach cancer and large bowel cancer, in populations in Europe, Latin America, Japan, and the North American continent indicated clearly that they have quite different

J. H. WEISBURGER ● Naylor Dana Institute for Disease Prevention, American Health Foundation, New York, New York. Supported in part by Grants CA 12376, CA 14298, and CA 15400 and Contract CP 43378 from the National Cancer Institute, NIH, U.S. Public Health Service.
G. M. WILLIAMS ● Fels Research Institute, Temple University School of Medicine, Philadelphia, Pennsylvania. Supported in part by Grant BC-133 from the American Cancer Society.

186
J. H.
WEISBURGER
AND
G. M.
WILLIAMS

causative and modifying elements, but both are associated mainly with dietary factors. Lung cancer, on the other hand, has been definitely traced to the personal habit of smoking cigarettes. In all of these instances, it is quite certain that specific types of chemicals or mixtures of chemicals are the determining factors. Thus, overall, the majority of human cancer may be due to specific types of synthetic chemicals, as is true for occupational disease, and to naturally occurring chemicals or mixtures, the nature of which remains to be defined in many instances.

The best way of controlling cancer is cancer prevention. This can be achieved by detection of the responsible carcinogens and their elimination. In addition, as will be developed in this chapter, many carcinogens are the so-called procarcinogens, that is, agents which require metabolic activation by the host in order to induce cancer. This sometimes complex process proceeds to different extents as a function of many variables such as species, strain, age, sex, diet, and other environmental conditions. Thus, understanding of this important activation process and its converse, detoxification and elimination, permits delineation of environmental conditions so that the risk for ultimate cancer development can be decreased.

## 2. Types of Chemical Carcinogens

Chemicals which can cause cancer (i.e., carcinogens) are classified into several types. They may have a chemical structure such that they do not require the participation of enzymes from the host organism to generate the key reactive intermediate, the ultimate carcinogen; these are sometimes labeled "direct-acting carcinogens". Or they may be of the type called "procarcinogens", which are active only after metabolic conversion by the host. Most direct-acting carcinogens are synthetic chemicals developed as laboratory tools for research; others are used in industry or as antitumor drugs. Some of these represent important occupational hazards, and potential risks to exposed patients. Because of their high reactivity they do not generally persist in the environment.

On the other hand, procarcinogens, which include most of the known chemical carcinogens, can exist in the environment in a relatively stable condition until taken in by an exposed individual and activated. Thus these chemicals appear to represent the greatest potential cancer threat to man. A hazard of a similar nature is also posed by chemicals which although not carcinogens themselves are precursors from which carcinogens can be synthesized in the body.

"Cocarcinogens" are agents which exhibit little if any carcinogenicity themselves, but augment, very considerably in some instances, the effect of either direct-acting carcinogens or procarcinogens. Shear, Berenblum, and Shubik pioneered in this area (see Berenblum, 1969; Van Duuren, et al., 1973; Hecker, 1971; Boutwell, 1974). They demonstrated that a dilute solution of croton oil enormously potentiated the effect of certain polycyclic aromatic hydrocarbons such as 3-methylcholanthrene in inducing skin tumors in mice. More recently it was established that this theoretically useful model has its counterpart with respect to cancer causation in man. Tobacco tar and tobacco smoke contain powerful cocarcinogenic or "promoting" agents (Wynder and Hoffmann, 1967). It is

suspected that other types of human cancer such as that in the large bowel may also stem from a combination of carcinogens and cocarcinogens (Narisawa *et al.*, 1974).

The metabolic fate of chemical carcinogens has been extensively studied in the attempts to understand their mode of action. There have been fewer studies with respect to promoting agents or cocarcinogens. Hecker (1971) and his school, Sivak and Van Duuren (1971), Boutwell (1974), and Kubinski *et al.* (1973) have developed information on the interaction of the classical agents of this type, croton oil and the active phorbol esters, with tissues, but more information is required as to the key metabolites derived from phorbol esters which exert the specific promoting effects.

While it has been known for some time that phenols also have a promoting effect under certain conditions, the nature of the metabolites responsible for this reaction is likewise obscure. Yet it seems important to understand these processes in detail, for not only does this class of chemicals possess intrinsic theoretical interest but it also appears that they are involved in potentiating lung cancer induction in animals, and probably in man, through their presence in sizable amounts in the smoke of tobacco products (Hoffmann and Wynder, 1971; Van Duuren *et al.*, 1973).

Data are beginning to appear that cancer of the large bowel may similarly stem from the cocarcinogenic or enhancing effect of certain bile acid metabolites. In this instance, these chemicals undergo metabolic reactions through the microflora in the gut, the composition and effectiveness of which appear to be mediated through diet (Hill *et al.*, 1971; Wynder and Reddy, 1973; Weisburger, 1973*b*). Diet also controls the conversion of cholesterol in the liver to bile acids through a number of mechanisms, including the intervention of the cytochrome P450 system, itself influenced in as yet unknown ways by ascorbic acid (Ginter, 1973).

Tannins present in a number of plants and extracts consumed by man are also complex phenolic substances, the fate of which has not been studied even though certain of them appear to be hepatotoxic and carcinogenic, to potentiate the carcinogenicity of 2-acetylaminofluorene, and possibly also to act as cocarcinogens (Weisburger, 1973*a*).

## 3. Metabolism of Chemical Carcinogens

Chemical carcinogens of various classes, whether primary direct-acting carcinogens, secondary procarcinogens, or cocarcinogenic promoters, undergo a variety of chemical or biochemical reactions when introduced into a living system. These reactions can be mediated simply by body water, by selective tissue or cell chemicals, or by enzymes from mammalian and microbiological cell systems. These reactions can lead to detoxification, that is, to less carcinogenic or less active products. They can also lead to more active metabolites or, indeed, to the key ultimate carcinogenic reactants (Miller and Miller, 1971). These reactions depend

188

J. H.
WEISBURGER
AND
G. M.
WILLIAMS

in part on the chemical structure of the agent, and are subject to many variables which are a function of this structure, of the species, age, dietary, and microbiological environment, and of the presence of other chemicals, and the like. Often these reactions are similar to the broader types of so-called drug metabolism systems which convert any exogenous chemical to a variety of metabolic products (Brodie and Gillette, 1971; Boyd and Smellie, 1972; Hathway, 1970, 1972; Hucker, 1973). They can be oxidative, as is true most of the time. Thus oxidation on aliphatic or aromatic carbon or nitrogen such as N- or O-dealkylation, hydroxylation, or epoxidation, including the "NIH shift," and oxidative deamination or dechlorination are the key reactions mediated by complex enzyme systems. Under some conditions, reductive reactions such as those involving nitro groups performed by mammalian or microbiological enzymes are important. Furthermore, there are a variety of conjugative or group transfer reactions, such as formation of glucuronic acid, sulfuric acid, or acyl derivatives, which participate in the metabolism of exogenous drugs, including carcinogens (Fishman, 1970). It is important to realize that these enzymes are concerned not just with the metabolism of the agent under study. The mere fact of introduction of such chemicals may change the operating level and potential of these very enzymes, not only for the chemical under study but also for a diversity of other chemicals such as hormones. Since a number of carcinogen-metabolizing enzymes are in turn affected by such endogenous components as hormones, there may be unexpected secondary metabolic, physiological, and, indeed, pathological reactions (Conney and Burns, 1972; Conney et al., 1973). Also, in many cases repeated or chronic administration, without immediate overt cellular damage, leads to appreciable changes in enzymatic operating potential. Thus the metabolism after chronic dosing may lead to qualitative and quantitative alteration in the products. Even diet as such, or diet containing traces of pesticides, for example, can affect the bias toward certain products under the control of metabolic enzyme systems. Metabolism studies in man are subject to many such variables, which include, for example, the smoking of cigarettes (cf. Pantuck et al., 1974).

Specific metabolic activation processes will be discussed in relation to each of the main types of chemical carcinogens. A few agents seem to undergo activation by a soluble enzyme system in the cytoplasm of the cell. Thus 4-nitroquinoline-N-oxide is reduced to the active hydroxylamino derivative by a reductase in the cytoplasm (Endo et al., 1971). However, most carcinogens requiring metabolic activation are transformed by enzyme systems located on the smooth membrane of the endoplasmic reticulum. Ultracentrifugation of a cell homogenate sediments the activity with the microsome fraction.

A detailed treatment of these enzyme systems is outside the scope of this review (see Brodie and Gillette, 1971). Briefly, there are a number of similar systems belonging to the family of cytochromes. Initially, they were labeled "cytochrome P450" because a reduced form treated with carbon monoxide exhibits an absorption peak at 450 nm. Now other cytochromes are known which show such properties but whose peak absorption is close to but not at 450 nm. All of these enzyme systems require NADPH as cofactor, and because most of these reactions

are oxidative they require oxygen. Just as isozyme variants are known for certain
soluble enzymes such as aldolase and lactic dehydrogenase, it may be that the family of cytochromes mediating the metabolism of carcinogens and drugs, and exogenous or endogenous chemicals generally, are isozymes bound to membranes.

### 3.1. Direct-Acting Carcinogens

Direct-acting carcinogens possess the proper reactivity inherent in their structure to take part in the key reactions with cellular and molecular receptors leading to cancer (Table 1). As the Millers have emphasized, this entails the generation of an electrophilic reagent or similar reactive entity (Miller and Miller, 1971). While these chemicals do not, therefore, require metabolic activation, some, depending on structure, may be chemically or enzymatically inactivated. For example, it has been shown that the mutagenicity of $N$-methyl-$N'$-nitro-$N$-nitrosoguanidine (MNNG) is reduced by the action of microsomal enzymes (Popper *et al.*, 1973; Sugimura *et al.*, 1973).

Also, some quite reactive chemicals do not appear to be highly carcinogenic. The underlying reason may be not only enzymatic detoxification but also simple reaction with cell constituents such as water, proteins, and peptides, which neutralizes their reactivity so that the amount of active agent available at target sites required for carcinogenicity is negligible. Even synthetically produced "ultimate" carcinogens, which serve as models for agents suspected of being derived metabolically from procarcinogens, have been found to be not carcinogenic or of lower carcinogenicity than was initially expected. These highly reactive chemicals given exogenously fail to reach key targets, but when produced intracellularly near the target they can lead to transformation and cancer. For example, synthetic epoxides of carcinogenic polycyclic aromatic hydrocarbons, long suspected of being the reactive intermediates, are less carcinogenic than the parent compounds (Miller and Miller, 1967). The sulfate ester of $N$-hydroxy-$N$-2-fluorenylacetamide fails to cause cancer in animals, yet there is strong evidence that agents such as this are metabolically produced active intermediates (Miller, 1970; Weisburger *et al.*, 1972). In part, this evidence was obtained by the *in vitro* activity of these agents in leading to cell transformations or to mutations (Miller and Miller, 1971).

Direct alkylating agents which do not require metabolic activation but do undergo biochemical detoxification can be detected under some conditions by their interaction with nitrobenzylpyridine, as developed by Preussmann *et al.* (1965) and by Sawicki and Sawicki (1969). However, there does not appear to be a direct relationship between this reactivity and carcinogenic risk, probably because tissues and cells contain many competing nucleophilic reactants.

There have been relatively few studies on the metabolism of direct-acting alkylating agents except insofar as attempts have been made to understand their action as drugs used in cancer chemotherapy. Some of these materials are also important carcinogens (Weisburger *et al.*, 1974). These materials not only

190

J. H.
WEISBURGER
AND
G. M.
WILLIAMS

TABLE 1
*Typical Direct-Acting Carcinogens*

| | |
|---|---|
| $\beta$-Propiolactone | $\begin{array}{cc} O\!\!-\!\!CO \\ \mid \quad \mid \\ CH_2\!\!-\!\!CH_2 \end{array}$ |
| 1,2,3,4-Diepoxybutane | $\begin{array}{cc} O \qquad O \\ \diagup \diagdown \qquad \diagup \diagdown \\ CH_2\!\!-\!\!CH \quad CH\!-\!CH_2 \end{array}$ |
| Ethyleneimine | $\begin{array}{c} NH \\ \diagup \diagdown \\ CH_2\!-\!CH_2 \end{array}$ |
| Propane sulfone | $\begin{array}{cc} O\!\!-\!\!\!-\!\!\!-\!\!SO_2 \\ \mid \qquad \mid \\ CH_2\!\!-\!\!CH_2\!\!-\!\!CH_2 \end{array}$ |
| Dimethyl sulfate | $CH_3OSO_2OCH_3$ |
| Methyl methanesulfonate | $CH_3SO_2OCH_3$ |
| Bis(2-chloroethyl)sulfide (mustard gas or yperite) | $\begin{array}{c} ClCH_2CH_2 \\ \diagdown \\ \qquad S \\ \diagup \\ ClCH_2CH_2 \end{array}$ |
| Nitrogen mustard ($HN_2$) | $\begin{array}{c} ClCH_2CH_2 \\ \diagdown \\ \qquad NCH_3 \\ \diagup \\ ClCH_2CH_2 \end{array}$ |
| Melphalan (sarcolysin) | $\begin{array}{c} ClCH_2CH_2 \\ \diagdown \\ \qquad N\text{-}p\text{-}L\text{-}C_6H_4CH_2CHCOOH \\ \diagup \qquad\qquad\qquad \mid \\ ClCH_2CH_2 \qquad\qquad NH_2 \end{array}$ |
| 2-Naphthylamine mustard (chlornaphazine) | $\begin{array}{c} ClCH_2CH_2 \\ \diagdown \\ \qquad N \\ \diagup \\ ClCH_2CH_2 \end{array}$ |
| Bis(chloromethyl)ether | $ClCH_2OCH_2Cl$ |
| Benzyl chloride | $C_6H_5CH_2Cl$ |
| Dimethylcarbamyl chloride | $(CH_3)_2NCOCl$ |

undergo oxidative enzymatic change but by virtue of their reactive centers also give rise to residues such as carbonium ions, often by a monomolecular $SN_1$ reaction or a bimolecular $SN_2$ interaction with a substrate (Jones and Edwards, 1973).

## 3.2. Procarcinogens

### 3.2.1. Metabolic Alteration by Mammalian Enzyme Systems

The metabolism of procarcinogens may take place in ways leading on the one hand to activation, i.e., the ultimate production of a reactive moiety (Fig. 1), or on the other hand to inactivation. The capacity to metabolize foreign chemicals is probably a consequence of the presence of enzyme systems for metabolizing similar endogenous molecules (Conney and Kuntzman, 1971). In view of the fact that the liver is involved in catabolism of many endogenous substances, it is not surprising that it also has the capacity to metabolize foreign carcinogens. Indeed, the liver possesses most of the specific activation systems to be discussed, and to our knowledge there is no carcinogen which cannot be metabolized by liver. This makes liver the logical source of enzyme preparations for studying *in vitro* metabolism.

In the past, many studies have dealt with drug- and carcinogen-metabolizing enzymes in liver. More recently, a beginning has been made to develop such information for other target organs in a variety of species, including man. Much more work along these lines is needed. Certainly the liver is an important metabolic organ. Not only can reactions therein lead to direct-acting ultimate carcinogens, but also additional reactions lead to conjugates which are transport forms, as noted above. Where specific tissues or cells have the enzymatic potential to split the active entities from their transport conjugates, cancer may result at such sites. Cancer in the urinary bladder most likely is due to the release of active carcinogens such as arylhydroxylamine derivatives from glucuronides.

The target organ affected may depend on a combination of complex interactions. For example, 2′,3-dimethyl-4-aminobiphenyl causes intestinal cancer in rats (Spjut, 1972) but urinary bladder cancer in hamsters (So and Wynder, 1972). Probably, a transport form of the agent is secreted in the bile and thus reaches the gut in the rat, but this occurs to a much lesser extent in the hamster. Biliary secretion of carcinogen metabolites in particular or drug metabolites in general is a function of molecular size, species, and other variables (Smith, 1973). This, in turn, controls whether metabolites are excreted into the gut via the bile or reach the kidneys via the blood for filtration and excretion in the urine. These processes are more common in rodents and some other species than in primates and man, a fact which needs consideration when extrapolating data obtained in rodents to man. Metabolites reaching the gut from bile may undergo further reaction due to the effect of microbial flora (Williams *et al.*, 1970; Hill *et al.*, 1971; Scheline, 1973). The products can be excreted in the stools or be resorbed (enterohepatic pathway) and are thus capable of further metabolism and interaction. These pathways may be important for the occurrence of certain types of cancer, such as that of the gall bladder, pancreas, and intestinal tract.

Metabolic enzymes are also present to lesser and varying degrees in most other organs, particularly kidney, lung, and gastrointestinal tract. The placenta contains a variety of enzyme systems capable of modifying drugs and thereby affecting transplacental passage (Gillette *et al.*, 1973; Conney *et al.*, 1973; Mirkin, 1970; Tomatis *et al.*, 1973a; Zachariah and Juchau, 1974; Juchau *et al.*, 1974). Enzymes metabolizing carcinogens are among those found in the placenta.

An organ such as mouse skin or subcutaneous tissue that contains enzyme systems for the activation of carcinogens like polycyclic aromatic hydrocarbons to yield epoxides, but that is poor in enzymes giving deactivated products or

192

J. H.
WEISBURGER
AND
G. M.
WILLIAMS

TYPICAL ACTIVATION REACTIONS

PROCARCINOGEN ⟶ PROXIMATE CARCINOGEN ⟶ ULTIMATE CARCINOGEN

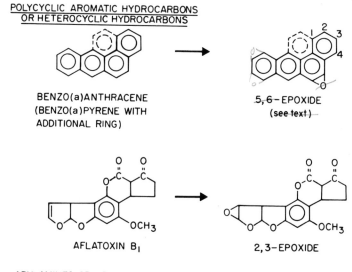

POLYCYCLIC AROMATIC HYDROCARBONS
OR HETEROCYCLIC HYDROCARBONS

BENZO(a)ANTHRACENE
(BENZO(a)PYRENE WITH
ADDITIONAL RING)

5,6-EPOXIDE
(see text)

AFLATOXIN B₁

2,3-EPOXIDE

ARYLAMINES OR ARYLAMIDES
HETEROCYCLIC AMINES

N-2-FLUORENYLACETAMIDE
(or 2-ACETYLAMINOFLUORENE)

N-HYDROXY
DERIVATIVE

ACTIVE ESTER
(SULFATE, ACETATE)
R=H OR —COCH₃

NITROARYL OR HETEROCYCLIC
COMPOUNDS

2-NITRONAPHTHALENE

2-HYDROXYLAMINO
NAPHTHALENE

3-HYDROXYXANTHINE

O ESTER

FIGURE 1. Schematic biochemical activation of typical procarcinogens. In some instances, several reactions are involved where a procarcinogen is converted to a proximate carcinogen, an intermediate, more active molecule which, however, does not have a structure such that it can interact directly with crucial macromolecular receptors in the cell. Nonetheless, in some instances, such as with the arylamines, this step is a controlling event since it is highly dependent on the structure of the chemical

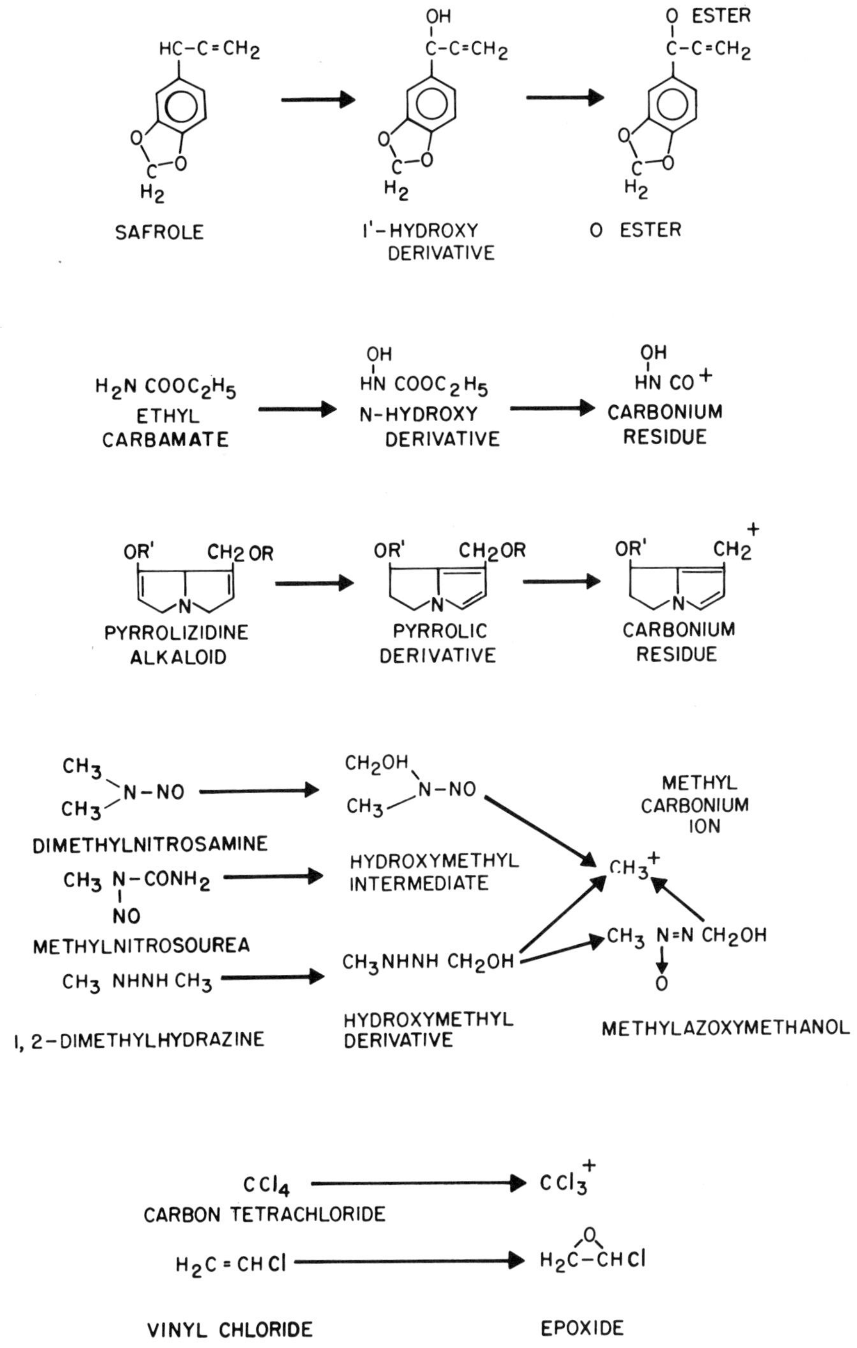

| | | |
|---|---|---|
| HC−C≡CH₂ | OH<br>C−C≡CH₂ | O ESTER<br>C−C≡CH₂ |
| SAFROLE | I'−HYDROXY<br>DERIVATIVE | O ESTER |

$H_2N\ COOC_2H_5$
ETHYL
CARBAMATE
→
OH
$HN\ COOC_2H_5$
N−HYDROXY
DERIVATIVE
→
OH
$HN\ CO^+$
CARBONIUM
RESIDUE

OR'    CH₂OR
PYRROLIZIDINE
ALKALOID
→
OR'    CH₂OR
PYRROLIC
DERIVATIVE
→
OR'    CH₂⁺
CARBONIUM
RESIDUE

$CH_3$
    N−NO
$CH_3$
DIMETHYLNITROSAMINE
→
$CH_2OH$
    N−NO
$CH_3$
HYDROXYMETHYL
INTERMEDIATE

$CH_3\ N−CONH_2$
    NO
METHYLNITROSOUREA

$CH_3\ NHNH\ CH_3$
I, 2−DIMETHYLHYDRAZINE
→
$CH_3NHNH\ CH_2OH$
HYDROXYMETHYL
DERIVATIVE

METHYL
CARBONIUM
ION

$CH_3^+$

$CH_3\ N=N\ CH_2OH$
        ↓
        O
METHYLAZOXYMETHANOL

$CCl_4$
CARBON TETRACHLORIDE
→
$CCl_3^+$

$H_2C=CHCl$
VINYL CHLORIDE
→
$H_2C-CHCl$ (epoxide)
EPOXIDE

and on the species, the strain, and certain environmental factors such as enzyme inducers or inhibitors. Formation of the ultimate carcinogen is also under enzymatic control. The exact nature of the ultimate carcinogen has not been fully documented in all cases. Because of the high reactivity of these chemicals, they cannot often be isolated. Their nature is usually elucidated on the basis of their precursors or their products of interaction.

194

J. H.
WEISBURGER
AND
G. M.
WILLIAMS

water-soluble conjugates, is extraordinarily sensitive to small amounts of such agents. On the other hand, an organ such as liver that is amply provided with such deactivating and conjugating enzymes is not sensitive, even though it may also be capable of synthesizing sizable amounts of the active epoxide intermediates.

Many carcinogens under certain experimental conditions and in the human situation possess specific affinity for certain target organs. For example, some aromatic amine carcinogens give rise to cancer of the urinary bladder in man, dog, and hamster, but liver cancer in the mouse (Weisburger et al., 1967). Among the carcinogenic nitrosamines, there appears to be organ specificity related to structure (Schmähl, 1970; Druckrey, 1973). The exact reason for this specificity has not been fully documented in all cases, but it is a reasonable assumption that the main effect depends on specific metabolic activation.

Under some conditions, the main target organ can be protected, in which case a secondary organ may be involved. For example, it has been known for more than 20 yr that administration of 3-methylcholanthrene together with 2-acetylaminofluorene protects rats against liver cancer induced by the latter, but more recently it has been noted that in hamsters there is an increased carcinogenic effect on the liver. The difference in response is due to a specific alteration of the ratio of activated vs. detoxified metabolites. Again, with 2-acetylaminofluorene, addition of tryptophan to the diet in part protects the liver, and urinary bladder cancer ensues (see Weisburger and Weisburger, 1973). In man, similar relationships may obtain through as yet unclear mechanisms. Heavy smokers may not necessarily develop lung cancer or heart disease, even though it is suspected that there is a genetically controlled metabolic difference in susceptibility (Kellermann et al., 1973a,b). Such individuals, however, may develop cancer in the urinary bladder after a longer latent period.

The use of enzyme preparations to study the metabolism of carcinogens in vitro offers many advantages. For the reasons indicated, liver is the usual source of these enzymes, although more effort is desirable to evaluate other tissues, especially target organs for selective carcinogens. The typical enzyme preparation consists of a postmitochondrial supernatant (Garner et al., 1971) or microsomal suspension (Grover and Sims, 1968; Gelboin, 1969) supplemented with an NADPH-regenerating system. The assay is usually for the production of a specific metabolite or of covalently bound carcinogen. Grover and Sims (1968) and Gelboin (1969) demonstrated that such a system could be used to measure the generation of reactive metabolites which covalently bind to macromolecules in the system. A number of laboratories are now using in vitro enzyme preparations to identify the ultimate reactive carcinogen metabolite (Selkirk et al., 1971; Garner, 1973; Swenson et al., 1973), to study factors affecting metabolism (Diamond and Gelboin, 1969; Hill and Shih, 1974), and to measure the metabolic activation of carcinogens to mutagens (Fukuda and Yamamoto, 1972; Ames et al., 1973a,b).

The study of carcinogenesis in cell culture is appealing because better control of dose, interval of exposure, and similar parameters can be obtained. Most of the available cell cultures are derived from fibroblasts. Few studies on metabolic capability have been performed except with the polycyclic hydrocarbon carcinogens, in which case important genetic parameters were discovered. Epithelial liver cell cultures which retain the capability of the organ have been sought, and Sullman *et al.* (1970) obtained human liver cell cultures which were sensitive to aflatoxin. Cultures of this sort may permit predictions of the sensitivity of humans to various carcinogens. Rat liver cells have been shown to possess arylhydroxylase (Gielen and Nebert, 1971) and to be sensitive to a variety of carcinogens (Montesano *et al.*, 1973; Williams *et al.*, 1973), but at present there is no reported culture which is known to possess all the *in vivo* carcinogen-metabolizing activities of liver.

The metabolism of polycyclic hydrocarbon carcinogens has been extensively studied by a number of groups (Gelboin *et al.*, 1972; Bast *et al.*, 1973; Bürkl *et al.*, 1973; Heidelberger, 1973; Kaufman *et al.*, 1973), and Nebert and Gelboin (1968) have described an inducible arylhydroxylase system in hamster fetus cells. Metabolism by epoxidation, discussed in detail below, and by alternate pathways, such as formation of one-electron oxidation, free radical or radical cation intermediates have been reviewed recently (Jerina and Daly, 1974; Ts'o and DiPaolo, 1974).

Cell culture offers many advantages in studying the mechanism of metabolism of carcinogens, particularly the effect of modifiers such as inducers or inhibitors. However, it is hazardous to postulate that these modifiers will have the same total effect in the organism as they do in culture. This is because if metabolism in the intact animal is blocked at one site it may be increased at another, such as has been described for dimethylnitrosamine in protein-deprived animals (Swann and McLean, 1971). Portions of the conjugating enzymes yielding inactive water-soluble metabolites often have low activity in cell culture, which needs consideration in relating *in vitro* to *in vivo* findings.

### 3.2.2. Metabolic Activation by Microorganisms

The intestines of all mammals are inhabited by a variety of bacteria. With respect to some carcinogens, their action has been felt to be decisive in the development of certain neoplasms, particularly those of the colon and rectum. However, the contribution of these organisms to metabolism of carcinogens has not been extensively studied. It is clear, especially in mutagenesis studies (Hollaender, 1971; Ames *et al.*, 1973a,b), that certain bacteria cannot activate procarcinogens; but they do possess the enzymes to hydrolyze conjugates such as glucuronides (Williams *et al.*, 1970) and glucosides (Laqueur, 1970). These activities are critical to the fate of some carcinogens. For example, cycasin, a constituent of the cycad nut, is a β-glucoside which is not carcinogenic until methylazoxymethanol, an aglycone, is generated. This is done only by intestinal flora which elaborate glucosidase. Thus in germ-free animals the glucoside is noncarcinogenic (Laqueur, 1970). Methylazoxymethanol is absorbed and further distributed in a manner similar to that of some nitrosamines, yielding liver and sometimes kidney tumors. In addition, colon cancers are induced in high frequency.

Bacterial β-glucuronidase can split the glucuronides of excreted carcinogen metabolites into the gut via the bile and thereby liberate an active moiety. The

196

J. H.
WEISBURGER
AND
G. M.
WILLIAMS

flora also has $N$-dehydroxylase, which inactivates $N$-hydroxy-FAA (Williams *et al.*, 1970), and reductases, which split azo dyes or reduce nitroaryl compounds. To be thus affected by gut bacterial enzymes, the chemicals must reach the large bowel. This is the case with poorly resorbed orally administered chemicals or with metabolites secreted in the bile (Gingell and Bridges, 1973; Williams, 1972; Albrecht and Manchon, 1973; Scheline, 1973; Yoshida and Miyakawa, 1973).

### 3.2.3. Metabolic Activation by Chemical Means, Including Endogenous Formation of Carcinogens

As noted, some procarcinogens are converted to active intermediates in the liver and further metabolized to transport forms which then enter the circulation. There are hydrolytic means, such as provided by tissue or bacterial enzymes like glucuronidase, which can hydrolyze conjugates with release of the active entities. The broad class of agents represented by alkylnitrosoureas or alkylnitroso-urethanes undergo hydrolytic reactions at neutral pH with release of the active electrophilic carcinogen (Sander, 1971; Mirvish, 1972; *IARC Monograph No. 4*, 1974). These reactions can be accelerated by some compounds such as those with SH groups. These alkylnitrosoureido chemicals are often powerful carcinogens because of their relative ease of hydrolysis. They are active at or near the site of introduction. However, they may have remote effects, depending on the rate of hydrolysis and transport. Ureido compounds, in particular, readily traverse the blood–brain barrier, and certain of these agents are therefore unique in leading to brain tumors. Chemicals with this structure need to be examined very carefully for their potential in leading to cancer at that site, especially if they have properties such that their residence time in the brain is sufficiently long. Furthermore, some of these agents readily cross the placenta and thus lead to cancer in the offspring when administered to pregnant animals.

Chemical carcinogens can also be formed in the host from suitable precursors. Sander (1971, 1973) noted that similar incidences of identical tumors could be formed when he administered nitrite and certain secondary amines separately as when the preformed nitrosamine was given. This discovery has led to a great deal of activity in many laboratories which has extended the original findings. In addition to the classical substrates, secondary amines, it has been found recently that some tertiary amines can also react with nitrite to produce a carcinogenic dialkylnitrosamine (Lijinsky, 1974). Inasmuch as many drugs and certain other environmental chemicals possess such structure, these reactions need to be studied in detail in order to delineate their importance in relation to the potential risk of carcinogenesis in man exposed to these agents and at the same time to nitrite. Some human foods, in particular certain types of meats such as ham, have been shown to contain small amounts, of the order of parts per billion, of dimethylnitrosamine (Bogovski *et al.*, 1972). Fried bacon may contain up to 80 ppb nitrosopyrrolidine, presumably derived from the nitrosation of proline followed by heat decarboxylation during frying. The importance of these reactions in causing human cancer is not known. Most fresh foods contain negligible amounts of nitrite. Meats treated with the legal amount of nitrite, 200 parts per million in the United States, contain low concentrations of about 5–20 ppm residual nitrite by the time they reach the consumer (Hustad *et al.*, 1973). Also, ascorbic acid and sulfhydryl compounds react with nitrite (Mirvish and Chu, 1973). It has been proposed to utilize this finding to decrease further the potential risk of endogenous nitrite–amine interaction leading to carcinogenic nitrosamines. However, Raineri and Weisburger (1974) have speculated about the importance of the previously practiced extensive curing of meats and other foods with large amounts of nitrite-containing salt and, of more importance, the formation of nitrite in foodstuffs that were cooked with water of high nitrate content and allowed to stand at room temperature. Ingestion of large amounts of nitrite, reacting with components of the food such as methylguanidine, may have led to the production in the stomach of nitrosamides, which are known gastric carcinogens. They attribute the declining incidence of stomach cancer in the United States over the last 40 yr to the decrease in curing of meats and the availability of mechanical refrigeration, leading to an overall reduction of nitrite intake.

### 3.3. Specific Activation and Metabolic Systems

There are a great diversity of chemical structures which have the specific and unique property of leading to neoplasia under certain well-defined conditions in animals and in man. Until recent years, it was not at all clear how chemicals as different as dimethylnitrosamine, safrole, 4-dimethylaminoazobenzene, carbon tetrachloride, ethionine, pyrrolizidine alkaloids, and 2-nitrofluorene all could lead to liver cancer in rodents, or why 3-methylcholanthrene could inhibit this process with some of these agents under some conditions but enhance it with others, or why powerful sarcoma-inducing polycyclic aromatic hydrocarbons did not usually cause cancer in the liver, or why some carcinogens were excellent mutagens in microbiological systems and other equally oncogenic agents were not.

Fortunately, considerable progress has been made in the last 20 yr in the field of biochemical pharmacology. Advances have occurred in the area of metabolism of drugs and their mode of action, but it can be said that, in part, advances in this broader field have stemmed from pioneering investigations on the metabolism and mode of action of chemical carcinogens. Conney *et al.* in 1956 were the first to unravel the mechanism by which the carcinogenic effect of the azo dye 4-dimethylaminoazobenzene was inhibited in animals fed the carcinogen 3-methylcholanthrene at the same time. They discovered that the latter agent induced enzymes which converted the azo dye to inactive metabolites. This marked the beginning of detailed studies on enzyme induction, first in relation to the carcinogenic process, then in pharmacology as a whole (Conney, 1967). Thus the current concepts of distinct classes of carcinogens was developed. Direct-acting carcinogens were found to have a molecular structure that gives them reactive alkylating properties. Because they can interact with significant

198

J. H.
WEISBURGER
AND
G. M.
WILLIAMS

TABLE 2

*Classes of Procarcinogens and Key Derived Active Metabolites*

| Procarcinogen | Actual or proposed proximate or ultimate carcinogen |
|---|---|
| Polycyclic aromatic hydrocarbons | Epoxide |
| | Radical ion? |
| Aflatoxin | Epoxide |
| Arylamine or amide; azo dyes | N-Hydroxylamino-O-esters; radical ion (?); epoxide (special case, cutaneous cancers) |
| Nitro aryl or heterocyclic compounds | N-Hydroxylamino-O-esters |
| 3-Hydroxyxanthine, related purines | O-Esters |
| Safrole | 1'-Hydroxy-O-ester |
| Urethan, alkylcarbamates | Active esters |
| Pyrrolizidine alkaloids | Pyrrolic esters |
| Alkynitrosamines or -amides, alkylhydrazines or -triazenes | Alkyl carbonium ion |
| Halogenated hydrocarbons | Haloalkyl carbonium ions |
| Vinyl halide or acetate | Epoxide? |

molecular targets such as DNA (Miller and Miller, 1971), they are mutagenic as well as carcinogenic. To do this, their reactivity must be such that they are not inactivated, mainly via a $SN_2$ process, with cellular nucleophils such as water or proteins not involved in the carcinogenic process. Since bacterial DNA seems less well shielded from such competing reactions, these agents are often highly mutagenic but of lower carcinogenicity.

The class of procarcinogens was found to require metabolic activation (Table 2). Without such activation they are not carcinogenic and not mutagenic. Since most of the activation reactions are oxidative in nature and most microbiological systems used as indicators to detect mutagenic events are poorly endowed with such oxidative enzymes, these chemicals were not usually known as mutagens. Incidentally, an understanding of this area now permits the use of certain mammalian activation systems to detect potential carcinogenic risk via a mutagenic event in a bacterial indicator system. Such tests are much more rapid than the classical carcinogen bioassays, although, to be sure, additional developmental work on them is required (Stoltz *et al.*, 1974). Another important by-product of advances in this field is that these tests can serve as collateral supporting evidence in the delineation of possible carcinogenic risks where the results of the classical rodent bioassays are not clear-cut or are controversial. Miller (1970) first generalized the concept that most procarcinogens are metabolized to electrophilic reagents, which appear to be the key intermediates for expression of carcinogenic activity. In some instances, the exact structure of the reagent derived from a chemical carcinogen is known, in others it can only be surmised, and additional efforts are required to properly document the process. Also, it has been proposed that the intermediate may have free radical character, and this equally reasonable point deserves further experimental proof. Some of the suggested intermediates, e.g., carbonium ions, have such an evanescent life that it is difficult to visualize how they could be produced at one place in the cell, say the endoplasmic reticulum, and then transported to the receptor such as DNA within the nucleus. It could be that these and maybe all such intermediates are produced in close proximity to the target, and perhaps a concerted three-point interaction between procarcinogen, activating enzyme, and reactive site needs to be considered. This could occur at the membrane interface between endoplasmic reticulum and nucleus.

### 3.3.1. Polycyclic and Heterocyclic Aromatic Hydrocarbons

Historically, polycyclic and heterocyclic aromatic hydrocarbons were the first pure chemical compounds that caused cancer in animal models. Thus investigations on their mode of action and metabolism have been almost a tradition. Even so, only quite recently has substantial progress toward the delineation of the activation process been made. These chemicals, typified by benz[a]anthracene, benzo[a]pyrene, dibenz[a,h]anthracene, 3-methylcholanthrene, and 7,12-dimethylbenz[a]anthracene, undergo numerous metabolic reactions (cf. Hathway, 1970, 1972). Boyland proposed in 1952 that the key activation reaction might be the formation of an epoxide. However, for many years the polycyclic aromatic hydrocarbons were considered to be direct acting, mainly because very small amounts applied to the skin or injected subcutaneously produced tumors. The elegant theoretical studies of the Pullmans and Daudels pinpointed an electronically reactive area in these molecules proposed as relevant to their carcinogenicity, the so-called K region (Bergmann and Pullman, 1969). However, it seemed that polycyclic hydrocarbons could not react well with molecular targets such as DNA. When Gelboin (1969) and Grover and Sims (1968) showed that these carcinogens combine to a significant extent with DNA in the presence of a microsomal oxidative system, the position changed. At the same time Witkop, Daly, and Jerina noted that benzenic hydrocarbons could undergo epoxidation with formation of arene oxides (Daly, 1971). These chemicals are chemically reactive and are also substrates for further enzymatic reactions such as dihydrodiol formation (Oesch, 1973) and conjugation with sulfhydryl amino acids or peptides like glutathione (Boyland, 1971; Booth et al., 1973).

Epoxidation of aryl structures appears to be a common metabolic reaction undergone not only by the carcinogenic polycyclic aromatic hydrocarbons but even by simple inactive mono- and dicyclic structures (Daly, 1971). These are not usually carcinogenic, probably because the epoxides of the smaller hydrocarbons are good substrates for hydrases and other detoxifying enzymes. Benzene itself has a leukemogenic effect in a few occupationally exposed individuals, perhaps because they, but not most populations, are genetically deficient in the detoxifying enzyme systems.

Synthetic methods developed mainly by Sims in London, and earlier by Newman in Columbus, permitted the preparation of epoxides of certain of the polycyclic aromatic hydrocarbons and the demonstration of their occurrence during metabolism (cf. Keysell et al., 1973; Stoming et al., 1973). In contrast to the parent hydrocarbons, they are mutagenic, readily cause cell transformations,

200

J. H.
WEISBURGER
AND
G. M.
WILLIAMS

interact rapidly with cellular macromolecules, and for the most part are carcinogenic (Heidelberger, 1973). Considering the complexity of the structure of the carcinogenic hydrocarbons and their heterocyclic analogues, it is not yet fully known which of the possible epoxides is primarily involved in the carcinogenic process. Perhaps for historical reasons the epoxides built on the K region were synthesized and studied most frequently, but other epoxides cannot at this time be ruled out as concerned with the oncogenic properties of polycyclic aromatic hydrocarbons. Several groups have demonstrated that the epoxides of polycyclic aromatic hydrocarbons are formed during metabolism (Grover *et al.*, 1973; Heidelberger, 1973; Keysell *et al.*, 1973; Stoming *et al.*, 1973; Waterfall and Sims, 1973), and newer techniques which permit detection of products of further metabolism such as dihydrodiols (Selkirk *et al.*, 1974) indicate the presence of a number of epoxide intermediates. Brookes' laboratory showed that the hydrolysis product of the adduct benz[*a*]anthracene-5,6-epoxide with pure DNA was different from the product isolated from mouse skin treated with benz[*a*]anthracene, and thus the epoxide produced *in vivo* may not be the 5,6-epoxide (Baird *et al.*, 1973). However, it could be that the material produced *in vivo* under a concerted type of reaction, perhaps in the presence of a carrier protein, interacts with DNA under steric and conformational conditions distinct from these when the epoxide is reacted with nude DNA.

Knowledge of the sequence of reactions of polycyclic aromatic hydrocarbons to epoxide, an activation step, followed by a series of possible detoxification steps, namely rearrangement to phenol (usually a toxic but probably not carcinogenic product), a dihydrodiol, or a sulfur amino acid conjugate, now allows a clearer understanding of differences in the oncogenicity of these compounds. They are highly carcinogenic to mouse skin or rodent subcutaneous tissue after application of minute amounts, mainly because these tissues are low in the enzymes such as epoxide hydrase and glutathione transferase that perform the detoxification steps (Boyland, 1971; Oesch, 1973). Primates appear to be much more "resistant" to these chemicals, perhaps because they have lower epoxide-forming potential, or because their detoxifying systems are more developed. This is probably true also with respect to rodent liver. Fetal or newborn mice and rats readily develop liver cancer on intake of polycyclic aromatic hydrocarbons, but older animals do not. This is probably because the hydrase- and glutathione-conjugating enzymes develop after birth (Oesch *et al.*, 1973), but the epoxide-forming system does so earlier. Through elegant *in vitro* and *in vivo* experimentation, it has been demonstrated that the reactions concerned with the metabolism of the polycyclic aromatic hydrocarbons are under genetic control (Gelboin *et al.*, 1972; Bürkl *et al.*, 1973; Kouri *et al.*, 1973; Nebert *et al.*, 1973; Kellermann *et al.*, 1973; Conney, 1973; Wiebel *et al.*, 1973). Inasmuch as polycyclic hydrocarbons are a component of cigarette smoke and tobacco tar, the possibility is being explored that a differential sensitivity to these agents exists in man. Development of more information might permit the assessment of the relative risk of cigarette smokers and thus provide an additional parameter in the worldwide efforts to reduce or prevent cancer (Wynder and Mabuchi, 1972).

### 3.3.2. Aflatoxin

Through the efforts of Büchi, Wogan, and their associates, the chemical structures of the aflatoxins, powerful carcinogenic mold products of environmental importance, were discovered (Wogan, 1973). Initially, four such chemicals were known. Aflatoxins $B_1$ and $G_1$ are characterized by a difuran ring system attached to a coumarin complex; the other two, aflatoxins $B_2$ and $G_2$, are similar but have a saturated double bond in the difurano ring. These latter chemicals are much less, if at all, carcinogenic. Aflatoxins $B_1$ and $G_1$ are potent liver carcinogens and also cause cancer at the point of application to mouse skin and subcutaneously in rats. Because of this, for many years it was thought that they might be direct acting, which drew attention to the lactone portion of the molecule. This turned out to be a false lead. Schoental (1970) and also Weisburger (1973$a$) proposed that the epoxide at the 2,3-position in the furane ring is the key carcinogenic intermediate, perhaps analogous to the carcinogenicity of the polycyclic hydrocarbons. This proposal was documented experimentally by the Millers' group who noted that the attachment to nucleic acids is indeed through that part of the molecule (Swenson $et$ $al.$, 1973) and more recently found that a synthetic 2,3-dichloro derivative acts as a powerful alkylating agent (Swenson $et$ $al.$, 1974). A microsome fraction converts aflatoxin $B_1$ to several derivatives, some of which inhibit molecular transcription and translation processes (Moulé and Frayssinet, 1972); aflatoxin $B_1$ itself is inactive. In view of the potent carcinogenicity of the aflatoxins to the liver of rats but not mice (except newborn mice; Vesselinovitch $et$ $al.$, 1972), it would seem that the 2,3-epoxide of aflatoxin $B_1$ is not a good substrate for detoxifying enzymes such as hydrase or glutathione transferase in the liver of rats and other sensitive species such as trout. Phenobarbital reduces the carcinogenic effect, perhaps by increasing detoxifying reactions (McLean and Marshall, 1971).

Another metabolite of aflatoxin $B_1$ that has been identified is aflatoxin $P_1$, a major excretion product in urine (Dalezios $et$ $al.$, 1971). It is the $O$-desmethyl derivative, and, like most phenolic products derived from aromatic compounds, it is probably not carcinogenic. Being a phenol, it appears only to a small extent as free compound, and is found mostly conjugated as a sulfate or glucuronide ester. Since it is the metabolite of aflatoxin $B_1$ excreted in urine as a large fraction of the dose, Wogan's group believe that aflatoxin $P_1$ may be a valuable tool for assessing aflatoxin intake in population groups, once sensitive procedures for specific analyses are available.

The metabolite aflatoxin M, so named because it was found in milk of lactating animals given aflatoxin $B_1$, also occurs in urine. It accounts for only a small portion of the dose, 1–4% (Campbell $et$ $al.$, 1970; Purchase $et$ $al.$, 1973). A microsome fraction from human liver is capable of oxidizing aflatoxin $B_1$ to the $M_1$ and $P_1$ metabolites. There are also some less polar metabolites whose structure is not known (Merrill and Campbell, 1974).

### 3.3.3. Aromatic Amines and Azo Dyes

The carcinogenic aromatic amines, azo dyes, and their derivatives and analogues do not usually cause cancer at the point of application. Thus they have been the

202

J. H.
WEISBURGER
AND
G. M.
WILLIAMS

prototypes of agents which require metabolic activation. Exceptions are 2-anthramine, which Bielschowsky (see Clayson, 1962) found to cause skin tumors on cutaneous application to rats. Also, 6-aminochrysene failed to induce visceral tumors when fed to rats (Lambelin *et al.*, 1967), but did cause tumors when applied to the skin of mice (Roncucci *et al.*, and Hoffmann *et al.*, personal communications). It is probable and needs to be shown that these chemicals are thus active, not because of the aromatic amino group directly, but because of epoxide formation at a position activated by the amino group. Hence these two and perhaps other aromatic amines are active through the aromatic hydrocarbon portion of their molecule. A preliminary report confirms this view, for no evidence of N-hydroxylation has been obtained, but the drug is excreted in relatively large amounts in the bile as a glucuronide (Grantham *et al.*, 1974a), and the blood levels drop rapidly (Franchi *et al.*, 1973).

Further evidence for this concept comes from the finding that fluorenylacetamide appears to cause more skin tumors, on promotion with croton oil, than the N-hydroxy metabolite (Miller *et al.*, 1964). Indirect support for an epoxy metabolite with arylamines is based on the isolation of some mercapturic acids derived from acetanilide (Grantham *et al.*, 1974b), although Calder *et al.* (1974) have provided data indicating that such intermediates could result from hydroxylamine derivatives. It is not known whether such epoxy intermediates are involved in extrahepatic carcinogenesis by certain arylamines such as 6-aminochrysene and benzidine in the breast, although with other arylamines a more conventional mechanism, the formation of electrophilic N-acetoxy-arylamines (see below), has been observed (Bartsch *et al.*, 1973).

It is now well established that a key activation reaction undergone by aromatic amines is hydroxylation on the nitrogen to form the corresponding hydroxylamino derivatives (see Miller and Miller, 1971; Thorgeirsson *et al.*, 1973; Uehleke, 1973; Weisburger and Weisburger, 1973; Arcos and Argus, 1974; Kriek, 1974). This reaction is stereospecific and takes place only when the amino group is on certain positions of the aromatic ring. Thus 2-naphthylamine, 2-fluorenamine, and 2-antramine are powerful carcinogens, whereas the pure 1-isomers are not. The groups of Radomski, Troll, and Gutmann have demonstrated that the hydroxylamines corresponding to the inactive 1-substituted arylamines are powerful carcinogens and mutagens. Just as in the case of the oxidation and further metabolism of the carcinogenic polycyclic aromatic hydrocarbons, the N-hydroxylation of aromatic amines likewise is probably under genetic control. Development of a simple clinical test for this property might permit selection of low risk individuals for employment where exposure to carcinogenic aromatic amines is possible. New techniques such as liquid chromatography might help (Gutmann, 1974).

With a number of aromatic amines, the effect noted is similar whether the chemical administered is the amine or an acylamide, especially if the acyl group is acetyl. It was known for many years, for example, that 2-fluorenamine and N-2-fluorenylacetamide have almost equivalent effects. However, the benzoyl has low carcinogenicity and the tosyl derivative even less, being inactive. At one time, it was felt that this difference rested on the ease of hydrolysis and liberation of the amine. Since the discovery of N-hydroxylation as a key activation reaction for aromatic amines, it appears more likely that the difference in activity rests on the relative ease of N-hydroxylation. In confirmation, Gutmann *et al.* (1967) have demonstrated that synthetic N-hydroxyacyl derivatives are carcinogenic even with bulky or complex acyl substituents.

Nonetheless, with certain other carcinogenic amines, there is a difference in carcinogenicity, such as the distinct effect of 2-naphthylamine and 2-naphthylacetamide in the dog. The dog may be unusual insofar as this species does not have acetyl transferase, and hence the equilibrium present in other species between acyl, specifically acetyl, derivatives and free amines does not hold. Gorrod (1973) has proposed that N-hydroxylation of acetamides occurs by a cytochrome P450–connected pathway, whereas free amines would be oxidized by a flavine adenine nucleotide-dependent enzyme complex. This interesting proposal deserves serious consideration and experimental documentation, for it does suggest clarification of certain currently obscure mechanisms.

The carcinogenic aromatic amines and acyl amides have distinct organotropic properties depending on their structure and on species, age, sex, and other variables. These properties are the result of the potential for sterospecific activation to the corresponding arylhydroxylamines as a function of these variables. However, even the arylhydroxylamines are not the ultimate carcinogenic entities in most cases. For rat liver, there is good evidence that a key activation step is conjugation to form the O-sulfate ester, mediated through a sulfotransferase (Miller and Miller, 1971; Weisburger and Weisburger, 1973). In addition, for rat liver and possibly other organs such as breast an acyl transferase, again yielding an active hydroxylamine ester, may be implicated (Lotlikar and Luha, 1971; Bartsch *et al.*, 1973; King and Olive, 1973). Additional activation mechanisms operating on the hydroxylamino compounds may be required, for these chemicals are carcinogenic under conditions where neither of these types of ester formation is necessarily involved. Peroxidases or other means for generating one-electron intermediates have been implicated (Bartsch and Hecker, 1971; Bartsch *et al.*, 1972; King *et al.*, 1973). Certain aromatic amines are carcinogenic to the urinary bladder through an intermediary hydroxylamine step by an as yet unknown specific activation mechanism (Lower and Bryan, 1973; Radomski *et al.*, 1973*a,b*).

In line with the concept that the higher molecular weight chemicals are more likely to be excreted in bile, more dichlorobenzidine than benzidine was found in the bile of dogs, whereas more benzidine was excreted in urine (Kellner *et al.*, 1973). In rhesus monkeys, the urine contained some unmetabolized 3,3'-dichlorobenzidine, whereas with benzidine only metabolites were noted, including N-acetyl derivatives. In certain strains of female rats, some aromatic amines and derivatives such as benzidine, N-2-fluorenylacetamide, and its N-hydroxy derivative are highly active carcinogens for the mammary gland. The mechanisms are not known. When both amine and hydroxylamino derivatives were tested, the latter were usually more active, suggesting that a hydroxylamino metabolite is

204

J. H.
WEISBURGER
AND
G. M.
WILLIAMS

involved (see Malejka-Giganti *et al.*, 1973). However, an epoxy compound is also possible, as discussed above, especially since breast tissue is an excellent target for polycyclic aromatic hydrocarbons.

The carcinogenic azo dyes, active mostly on rodent liver and in some instances on hamster and dog urinary bladder, undergo activation via mechanisms similar to those described for the aromatic amines (Miller and Miller, 1971; Terayama, 1967). The prototype, 4-dimethylaminoazobenzene, requires an *N*-methyl group, and despite many efforts the corresponding *N*-methyl-*N*-hydroxy derivative has not been synthesized. However, the corresponding synthetic *N*-methylben-zoyloxy compound assumes all the properties of an ultimate carcinogen. The suggestion that *N*-*O*-ester is the reactive entity with the azo dyes is plausible. Certain azo dyes, such as *o*-aminoazotoluene, are carcinogenic even though they do not have an *N*-methyl substitution. While there have been no detailed investigations of their metabolism, it is probable that they are activated as if they were classical carcinogenic aromatic amines. However, special mechanisms may relate to the *o*-methylamino substitution (Weisburger, unpublished observations).

In addition, carcinogenic azo dyes undergo detoxification reactions through reductive splitting of the azo link and through hydroxylation on the ring system. Reduction of the azo bond is also mediated to a considerable extent by the bacterial flora (Scheline, 1973). For this reason, feces usually do not contain azo dye, or metabolites with the azo bond intact, even though such chemicals are known to be excreted into the gut via the bile. Complex azo dyes containing carcinogenic components such as benzidine may be hazardous because of metabolic release and resorption of carcinogenic intermediates from the gut.

### 3.3.4. Nitro Aryl Compounds

The nitro analogues of the carcinogenic aromatic amines are usually also carcinogenic, mostly to the same target organs as the corresponding amines. In addition, however, most of them induce cancer in the forestomach of rodents on oral ingestion. It would seem that these nitro aryl derivatives are reduced in susceptible organs to the corresponding arylhydroxylamines, which undergo further activation, as described above, as a function of structure, species, target organ, and the like (Gillette, 1971; Weisburger and Weisburger, 1973; Poirier and Weisburger, 1973). Inasmuch as the reduction of nitroaryl derivatives appears to be less stereospecific than the oxidation of the corresponding aromatic amines, it could be that such chemicals are more generally carcinogenic than the corresponding amines. This point remains to be proven. It is important because some of these, such as 1-nitronaphthalene, have assumed increasing industrial importance as a result of the desirable progressive elimination from commerce of the carcinogenic aromatic amines like 2-naphthylamine. Often the nitroaryl derivatives are not as soluble. Therefore, they are sometimes less carcinogenic because of poor absorption.

There have been few specific studies on the mechanism of reduction of carcinogenic nitroaryl compounds (see Gillette, 1971). It would appear that there are two distinct enzyme systems, one membrane bound and the other in the

cytoplasm. In many instances, the membrane-bound system, requiring NADPH
and oxygen, is more active. It is presumed that the mechanism involved is an
oxidation of NADPH by the nitroaryl compound. The soluble enzyme also
functions with NADH and may be similar to Ernster's enzyme, which in turn
may be similar to xanthine oxidase. 4-Nitroquinoline-N-oxide and related carcinogens are reduced very effectively to a cytoplasmic enzyme similar to Ernster's
system (Sugimura et al., 1966; see Endo et al., 1971). In this instance, the nitro
derivative is an excellent substrate, but the corresponding hydroxylamino derivative a poor one. Consequently, the active carcinogenic intermediate hydroxylamino derivative accumulates. In fact, even the unstable 4-nitrosoquinoline-N-
oxide can be detected (Matsuyama and Nagata, 1973). This is not so with other
carcinogenic nitroaryl compounds, where the arylhydroxylamine seems to be a
good substrate; they are difficult to visualize by *in vitro* assays (Poirier and
Weisburger, 1973). In addition to mammalian enzymes, bacterial enzymes from
the gut flora may play an important role in reducing aromatic nitro groups
(Zachariah and Juchau, 1974) and also aromatic N-hydroxylamino derivatives
(Williams et al., 1970).

Bryan, Price, and associates discovered a series of nitrofurano thiazolyl derivatives which are carcinogenic for a number of sites in rodents. While the exact
mode of action of these agents has not been delineated, it would appear that they
can be considered heterocyclic analogues of benzidine or more accurately of
4-nitro-4'-aminobiphenyl. In rats and in mice, the major portion of the dose is
excreted in the urine and much of the remainder in the stools in 4 days after a
single dose (Cohen et al., 1973). A small portion of the urinary radioactivity is
accounted for by the drug administered. The balance of the metabolites remain to
be identified. In accordance with the fate of other chemicals with similar
structures, reduction of the nitro group to the hydroxylamino constituent should
yield an active intermediate. However, such structures may be somewhat unstable,
and thus special techniques may be necessary to demonstrate their transitory
existence (Yahagi et al., 1974).

### 3.3.5. Safrole

Safrole, a natural product and also a formerly used synthetic food additive, has
caused cancer in rats when administered at high dose levels for extended periods
of time. It has therefore been banned. As a methylenedioxy compound, its
structure has certain similarities to that of piperonyl butoxide, an insecticide
synergist capable of modifying the metabolism of specific insecticides. It was
demonstrated recently that the carcinogenicity of safrole is not related to the
presence of the methylenedioxy group, even though this structure provides the
necessary groups to constitute a bicyclic molecule.

The key metabolic reaction is a biochemical hydroxylation at the 1'-position in
the allyl side-chain (Borchert et al., 1973). 1'-Hydroxysafrole is excreted in urine
as a small fraction of the dose in rats, guinea pigs, and hamsters, and in larger
amounts in mice. Pretreatment of rats with an enzyme inducer, phenobarbital or

206

J. H.
WEISBURGER
AND
G. M.
WILLIAMS

3-methylcholanthrene, increases the excretion considerably. However, this is not seen in guinea pigs or hamsters. 1'-Hydroxysafrole appears to be a carcinogenic intermediate, for it causes tumors much faster at lower dose levels than safrole. Also, it causes tumors at the point of application or at the point of ingestion, the forestomach. However, 1'-hydroxysafrole appears to require additional activation, perhaps by esterification as with the corresponding aromatic amines and their N-hydroxy derivatives. Thus 1'-acetoxysafrole is a potent local-acting oncogen. Also, 1'-hydroxysafrole fails to interact *in vitro* with model molecular receptors, whereas the 1'-acetoxy compound does. Another metabolite possibly involved is 1'-ketosafrole, which also seems to be a reactive intermediate. More developments in this area will, it is hoped, fully account for the carcinogenicity of safrole.

### 3.3.6. 3-Hydroxyxanthine and Related Purine-N-Oxides

While studying the biological and biochemical properties of certain purine derivatives, Brown (1968) discovered the carcinogenicity of certain purine-N-oxides. These chemicals cause cancer at the point of application, but some of them are also active at remote sites, mainly in the liver. It has now been demonstrated that certain of these hydroxylated derivatives are substrates for sulfotransferase, just as are the hydroxy derivatives of certain carcinogenic aromatic amines (McDonald *et al.*, 1973). However, there does not seem to be a relationship between the sulfoacceptor activity and oncogenicity. It might be important to relate this biochemical parameter to the ease of liver tumor formation, inasmuch as sulfate ester formation appears to be involved mainly with carcinogenesis in the liver. Other reactions to be identified relate to sarcomagenicity and even mutagenicity (McCuen *et al.*, 1974). Stöhrer *et al.* (1973) have identified the reaction product of the model activated oncogen 3-acetoxyxanthine and tryptophan as a material attached to the 3-carbon of tryptophan through the 8-position of xanthine. A similar product appears to be excreted in urine of rats injected intraperitoneally with labeled 3-hydroxyxanthine.

### 3.3.7. Urethan and Carcinogenic Carbamates

Urethan is a classic carcinogen which, when administered as a single dose or repeatedly in smaller doses, induces pulmonary tumors in mice, the effect depending in part on strain, and diverse tumors in other rodents after longer latent periods such as melanomas in hamsters. It seems fairly well established that urethan, as such, is not carcinogenic and requires biochemical activation (see Mirvish, 1968; Yamamoto *et al.*, 1971). N-Hydroxyurethan, a candidate metabolite, has never been detected reliably. This chemical, however, appears more reactive than the parent compound, but possibly not through the hydroxylamino group directly. It has been thought, however, that the hydroxylamino group might confer reactive properties on the molecule, with the carbethoxy function as a leaving group. In this sense, it might be similar to the interesting, more complex carbamates discovered by Harris *et al.* (1970), or the pyrrolizidine alkaloids described below.

The pyrrolizidine or *Senecio* alkaloids are a family of naturally occurring highly hepatotoxic and carcinogenic chemicals (McLean, 1970; Miller, 1973). Their effect is modified by diet (Newberne, 1974). The key activation process of this class of agents is enzymatic dehydrogenation to pyrrolic metabolites which exhibit high reactivity, accounted for as a redistribution of charges within the molecule (Jago *et al.*, 1970; Mattocks and White, 1973; Hsu *et al.*, 1973). Thus results a leaving group, and conversion to a carbonium ion or similar electrophilic reagent. Younger rats produce more pyrrolic metabolites than adults. Also, whereas in young rats there is little effect of sex, in older animals males form more pyrrolic metabolites. These metabolic conversions appear to account for the toxic effects of the alkaloids.

The tissue distribution of another hepatotoxin, luteoskyrin, has been reported by Uraguchi *et al.* (1972). In the mouse, this chemical is eliminated progressively, more in feces than in urine. A relationship has been found among toxicity, uptake by organs, and elimination.

### 3.3.9. Carcinogenic Nitrosamines and Related Compounds

Carcinogenic nitrosamines and related compounds have been the subject of study for only about 20 yr. Dimethylnitrosamine, formerly an important industrial intermediate, was first found to cause cancer by Magee and Barnes in 1956 (see Magee *et al.*, 1974). Since that time, many different types of this broad class of chemicals have been synthesized and their carcinogenicity studied (see Schmähl, 1970; Druckrey, 1973; Weisburger, 1973*a*). Virtually all of them exhibit some degree of carcinogenicity, except when there is no alkyl group, as in diphenylnitrosamine. As a function of structure, species, dose rate, and other variables, these chemicals exhibit exquisite target specificity. A beginning has been made toward understanding this important tissue affinity on the basis of specific metabolic reactions (Druckrey, 1973; Magee *et al.*, 1974).

Current concepts visualize the production of a reactive electrophilic intermediate. With the simplest of the nitrosamines, dimethylnitrosamine, this has been described as $CH_3^+$. In view of the very short half-life of such structures predicted by classical organic chemistry, it is possible that they are produced transitorily during a concerted reaction among substrate, enzyme system, and target. Data on this point require further refinement, perhaps through the study of kinetics. Care must be taken to account for isotope effects in the metabolism of such small molecules (Keefer *et al.*, 1973). The complexity of the conversion of even simple prototypes in this class of compounds is attested to by the fact that dimethylnitrosamine is much more toxic than the diethyl higher homologue but the latter appears to be somewhat more carcinogenic. As noted elsewhere in this volume, dimethylnitrosamine yields much higher levels of 7-methylguanine, a cellular product obtained on hydrolysis of RNA, than the ethyl homologue does of 7-ethylguanine.

208

J. H.
WEISBURGER
AND
G. M.
WILLIAMS

With the more complex longer-chain aliphatic nitrosamines such as the dipropyl or dibutyl derivatives, or with cyclic nitrosamines such as nitrosopyrrolidine or nitrosopiperidine, the exact activation reactions have not yet been delineated. They are certainly oxidative. Many species, including primates and man, possess these enzymes. Thus these chemicals are reliably carcinogenic in primates, although in man there has been no case of cancer unambiguously related to exposure (O'Gara and Adamson, 1972; Montesano and Magee, 1974; Weisburger, 1974).

The first step in the metabolism of an alkylnitrosamine appears to be a classical C-hydroxylation. Thus with dimethylnitrosamine the reaction sequence is as follows (Druckrey, 1973):

$$O{=}N{-}N\overset{\displaystyle CH_3}{\underset{\displaystyle CH_3}{\Big\langle}} \;\rightarrow\; O{=}N{-}N\overset{\displaystyle CH_3}{\underset{\displaystyle CH_2OH}{\Big\langle}} \;\rightarrow\; O\overset{\displaystyle N{=}N{-}CH_3}{\underset{\displaystyle H{-}O}{\Big\langle}}CH_2$$

$$CH_2O + \overset{\displaystyle CH_3}{\underset{\displaystyle -OH}{N{=}N}} \xrightarrow{H^+} CH_3^+ + N_2 + H_2O$$

The eventual product postulated is a methyl carbonium ion.

With a more complex alkyl group, the question is whether hydroxylation occurs proximate to the nitrogen on the $\alpha$-position, as proposed initially (Druckrey, 1973), or through a $\beta$-oxidation as in fatty acids, as visualized by Krüger (1971; Krüger and Bertram, 1973; Althoff et al., 1973). With longer-chain alkylnitrosamines, $\omega$-hydroxylation can also occur (Druckrey et al., 1964; Okada and Suzuki, 1972; Blattmann and Preussmann, 1973; Ito et al., 1973). There is evidence that all of these intermediates are metabolites and that some of them are carcinogens. More recently, Schoental (1973) has proposed an intermediate with an aldehyde or keto functional group. Attempts have been made to understand these problems with cyclic nitrosamines, which are powerful carcinogens, but no unambiguous mechanism has emerged (Krüger, 1973; Lijinsky et al., 1973). Neunhoeffer et al. (1970) have postulated an enzymatically controlled rearrangement to hydroxamic acid derivatives.

In vitro studies, utilizing tissue slices or homogenates and subcellular fractions, have developed a certain relationship between rate of metabolism and carcinogenicity. The metabolism was often measured by $CO_2$ or aldehyde evolution, or combination of radioactivity from the tagged carcinogens with cellular macromolecules such as RNA or DNA (Rao and Vesselinovitch, 1973; Montesano and Magee, 1974).

Along these lines, Czygan et al. (1973) have demonstrated the conversion in vitro of dimethylnitrosamine by a microsome fraction of mouse liver to a mutagen detected in the system of Ames. The reaction is inhibited by carbon monoxide and appears to be cytochrome P450 dependent.

Just as the aliphatic or alkylaryl nitrosamines exhibit quite specific and selective organ affinity, in part a function of dose and other variables, probably owing to differences in metabolism related to them, the cyclic and heterocyclic nitrosamines do the same, but to an even more pronounced extent. To date, there have been few studies to determine the specific metabolites derived from such agents.

Small amounts of cyclic nitrosamines, such as nitrosomorpholine and dinitrosopiperazine, are excreted in urine. The amount excreted, as such, appears to be enhanced through increasing diuresis (Sander *et al.*, 1973).

Treatment of rats and mice with 3-methylcholanthrene decreases the carcinogenic effect of dimethylnitrosamine in the liver in rats but causes more extrahepatic tumors, especially in the lung (Hoch-Ligeti *et al.*, 1968). Venkatesan *et al.* (1970) found a decreased liver microsomal demethylation of dimethylnitrosamine on pretreatment with 3-methylcholanthrene or with phenobarbital. In mice, tumors at various sites were induced faster, especially in the lung and kidneys, by the mixture of dimethylnitrosamine and methylcholanthrene, but no data on metabolism under these conditions are available (Cardesa *et al.*, 1973). In rats, phenobarbital has little effect on metabolism (Kato *et al.*, 1967) and on carcinogenicity (Kunz *et al.*, 1969). On the other hand, aminoacetonitrile inhibits both metabolism and carcinogenicity (Fiume *et al.*, 1970; Hadjiolov, 1971; Mirvish and Sidransky, 1971). The dialkyltriazenes are related to the nitrosamines because, presumably, they form similar reactive intermediates during metabolism (see Druckrey, 1973). Except for the demonstration that labeled alkyltriazenes yield altered nucleic acids, with radioactivity attached to the guanylic acid in RNA, there have been no studies on the overall metabolism of these agents, some of which are related to dyestuff intermediates. It is obvious, however, that the key reaction is hydroxylation of the dialkyl groups attached to nitrogen, leading eventually to the production of a highly reactive intermediate.

4(5)-3,3-Dimethyl-1-triazenoimidazole-5(4)-carboxamide (DIC) was developed as a drug useful in chemotherapy of certain neoplasms. As might be expected on the basis of its structure, containing a dialkyltriazeno residue, this chemical is also a powerful carcinogen. Metabolism in animals and man leads to microsomal dealkylation, with production of a residue described as a methylcarbonium ion similar to what is seen during the metabolism of dimethylnitrosamine or the 1-aryl-3,3-dialkyltriazenes, described above. The remainder of the DIC molecule, namely 4(5)-aminoimidazole-5(4)-carboxamide, is found in urine of rodents and man (Skibba *et al.*, 1970*a,b*).

### 3.3.10. *Alkylnitrosoureido Compounds*

Alkylnitrosoureido compounds do not seem to require enzymatic metabolic activation, although such a reaction is not ruled out and could possibly account for their high local reactivity and carcinogenicity. Nonetheless, these chemicals do react at neutral pH with macromolecular and cellular receptors, and also with

210

J. H.
WEISBURGER
AND
G. M.
WILLIAMS

sulfhydryl compounds. They have limited half-life in aqueous media, especially above pH 6. Thus it is not expected that such chemicals persist in the environment. However, they can be readily formed from precursors and nitrite (Sander, 1971; Mirvish, 1972; Mirvish and Chu, 1973; Preussmann, 1974).

Kawachi et al. (1970) have described an enzyme system which removes the nitroso group and thus leads to an inactive compound. They ascribe the predominantly local action of this class of compounds to such an inactivating reaction. However, large doses of such compounds may exhibit a remote effect, presumably because they exceed the capacity of the enzyme removing the nitroso group. Bralow et al. (1973) have reported that N-methyl-N'-nitro-N-nitrosoguanidine (MNNG), a highly active gastric carcinogen in the Wistar rat, is inactive in several inbred rat strains. It might be that these strains have high levels of the inactivating enzyme system.

Intrarectal administration of MNNG in rats readily induces colorectal cancer but no other lesions (Narisawa et al., 1973; So et al., 1973). However, the related nitrosomethylurea in mice leads not only to colorectal cancers but at high dose levels also to leukemias and lung tumors, indicating that this chemical can be absorbed from the large bowel (this laboratory, unpublished data) and suggesting also that it is not denitrosated as readily as MNNG.

Methylureido derivatives, such as N-methylnitrosourea, even though administered intravenously, exhibit a selective carcinogenic effect on some organs, including the brain and nervous system. Shortly after injection of radioactive methylnitrosourea, radioactivity is found distributed in many organs, including the brain, in a uniform manner (Kleihues and Patzschke, 1971; Goth and Rajewsky, 1972). Thus the distribution of carcinogenicity under these conditions does not seem to account for the significant organotropic effect. Along these same lines, orally administered methylnitrosourethan causes cancer in the stomach and to some extent in the exocrine pancreas in guinea pigs (Druckrey et al., 1968; J. K. Reddy et al., 1974). Even so, liver nucleic acids are alkylated to a greater extent than pancreatic nucleic acids, perhaps a reflection of relative rates of metabolism (Alarif and Epstein, 1974). These and similar data suggest that a much more detailed approach to the metabolism of these powerful carcinogenic and mutagenic agents is necessary in order to account for their selective effect.

The fact needs to be considered in all these models that alkylnitrosoureas and related chemicals are powerful carcinogens under virtually all conditions. With these compounds there have been proven chemical reactions in which the alkyl group is transferred to a macromolecular receptor. Even here, however, it can be stated that specificity toward an organ under certain experimental conditions is not matched a priori with a similar biochemical specificity (Kleihues and Patzschke, 1971).

The nitroso group is certainly essential for the carcinogenicity of this type of chemical. Interestingly, there is differential tissue labelling, depending on whether the material studied has carbon labeled in the methyl or alkyl group, or in the guanidino portion (Tanaka and Sano, 1971; Sugimura et al., 1973; Schmall et al., 1973). Furthermore, the alkyl group appears to combine predominantly with nucleic acids, whereas the guanidino residue and metabolites thereof are found in proteins.

### 3.3.11. Dialkylhydrazines, Azoxyalkanes, and Cycasin

Laqueur (1970) discovered the carcinogenicity of the plant product cycasin, the β-glucoside of methylazoxymethanol, to small and large bowel, liver, and kidney. He demonstrated that this product undergoes hydrolysis, mainly through enzymes provided by the intestinal microflora of rodents, with release of the aglycone. The tissues of infant animals apparently have a β-glucosidase capable of splitting cycasin, but this enzyme is repressed during development (Matsumoto *et al.*, 1972). Thus cycasin exhibits toxic and carcinogenic effects in older animals only when administered by a route leading to contact with and enzymatic activation by gut microflora.

Cycasin is apparently not secreted appreciably in the bile, for parenteral injection has no pathological effect, indicating that the chemical does not reach the gut in significant amounts. It is excreted unchanged in urine. Given orally, however, it is highly toxic, as is the aglycone methylazoxymethanol. Under these conditions, only about 50% cycasin is recovered from urine (Kobayashi and Matsumoto, 1965; Laqueur, 1970). Similar parenteral injections of methylazoxymethanol have induced cancer in the liver, kidney, gall bladder, and large bowel, suggesting that this chemical can reach these sites. From the fact that cancer is seen in the gall bladder (Laqueur, 1970), the conclusion can be drawn that sufficient material is secreted in the bile.

The experiments of Wittig, of Gennaro, and of Druckrey (see Weisburger, 1973*b*) suggest that the mechanism proposed previously—conversion of 1,2-dimethylhydrazine to methylazoxymethanol or a glucuronide thereof in the liver, secretion in the bile, and release of an active intermediate by bacterial flora in the gut—may be relevant only to the induction, under certain conditions, of tumors in the small intestine. Tumors in the large bowel may stem from a direct specific oxidation of 1,2-dimethylhydrazine by the tissue, a concept we are currently examining experimentally. Further support for this view comes from the finding of B. S. Reddy *et al.* (1974*b*) that this agent causes cancer in the large bowel in germ-free rats.

Druckrey (1973) proposed that 1,2-dimethylhydrazine is oxidized in a concerted manner by mixed-function oxidases via azoxymethane to methylazoxymethanol and thence to an active methyldiazonium salt. Magee *et al.* (1973) observed that only small amounts of a dose of labeled 1,2-dimethylhydrazine are excreted in bile or feces. Extensive experimentation currently under way confirms this preliminary finding, and shows further that the major portion of a single dose is exhaled (this laboratory, unpublished data). A small portion of the respiratory radioactivity is in the form of $CO_2$, but, interestingly, the major part is in the form of basic compounds trapped by dilute acid, tentatively identified as methylhydrazine, and perhaps methylamine. Administration of tritiated dimethylhydrazine leads to concentration of radioactivity in liver, kidney, and intestinal tract, organs

212

J. H.
WEISBURGER
AND
G. M.
WILLIAMS

sensitive to cancer induction with this agent. On the other hand, with the diethyl analogue, radioactivity is noted in the hematopoietic system in the brain, again the target organ with these agents (Pozharisski *et al.*, 1974).

More complex 1,2-dialkylhydrazines, including 1-methyl-2-benzylhydrazine and procarbazine, are also carcinogenic. They undergo a series of metabolic reactions like those of the prototype 1,2-dimethylhydrazine, including oxidation to active intermediates. Toth and Shimizu (1973) have described the carcinogenicity of 1,1-dimethylhydrazine and related chemicals. There is little information on their metabolism except that they produce formaldehyde with a microsome fraction of liver from various species. This reaction is increased by enzyme inducers (Prough *et al.*, 1970; Kreis, 1970). Another metabolite of methylhydrazine is methane. With a higher homologue such as ethyl- or butylhydrazine, ethane or butane is found.

### 3.3.12. *Halogenated Hydrocarbons*

Carbon tetrachloride has been known for almost 30 yr to induce liver tumors in mice. This chemical is highly hepatotoxic in virtually all species, including man. Reuber and Glover (1970) showed that it is also carcinogenic in some strains of rats in which this agent tends to give only a moderate cirrhosis. Chloroform appears to be less active as a hepatotoxin or carcinogen. Other chlorinated hydrocarbons lead to liver damage and in some cases liver tumors in rodents (Tomatis *et al.*, 1973*b*; *IARC Monograph No. 5*, 1974). Also, ethylene bromide has recently been found to be carcinogenic (Olson *et al.*, 1973).

A number of investigators have observed that these chlorinated hydrocarbons undergo metabolic activation leading to production of intermediates which can combine covalently with cellular macromolecules and which are thought to be required for the expression of toxic and carcinogenic effects (see Recknagel, 1967; Fowler, 1969; Smuckler, 1972; Gandolfi and Van Dyke, 1973; Ilett *et al.*, 1973; Uehleke *et al.*, 1973).

The dehydrohalogenation is potentiated *in vitro* and *in vivo* by enzyme inducers such as 3-methylcholanthrene and phenobarbital. In fact, McLean *et al.* (1969) have described a method for inducing instant cirrhosis in rats by administering phenobarbital together with carbon tetrachloride (see also Cornish *et al.*, 1973). Recknagel (1967) developed the concept of carbon tetrachloride-mediated peroxide production, which he thought was the mechanism of hepatotoxicity. On the other hand, antioxidants protect against the hepatotoxicity of halogenated hydrocarbons, ethanol, and hydrazine (DiLuzio *et al.*, 1973). Some antioxidants induce liver enzymes, as does phenobarbital, and it would seem that the metabolite responsible for hepatotoxicity is rapidly transformed further under these conditions. Similar findings have been obtained with respect to protection against other carcinogens (see Grantham *et al.*, 1973; Wattenberg, 1973).

Bromobenzene is also a hepatotoxin whose effect is moderated by enzyme inducers such as 3-methylcholanthrene. The effect appears to rest on an induction of the detoxification pathway in the form of epoxide hydrase (Zampaglione *et al.*,

1973). A similar action underlies the effect of acetaminophen (Mitchell *et al.*, 1973).

Maltoni and Lefemine (1974) have described the carcinogenicity of vinyl chloride in rats and mice, leading to a variety of tumors, including rarely seen angiosarcomas in the liver. Similar liver tumors have been observed as an occupational risk in workmen engaged in the production of vinyl chloride– and perhaps vinyl acetate–based polymers (Selikoff and Hammond, 1974). A number of groups are currently studying the metabolism of vinyl chloride to determine the active intermediates. On the basis of present background, it appears that the epoxide, formed in cells poorly endowed with the corresponding detoxification systems such as epoxide hydrase or glutathione transferase, would be sensitive.

### 3.3.13. Dioxane

Dioxane leads to liver tumors in rats and guinea pigs. Tumors of the nasal cavity, as well as alterations in the kidney, are also noted. There are no data on the metabolite responsible for these effects. However, pretreatment of rats with 3-methylcholanthrene increases the toxicity of dioxane, suggesting that a metabolite is involved in the pathological effect of this agent (Argus *et al.*, 1973). Peroxides are apparently not responsible for this effect.

### 3.3.14. Thioacetamide and Acetamide

Thioacetamide, a powerful hepatotoxin and carcinogen to the liver of rodents in relatively small doses, has not been explored in detail with respect to metabolism or the specific metabolites which might be responsible for its effects. Other thioamides, such as thiouracil, act similarly, and this entire group deserves study.

Acetamide is also hepatotoxic and carcinogenic, but this chemical probably is not an intermediate in the action of the thio analogues, mainly because much higher dose levels are required. The effect of acetamide is antagonized by arginine glutamate (Weisburger *et al.*, 1969), suggesting that the metabolism of ammonia is somehow involved (Visek, 1972). The alternative possibility of N-hydroxylation has been explored in a preliminary way with inconclusive results (Dr. James Miller, personal communication).

### 3.3.15. Ethionine

Ethionine, an antimetabolite to methionine, causes liver tumors in rats but not hamsters when relatively large amounts are fed chronically. Also, it is a tool for induction of experimental pancreatitis. Ethionine seems to undergo metabolism similar to that of methionine, including ATP-mediated incorporation into nucleic acids via S-adenosylethionine (Farber, 1973a; Miller, 1973). This metabolite is also excreted in urine of rats fed a diet containing 0.2% ethionine (Smith and Pollard, 1969). Ethionine sulfoxide is another urinary metabolite present in detectable amounts only after chronic feeding of ethionine, but not after a single dose. The precise mechanism whereby this agent, produced by certain microorganisms,

214

J. H.
WEISBURGER
AND
G. M.
WILLIAMS

leads to cancer has not yet been clarified. Farber (1973*a,b*), the main contributor to this field along with Novelli and the late J. Stekol, has summarized the early carcinogenic process.

### 3.3.16. Diethylstilbestrol

Diethylstilbestrol (DES) has induced cancer in the endocrine system in animals under some conditions. Also, it has led to a rare type of vaginal cancer in young prepubertal girls consequent to the administration of large amounts of this drug to their mothers during gestation, but not when small amounts were given. The mechanism is unclear, but may be associated with the induction of a chronic hormonal imbalance in the offspring through the passage of the drug itself or unknown metabolites across the placenta. As a model, Fischer *et al.* (1973) have observed that labeled DES is absorbed more readily than the glucuronide from the intestine in weanling rats. However, in 5-day-old rats the glucuronide may be absorbed intact, whereas in older animals bacterially mediated hydrolysis of the glucuronic acid conjugate precedes resorption. DES induces renal cancer in male but not female hamsters, and not in male or female rats. Gabaldon and Lacomba (1972) noted much higher glucuronyl transferase activity for DES in hamsters than in rats but felt that this finding alone does not account for the carcinogenicity of DES in hamster kidney.

## 4. Variation in Carcinogen Metabolism

As is apparent from the detailed description of the metabolic processes operating on chemical carcinogens, these are general systems akin to those that apply to exogenous chemicals and drugs in general and, indeed, also to certain endogenous products such as steroid hormones. There are rather specific activation reactions and also fairly broad detoxification processes mediated by cellular mammalian enzymes, as well as by microbiological systems. Whether or not a given carcinogen is active under certain conditions, the degree and extent of its activity, the site affected, and under some conditions the time required to elicit the effect depend more on the ratio of activation reactions vs. detoxification reactions than on virtually any other currently known parameter controlling the overall carcinogenic process (Weisburger, 1973*a*). It is important, therefore, to understand fully the variables controlling this ratio, so that if a sensitive bioassay system is desired the ratio can be maximized, or if human cancer prevention is the goal it can be minimized.

These reactions depend on species, strain (and in man, a truly heterogeneous population, on individuals), age, sex, endocrine status, diet, and intestinal flora, on the presence of other chemicals, synthetic or naturally occurring, on the mode and frequency of exposure, and on numerous other parameters. Full discussion of these variables for each type of carcinogen is properly the subject of a separate monograph. Only a few essential and striking examples will be noted here.

## 4.1. Species and Strain

We have developed elsewhere in this chapter the point that metabolic activation or detoxification with different chemical carcinogens under varied environmental conditions is a key controlling element as to whether the individual concerned, whether man or animal model, develops cancer. Thus it seems desirable to be in a position to assess the risk through appropriate experimental approaches. Recently, the genetically mediated differences in inducibility of aryl hydrocarbon hydroxylase have been made the basis for a preliminary screen which, when fully developed, may be the basis for selection of individuals at high and low risk of developing cancer when exposed to compounds such as are present in cigarette smoke (Kellermann *et al.*, 1973*a,b*). Inasmuch as aryl hydrocarbon hydroxylase belongs to the family of mixed-function oxidases, it will be interesting and important to delineate the generality of this finding with respect to the metabolism and inducibility toward other substrates which may also present carcinogenic risks. There is hope for future exploitation of such reactions, for the metabolism of carcinogens is genetically determined and varies greatly among species (Patterson, 1973), as does the metabolism of other exogenous chemicals (Hucker, 1970; Weisburger and Rall, 1972). This has been useful in elucidating steps in activation reactions. For example, the guinea pig does not develop cancer after exposure to *N*-2-fluorenylacetamide, whereas the rat does. When it was suspected that *N*-hydroxylation was involved in the activation of *N*-2-fluorenylacetamide, the finding that the guinea pig could not *N*-hydroxylate confirmed the significance of this reaction (Miller and Miller, 1971; Weisburger and Weisburger, 1973).

Some carcinogens, such as the nitrosamines, appear to be actively metabolized by most species, including man (Magee *et al.*, 1974; Weisburger, 1974). Although there are no proven data for the carcinogenicity of nitrosamines in man, they are active in all other species tested, in agreement with the metabolic parameters. On the other hand, hydrazine and asymmetrical hydrazines seem active predominantly in mice and hamsters. It will be useful to relate these findings to information on metabolism as a function of species.

The species difference may be manifested primarily as a sex difference. For example, in the rat, metabolism of certain drugs is less active in males, whereas there is no sex difference in other species. Such differences extend even to strains or to breeds within a species.

## 4.2. Sex and Endocrine Status

For most experimental species, males are more susceptible to some of the aromatic amine liver carcinogens than are females. On the other hand, female mice have been found to be more sensitive to carbon tetrachloride and *o*-aminoazotoluene and female rats and mice more sensitive to diethylnitrosamine.

The basis for these various sex differences is not yet fully documented. In some special cases it could be that steroid hormones compete with carcinogens for

216

J. H.
WEISBURGER
AND
G. M.
WILLIAMS

metabolism or some other reaction such as binding. The more general and plausible reason relates to differences in the amount or activity of activating vs. deactivating enzymes.

Williams and Rabin (1971) have shown that a variety of carcinogens inhibit the steroid hormone–mediated association of ribosomes with endoplasmic membranes. The cytosolic protein which binds corticosteroids also binds 4-dimethylaminoazobenzene and 3-methylcholanthrene. However, there is no significant competition between carcinogens and steroids for binding sites (Litwak et al., 1972; Keightly and Okey, 1973). These results may indicate that the covalent binding of activated carcinogens may be at a different site on the binding molecule than the noncovalent binding of steroids. On the other hand, steroids do compete with carcinogens for metabolism. Thus steroids inhibit the metabolism of benzo[a]pyrene (Nebert et al., 1970), aflatoxin (Patterson and Roberts, 1972; Schwartz, 1974), and 7,12-dimethylbenz[a]anthracene (Booth et al., 1974).

The other main possibility, that there are sex differences in the amount or activity of metabolizing enzymes, has not been extensively studied. It is well known that in rats metabolism of many drugs is more active in males than in females (Conney, 1967; Conney and Burns, 1972).

The fact that N-2-fluorenylacetamide is more hepatocarcinogenic in certain strains of rats to males than to females rests on the level of sulfotransferase (Miller and Miller, 1971; Gutmann et al., 1972). Diethylnitrosamine usually is slightly more active in female rats, but in mice, males respond better, a reflection of metabolism (Kato et al., 1967; Rao and Vesselinovitch, 1973; Magee et al., 1974).

Whenever experiments in chemical carcinogenesis reveal a difference in response between male and female animals, investigation of the underlying differences in enzymes concerned with activation and deactivation reactions contributes the key to the endocrine effect. However, in several instances when a carcinogen is administered to a sexually immature animal, or even a newborn animal, with no further treatment during the adult sexually differentiated stage, there still appears to be a sex-linked incidence of cancer, not only as might be expected in endocrine-responsive organs such as breast, but also in liver and other tissues (see Toth, 1968).

## 4.3. Age

Newborn and young animals have been shown to be more susceptible to tumor induction at several sites than older animals (Toth, 1968; Tomatis et al., 1973a). In some cases, this is probably because of the higher levels of cell proliferation in the affected organ, since susceptibility in older animals can be heightened by inducing cell replication. Drug-metabolizing enzymes are usually very low in newborn animals (Brodie and Gillette, 1971), and this seems to be true of those involved with detoxification of chemical carcinogens, but perhaps is not so for activating enzymes. For example, the rate of total body clearance of 9,10-dimethyl-1,2-benzanthracene (7,12-dimethylbenz[a]anthracene) is lower for newborn mice than for adults (Domsky et al., 1963).

There is considerable concern about the possible effect of environmental carcinogens on unborn fetuses through placental transmission and possible fetal metabolism. It is apparent that many of the ultimate carcinogens derived from procarcinogens through metabolic activation are highly reactive entities. Unless these are stabilized to a transport form which can subsequently be released in the fetus, it seems unlikely that activation to a final carcinogenic product in the mother would lead to the expression of carcinogenicity in the fetus. Thus the question is whether placental transfer of a procarcinogen or a proximate but not ultimate carcinogen might lead to cancer in the offspring if the fetus possesses the necessary enzymatic potential to produce the ultimate carcinogenic metabolite. In recent years, a number of studies on the capability of fetuses to carry out such reactions have been performed (Pelkonen *et al.*, 1973; Gillette *et al.*, 1973; Tomatis *et al.*, 1973*a*).

From animal systems and from experiments with human fetuses in societies where this is considered permissible, useful comparative data have been obtained. Much more needs to be learned about the capability of fetuses of various species to perform biochemical alterations on substrates such as drugs and carcinogens as a function of fetal age. It would seem that in most cases the fetus has lower enzymatic potential than the adult. However, fetuses do have many of the enzymes concerned with activation reactions, such as those that epoxidize polycyclic aromatic hydrocarbons (and perhaps aflatoxin, not yet studied) and nitroreductases, but seem to be deficient in the detoxification steps such as conjugation with glucuronic acid or epoxide hydrase (Brodie and Gillette, 1971). Thus, on balance, the fetus may be more sensitive for this reason, as is also documented by the demonstration that fetuses or certainly newborn animals are exquisitely sensitive to a variety of chemical carcinogens.

## 5. Modification of Carcinogen Metabolism

A number of factors have been found which alter the induction of cancer by certain carcinogens. Most of these factors are effective by virtue of altering metabolism. The host may be completely protected if the modifier inhibits activation while deactivation proceeds unimpaired in the same or another organ.

The enzymes concerned with the metabolism of carcinogens are in a dynamic equilibrium between synthesis and degradation. Thus the level of these enzymes depends on a number of endogenous and, more importantly, exogenous elements. These include the agent itself, other chemicals, carcinogenic or not, enzyme inducers or inhibitors, and also, to some extent, the diet. More subtle effects relate to stresses such as temperature and crowding. For many reasons, including the central importance of the organ and also the ease of isolating cellular and molecular entities, liver enzymes have received extensive study. However, because of the need to understand carcinogen activation and detoxification at target sites other than the liver, such as the lung, the breast, the kidney, and the intestinal tract, a beginning has been made to understand enzymes in these

218

J. H.
WEISBURGER
AND
G. M.
WILLIAMS

organs in relation to environmental modifiers (Dao and Libby, 1972; Janss *et al.*, 1972; Wattenberg, 1972; Gram, 1973).

## 5.1. Diet

Many types of cancer in man are mediated by diet in an as yet unclear manner. These include cancer of the digestive tract and of certain endocrine-sensitive organs such as the breast (Wynder and Mabuchi, 1972). Diet components, e.g., protein, do affect liver enzymes (Rumack *et al.*, 1973). The importance of diet in human cancer development is undeniable and has been studied in some model systems. Metabolism of benzo[*a*]pyrene is reduced by a protein-deficient diet (Paine and McLean, 1973). Also, with dimethylnitrosamine a protein-free diet results in a decrease of activating *N*-demethylation and a lower yield of liver tumors following exposure. Interestingly, the kidney activation is not greatly affected and the incidence of renal tumors increases (Swann and McLean, 1971). This illustrates the important point that metabolism in different organs may be regulated differently. However, more data are needed on the specific enzymatic pattern dealing with carcinogen metabolism under these conditions. Fat is a key dietary component in international metabolic epidemiological comparisons (Wynder and Mabuchi, 1972) which needs study (Chan and Cohen, 1974; B. S. Reddy *et al.*, 1974*a*; Rogers *et al.*, 1974). Diet also affects the intestinal microflora, which can be an important factor in the metabolism of certain carcinogens (see Hill, 1974; Weisburger, 1973*b*). The microflora also affects hepatic enzymes, perhaps through a feedback process of certain metabolites (Reddy *et al.*, 1973).

Discovery of the involvement of micronutrients such as riboflavin in the metabolism of the carcinogenic azo dyes, controlling a deactivation process through an effect on azo dye reductase, is a classic in this field. More recently, riboflavin has been assigned additional roles in the carcinogenic process (Chan *et al.*, 1972; Yang, 1973; Rivlin, 1973) Vitamin A and perhaps vitamin E participate in metabolism of carcinogens, but only a beginning has been made in understanding the precise site of their involvement (Nair and Kayden, 1972; Becking, 1973; Yeh and Johnson, 1973; Genta *et al.*, 1974).

## 5.2. Effect of Mode and Frequency of Exposure

With a number of carcinogens distinct effects are noted as a function of mode of introduction. As already mentioned, cycasin is active when given by mouth but not when injected parenterally because this agent requires enzymatic hydrolysis mediated by gut flora. Dibutylnitrosamine induces mainly urinary bladder cancers on subcutaneous injection, but also liver and pulmonary tumors on oral intake. The reasons apparently are distinct concentration effects in the liver and metabolism therein when administered by these two routes. It is well known that in many strains of mice small amounts of some polycyclic aromatic hydrocarbons are highly carcinogenic when applied cutaneously but not much so when given by mouth. The difference again rests on activating and detoxifying enzymes at these two sites. *and* TRANSPORT!!

Some carcinogens such as polycyclic hydrocarbons are more active when the same total amount is administered subcutaneously in fractionated doses than when a single large dose is given. This is because the latter mode leads to extensive *transport away from the site.* formation of detoxified metabolites. With some nitrosamines, the target organ depends on dose rate (Nemoto and Takayama, 1973; Magee *et al.*, 1974). Some carcinogens such as most aromatic amines and azo dyes must be administered for a minimal amount of time to accumulate the necessary increasing amounts of active carcinogen in the form of *N*-hydroxy derivatives (see Weisburger and Weisburger, 1973).

## 5.3. Effect of Other Agents

It is a truism to state that the environment is very complex. Thus the induction of cancer in man and in animal models requires careful analysis to dissect the manifold elements which eventually control whether a neoplasm does or does not occur. In animal models and with powerful carcinogens, such elements as quality and quantity of diet, including the possible presence of traces of pesticides and hormones as well as the amount of roughage, may not play a decisive role. With lower dose levels or weaker carcinogens, they may. The effect may hinge on the relative activity of enzymes concerned with the metabolism of the carcinogen, but more data in this area are required.

There are more than 200 chemicals known to stimulate the activity of microsomal enzymes (Conney, 1967; Brodie and Gillette, 1971). Many are compounds which are themselves metabolized by microsomal enzymes. Among the most studied are phenobarbital, polycyclic aromatic hydrocarbons such as 3-methylcholanthrene, benzo[*a*]pyrene, and benzo[*a*]anthracene, and certain flavones. These may either enhance or decrease the tumorigenicity of a carcinogen according to whether they induce activating or deactivating enzymes. It is now established for several of these inducers that they promote synthesis of new enzymes.

In the case of carcinogens which are primarily inactivated by metabolism, inhibition of metabolism may actually increase the activity. The direct-acting carcinogen *N*-methyl-*N'*-nitro-*N*-nitrosoguanidine is also mutagenic, as are many carcinogens (see below). *In vitro* microsomal metabolism produces a loss of its mutagenicity (Popper *et al.*, 1973) and a protein-deficient diet decreases the microsomal inactivation (Czygan *et al.*, 1974). The toxicity and probably also the carcinogenicity of direct-acting alkylating agents such as nitrogen mustards are decreased by enzyme induction (Belitsky and Yaguzhinsky, 1972).

While the activation reactions for some types of carcinogens have been understood for some time now, for example, the aromatic amines and azo dyes, background data for these processes with other agents are of recent date and their modulation by enzyme inducers and inhibitors is not as well documented. This is especially true for extrahepatic sites.

220

J. H.
WEISBURGER
AND
G. M.
WILLIAMS

Many of the detoxification steps, such as conjugation reactions with glucuronic acid, are inducible. The outcome of a carcinogenicity experiment will depend on the relative increases of the activation step compared to the detoxification step. An extensively studied example is that of the carcinogen N-2-fluorenylacetamide. Methylcholanthrene decreases carcinogenicity in the rat and increases it in the hamster. In both species, there is an increased formation of the proximate carcinogen, the N-hydroxy derivative. However, in the rat there is a more pronounced increase in glucuronyl transferase, leading to detoxified metabolites (Irving, 1970). Antioxidants such as butylated hydroxytoluene have similar effects (Grantham et al., 1973). Peraino et al. (1971) discovered that phenobarbital given together with this carcinogen reduced the carcinogenic effect—again for a similar reason, increased detoxification through glucuronide formation (Matsushima et al., 1972). Interestingly, for reasons that are not yet clear, phenobarbital given after the carcinogen increased carcinogenicity. We, and in part Kunz et al. (1969), have confirmed this effect with another hepatocarcinogen, diethylnitrosamine. These studies have more than theoretical importance, for Wattenberg (1972, 1973) has described the occurrence in foods consumed by man of materials such as flavones which are potent enzyme inducers and which can modify response of carcinogens.

If the ultimate carcinogens in the form of electrophilic reactants or radical ions are the key intermediates produced on metabolism of many if not all chemical carcinogens, it would seem that their effect would be reduced or even abolished by providing competitive concentrations of nucleophilic trapping agents to interfere with their reaction with key cellular targets. A beginning success along these lines has been achieved, and more effort is warranted (Miller and Miller, 1972).

## 5.4. Chemical Carcinogens and Mutagens

Until recently there was much controversy about whether mutagens were carcinogenic, or carcinogens mutagenic (Hollaender, 1971). With the insight provided by the understanding of metabolic activation of chemical carcinogens to highly reactive products, it is now quite apparent that such ultimate carcinogens are also mutagenic. It would appear, however, that not all mutagens are carcinogenic, perhaps because such agents introduced in the microbiological system are not detoxified readily, whereas in a mammalian system they are. Examples are hydroxylamine and 8-hydroxyquinoline. From a practical point of view, newer methods can now be devised to assess, in preliminary way, the potential carcinogenic risk of chemicals or mixtures by determining their mutagenic potential (see Ames et al., 1973a,b; Duncan and Brookes, 1973; Heidelberger, 1973; Stoltz et al., 1974). Care must be taken to secure proper and reliable enzymatic activation processes. This can be accomplished through an in vitro system, for example, a microsomal preparation or a host-mediated system (Fahrig, 1973; Legator, 1973; Nakajima and Iwahara, 1973). Similar considerations apply to cell transformation as an end point and indication of carcinogenicity

(see DiPaolo *et al.*, 1973; Huberman and Sachs, 1973; Nebert *et al.*, 1973).
Needless to say, the results obtained warrant careful interpretation in the light of current knowledge.

Another method whereby metabolites of carcinogens in body fluids or in urine may give an indication of exposure has been developed in a preliminary way by Durston and Ames (1974), who detected materials possibly capable of inducing mutation in sensitive microorganisms. This system, when further developed, could serve to monitor exposure of individuals to certain carcinogens, both voluntary exposure as in cigarette smoking and involuntary exposure as in diet and occupation. With newer methods, which are highly sensitive and selective, perhaps other metabolites of carcinogens can be detected, as was done, for example, with industrial chemicals by Imamura and Ikeda (1973).

 ## 6. Concluding Remarks and Prospects

Thirty years ago, the field of chemical carcinogenesis was concerned with the description of a few types of chemicals, mainly polycyclic aromatic hydrocarbons, aromatic amines and azo dyes, and several miscellaneous agents such as urethan. Their mechanism of action was obscure. In the intervening years, a number of additional classes of chemical carcinogens have been discovered. Included are the important nitrosamine derivatives, certain mycotoxins, other natural products such as safrole, and commercial chemicals such as vinyl chloride, asbestos, and chromates. Some of these chemicals are laboratory curiosities, others are tonnage industrial products which have caused cancer not only in animals but also in man. Efforts have been and are being made to discover the carcinogenic principles responsible for certain human cancers (Wynder, 1974).

However, the exciting development in the study of chemical carcinogens is insight into their mode of action. The question of why such heterogeneous chemicals as polycyclic aromatic hydrocarbon, aromatic amine, nitrosamine, mycotoxin, *Senecio* alkaloid, and safrole should cause cancer was, indeed, most puzzling. Now, a unified lead has been derived from detailed understanding of the metabolism of these agents—the realization that they can undergo metabolic conversion to the highly reactive carcinogenic intermediates that Miller and Miller (1971) have termed "ultimate carcinogens." To be carcinogenic, an agent needs to be converted to such a form. It is these metabolites which react with key cellular and molecular, probably macromolecular, receptors, discussed elsewhere in this treatise. However, there are a few chemical carcinogens, for example, acetamide, hydrazine, and some of the inorganic carcinogenic chemicals (Sunderman, 1971), for which there are no data on activated forms.

The knowledge that chemical carcinogens are converted to such activated forms is being utilized currently to devise short-term bioassay systems. These should permit pretesting of the large number of environmental chemicals, and also act as realistic tracers for the isolation and purification of endogenous agents responsible for cancer in man (Stoltz *et al.*, 1974). Once the specific chemicals and

222

J. H.
WEISBURGER
AND
G. M.
WILLIAMS

situations which lead to human cancer have been pinpointed, the goal of much of the research on the etiology of cancer, it may be possible to devise conditions realistically applicable to man which would increase detoxification reactions and minimize activation. Thus, short of the capability of eliminating chemical carcinogens from the environment altogether, application of the background of information on metabolic fate could provide the clues to reduce the incidence of or, indeed, prevent cancer in man.

ACKNOWLEDGMENTS

We are grateful for excellent editorial and secretarial support to M. Mervis, B. Miller, W. Chernis, and D. Peetsch.

## 7. References

ALARIF, A., AND EPSTEIN, S. S., 1974, The metabolism of the pancreatic carcinogens $N\text{-}^{14}C$-methyl-$N$-nitrosourethane and methylnitrosourea in guinea pigs, and their *in vitro* metabolism in the guinea pig and human pancreas, *Proc. Am. Assoc. Cancer Res.* **15**:68.

ALBRECHT, R., AND MANCHON, P., 1973, Metabolisme et toxicité des colorants azoiques, *Ann. Nutr. Aliment.* **27**:1–9.

ALTHOFF, J., KRUEGER, F. W., AND MOHR, U., 1973, Carcinogenic effect of dipropylnitrosamine and compounds related by $\beta$-oxidation, *J. Natl. Cancer Inst.* **51**:287–288.

AMES, B. N., SIMS, P., AND GROVER, P. L., 1972, Epoxides of carcinogenic polycyclic hydrocarbons are frameshift mutagens, *Science* **176**:47–49.

AMES, B. N., DURSTON, W. E., YAMASAKI, E., AND LEE, F. D., 1973a, Carcinogens are mutagens: A simple test system combining liver homogenates for activation and bacteria for detection, *Proc. Natl. Acad. Sci.* **70**:2281–2285.

AMES, B. N., LEE, F. D., AND DURSTON, W. E., 1973b, An improved bacterial test system for the detection and classification of mutagens and carcinogens, *Proc. Natl. Acad. Sci.* **70**:782–786.

ARCOS, J. C. AND ARGUS, M. F., 1974, *Chemical Induction of Cancer*, Academic Press, New York and London.

ARGUS, M. F., SOHAL, R. S., BRYANT, G. M., HOCH-LIGETI, C., AND ARCOS, J. C., 1973, Dose–response and ultrastructural alterations in dioxane carcinogenesis, *Europ. J. Cancer* **9**:237–243.

BAIRD, W. M., DIPPLE, A., GROVER, P. L., SIMS, P. AND BROOKES, P., 1973, Studies on the formation of hydrocarbon-deoxyribonucleoside products by the binding of derivatives of 7-methylbenz(a)anthracene to DNA in aqueous solution and in mouse embryo cells in culture, *Cancer Research* **33**:2386–2392.

BARTSCH, H., AND HECKER, E., 1971, On the metabolic activation of the carcinogen $N$-hydroxy-$N$-2-acetylaminofluorene. III. Oxidation with horseradish peroxidase to yield 2-nitrosofluorene and $N$-acetoxy-$N$-2-acetylaminofluorene, *Biochim. Biophys. Acta* **237**:567.

BARTSCH, H., MILLER, J. A., AND MILLER, E. C., 1972, $N$-Acetoxy-$N$-acetylaminoarenes and nitrosoarenes: One-electron non-enzymatic and enzymatic oxidation products of various carcinogenic aromatic acetylhydroxamic acids, *Biochim. Biophys. Acta* **273**:40.

BARTSCH, H., DWORKIN, C., MILLER, E. C., AND MILLER, J. A., 1973, Formation of electrophilic $N$-acetoxyarylamines in cytosols from rat mammary gland and other tissues by transacetylation from the carcinogen $N$-hydroxy-4-acetylaminobipheryl, *Biochim. Biophys. Acta* **304**:42–55.

BAST, R. C., JR., SHEARS, B. W., RAPP, H. J., AND GELBOIN, H. V., 1973, Aryl hydrocarbon (benzo(a)pyrene) hydroxylase in guinea pig peritoneal macrophages: Benz(a)anthracene-induced increase of enzyme activity *in vivo* and in cell culture, *J. Natl. Cancer Inst.* **51**:675–678.

BECKING, G. C., 1973, Vitamin A status and hepatic drug metabolism in the rat, *Canad. J. Physiol. Pharmacol.* **51**:6–11.

BELITSKY, G. A., and YAGUZHINSKY, L. S., 1972, The effect of benz(a)anthracene as an inductor of multipurpose oxidases on the toxic and antiblastomic action of N,N-bis(chloroethyl)aniline, *Voprosy Onkol.* **18(6)**:72–74.

BERENBLUM, I., 1969, A re-evaluation of the concept of cocarcinogenesis, *Prog. Exp. Tumor Res.* **2**:21–30.

BERGMANN, E. D., AND PULLMAN, B., eds., 1969, *Physicochemical Mechanism of Carcinogenesis*, Israel Academy of Sciences and Humanities, Jerusalem.

BLATTMANN, L., AND PREUSSMANN, R., 1973, Struktur von metaboliten Carcinogener Dialkylnitrosamine im Rattenurin, *Z. Krebsforsch.* **79**:3–5.

BOGOVSKI, P., PREUSSMANN, R., WALKER, E. A., AND DAVIS, W., eds., 1972, *N-Nitroso Compounds: Analysis and Formation*, Scientific Publication No. 3, International Agency for Research on Cancer, Lyon.

BOOTH, J., KEYSELL, G. R., AND SIMS, P., 1973, Formation of glutathione conjugates as metabolites of 7,12-dimethylbenz(a)anthracene by rat liver homogenates, *Biochem. Pharmacol.* **22**:1781–1791.

BOOTH, J., KEYSELL, G. R., AND SIMS, P., 1974, Effect of oestradiol on the *in vitro* metabolism of 7,12-dimethylbenz(a)anthracene and its hydroxymethyl derivatives, *Biochem. Pharmacol.* **23**:735–744.

BORCHERT, P., WISLOCKI, P. G., MILLER, J. A., AND MILLER, E. C., 1973a, The metabolism of the naturally occurring hepatocarcinogen safrole to 1'-hydroxysafrole and the electrophilic reactivity of 1'-acetoxysafrole, *Cancer Res.* **33**:575–589.

BORCHERT, P., MILLER, J. A., MILLER, E. C., AND LAIRES, T. K., 1973b, 1'-Hydroxysafrole: A proximate carcinogenic metabolite of safrole in the rat and mouse, *Cancer Res.* **33**:590–600.

BOUTWELL, R. K., 1974, The function and mechanism of promoters of carcinogenesis, *CRC Crit. Rev. Toxicol.* **2**:419–443.

BOYD, J. S., AND SMELLIE, R. M. S., eds., 1972, *Biological Hydroxylation Mechanisms*, Academic Press, New York.

BOYLAND, E., 1952, Different types of carcinogens and their possible modes of action, *Cancer Res.* **12**:77–84.

BOYLAND, E., 1971, Mercapturic acid conjugation, in: *Concepts in Chemical Pharmacology*, Part II (B. B. Brodie and J. R. Gillette, eds.), pp. 401–421, Springer, New York.

BRALOW, S. P., GRUENSTEIN, M., AND MERANZE, D. R., 1973, Host resistance to gastric adenocarcinomatosis in three strains of rats ingesting N-methyl-N'-nitro-N-nitrosoguanidine, *Oncology* **27**:168.

BRODIE, B. B., AND GILLETTE, J. R., eds., 1971, *Concepts in Chemical Pharmacology*, Part II, Springer, New York.

BROWN, J. B., 1968, Purine N-oxides as antimetabolites and oncogens, in: *Frontiers of Biology*, Vol. 10, pp. 237–259, North-Holland, Amsterdam.

BÜRKL, K., LIEBELT, A. G., AND BRESNICK, E., 1973, Expression of aryl hydrocarbon hydroxylase induction in mouse tissues *in vivo* and in organ culture, *Arch. Biochem. Biophys.* **158**:641–649.

CALDER, I. C., CREEK, M. J., AND WILLIAMS, P. J., 1974, N-Hydroxyphenacetin as a precursor of 3-substituted 4-hydroxyacetanilide metabolites of phenacetin, *Chem.-Biol. Interact.* **8**:87–90.

CAMPBELL, T. C., CAEDO, J. P., JR., BULATAO-JAYME, J., SALAMAT, L., AND ENGEL, R. W., 1970, Aflatoxin M₁ in human urine, *Nature (Lond.)* **227**:403.

CARDESA, A., POUR, P., RUSTIA, M., ALTHOFF, J., AND MOHR, U., 1973, The syncarcinogenic effect of methylcholanthrene and dimethylnitrosamine in Swiss mice, *Z. Krebsforsch.* **79**:98–107.

CHAN, P. C., AND COHEN, L. A., 1974, Effect of dietary fat, antiestrogen, and antiprolactin on the development of mammary tumors in rats, *J. Natl. Cancer Inst.* **52**:25–30.

CHAN, P. C., OKAMOTO, T., AND WYNDER, E. L., 1972, Possible role of riboflavin deficiency in epithelial neoplasia. III. Induction of. microsomal aryl hydrocarbon hydroxylase, *J. Natl. Cancer Inst.* **48**:1341–1345.

CLAYSON, D. B., 1962, *Chemical Carcinogenesis*, Little, Brown, Boston.

COHEN, S. M., ALTER, A., AND BRYAN, G. T., 1973, Distribution of radioactivity and metabolism of formic acid 2-(4-(5-nitro-2-furyl)-2-¹⁴C-2-thiazolyl) hydrazide following oral administration of rats and mice, *Cancer Res.* **33**:2802–2809.

CONNEY, A. H., 1967, Pharmacological implications of microsomal enzyme induction, *Pharmacol. Rev.* **19**:317–366.

224

J. H.
WEISBURGER
AND
G. M.
WILLIAMS

CONNEY, A. H., 1973, Carcinogen metabolism and human cancer, *New Engl. J. Med.* **289**:971–973.

CONNEY, A. H., AND BURNS, J. J., 1972, Metabolic interactions among environmental chemicals and drugs, *Science* **178**:576–586.

CONNEY, A. H., AND KUNTZMAN, R., 1971, Metabolism of normal body constituents by drug metabolizing enzymes in liver microsomes, in: *Concepts in Chemical Pharmacology*, Part 2 (B. B. Brodie and J. R. Gillette, eds.), pp. 401–421, Springer, New York.

CONNEY, A. H., LEVIN, W., JACOBSON, M., AND KUNTZMAN, R., 1973, Effect of drugs and environmental chemicals on steroid metabolism, *Clin. Pharmacol. Ther.* **14**:727–741.

CORNISH, H. H., LING, B. P., AND BARTH, M. L., 1973, Phenobarbital and organic solvent toxicity, *Am. Ind. Hyg. Assoc. J.* **34**:487–492.

CRADDOCK, V. M., 1971, Liver carcinomas induced in rats by single administration of dimethylnitrosamine after partial hepatectomy, *J. Natl. Cancer Inst.* **47**:889–907.

CZYGAN, P., GREIM, H., GARRO, A. J., HUTTERER, F., SCHAFFNER, F., POPPER, H., ROSENTHAL, O., AND COOPER, D. Y., 1973, Microsomal metabolism of dimethylnitrosamine and the cytochrome P-450 dependency of its activation to a mutagen, *Cancer Res.* **33**:2983–2986.

CZYGAN, P., GREIM, H., GARRO, A., SCHAFFNER, F., AND POPPER, H., 1974, The effect of dietary protein deficiency on the ability of isolated hepatic microsomes to alter the mutagenicity of a primary and a secondary carcinogen, *Cancer Res.* **34**:119–123.

DALEZIOS, J., WOGAN, G. N., AND WEINREB, S. M., 1971, Aflatoxin $P_1$: A new aflatoxin metabolite in monkeys, *Science* **171**:584–585.

DALY, J., 1971, Enzymatic oxidation at carbon, in: *Concepts in Chemical Pharmacology*, Part II (B. B. Brodie and J. R. Gillette, eds.), pp. 285–311, Springer, New York.

DAO, T. L. AND LIBBY, P. R., 1972, Steroid sulphate formation in human breast tumors and hormone dependency, in: *Estrogen Target Tissues and Neoplasia* (T. L. Dao, ed.), pp. 181–200, Chicago University Press, Chicago.

DIAMOND, L., AND GELBOIN, H. V., 1969, Alpha-naphthoflavone: An inhibitor of hydrocarbon cytotoxicity and microsomal hydroxylase, *Science* **7**:1023–1025.

DiLUZIO, N. R., STEGE, T. E., AND HOFFMAN, E. O., 1973, Protective influence of diphenyl-*p*-phenylenediamine on hydrazine induced lipid peroxidation and hepatic injury, *Exp. Mol. Pathol.* **19**:284–292.

DiPAOLO, J. A., NELSON, R. L., DONOVAN, P. J., AND EVANS, C. H., 1973, Host-mediated *in vivo–in vitro* assay for chemical carcinogenesis, *Arch. Pathol.* **95**:380–385.

DIPPLE, A., AND SLADE, T. A., 1970, Structure and activity in chemical carcinogenesis: Reactivity and carcinogenicity of 7-bromomethylbenz(a)anthracene and 7-bromomethyl-12-methyl-benz(a)anthracene, *Europ. J. Cancer* **6**:417–423.

DOMSKY, I. I., LIJINSKY, W., SPENCER, K., AND SHUBIK, P., 1963, Rate of metabolism of 9,10-dimethyl-1,2-benzanthracene in newborn and adult mice, *Proc. Soc. Exp. Biol. Med.* **113**:110–112.

DRUCKREY, H., 1973, Specific carcinogenic and teratogenic effects of "indirect" alkylating methyl and ethyl compounds, and their dependency on stages of ontogenic developments, *Xenobiotica* **3**:271–303.

DRUCKREY, H., PREUSSMANN, R., IVANKOVIC, S., SCHMIDT, C. H., MENNEL, H. D., AND STAHL, K. W., 1964, Selektive Erzeugung von Blasenkrebs an Ratten durch Dibutyl- und *N*-Butyl-*N*-butanol(4)-nitrosamin, *Z. Krebsforsch.* **66**:280.

DRUCKREY, H., IVANKOVIC, S., BÜCHELER, J., PREUSSMANN, R., AND THOMAS, C., 1968, Erzeugung von Magen- und Pankreas-Krebs beim Meerschweinchen durch Methylnitrosoharnstoff und-urethan, *Z. Krebsforsch* **71**:167–182.

DUNCAN, M. E., AND BROOKES, P., 1973, The induction of azaguanine-resistant mutants in cultured Chinese hamster cells by reactive derivatives of carcinogenic hydrocarbons, *Mutation Res.* **21**:107–118.

DURSTON, W. E. AND AMES, B. N., 1974, A simple method for the detection of mutagens in urine studies with the carcinogen 2-acetylaminofluorene, *Proc. Natl. Acad. Sci.* **71**:737–741.

ENDO, H., AND TAKAHASHI, K., 1973, Methylguanidine, a naturally occurring compound showing mutagenicity after nitrosation in gastric juice, *Nature (Lond.)* **245**:325–326.

ENDO, H., ONO, T., AND SUGIMURA, T., eds., 1971, *Chemistry and Biological Actions of 4-Nitroquinoline-1-oxide*, Springer, New York.

FAHRIG, R., 1973, Metabolic activation of mutagens in mammals: Host-mediated assay utilizing the induction of mitotic gene conversion in *Saccharomyces cerevisiae*, *Agents Actions* **3**:99–110.

FARBER, E., 1973*a*, Hyperplastic liver nodules, in: *Methods in Cancer Research*, Vol. VII, Academic Press, New York.

FARBER, E., 1973b, Carcinogenesis—Cellular evolution as a unifying thread, *Cancer Res.* **33:**2537–2550.

FISCHER, L. J., KENT, J. H., AND WEISSINGER, J. L., 1973, Absorption of diethylstilbestrol and its glucuronide conjugate from the intestine of five- and twenty-five-day-old rats, *J. Pharmacol. Exp. Ther.* **185:**163–170.

FISHMAN, W. H., 1970, *Metabolic Conjugation and Metabolic Hydrolysis*, Vols. I and II, Academic Press, New York.

FIUME, L., CAMPADELLI-FIUME, G., MAGEE, P. N., AND HOLSMAN, J., 1970, Cellular injury and carcinogenesis: Inhibition of metabolism of dimethylnitrosamine by aminoacetonitrile, *Biochem. J.* **120:**601–605.

FOWLER, J. S. L., 1969, Carbon tetrachloride metabolism in the rabbit, *Brit. J. Pharmacol.* **37:**733–737.

FRANCHI, G., FORGIONE, A., FILIPPESCHI, S., CSETENYI, J., AND GARATTINI, S., 1973, A spectrophotometric method for the estimation of the carcinostatic agent 6-chrysenamine (F.O.R.T.C. 116) in biological fluids and tissues, *Europ. J. Cancer* **9:**591–595.

FUKUDA, S., AND YAMAMOTO, N., 1972, Detection of activating enzymes for 4-nitroquinoline-1-oxide activation with a microbial assay system, *Cancer Res.* **32:**735–439.

GABALDON, M., AND LACOMBA, J., 1972, Glucuronyltransferase activity towards diethylstilbestrol in rat and hamster: Effect of activators, *Europ. J. Cancer* **8:**275–279.

GANDOLFI, A. J., AND VAN DYKE, R. A., 1973, Dechlorination of chloroethane with a reconstituted liver microsomal system, *Biochem. Biophys. Res. Commun.* **53:**687–692.

GARNER, R. C., 1973, Chemical evidence for the formation of a reactive aflatoxin $B_1$ metabolite by hamster liver microsomes, *FEBS Letters* **36:**261–264.

GARNER, R. C., MILLER, E. C., MILLER, J. A., GARNER, J. V., AND HAMSON, R. S., 1971, Formation of a factor lethal for *S. typhimurium* TA 1530 and TA 1531 on incubation of aflatoxin $B_1$ with rat liver microsomes, *Biochem. Biophys. Res. Commun.* **45:**774–780.

GELBOIN, H. V., 1969, A microsome-dependent binding of benzo(a)pyrene to DNA, *Cancer Res.* **29:**1272–1276.

GELBOIN, H. V., KINOSHITA, N., AND WIEBEL, F. J., 1972, Microsomal hydroxylases: Induction and role in polycyclic hydrocarbon carcinogenesis and toxicity, *Fed. Proc.* **31:**1298–1309.

GENTA, V. M., KAUFMAN, D. G., HARRIS, C. C., SMITH, J. M., SPORN, M. B., AND SAFFIOTTI, U., 1974, Vitamin A deficiency enhances binding of benzo(a)pyrene to tracheal epithelial DNA, *Nature(Lond.)* **247:**48–49.

GIELEN, J. E., AND NEBERT, D. W., 1971, Microsomal hydroxylase induction in liver cell culture by phenobarbital, polycyclic hydrocarbons and p,p'-DDT, *Science* **172:**167–169.

GILLETTE, J. R., 1971, Reductive enzymes, in: *Concepts in Biochemical Pharmacology, Part 2* (B. B. Brodie and J. R. Gillette, eds.), pp. 349–361, Springer, New York.

GILLETTE, J. R., MENARD, R. H., AND STRIPP, B., 1973, Active products of fetal drug metabolism, *Clin. Pharmacol. Ther.* **14:**680–692.

GINGELL, R., AND BRIDGES, J. W., 1973, Intestinal azo-reduction and glucuronide conjugation of prontosil, *Xenobiotica* **3:**599–604.

GINGELL, R., BRIDGES, J. W., AND WILLIAMS, R. T., 1971, The role of the gut flora in the metabolism of prontosil and neoprontosil in the rat, *Xenobiotica* **1:**143–156.

GINTER, E., 1973, Cholesterol: Vitamin C controls its transformation to bile acids, *Science* **1791:**702–704.

GORROD, J. W., 1973, Differentiation of various types of biological oxidation of nitrogen in organic compounds, *Chem.-Biol. Interact.* **7:**289–303.

GOTH, R. AND RAJEWSKY, M. F., 1972, Ethylation of nucleic acids by ethylnitrosourea-1-$^{14}$C in the fetal and adult rat, *Cancer Res.* **32:**1501–1505.

GRAM, T. E., 1973, Comparative aspects of mixed function oxidation by lung and liver of rabbits, *Drug Metab. Rev.* **2:**1–32.

GRANTHAM, P. H., WEISBURGER, J. H., AND WEISBURGER, E. K., 1973, Effect of the antioxidant butylated hydroxytoluene (BHT) on the metabolism of the carcinogens N-2-fluorenylacetamide and N-hydroxy-N-2-fluorenylacetamide, *Food Cosmet. Toxicol.* **11:**209–217.

GRANTHAM, P. H., GIAO, NG. B., MOHAN, L. C., WEISBURGER, E. K., BUU-HOI, NG. P., AND RONCUCCI, R., 1974a, Metabolism of 6-aminochrysene in the rat, *Toxicol. Appl. Pharmacol.* **29:**95.

GRANTHAM, P. H., MOHAN, L. C., WEISBURGER, E. K., FALES, H. M., SOKOLOSKI, E. A., AND WEISBURGER, J. H., 1974b, Identification of new water soluble metabolites of acetanilide, *Xenobiotica* **4:**69–76.

226

J. H.
WEISBURGER
AND
G. M.
WILLIAMS

GROVER, P. L., AND SIMS, P., 1968, Enzyme-catalysed reaction of polycyclic hydrocarbons with deoxyribonucleic acid and protein *in vitro, Biochem. J.* **110:**159–160.

GROVER, P. L., HEWER, A., AND SIMS, P., 1973, K-region epoxides of polycyclic hydrocarbons: Formation and further metabolism of benz(a)anthracene-5,6-oxide by human lung preparations, *FEBS Letters* **34:**63–68.

GUTMANN, H. R., 1974, Isolation and identification of the carcinogen N-hydroxy-2-fluorenylacetamide and related compound by liquid chromatography, *Anal. Biochem.* **58:**469–478.

GUTMANN, H. R., GALITSKI, S. B., AND FOLEY, W. A., 1967, The conversion of noncarcinogenic aromatic amides to carcinogenic arylhydroxamic acids by synthetic N-hydroxylation, *Cancer Res.* **27:**1443–1455.

GUTMANN, H. R., MALEJKA-GIGANTI, D., BARRY, E. J., AND RYDELL, R. C., 1972, On the correlation between the hepatocarcinogenicity of the carcinogen N-2-fluorenylacetamine and the metabolic activation by the rat, *Cancer Res.* **32:**1554–1561.

HADJIOLOV, D., 1971, The inhibition of dimethylnitrosamine carcinogenesis in rat liver by aminoacetonitrile, *Z. Krebsforsch.* **76:**91–92.

HARRIS, P. N., GIBSON, W. R., AND DILLARD, R. D., 1970, The oncogenicity of two 1,1-diaryl-2-propynyl-N-cycloalkylcarbamates, *Cancer Res.* **30:**2952–2954.

HATHWAY, D. E., 1970, *Foreign Compound Metabolism in Mammals*, Vol. I, The Chemical Society, Burlington House, London.

HATHWAY, D. E., 1972, *Foreign Compound Metabolism in Mammals*, Vol. II, The Chemical Society, Burlington House, London.

HECKER, E., 1971, Isolation and characterization of cocarcinogenic principles from croton oil, in: *Methods in Cancer Research* (H. Busch, ed.) Vol. 6, pp. 439–484, Academic Press, New York.

HEIDELBERGER, C., 1973, Current trends in chemical carcinogenesis, *Fed. Proc.* **32:**2154–2161.

HIGGINSON, J. AND MUIR, C. S., 1973, Epidemiology, in: *Cancer Medicine* (J. F. Holland and E. Frei, III, eds.), pp. 241–306, Lea and Febiger, Philadelphia.

HILL, M. J., 1974, Bacteria and the etiology of colonic cancer, *Cancer* **34:**815–818.

HILL, D. L. AND SHIH, T. W., 1974, Vitamin A compounds and analogs as inhibitors of mixed function oxidases that metabolize carcinogenic polycyclic hydrocarbons and other compounds, *Cancer Res.* **34:**564–570.

HILL, M. J. AND ARIES, V. C., 1971, Faecal steroid composition and its relationship to cancer of the large bowel, *J. Pathol.* **104:**129–139.

HILL, M. J., DRASAR, B. S., ARIES, V., CROWTHER, J. S., HAWKSWORTH, G., AND WILLIAMS, R. E. O., 1971, Bacteria and aetiology of cancer of large bowel, *Lancet* **1:**95–100.

HOCH-LIGETI, C., ARGUS, M. F., AND ARCOS, J. C., 1968, Combined carcinogenic effects of dimethylnitrosamine and 3-methylcholanthrene in the rat, *J. Natl. Cancer Inst.* **40:**535–549.

HOFFMANN, D., AND WYNDER, E. L., 1971, A study of tobacco carcinogenesis. XI. Tumor initiators, tumor accelerators and tumor promoting activity of condensate fractions, *Cancer* **27:**848–864.

HOLLAENDER, A., ed., 1971, *Chemical Mutagens: Principles and Methods for Their Detection*, Plenum Press, New York.

HSU, I. C., SHUMAKER, R. C., AND ALLEN, J. R., 1973, Tissue distribution of tritum-labeled dehydroretronecine, *Chem.-Biol. Interact.* **8:**163–170.

HUBERMAN, E., AND SACHS, L., 1973, Metabolism of the carcinogenic hydrocarbon benzo(a)pyrene in human fibroblast and epithelial cells, *Int. J. Cancer* **11:**412–418.

HUCKER, H. B., 1970, Species differences in drug metabolism, *Ann. Rev. Biochem.* **10:**99–118.

HUCKER, H. B., 1973, Intermediates in drug metabolism reaction, *Drug Metab. Rev.* **21:**33–56.

HUSTAD, G. O., CERVENY, J. G., TRENK, H., DEIBEL, R. H., KAULTER, D. A., FAZIO, T., JOHNSTON, R. W., AND KOLARI, O. E., 1973, Effect of sodium nitrite and sodium nitrate on botulinal toxin production and nitrosamine formation in wieners, *Appl. Microbiol.* **26:**22–26.

*IARC Monograph No. 4 on the Evaluation of Carcinogenic Risk of Chemicals to Man*, 1974, International Agency for Research on Cancer, Lyon.

*IARC Monograph No. 5 on the Evaluation of Carcinogenic Risk of Chemicals to Man*, 1974, International Agency for Research on Cancer, Lyon.

ILETT, K. F., REID, W. D., SIPES, I. G., AND KRISHNA, G., 1973, Chloroform toxicity in mice: Correlation of renal and hepatic necrosis with covalent binding of metabolites to tissue macromolecules, *Exp. Mol. Pathol.* **19:**215–229.

IMAMURA, T., AND IKEDA, M., 1973, Lower fiducial limit of urinary metabolite level as an index of excessive exposure to industrial chemicals, *Brit. J. Ind. Med.* **30:**289–292.

IRVING, C. C., 1970, Conjugates of N-hydroxy compounds, in: *Metabolic Conjugation and Metabolic Hydrolysis*, Vol. I, (W. H. Fishman, ed.), pp. 53–119, Academic Press, New York.

ITO, N., HIASA, Y., TOYOSHIMA, K., OKAJIMA, E., KAMAMOTO, Y., MAKIURA, S., YOKOTA, Y., SUGIHARA, S., AND MATAYOSHI, K., 1973, Rat bladder tumors induced by N-butyl-N-(4-hydroxybutyl)nitrosamine, in: *Topics in Chemical Carcinogenesis* (W. Nakahara, S. Takayama, T. Sugimura, and S. Odashima, eds.), p. 175, University Park Press, Baltimore.

JAGO, M. V., EDGAR, J. A., SMITH, L. W., AND CULVENOR, C. C. J., 1970, Metabolic conversion of heliotridine-based pyrrolizidine alkaloids to dehydroheliotridine, *Mol. Pharmacol.* **6:**402–406.

JANSS, D. H., MOON, R. C., AND IRVING, C. C., 1972, The binding of 7,12-dimethylbenz(a)anthracene to mammary parenchyma DNA and protein *in vivo*, *Cancer Res.* **32:**254–258.

JERINA, D. M. AND DALY, J. W., 1974, Arene oxides: A new aspect of drug metabolism, *Science* **185:**573–582.

JONES, A. R., AND EDWARDS, K., 1973, Alkylating esters. VII. The metabolism of iso-propyl methanesulphonate and iso-propyl iodide in the rat, *Experientia* **29:**538–539.

JUCHAU, M. R., ZACHARIAH, P. K., COLSON, J., SYMMS, K. G., KRAMER, J., AND JAFFE, S. J., 1974, Studies on human placental carbon monoxide–binding cytochrome, *Drug Metab. Disposition* **2:**79–86.

KAMATAKI, J., KITADA, M., AND KITAGAWA, H., 1973, Difference in the substrate specificities of drug metabolizing enzymes in human term placenta and fetal liver, *Chem. Pharm. Bull.* **21:**2329–2331.

KATO, R., SHOJI, H., AND TAKANAKA, A., 1967, Metabolism of carcinogenic compounds. I. Effect of phenobarbital and methylcholanthrene on the activities of N-demethylation of carcinogenic compounds by liver microsomes of male and female rats, *Gann* **58:**467–469.

KAUFMAN, D. G., GENTA, V. M., HARRIS, C. C., SMITH, J. M., SPORN, M. B., AND SAFFIOTTI, U., 1973, Binding of $^3$H-labeled benzo(a)pyrene to DNA in hamster trachea epithelial cells, *Cancer Res.* **33:**2837–2841.

KAWACHI, T., KOGURE, K., KAMIJO, Y., AND SUGIMURA, T., 1970, The metabolism of N-methyl-N'-nitro-N-nitrosoguanidine in rats, *Biochim. Biophys. Acta* **222:**409–415.

KEEFER, L. K., LIJINSKY, W., AND GARCIA, H., 1973, Deuterium isotope effect on the carcinogenicity of dimethylnitrosamine in rat liver, *J. Natl. Cancer Inst.* **51:**299–302.

KEIGHTLY, D. D., AND OKEY, A. B., 1973, Effects of dimethylbenz(a)anthracene and dihydrotestosterone on estradiol-17β binding in rat mammary cytosol fraction, *Cancer Res.* **33:**2637–2642.

KELLERMANN, G., SHAW, C. R., AND LUYTEN-KELLERMANN, M., 1973a, Aryl hydrocarbon hydroxylase inducibility and bronchogenic carcinoma, *N. Engl. J. Med.* **289:**934–937.

KELLERMANN, G., LUYTEN-KELLERMANN, M., AND SHAW, C. R., 1973b, Metabolism of polycyclic aromatic hydrocarbons in cultured human leukocytes under genetic control, *Humangenetik* **20:**257–263.

KELLNER, H. M., CARIST, O. E., AND LOTZSCH, K., 1973, Animal studies on the kinetics of benzidine and 3,3'-dichlorobenzidine, *Arch. Toxikol.* **31:**61–79.

KEYSELL, G. R., BOOTH, J., GROVER, P. L., HEWER, A., AND SIMS, P., 1973, The formation of "K-region" epoxides as hepatic microsomal metabolite of 7-methylbenz(a)anthracene and 7,12-dimethylbenz(a)anthracene and their 7-hydroxymethyl derivatives, *Biochem. Pharmacol.* **22:**2853–2867.

KING, C. M., AND OLIVE, C. W., 1973, Comparative effects of age, strain and species on the activation of N-hydroxy-2-fluorenylacetamide (N-hydroxy-FAA) by soluble acyltransferases, *Proc. Am. Assoc. Cancer Res.* **14:**41.

KING, C. M., BEDNAR, T. W., AND LINSMAIER-BEDNAR, E. M., 1973, Activation of the carcinogen N-hydroxy-2-fluorenylacetamide: Insensitivity to cyanide and sulfide of the peroxidase $H_2O_2$ induced formation of nucleic adducts, *Chem.-Biol. Interact.* **7:**185–188.

KLEIHUES, P., AND PATZSCHKE, K., 1971, Verteilung von N-($^{14}$C) Methyl-N-nitroharnstoff in der Ratte nach systemischer Applikation, *Z. Krebsforsch.* **75:**193–200.

KOBAYASHI, A., AND MATSUMOTO, H., 1965, Studies on methylazoxymethanol, the aglucone of cycasin, *Arch. Biochem. Biophys.* **110:**373–380.

KOURI, R. E., RATRIE, H., AND WHITMORE, C. E., 1973, Evidence of a genetic relationship between susceptibility to 3-methylcholanthrene-induced subcutaneous tumors and inducibility of aryl hydrocarbon hydroxylase, *J. Natl. Cancer Inst.* **51:**197–200.

KRIEK, E., 1974, Carcinogenesis by aromatic amines, *Biochimica et Biophysica Acta* **355:**177–203.

KREIS, W., 1970, Metabolism of an antineoplastic methylhydrazine derivative in a P815 mouse neoplasm, *Cancer Research* **30:**82–89.

KRÜGER, F. W., 1971, Metabolism von Nitrosaminen *in vivo*, *Z. Krebsforsch.* **76:**145–154.

228

J. H.
WEISBURGER
AND
G. M.
WILLIAMS

KRÜGER, F. W., 1973, New aspects in metabolism of carcinogenic nitrosamines, in: *Topics in Chemical Carcinogenesis* (W. Nakahara, S. Takayama, T. Sugimura, and S. Odashima, eds.), pp. 213–235, University Park Press, Baltimore.

KRÜGER, F. W., AND BERTRAM, B., 1973, Metabolism of nitrosamines *in vivo*, *Z. Krebsforsch.* **80:**189–196.

KUBINSKI, H., STRANGSTALIEN, M. A., BAIRD, W. M., AND BOUTWELL, R. K., 1973, Interactions of phorbol esters with cellular membranes *in vitro*, *Cancer Res.* **33:**3103–3107.

KUNZ, W., SCHAUDE, G., AND THOMAS, C., 1969, Die Beeinflussung der Nitrosamincarcinogenese durch Phenobarbital und Halogenkohlenwasserstoffe, *Z. Krebsforsch.* **72:**291–304.

LAMBELIN, G., MEES, G., AND BUU-HOI, NG. P., 1967, Chronic toxicity of 6-aminochrysene in the rat, *Arzneimittel-Forschung* **17:**117–1121.

LAQUEUR, G. L., 1970, Contribution of intestinal macroflora and microflora to carcinogenesis, in: *Carcinoma of the Colon and Antecedent Epithelium*, (W. J. Burdette, ed.), pp. 305–313, Thomas, Springfield, Ill.

LEGATOR, M. S., 1973, Procedure for conducting the host-mediated assay utilizing bacteria (*Salmonella typhimurium*), *Agents Actions* **3:**111–115.

LIJINSKY, W., 1974, Reaction of drugs with nitrous acid as a source of carcinogenic nitrosamies, *Cancer Res.* **34:**255–258.

LIJINSKY, W., KEEFER, L., LOO, J., AND ROSS, A. E., 1973, Studies of alkylation of nucleic acids in rats by cyclic nitrosamines, *Cancer Res.* **33:**1634–1641.

LITWAK, G., MOREY, K. S., AND KETTERER, B., 1972, Corticosteroid binding proteins of liver cytosol and interactions with carcinogens, in: *Effects of Drugs on Cellular Control Mechanisms* (B. R. Rabin and R. B. Freedman, eds.), pp. 105–130, Macmillan, London.

LOTLIKAR, P. D., AND LUHA, L., 1971, Acetylation of the carcinogen N-hydroxy-2-acetylaminofluorene by acetyl coenzyme A to form a reactive ester, *Mol. Pharmacol.* **7:**381–388.

LOWER, G. M., AND BRYAN, G. T., 1973, Enzymatic N-acetylation of carcinogenic aromatic amines by liver cytosol of species displaying different organ susceptibilities, *Biochem. Pharmacol.* **22:**1581–1588.

MAGEE, P. N., HAWKS, A., STEWART, B. W., AND SWANN, P. F., 1973, Mechanisms of carcinogenesis by alkylnitrosamine and related compounds, in: *Proceedings of the 5th International Congress of Pharmacology*, Vol. 2, pp. 140–149, Karger, S., Basel and New York.

MAGEE, P. N., MONTESANO, R., AND PREUSSMANN, R., 1974, in: *Chemical Carcinogens* (C. Searle, ed.), American Chemical Society Monograph, Washington, D.C., in press.

MALEJKA-GIGANTI, D., GUTMANN, H. R., AND RYDELL, R. E., 1973, Mammary carcinogenesis in the rat by topical application of fluorenylhydroxamic acids, *Cancer Res.* **33:**2489–2497.

MALTONI, C., AND LEFEMINE, G., 1974, Le potenzialita dei saggi sperimentali nella predizione dei rischi oncogeni ambientali. Un esempio: Il cloruro di vinile, *Lincei-Rend. Sci. Fis. Mat. Nat.* **56:**1–11.

MATSUMOTO, H., NAGATA, Y., NISHIMURA, E. T., BRISTOL, R., AND HABER, M., 1972, β-Glucosidase modulation in preweanling rats and its association with tumor induction by cycasin, *J. Natl. Cancer Inst.* **49:**423–434.

MATSUSHIMA, T., GRANTHAM, P. H., WEISBURGER, E. K., AND WEISBURGER, J. H., 1972, Phenobarbital-mediated increase in ring- and N-hydroxylation of the carcinogen N-2-fluorenylacetamide, and decrease in amounts bound to liver deoxyribonucleic acid, *Biochem. Pharmacol.* **21:**2043–2051.

MATSUYAMA, A., AND NAGATA, C., 1973, Detection of the unstable intermediate 4-nitrosoquinoline 1-oxide, in: *Topics in Chemical Carcinogenesis* (W. Nakahara, S. Sakayama, T. Sagimura and S. Odashima, eds.), pp. 35–51, University Park Press, Baltimore.

MATTOCKS, A. R., AND WHITE, I. N. H., 1973, Toxic effects and pyrrolic metabolites in the liver of young rats given the pyrrolizidine alkaloid retrosine, *Chem.-Biol. Interact.* **6:**297–306.

MCCUEN, R. W., STÖHRER, G., AND SIROTNAK, F. M., 1974, Mutagenicity of derivatives of the oncogenic purine-N-oxides, *Cancer Res.* **34:**378–384.

MCDONALD, J. J., STÖHRER, G., AND BROWN, G. B., 1973, Oncogenic purine N-oxide derivatives as substrates for sulfotransferase, *Cancer Res.* **33:**3319–3323.

MCLEAN, A. E. M., 1970, The effect of protein deficiency and microsomal enzyme induction by DDT and phenobarbitone on the acute toxicity of chloroform and a pyrrolizidine alkaloid, retrosine, *Brit. J. Exp. Pathol.* **51:**317–321.

MCLEAN, A. E. M., AND MAGEE, P. N., 1970, Increased renal carcinogenesis by dimethylnitrosamine in protein deficient rats, *Brit. J. Exp. Pathol.* **51:**587–590.

MCLEAN, A. E. M., AND MARSHALL, A., 1971, Reduced carcinogenic effect of aflatoxin in rats given phenobarbitone, *Brit. J. Exp. Pathol.* **52:**322–329.

MCLEAN, E. K., MCLEAN, A. E. M., AND SUTTON, P. M., 1969, Instant cirrhosis, *Brit. J. Exp. Pathol.* **50**:502–506.

MILLER, E. C., AND MILLER, J. A., 1967, Low carcinogenicity of the K-region epoxides of 7-methylbenz(a)anthracene and benz(a)anthracene in the mouse and rat, *Proc. Soc. Exp. Biol. Med.* **124**:915–919.

MILLER, E. C., AND MILLER, J. A., 1971, The mutagenicity of chemical carcinogens: Correlations, problems, and interpretations, in: *Chemical Mutagens* (A. Hollaender, ed.), pp. 83–119, Plenum Press, New York.

MILLER, E. C., AND MILLER, J. A., 1972, Approaches to the mechanisms and control of chemical carcinogenesis, in: *Environment and Cancer*, pp. 5–39, Williams and Wilkins, Baltimore.

MILLER, E. C., MILLER, J. A., AND ENOMOTO, M., 1964, The comparative carcinogenicities of 2-acetylaminofluorene and its N-hydroxy metabolite in mice, hamsters, and guinea pigs, *Cancer Res.* **24**:2018–2031.

MILLER, J. A., 1970, Carcinogenesis by chemicals: An overview, *Cancer Res.* **30**:559–576.

MILLER, J. A., 1973, Naturally occurring substances that can induce tumors, in: *Toxicants Occurring Naturally in Foods*, pp. 509–548, National Academy of Sciences, Washington, D.C.

MILLER, J. A., AND MILLER, E. C., 1971, Chemical carcinogenesis: Mechanisms and approaches to its control, *J. Natl. Cancer Inst.* **47**:V–XIII.

MIRKIN, B. L., 1970, Developmental pharmacology, *Ann. Rev. Pharmacol.* **10**:255–272.

MIRVISH, S. S., 1968, The carcinogenic action and metabolism of urethan and N-hydroxyurethan, *Advan. Cancer Res.* **11**:1–42.

MIRVISH, S. S., 1972, Kinetics of N-nitrosation reactions in relation to tumorigenesis experiments with nitrite plus amines or ureas, in: *N-Nitroso Compounds: Analysis and Formation*, pp. 104–108, International Agency for Research on Cancer, Lyon.

MIRVISH, S. S., AND CHU, C., 1973, Chemical determination of methylnitrosourea and ethylnitrosourea in stomach content of rats, after intubation of the alkylureas plus sodium nitrite, *J. Natl. Cancer Inst.* **50**:745–750.

MIRVISH, S. S., AND SIDRANSKY, H., 1971, Labeling *in vivo* of rat liver proteins by tritium-labeled dimethylnitrosamine, *Biochem. Pharmacol.* **20**:3493–3499.

MITCHELL, J. R., JOLLOW, D. J., POTTER, W. Z., DAVIS, D. C., GILLETTE, J. R., AND BRODIE, B. B., 1973, Acetaminophen-induced hepatic necrosis. I. Role of drug metabolism, *J. Pharmacol. Exp. Ther.* **187**:185–194.

MONTESANO, R., AND MAGEE, P. N., 1974, Comparative metabolism *in vitro* of nitrosamines in various animal species including man, in: *Chemical Carcinogenesis Essays* (R. Montesano, L. Tomatis, and W. Davis, Eds.), pp. 39–56, International Agency for Research on Cancer, Lyon.

MONTESANO, R., SAINT VINCENT, L., AND TOMATIS, L., 1973, Malignant transformation *in vitro* of rat liver cells by dimethylnitrosamine and N-methyl-N'-nitro-N-nitrosoguanidine, *Brit. J. Cancer* **28**:215–220.

MOULÉ, Y., AND FRAYSSINET, C., 1972, Enzymic conversion of aflatoxin $B_1$ to a derivative inhibiting *in vitro* transcription, *FEBS Letters* **25**:52–56.

NAIR, P. P., AND KAYDEN, H. J., 1972, International conference on vitamin E and its role in cellular metabolism, *Ann. N.Y. Acad. Sci.* **203**:1–247.

NAKAJIMA, T., AND IWAHARA, S., 1973, Mutagenicity of dimethylnitrosamine in the metabolic process by rat liver microsomes, *Mutation Res.* **18**:121–127.

NARISAWA, T., NAKANO, H., HAYAKAWA, M., SATO, T., AND SAKUMA, A., 1973, Tumors of the colon and rectum induced by N-methyl-N'-nitro-N-nitrosoguanidine, in: *Topics in Chemical Carcinogenesis* (W. Nakahara, S. Takayama, T. Sugimura, and S. Adashima, eds.), p. 145, University Park Press, Baltimore.

NARISAWA, T., MAGADIA, N. E., WEISBURGER, J. H., AND WYNDER, E. L., 1974, Promoting effect of bile acid on colon carcinogenesis after intrarectal instillation of N-methyl-N-nitro-N-nitroso-guanidine in rats, *J. Natl. Cancer Inst.* **53**:1093–1097.

NEBERT, D. W., AND GELBOIN, H. V., 1968, Substrate-inducible microsomal aryl hydroxylase in mammalian cell culture, *J. Biol. Chem.* **243**:6242–6249.

NEBERT, D. W., BAUSSERMAN, L. L., AND BATES, R. R., 1970, Effect of 17β-estradiol and testosterone on aryl hydrocarbon hydroxylase activity in mouse tissues *in vivo* and in cell culture, *Int. J. Cancer* **6**:470–475.

NEBERT, D. W., CONSIDINE, N., AND OWENS, S. S., 1973, Genetic expression of aryl hydrocarbon hydroxylase induction. VI. Control of other aromatic hydrocarbon–inducible mono-oxygenase activities at or near the same genetic locus, *Arch. Biochem. Biophys.* **157**:148–159.

230

J. H.
WEISBURGER
AND
G. M.
WILLIAMS

NEMOTO, N., AND TAKAYAMA, S., 1973, Formation of $N^7$-methylguanidine in nuclear DNA and cytoplasmic RNA in mice on continuous oral administration of dimethylnitrosamine-$^3$H solution, *Z. Krebsforsch.* **80:**113–125.

NEUNHOEFFER, O., WILHELM, G., AND LEHMANN, G., 1970, Eine enzymatische Umlagerung cancerogener Nitrosamine, *Z. Naturforsch.* **25:**302–307.

NEWBERNE, P. M., 1974, Section 3, Report of discussion group No. 2 Diets in: *Carcinogenesis Testing of Chemicals* (L. Golberg, ed.) pp. 17–20, CRC Press, Cleveland, Ohio.

OESCH, F., 1973, Mammalian epoxide hydrases: Inducible enzymes catalysing the inactivation of carcinogenic and cytotoxic metabolites derived from aromatic and olefinic compounds, *Xenobiotica* **3:**305–340.

OESCH, F., JERINA, D. M., DALY, J. W., AND RICE, J. M., 1973, Induction, activation and inhibition of epoxide hydrase: An anomalous prevention of chlorobenzene-induced hepatotoxicity by an inhibitor of epoxide hydrase, *Chem.-Biol. Interact.* **6:**189–202.

O'GARA, R. W., AND ADAMSON, R. H., 1972, Spontaneous and induced neoplasms in nonhuman primates, in: *Pathology of Simian Primates*, Part I, pp. 190–238, Karger, Basel.

OKADA, M., AND SUZUKI, E., 1972, Metabolism of butyl(4-hydroxybutyl)-nitrosamine in rats, *Gann* **63:**391.

OLSON, W. A., HABERMANN, R. T., WEISBURGER, E. K., WARD, J. M., AND WEISBURGER, J. H., 1973, Induction of stomach cancer in rats and mice by halogenated aliphatic fumigants, *J. Natl. Cancer Inst.* **51:**1993–1995.

PAINE, A. J., AND McLEAN, A. E. M., 1973, The effect of dietary protein and fat on the activity of aryl hydrocarbon hydroxylase in rat liver, kidney and lung, *Biochem. Pharmacol.* **22:**2875–2880.

PANTUCK, E. J., HSAIO, K. C., MAGGIS, A., NAKAMURA, K., KUNTZMAN, R., AND CONNEY, A. H., 1974, Effect of cigarette smoking on phenacetin metabolism, *Clin. Pharmacol. Ther.* **15:**9–17.

PATTERSON, D. S. P., 1973, Metabolism as a factor in determining the toxic action of the aflatoxins in different animal species, *Food Cosmet. Toxicol.* **11:**287–294.

PATTERSON, D. S. P., AND ROBERTS, B. A., 1972, Steroid sex hormones as inhibitors of aflatoxin metabolism in liver homogenates, *Experientia*, 929–930.

PELKONEN, O., KALTIALA, E. O., LARMI, T. K. I., AND KÄRKI, N. T., 1973, Comparison of activities of drug metabolizing enzymes in human fetal and adult livers, *Clin. Pharmacol. Ther.* **14:**840–846.

PERAINO, C., FRY, R. J., AND STAFFELDT, E., 1971, Reduction and enhancement by phenobarbital of hepatocarcinogenesis induced in the rat by 2-acetylaminofluorene, *Cancer Res.* **31:**1506–1512.

POIRIER, L. A., AND WEISBURGER, J. H., 1973, Enzymic reduction of carcinogenic aromatic nitro compounds by rat and mouse liver fractions, *Biochem. Pharmacol.* **23:**661–669.

POPPER, H., CZYGAN, P., GREIM, H., SCHAFFNER, F., AND GANO, A. J., 1973, Mutagenicity of primary and secondary carcinogens altered by normal and induced hepatic microsomes, *Proc. Soc. Exp. Biol. Med.* **142:**727–729.

POUND, A. W., LAWSON, T. A., AND HORN, L., 1973, Increased carcinogenic action of dimethylnitrosamine after prior administration of carbon tetrachloride, *Brit. J. Cancer* **27:**451–459.

POZHARISSKI, K. M., KAPUSTIN, J. M., LIKHACHEV, A. Y., AND SHAPOSHNIKOV, Y. D., 1974, The dynamics of the rat tissue methylation in symmetric dimethylhydrazine-$^3$H administration, *Voprosy Onkol.* **20(1):**69–76. .

PREUSSMANN, R., 1974, Formation of carcinogens from precursors occurring in the environment: New aspects of nitrosamine-induced tumorigenesis, in: *Special Topics in Carcinogenesis* (E. Grundmann, ed.) Vol. 44, pp. 9–15, Springer-Verlag, New York, Heidelberg, Berlin.

PREUSSMANN, R., HENGY, H., AND DRUCKREY, H., 1965, Studies on the detection of alkylating agents. I. Spectrophotometric determination of diazoalkanes with 4-(4-nitrobenzyl)pyridinium perchlorate, *Chem. Ann.* **684:**57.

PROUGH, R. A., WITTKOP, J. A., AND REED, D. J., 1970, Further evidence on the nature of microsomal metabolism of procarbazine and related alkylhydrazones, *Arch. Biochem. Biophys.* **140:**450–458.

PURCHASE, I. F. H., STEYN, M., AND GILFILLAN, T. C., 1973, Metabolism and acute toxicity to aflatoxin $B_1$ in rats, *Chem.-Biol. Interact.* **7:**283–287.

RADOMSKI, J. L., CONZELMAN, G. M., JR., REY, A. A., AND BRILL, E., 1973a, The N-oxidation of certain aromatic amines, acetamides and nitro compounds by monkeys and dogs, *J. Natl. Cancer Inst.* **50:**989–995.

RADOMSKI, J. L., REY, A. A., AND BRILL, E., 1973b, Evidence for a glucuronic acid conjugate of N-hydroxy-4-aminobiphenyl in the urine of dogs given 4-aminobiphenyl, *Cancer Res.* **33:**1284–1289.

RAINERI, R., AND WEISBURGER, J. H., 1974, Role of the reduction of dietary nitrate to nitrite in the etiology of gastric cancer, *Proc. Am. Assoc. Cancer Res.* **15**:39.

RAO, K. V. N., AND VESSELINOVITCH, S. D., 1973, Age- and sex-associated diethylnitrosamine dealkylation activity of the mouse liver and hepatocarcinogenesis, *Cancer Res.* **33**:1625–1627.

RECKNAGEL, R. O., 1967, Carbon tetrachloride hepatotoxicity, *Pharmacol. Rev.* **19**:145–208.

REDDY, B. S., PLEASANTS, J. R., AND WOSTMANN, B. S., 1973, Metabolic enzymes in liver and kidney of the germfree rat, *Biochim. Biophys. Acta* **320**:1–8.

REDDY, B. S., WEISBURGER, J. H., AND WYNDER, E. L., 1974a, Effects of dietary fat level and dimethylhydrazine on fecal acid and neutral sterol excretion and colon carcinogenesis in rats, *J. Natl. Cancer Inst.* **52**:507–511.

REDDY, B. S., WEISBURGER, J. H., NARISAWA, T., AND WYNDER, E. L., 1974b, Colon carcinogenesis in germfree rats with 1,2-dimethylhydrazine and N-methyl-N'-nitro-N-nitrosoguanidine, *Cancer Res.*, **34**:2368–2372.

REDDY, J. K., SVOBODA, D. J., AND RAO, M. S., 1974, Susceptibility of an inbred strain of guinea pigs to the induction of pancreatic adenocarcinoma by N-methyl-N-nitrosourea, *J. Natl. Cancer Inst.* **52**:991–993.

REUBER, M. D., AND GLOVER, E. L., 1970, Cirrhosis and carcinoma of the liver in male rats given subcutaneous carbon tetrachloride, *J. Natl. Cancer Inst.* **44**:419–427.

RICE, J. M., 1973, An overview of transplacental chemical carcinogenesis, *Teratology* **8**:113–126.

RIVLIN, R. S., 1973, Riboflavin and cancer: A review, *Cancer Res.* **33**:1977–1986.

ROGERS, A. E., SANCHEZ, O., FEINSOD, F. M., AND NEWBERNE, P. M., 1974, Dietary enhancement of nitrosamine carcinogenesis, *Cancer Res.* **34**:96–99.

RUMACK, B. H., HOLTZMAN, J., AND CHASE, H. P., 1973, Hepatic drug metabolism and protein malnutrition, *J. Pharmacol. Exp. Ther.* **186**:441–446.

SANDER, J., 1971, Untersuchungen über die Entstehung cancerogener Nitrosoverbindungen im Magen von Versuchstieren und ihre Bedeutung für den Menschen, *Arzneimittel-Forschung* **21**:1572–1580, 1707–1713, 2034–2039.

SANDER, J., 1973, The formation of N-nitroso compounds in the stomach of animal and man and in the diet, in: *Transplacental Carcinogensis*, International Agency for Research on Cancer, Lyon.

SANDER, J., SCHWEINSBERG, F., LADENSTEIN, M., BENZING, H., AND WAHL, S. A., 1973, Messung der renalen Nitrosaminausscheidung am Hund zum Nachweis einer Nitrosaminbildung *in vivo*, *Hoppe-Seylers Z. Physiol. Chem.* **354**:384–390.

SAWICKI, E., AND SAWICKI, C. R., 1969, Analysis of alkylating agents: Applications to air pollution, *Ann. N.Y. Acad. Sci.* **163**:895–920.

SCHELINE, R. R., 1973, Metabolism of foreign compounds by gastrointestinal microorganisms, *Pharmacol. Rev.* **24**:451–523.

SCHMÄHL, D., 1970, *Entstehung, Wachstum und Chemotherapie maligner Tumoren*, Cantor, Aulendorf.

SCHMALL, B., CHENG, C. J., FUJIMURA, S., GERSTEIN, N., GRUNBERGER, D., AND WEINSTEIN, I. B., 1973, Modification of proteins by 1-(2-chloroethyl)-3-cyclohexyl-1-nitrosourea (NSC 79037) *in vitro*, *Cancer Res.* **33**:1921–1924.

SCHOENTAL, R., 1970, Hepatotoxic activity of retrorsine, senkirkine and hydroxysenkirkine in newborn rats, and the role of epoxides in carcinogenesis by pyrrolizidine alkaloids and aflatoxins, *Nature (Lond.)* **227**:401–402.

SCHOENTAL, R., 1973, The mechanisms of action of the carcinogenic nitroso and related compounds, *Brit. J. Cancer* **28**:436–439.

SCHWARTZ, A. G., 1974, Protective effect of benzoflavone and estrogen against 7,12-dimethylbenz(a)anthracene- and aflatoxin-induced cytotoxicity in cultured liver cells, *Cancer Res.* **34**:10–15.

SELIKOFF, I. J., AND HAMMOND, E. C., 1974, Working group: Toxicity of vinyl chloride—Polyvinyl chloride, New York Academy of Sciences meeting. *Ann. N.Y. Acad. Sci.*, in press.

SELKIRK, J. K., HUBERMAN, E., AND HEIDELBERGER, C., 1971, An epoxide is an intermediate in the microsomal metabolism of the chemical carcinogen, dibenz(a,h)anthracene, *Biochem. Biophys. Res. Commun.* **43**:1010–1016.

SELKIRK, J. K., CROG, R. G., AND GELBOIN, H. V., 1974, Benzo(a)pyrene metabolites: Efficient and rapid separation by high-pressure liquid chromatography, *Science* **184**:169–171.

SIVAK, A., AND VAN DUUREN, B. L., 1971, Cellular interactions of phorbol myristate acetate in tumor promotion, *Chem.-Biol. Interact.* **3**:401–411.

232

J. H.
WEISBURGER
AND
G. M.
WILLIAMS

Skibba, J. L., Beal, D. D., Ramirez, G., and Bryan, G. T., 1970a, N-Demethylation of the antineoplastic agent 4(5)-(3,3-dimethyl-1-triazeno)imidazole-5(4)-carboxamide by rats and man, Cancer Res. 30:147–150.

Skibba, J. L., Ramirez, G., Beal, D. D., and Bryan, G. T., 1970b, Metabolism of 4(5)-(3,3-dimethyl-1-triazeno)imidazole-5(4)-carboxamide to 4(5)-aminoimidazole-5(4)-carboxamide in man, Biochem. Pharmacol. 19:2043–2051.

Smith, R. C., and Pollard, D. R., 1969, Excretion of S-adenosylethionine in the urine of rats fed a diet containing ethionine, Biochim. Biophys. Acta 184:397–403.

Smith, R. L., 1973, The Excretory Function of Bile, Chapman and Hall, London.

Smuckler, E. A., 1972, The pathology of halogenated hydrocarbons and halothane: A brief review and speculation, in: Cellular Biology and Toxicity of Anaesthetics (B. R. Fink, ed.), pp. 221–237, Williams and Wilkins Co., Baltimore.

So, B. T., and Wynder, E. L., 1972, Induction of hamster tumors of the urinary bladder by 3,2′-dimethyl-4-aminobiophenyl, J. Natl. Cancer Inst. 48:1733–1738.

So, B. T., Magadia, N. E., and Wynder, E. L., 1973, Induction of carcinomas of the colon and rectum in rats by intrarectal instillation of N-methyl-N′-nitro-N-nitrosoguanidine, J. Natl. Cancer Inst. 50:927–932.

Spjut, H. J., 1972, Newer concepts of cancer of the colon and rectum: Similarities between human and experimentally induced tumors of the large intestine, Dis. Colon Rectum 15:94–99.

Stöhrer, G., Salemnick, G., and Brown, G. B., 1973, A chemical adduct of tryptophan and the oncogen 3-acetoxyxanthine, Biochemistry 12:5084–5086.

Stoltz, D. R., Poirier, L. A., Irving, C. C., Stich, H. F., Weisburger, J. H., and Grice, H. C., 1974, Evaluation of short term tests for carcinogenicity, Toxicol. Appl. Pharmacol. 29:157–180.

Stoming, T., Knapp, D., and Bresnick, E., 1973, Gas chromatographic separation of K-region epoxide and of the cis- and-trans-11,12-diol derivatives of 3-methylcholanthrene, Life Sci. 12:425–429.

Sugimura, T., Okabe, T., and Nagao, M., 1966, Metabolism of 4-nitroquinoline 1-oxide, a carcinogen. III. Enzyme catalyzing the conversion of 4-nitroquinoline 1-oxide to 4-hydroxyaminoquinoline 1-oxide in rat liver and heptomas, Cancer Res. 27:1717–1721.

Sugimura, T., Kawachi, T., Kogura, K., Nagao, M., Tanaka, N., Fujimura, S., Takayama, S., Shimosato, Y., Noguchi, M., Kuwabara, N., and Yamada, T., 1973, Induction of stomach cancer by N-methyl-N′-nitro-N′nitrosoguanidine: Experiments in dogs as clinical models and the metabolism of this carcinogen, in: Topics in Chemical Carcinogenesis (W. Nakahara, S. Takayama, T. Sugimura, and S. Odashima, eds.), pp. 105–119, University Park Press, Baltimore.

Sullman, S. F., Armstrong, S. J., Zuckerman, A. J., and Rees, K. R., 1970, Further studies on the toxicity of the aflatoxins on human cell cultures, Brit. J. Exp. Pathol. 51:314–316.

Sunderman, F. W., Jr., 1971, Metal carcinogenesis in experimental animals, Food Cosmet. Toxicol. 9:105–120.

Swann, P. F., and McLean, A. E. M., 1971, The effect of a protein-free high-carbohydrate diet on the metabolism of dimethylnitrosamine in the rat, Biochem. J. 124:283–288.

Swenson, D. H., Miller, J. A., and Miller, E. C., 1973, 2,3-Dihydro-2,3-dihydroxy-aflatoxin $B_1$: An acid hydrolysis product of an RNA–aflatoxin $B_1$ adduct formed by hamster and rat liver microsomes in vitro, Biochem. Biophys. Res. Commun. 53:1260–1267.

Swenson, H., Miller, J. A., and Miller, E. C., 1974, Aflatoxin $B_1$-2,3-dichloride: A toxic and reactive derivative of aflatoxin $B_1$, Proc. Am. Assoc. Cancer Res. 15:43.

Tanaka, A., and Sano, T., 1971, Metabolism of N-methyl-N′-nitro-N-nitrosoguanidine in rats, Experientia 27:1007–1008.

Terayama, H., 1967, Aminoazo carcinogenesis—Methods and biochemical problems, Meth. Cancer Res. 1:399–449.

Thorgeirsson, S. S., Jollow, D. J., Sasame, H. A., Green, I., and Mitchell, J. R., 1973, The role of cytochrome P-450 in N-hydroxylation of 2-acetylaminofluorene, Mol. Pharmacol. 9:398–404.

Tomatis, L., Mohr, U., and Davis, W., 1973a, Transplacental Carcinogenesis, International Agency for Research on Cancer, Lyon.

Tomatis, L., Partensky, C., and Montesano, R., 1973b, The predictive value of mouse liver tumor induction in carcinogenicity testing—A literature survey, Int. J. Cancer 12:1–20.

Toth, B., 1968, A critical review of experiments in chemical carcinogenesis using newborn animals, Cancer Res. 28:727–738.

Toth, B., and Shimizu, H., 1973, Methylhydrazone tumorigenesis in Syrian golden hamsters and the morphology of malignant histiocytomas, Cancer Res. 33:2744–2753.

Ts'o, P. O. P., and DiPaolo, J. A., eds., 1974, *Chemical Carcinogenesis*, Marcel Dekker, Inc., New York.

Uehleke, H., 1973, The role of cytochrome P-450 in the N-oxidation of individual amines, *Drug Metab. Disposition* **1**:299–313.

Uehleke, H., Hellmer, K. H., and Tabarelli, S., 1973, Binding of $^{14}$C-carbon tetrachloride to microsomal proteins *in vitro* and formation of CHCl$_3$ by reduced liver microsomes, *Xenobiotica* **3**:1–11.

Uraguchi, K., Ueno, I., Ueno, Y., and Komai, Y., 1972, Absorption, distribution and excretion of luteoskyrin with special reference to the selective action on the liver, *Toxicol. Appl. Pharmacol.* **21**:335–347.

Van Duuren, B. L., Katz, C., and Goldschmidt, B. M., 1973, Cocarcinogenic agents in tobacco carcinogenesis, *J. Natl. Cancer Inst.* **51**:703–705.

Venkatesan, N., Argus, M. F., and Arcos, J. C., 1970, Mechanism of 3-methylcholanthrene-induced inhibition of dimethylnitrosamine demethylase in rat liver, *Cancer Res.* **30**:2556–2562.

Vesselinovitch, S. D., Mihailovich, N., Wogan, G. N., Lombard, L. S., and Rao, V. N., 1972, Aflatoxin B$_1$, a hepatocarcinogen in the infant mouse, *Cancer Res.* **32**:2289–2291.

Visek, W. J., 1972, Effects of urea hydrolysis on cell lifespan and metabolism, *Fed. Proc.* **31**:1178–1193.

Waterfall, J. F., and Sims, P., 1973, The metabolism of dibenzo(a,h)pyrene and dibenzo(a,i)pyrene and related compounds by liver preparations and their enzyme induced binding to cellular macromolecules, *Biochem. Pharmacol.* **22**:2469–2483.

Wattenberg, L. W., 1972, Dietary modification of intestinal and pulmonary aryl hydrocarbon hydroxylase activity, *Toxicol. Appl. Pharmacol.* **23**:741–748.

Wattenberg, L. W., 1973, Inhibition of chemical carcinogen–induced pulmonary neoplasia by butylated hydroxyanisole, *J. Natl. Cancer Inst.* **50**:1541–1544.

Weisburger, J. H., 1973a, Chemical carcinogenesis, in: *Cancer Medicine* (J. F. Holland and E. Frei, eds.), pp. 45–91, Lea and Febiger, Philadelphia.

Weisburger, J. H., 1973b, Chemical carcinogenesis in the gastrointestinal tract, in: *Seventh National Cancer Proceedings*, pp. 465–473, American Cancer Society, New York.

Weisburger, J. H., 1974, Assessment of human exposure and response to N-nitroso compounds: A new view on the etiology of digestive tract cancers, *Toxicol. Appl. Pharmacol.*, in press.

Weisburger, J. H., and Rall, D. P., 1972, Do animal models predict carcinogenic hazards for man? in: *Environment and Cancer*, pp. 437–452, Williams and Wilkins, Baltimore.

Weisburger, J. H., and Weisburger, E. K., 1973, Biochemical formation and pharmacological, toxicological, and pathological properties of hydroxylamines and hydroxamic acids, *Pharmacol. Rev.* **25**:1–66.

Weisburger, J. H., Hadidian, Z., Frederickson, T. N., and Weisburger, E. K., 1967, Host properties determine target, bladder or liver in chemical carcinogenesis, in: *Bladder Cancer: A Symposium* (W. B. Deichmann and K. F. Lampe, eds.), pp. 45–57, Aesculapius, Birmingham, Ala.

Weisburger, J. H., Yamamoto, R. S., Glass, R. M., and Frankel, H. H., 1969, Prevention by arginine glutamate of the carcinogenicity of acetamide in rats, *Toxicol. Appl. Pharmacol.* **14**:163–175.

Weisburger, J. H., Yamamoto, R. S., Williams, G. M., Grantham, P. H., Matsushima, T., and Weisburger, E. K., 1972, On the sulfate ester of N-hydroxy-N-2-fluorenylacetamide as a key ultimate hepatocarcinogen in the rat, *Cancer Res.* **32**:491–500.

Weisburger, J. H., Griswold, D. P., Jr., Prejean, J. D., Casey, A. E., Wood, H. B., Jr., and Weisburger, E. K., 1974, The carcinogenic properties of some of the principal drugs used in clinical cancer chemotherapy, *Rec. Results Cancer Res.*, in press.

Wiebel, F. J., Leutz, J. C., and Gelboin, H. V., 1973, Aryl hydrocarbon (benzo(a)pyrene) hydroxylase: Inducible in extrahepatic tissues of mouse strains, not inducible in liver, *Arch. Biochem. Biophys.* **154**:292–294.

Williams, D. J., and Rabin, B. R., 1971, Distribution by carcinogens of the hormone dependent association of membranes with polysomes, *Nature* **232**:102–105.

Williams, G. M., Elliot, J. M., and Weisburger, J. H., 1973, Carcinoma after malignant conversion *in vitro* of epithelial like cells from rat liver following exposure to chemical carcinogens, *Cancer Res.* **33**:606–612.

Williams, J. R., Jr., Grantham, P. H., Marsh, H. H., III, Weisburger, J. H., and Weisburger, E. K., 1970, The participation of liver fractions and of intestinal bacteria in the metabolism of N-hydroxy-N-2-fluorenylacetamide in the rat, *Biochem. Pharmacol.* **19**:173–188.

Williams, R. T., 1972, Toxicological implications of biotransformation by intestinal microflora, *Toxicol. Appl. Pharmacol.* **23**:769–781.

234

J. H.
WEISBURGER
AND
G. M.
WILLIAMS

WOGAN, G. N., 1973, Aflatoxin carcinogenesis, in: *Methods in Cancer Research*, Vol. VII, pp. 309–344, Academic Press, New York.

WYNDER, E. L., 1974, Working groups in cancer etiology, *Cancer Res.* **34**:1516–1518.

WYNDER, E. L., AND HOFFMANN, D., 1967, *Tobacco and Tobacco Smoke*, Academic Press, New York.

WYNDER, E. L., AND MABUCHI, K., 1972, Etiological and preventive aspects of human cancer, *Preventive Med.* **1**:300–334.

WYNDER, E. L., AND REDDY, B. S., 1973, Studies in large-bowel cancer: Human leads to experimental application, *J. Natl. Cancer Inst.* **50**:1099–1106.

YAHAGI, T., NAGAO, M., HARA, K., MATSUSHIMA, T., SUGIMURA, T., AND BRYAN, G. T., 1974, Relationship between the carcinogenic and mutagenic or DNA-modifying effects of nitrofuran derivatives, including AF-2, a food additive widely used in Japan, *Cancer Res.* **34**: 2266–2273.

YAMAMOTO, R. S., WEISBURGER, J. H., AND WEISBURGER, E. K., 1971, Controlling factors in urethan carcinogenesis in mice: Effect of enzyme inducers and metabolic inhibitors, *Cancer Res.* **31**:483–486.

YANG, C. S., 1973, Alterations of the aryl hydrocarbon hydroxylase system during riboflavin depletion and repletion, *Arch. Biochem. Biophys.* **160**:623–630.

YEH, Y.-Y., AND JOHNSON, R. M., 1973, Vitamin E deficiency in the rat. IV. Alteration in mitochondrial membrane and its relation to respiratory decline, *Arch. Biochem. Biophys.* **159**:821–831.

YOSHIDA, O., AND MIYAKAWA, M., 1973, Etiology of bladder cancer: "Metabolic" aspects, in: *Analytic and Experimental Epidemiology of Cancer* (W. Nakahara, T. Hirayama, K. Nishioka, and H. Sugano, eds.), pp. 31–39, University Park Press, Baltimore.

ZACHARIAH, P. K., AND JUCHAU, M. R., 1974, The role of gut flora in the reduction of aromatic nitro-groups, *Drug Metab. Disposition* **2**:74–78.

ZAMPAGLIONE, N., JOLLOW, D. J., MITCHELL, J. R., STRIPP, B., HAMRICK, M., AND GILLETTE, J. R., 1973, Role of detoxifying enzymes in bromobenzene-induced liver necrosis, *J. Pharmacol. Exp. Ther.* **187**:218–227.

# 8

# Chemical Carcinogenesis: Interactions of Carcinogens with Nucleic Acids

D. S. R. Sarma, S. Rajalakshmi, and
Emmanuel Farber

## 1. Introduction

Two of the major conceptual advances in chemical carcinogenesis made during the past several years have been the discovery of (1) the enzymatic activation of procarcinogens to reactive ultimate carcinogens and (2) the chemical interactions of the active metabolites of many carcinogens with a variety of tissue nucleophils including RNA, DNA, and protein. This chapter is concerned with the interactions of chemical carcinogens and their activated metabolites, proximate and ultimate carcinogens, with nucleic acids, both DNA and RNA.

Two important aspects of the interaction of carcinogens with nucleic acids are the nature and fate of the chemical products and their significance in carcinogenesis. Major emphasis will naturally be given to the first, since this is our area of major knowledge. Although the second, relevance to carcinogenesis, is the most important from the point of view of cancer, this must of necessity remain speculative today, until new ways are found for its scientific analysis.

This chapter will summarize our current knowledge in regard to (1) the nature of the interactions between chemical carcinogens and nucleic acids, both DNA and RNA, with emphasis on those interactions occurring *in vivo*; (2) the nature of the resultant structural and functional alterations of these macromolecules; and

D. S. R. Sarma, S. Rajalakshmi, and Emmanuel Farber ● Fels Research Institute and Departments of Pathology and Biochemistry, Temple University of Medicine, Philadelphia, Pennsylvania.

236

D. S. R. SARMA,
S. RAJALAKSHMI
AND
EMMANUEL
FARBER

(3) the mechanisms by which the cell attempts to repair the altered macromolecules in order to restore normal function. In addition, some general considerations concerning the possible relevance of alterations in nucleic acids to the initiation phase of carcinogenesis and to the subsequent development and evolution of cancer will be presented.

## 2. Interaction of Chemical Carcinogens with DNA

### 2.1. Covalent Interactions

#### 2.1.1. General

Most chemical carcinogens either as such or after suitable metabolic conversion are highly reactive and lead to some type of covalent interactions with DNA. It is becoming evident that all four bases of DNA and in some instances the phosphodiester backbone are targets for one or more carcinogens under some circumstances. By far the most reactive groups are the purine nitrogens (Fig.

FIGURE 1(A,B). Sites of interaction of chemical carcinogens with DNA *in vivo* and *in vitro*.

1A,B). Except for those present at positions 3 and 7, the other functional groups **237**

INTERAC-
TIONS OF
CARCINOGENS
WITH NUCLEIC
ACIDS
are engaged in either covalent bonding or hydrogen bonding. The N-7 of guanine
appears to be the most reactive site, followed by the N-3 and N-7 positions of
adenine (Shapiro, 1969). This reactivity of N-7 of guanine has been attributed to
its position peripherally in the wide groove of the Watson–Crick model of the
double helix (Reiner and Zamenhof, 1957). Another possible basis for the high
nucleophilic activity of N-7 of guanine is the role of guanine as a hydrogen bond
donor. It donates two bonds and accepts only one, thereby generating an increase
in electron density over the guanine ring; this in turn may be reflected in the
increased reactivity of the N-7 position. The increased nucleophilic activity of N-7
of guanine has also been suggested from wave-mechanical studies (Pullman and
Pullman, 1959). It should be pointed out that chemical carcinogens interact at
several other positions in the purines and pyrimidines of DNA to a considerably
lesser degree. To date, interactions at the following sites have been reported: N-7,
O-6, N-3, 2-NH$_2$, and C-8 of guanine; 6-NH$_2$, N-1, N-3, and N-7 of adenine; N-1,
N-3, and C-5 of cytosine; and O-4 and C-6 of thymine (Fig. 1A,B). Thus there are
very few positions of the four bases of DNA that have not been reported to be
attacked by chemical carcinogens *in vivo* or *in vitro*. Much of this work has been
reviewed recently (Lawley, 1966, 1972 *a,b*; E. C. Miller and Miller, 1971; Irving,
1973).

### 2.1.2. Alkylating Agents

The alkylating agents are a large and chemically diverse group of compounds
which include ethyleneimines, methanesulfonates, epoxides, nitrogen and sulfur
mustards, and certain lactones, nitrosamines, and nitrosamides.

There are two generally recognized mechanisms for alkylation, the SN$_1$
(unimolecular nucleophilic substitution) and SN$_2$ (bimolecular nucleophilic substitution) reactions (for details on SN$_1$ and SN$_2$ reactions, refer to Ingold, 1970;
Pauling, 1970; Benfey, 1970). The positive or electrophilic atom in the ultimate
reactive form of the carcinogen reacts with the relatively negative or nucleophilic
atoms of the molecules attacked. In SN$_2$ reactions, the compounds react with each
nucleophilic center to a different extent depending on the degree of nucleophilic
activity. In SN$_1$ reactions, the compounds tend to react with all nucleophils to a
more equal extent. For example, N-methylnitrosourea (MNU) and dimethylnitrosamine (DMN) (SN$_1$-type compounds) yield both *O*- and *N*-substituted
guanine products, whereas methyl methanesulfonate (MMS) and dimethylsulfate
(DMS) (SN$_2$ type) yield mainly *N*-substituted products.

Among the potent alkylating carcinogens are nitroso compounds. In general,
these compounds are either alkylating agents *per se* (nitrosamides and nitrosamidines) or are converted metabolically to such agents. The ultimate alkylating
species are most probably carbonium ions (Magee and Schoental, 1964; Druckrey
*et al.*, 1967a). The lowest alkyl homologues, dimethyl- and diethylnitrosamine (DEN), produce 7-methyl- or 7-ethylguanine as a major product and
a variety of other less abundant derivatives at other sites (Fig. 1A,B and Table 1).

D. S. R. SARMA,
S. RAJALAKSHMI
AND
EMMANUEL
FARBER

TABLE 1

Patterns of Methylation of DNA in Intact Cells or in Isolated DNA by Methylating Agents[a]

Molar percentage of methylation of DNA by

| Product | MMS in vitro | DMS in vitro | DMS in vivo | MNNG in vitro | MNNG in vivo | MNU in vitro | DMN in vivo | MAM-acetate in vitro | MAM-acetate in vivo |
|---|---|---|---|---|---|---|---|---|---|
| N-7-MeG | 78–91[b] | 76[c] | 71–84[c] | 67–76[c] | 70–71[c] | Major product[c] | 77–82[d] | Major product[e] | Major product[f] 61[g] |
| N-3-MeG | 0.68[h] | 1[i] (poly G) | | 2[i] (poly G) | | 1[i] | 0.3–1.0[l] | | |
| O-6-MeG | 0.32[h] | 0.2[c] | 0.5–1c | 6–7[c] | 6[c] | 7[i] | 6[j,k] | | |
| N-1-MeA | Not detectable[j] | 3[c] | | 1[c] | 1[c] | | 1.2–7[d,j] | | |
| N-3-MeA | 1–5[b] | 15–19[c] | 11–15[c] | 3–12[c] | 7[c] | | 2.6–9[d,j] | | |
| N-1-MeC | 8–20[b] | 2[c] | | 2[c] | 2[c] | | 1–7 | | |
| O-4-MeT | 1[b] | | | | | Small concentration[l] | | | |
| Phosphotriester | 1 or less[n] | | | | | 18[m] | | | |

[a] In vitro signifies reaction with isolated DNA (e.g., salmon sperm or calf thymus). In vivo signifies reaction with DNA in an intact cell. The cells used varied considerably—E. coli, T bacteriophages, rat liver (intact animal), hamster embryo cells, and mouse L cells.
[b] Lawley and Brookes (1963).
[c] Lawley and Thatcher (1970).
[d] Lawley et al. (1968).
[e] Matsumoto and Higa (1966).
[f] Shank and Magee (1967).
[g] Nagata and Matsumoto (1969).
[h] Lawley and Shah (1972b).
[i] Lawley et al. (1971/1972).
[j] O'Connor et al. (1973).
[k] Craddock (1973).
[l] Lawley et al. (1973).
[m] Lawley (1973).
[n] Bannon and Verly (1972).

239

INTERAC-
TIONS OF
CARCINOGENS
WITH NUCLEIC
ACIDS

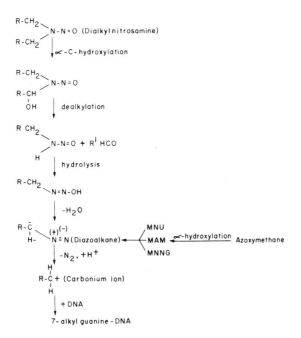

FIGURE 2. Probable mechanism for the formation of reactive alkylating
intermediate from dialkylnitrosamines and dialkylnitrosamides.

Presumably, the intermediate active derivative is the product of oxidative
dealkylation (Fig. 2).

The nature of the ultimate reactive form is not clearly established. Some
authors have suggested that diazomethane is the reactive intermediate (Fig. 2)
(Heath, 1961; Magee and Hultin, 1962), although this intermediate has never
been demonstrated. On the contrary, Lijinsky et al. (1968), using CD$_3$-labeled
DMN in vivo, have demonstrated that the methyl group enters 7-methylguanine
intact. Similar conclusions were reached using N-methyl-N'-nitro-N-
nitrosoguanidine (MNNG) and DNA in Escherichia coli (Lingens et al., 1971) and
MNU and DNA from salmon sperm (Lawley and Shah, 1973). These results
suggest that diazomethane may not be the intermediate.

Unlike dialkylnitrosamines, the nitrosamides and nitrosamidines such as MNU,
N-methylnitrosourethan (MNUT), and MNNG do not require enzyme activation.
The decomposition of MNNG to alkyl intermediates is stimulated by thiols
(McCalla et al., 1968; Schulz and McCalla, 1969; Lawley and Thatcher, 1970),
while that of MNU is not (Lawley, 1972b).

7-Methylguanine has been detected also as the major product in nucleic acids
after the administration of 1-$^{14}$C-di-n-propyl- or 1-$^{14}$C-di-n-butylnitrosamine but
not when DEN or 2-$^{14}$C-di-n-propylnitrosamine is given. This suggests that higher
di-n-alkylnitrosamines are metabolically converted to methyl-alkyl- or dimethylnitrosamine by a pathway analogous to fatty acid degradation. In support of this

240

D. S. R. SARMA,
S. RAJALAKSHMI
AND
EMMANUEL
FARBER

hypothesis is the *in vivo* formation of 7-methylguanine in rat liver DNA and RNA after the administration of the probable intermediates of $\beta$-oxidation of di-*n*-propylnitrosamine such as 1-($^{14}$C)-$\beta$-hydroxypropyl propylnitrosamine, $^{3}$H-(2-oxopropyl)propylnitrosamine, and ($^{3}$H-methyl)propylnitrosamine (Krüger, 1973; Krüger and Bertram, 1973). Further, DEN or 2-1-$^{14}$C-di-*n*-propylnitrosamine does not generate any 7-methylguanine.

7-Methylguanine is not obtained with the cyclic 2,5-$^{14}$C- and 3,4-$^{14}$C-*N*-nitrosopyrrolidine, thus indicating that the hypothesis implicating $\beta$-oxidation may not apply to all complex nitroso compounds (Krüger, 1972). However, 7-methylguanine was reported by Lee and Lijinsky (1966) to be produced from tritium-labeled nitrosopyrrolidine. Although a number of cyclic nitrosamines, such as *N*-nitrosomorpholine, *N*-nitrosodihydrouracil, *N*-nitrosopiperidine, and *N,N*-nitrosopiperazine, are carcinogens, very little is known regarding the mechanism of action of these agents. Circumstantial evidence exists to indicate that at least with *N*-nitrosomorpholine (Stewart and Magee, 1972) and with *N*-nitrosopyrrolidine (Krüger, 1972) ring opening occurs and one or more derivatives interact with nucleic acids. In studies with *N*-nitroso-3-$^{14}$C-morpholine, radioactive $CO_2$ was produced linearly for 30 h and at least six radioactive compounds were found on acid hydrolysis of liver DNA, one of which proved to be 7-(2-hydroxyethyl)guanine (Stewart, Swan, Holswon, and Magee, personal communication).

Many alkylating agents in general, be they methylating or ethylating, produce 7-alkylguanine as the major product in DNA (over 70%) (Table 1). However, many other reaction products of lesser quantities have been reported with alkylating carcinogens, such as substitutions on O-6, N-3, and 2-NH$_2$ of guanine; N-1, N-3, N-7, and 6-NH$_2$ of adenine; N-1, N-3, and C-5 of cytosine; and O-4 of thymine (Table 1). The quantitative and qualitative nature of the alkylation products varies with the agent, the type of DNA (single or double strand), and the organism used. For example, very little guanine methylated at O-6 is found with MMS, while approximately 6% of the methylation with DMN or MNU is at this position. Furthermore, methylation at O-4 of thymine has been reported to occur with MNU (Lawley *et al.*, 1973).

Formation of phosphotriesters as a result of interaction between DNA and alkylating agents has been demonstrated (Elmore *et al.*, 1948; Alexander, 1952; Stacey *et al.*, 1957/1958; Lett *et al.*, 1962; Rhaese and Freese, 1969; Bannon and Verly, 1972; Walker and Ewart, 1973; Lawley, 1973). Lett *et al.* (1962) have suggested that alkylating agents react primarily with phosphates in DNA and have presented spectrophotometric evidence for transalkylation from triester phosphates to bases in the DNA. However, Lawley and Brookes (1963) indicated that phosphate alkylation is negligible. Bannon and Verly (1972) have shown that with ethyl methanesulfonate (EMS), 15% of the DNA alkylation is on the phosphate while with MMS only 1% is on the phosphate. Lawley (1973), using MNU, has shown that 19% of the DNA alkylation is on the phosphodiester. It may be that the alkylation of phosphodiesters, like alkylation of O-6 of guanine, is associated mainly with the alkylating agents which are of the SN$_1$ type.

241

INTERAC-
TIONS OF
CARCINOGENS
WITH NUCLEIC
ACIDS

*a. β-Propiolactone.* β-Propiolactone, a highly strained four-membered car- cinogenic lactone, does not require metabolic activation (Walpole *et al.*, 1954). The hydrolysis product, β-hydroxypropionic acid, is not carcinogenic, thus indicating the need for the intact lactone ring for carcinogenesis (Dickens and Jones, 1963). Roberts and Warwick (1963) have shown that β-propiolactone interacts with RNA to yield 7-(2-carboxyethyl)guanine. Similar products are obtained by interaction of β-propiolactone with mouse skin DNA (Boutwell *et al.*, 1969).

*b. 1,2-Dimethylhydrazine.* 1,2-Dimethylhydrazine (1,2-DMH) is carcinogenic to colon and rectum of rat (Preussmann *et al.*, 1967; Druckrey *et al.*, 1967b). This compound appears to require metabolic activation and yields 7-methylguanine in DNA of both colon and liver of mice (Hawks *et al.*, 1972).

*c. Methylazoxymethanol.* Cycasin, a naturally occurring carcinogen, is the β-glucoside of methylazoxymethanol (MAM) (Spatz and Laqueur, 1967; Lac- queur and Spatz, 1968). On oral administration, cycasin is hydrolyzed by bacterial β-glucosidase in the intestine to yield the actual carcinogen, MAM. Nonenzymatic methylation of DNA by MAM has been demonstrated, and the major reaction product is N-7-methylguanine (Matsumoto and Higa, 1966). A similar pattern of alkylation of DNA by MAM and DMN was observed in the intact rat (Shank and Magee, 1967). It has been suggested that MAM may yield methyldiazonium ion (Nagasawa *et al.*, 1972), which on losing nitrogen yields a carbonium ion (Fig. 2).

*d. Azoxymethane.* Like 1,2-dimethylhydrazine, azoxymethane is a colon car- cinogen (Druckrey, 1970). This agent may undergo enzymatic α-hydroxylation to yield MAM (Druckrey, 1972) (Fig. 2).

*e. Urethan.* Urethan (ethylcarbamate), an aliphatic amide, is a multipotential carcinogen (Mirvish, 1968) and a "promoting" agent (Kawamoto *et al.*, 1958; Berenblum and Trainin, 1960). Urethan does not react with DNA directly, but requires metabolic activation. The initial step may be N-hydroxylation to form N-hydroxyurethan, which may in turn be esterified (Boyland and Nery, 1965; Nery, 1968). The ester may result in the formation of an ethoxycarboxylating agent and by subsequent loss of carbon dioxide may form the ethylating species (Nery, 1968, 1969; Williams and Nery, 1971). Administration of 1-[14]C- ethylcarba- mate or ethyl(carboxyl-[14]C)carbamate results in the formation of a single radioac- tive compound in the RNA of mouse liver, which has been identified as the ethyl ester of cytosine-5-carboxylate (Boyland and Williams, 1969). It is not clear whether such a compound is formed in DNA of such urethan-treated animals. Several unidentified labeled components have been detected in the DNA of rats following the administration of 1-[14]C- or 2-[3]H-urethan (Prodi *et al.*, 1970a).

*f. Ethionine.* Ethionine, the ethyl analogue of methionine, is a hepatocar- cinogen (Farber, 1963). *In vivo*, it is metabolized in a manner similar to that of methionine, yielding S-adenosylethionine. Administration of large doses of

242

D. S. R. SARMA,
S. RAJALAKSHMI
AND
EMMANUEL
FARBER

ethionine results in the ethylation of rat liver DNA (Stekol, 1965). The major product appears to be 7-ethylguanine (Swann *et al.*, 1971; Cox and Farber, 1972). *In vivo*, S-adenosyl-L-ethionine can substitute for S-adenosine-L-methionine in several reactions. However, so far the normal analogue of 7-ethylguanine, 7-methylguanine, has not been found in liver DNA. Swann *et al.* (1971) suggest that ethylation of DNA by ethionine may possibly not be by the action of a methyltransferase using S-adenosyl-L-ethionine as the ethyl-group donor.

*g. Nitrogen and Sulfur Mustards.* There are a great variety of monofunctional and bifunctional alkylating derivatives of nitrogen and sulfur mustards. Elmore *et al.* (1948) and later Alexander (1952) observed that mustard gas esterifies the primary phosphate groups of DNA. Using $^{35}$S-sulfur mustard and DNA at low levels of reaction, about 1 mmole/mole DNA-P, Brookes and Lawley (1961) identified a reaction product as di(guanine-7-ethylsulfide). Bifunctional alkylating agents thus can interact with two nucleophilic centers, especially N-7 of guanine, to form a bridge between them. The covalent crosslinking of DNA can be intra- or interstrand or between two separate duplex structures.

Denatured DNA yields a lower proportion of diguaninyl product than does double-stranded DNA (Brookes and Lawley, 1961), thus suggesting that such a product arises preferentially from interstrand rather than intrastrand crosslinking. About 25% of the guanine alkylations in DNA by mustard gas is the diguaninyl product (Brookes and Lawley, 1961). The amount of diguaninyl product formed varies with the GC content of DNA (Lawley, 1966). For example, DNA from *Pseudomonas aeruginosa* (GC 67%) gave 26% diguaninyl product, that from *Escherichia coli* (GC 50%) 20%, and that from *Bacillis cereus* (GC 34%) 13%.

### 2.1.3. Aromatic Amines and Amides

*a. 2-Acetylaminofluorene and Related Compounds.* Aromatic amines and amides appear to require metabolic activation to the N-hydroxy derivatives as the initial step in their interaction with DNA (E. C. Miller and Miller, 1969; Irving, 1970; Weisburger and Weisburger, 1973). It appears that, at least in the rat liver and with 2-acetylaminofluorene (2-AAF), a second step is necessary, esterification of N-hydroxy derivative (see J. A. Miller, 1970; Weisburger and Weisburger, 1973). Glucuronide (Irving *et al.*, 1969; Irving and Russell, 1970; Irving, 1971) and sulfate (DeBaun *et al.*, 1970; Weisburger *et al.*, 1972) esters of N-hydroxy-2-AAF have been reported. Nonenzymatic acylation of N-hydroxy-2-AAF by acetyl coenzyme A, carbamoylphosphate, or acetylphosphate has also been demonstrated (Lotlikar and Luha, 1971a,b). It is not clear which of these esters is involved in the *in vivo* binding of N-hydroxy-2-AAF with DNA of the target tissue. Although the sulfate conjugate of N-hydroxy-2-AAF is a likely key metabolite in the induction of liver cancer by 2-AAF in rats (DeBaun *et al.*, 1970), it may not be involved in the binding of these carcinogens (2-AAF or N-hydroxy-2-AAF) to rat liver DNA *in vivo* (Irving *et al.*, 1969; Irving, 1971). Further, N-hydroxy-2-AAF sulfotransferase activity is not detectable in two tissues of rat susceptible to carcinogenesis by N-hydroxy-2-AAF: Zymbal's gland (the sebaceous gland of the external auditory canal) and the mammary gland (Irving *et al.*, 1971).

243

INTERAC-
TIONS OF
CARCINOGENS
WITH NUCLEIC
ACIDS

The glucuronide conjugate of N-hydroxy-2-AAF has been suggested to be involved in the binding of the carcinogen to rat liver DNA (Irving *et al.*, 1969; Irving, 1971; Irving and Russell, 1970), although this is by no means established *in vivo* (J. A. Miller *et al.*, 1970). More recently, involvement of O-acetyl derivatives has been suggested (King and Phillips, 1972; Bartsch *et al.*, 1972).

The covalent interaction between the active derivative of N-hydroxy-2-AAF and DNA *in vivo* occurs at the C-8 position of guanine (Kriek *et al.*, 1967; Kriek, 1968; Irving and Veazey, 1969). It has been suggested that there are two types of reactions of N-acetoxy-2-AAF with guanine in DNA: a major product (80%), N-(deoxyguanosine-8-yl)-2-fluorenylacetamide, and a minor one (Kriek, 1972). The exact chemical nature of the minor component(s) (20%) is not known other than that it is a derivative of guanine. It has been suggested that it may be the result of an interaction at the 1- or 3-position of the fluorene ring, rather than through the amino nitrogen (Kriek, 1972).

Based on the studies with circular dichroism, proton magnetic resonance spectroscopy, and computer-generated molecular models of oligonucleotides containing bound 2-AAF, Nelson *et al.* (1971) have suggested an interesting model. After interaction with 2-AAF, the guanine base rotates around the glycosidic bond at N-9. This allows an interaction of the fluorene compound with the adjacent base in the nucleotide chain, producing a type of intercalation. One would anticipate localized regions of denaturation of the DNA at some sites of interaction with 2-AAF. Conceivably, the regions of denaturation of DNA observed on electron microscopic examination of DNA from livers of animals fed a regimen containing 2-AAF (Epstein *et al.*, 1969/1970) might be grosser manifestations of such an effect on DNA.

*b. 2-Naphthylamine and Related Compounds.* The single administration of tritiated 2-naphthylamine to mouse yields bound metabolite(s) with liver DNA (Hughes and Pilczyk, 1969/1970). Assuming that 2-amino-1-naphthol is the proximate carcinogenic metabolite of 2-naphthylamine (an assumption that is debatable; Anderson *et al.*, 1964), Troll *et al.* (1963) have studied the *in vitro* binding of 8-$^{14}$C-2-aminonaphthol with DNA. Incubating labeled 2-amino-1-naphthol with salmon sperm DNA at pH 7.5 and 37°C for several days resulted in the incorporation of the radioactivity into DNA and a decrease in the transition midpoint ($T_m$). This aspect requires further experimentation, since King and Kriek (1965) were unable to confirm the reduction in $T_m$ on incubation of DNA with 2-amino-1-naphthol under the conditions employed by Troll *et al.* (1963).

*c. p-Dimethylaminoazobenzene and Derivatives.* Relatively little is known about the mechanism involved in the binding of azo dyes to DNA *in vivo*. The Millers and coworkers have proposed that the activation of carcinogenic azo dyes may be similar to the activation of other aromatic amines (Poirier *et al.*, 1967; E. C. Miller and Miller, 1969; J. A. Miller and Miller, 1969). Thus the *in vivo* activation of

244

D. S. R. SARMA,
S. RAJALAKSHMI
AND
EMMANUEL
FARBER

4-dimethylaminoazobenzene (DAB) may involve the following series of reactions: (1) mono-N-demethylation, (2) N-hydroxylation, and (3) conjugation as a sulfate ester (Poirier *et al.*, 1967) or transacetylation (Bartsch *et al.*, 1972). However, in the case of ring-methylated azo dyes such as 3'-methyl-DAB, hydroxylation of the ring-methyl group followed by conjugation (e.g., as sulfate) may occur. This may lead to the formation of a carbonium ion by a route analogous to that hypothesized for methylated polycyclic aromatic hydrocarbons (Dipple, 1972). Roberts and Warwick (1961), using N, N'-dimethyl-4-aminoazobenzene labeled with tritium in the prime or aniline ring, have observed the incorporation of tritium into rat liver DNA. The specific activity is approximately 3% that found in hepatic proteins. More recently J. A. Miller *et al.* (1970), using tritiated N-methyl-4-aminoazobenzene (radioactivity in the prime ring), have obtained rat liver DNA with radioactivity. Degradation of such DNA yields a product chromatographically identical to N-(deoxyguanosine-8-yl)-N-methyl-4-aminoazobenzene.

It is of interest to note that the binding to DNA of another azo dye, 2-methyl-DAB, at least a weak carcinogen, following a single administration, is higher than can be obtained with the carcinogen DAB (Warwick, 1969). However, on continuous feeding, the level of binding of 2-methyl-DAB to liver DNA is somewhat lower than in the case of DAB (Roberts, 1969). 2-Methyl-DAB has been reported to induce liver cancer when fed to animals subjected to partial hepatectomy (Warwick, 1967).

*d. Ortho-aminoazotoluene.* o-Aminoazotoluene (o-AAT) is the first azo dye shown to induce liver cancer in rats (Sasaki and Yoshida, 1935). Intragastric administration of tritiated o-AAT to C57 mice results in liver DNA with covalently bound radioactivity (Lawson and Clayson, 1969). The nature of the interaction is not known.

*2.1.4. Polycyclic Aromatic Hydrocarbons*

Felix Bergmann (1942) was the first to suggest that, in addition to aromaticity, geometry of the molecule is involved in hydrocarbon carcinogenicity. Since then, from time to time, intercalation and other noncovalent interactions between DNA and certain planar polycyclic hydrocarbons such as benzo[a]pyrene (BP) and 3-methylcholanthrene (3-MC) (Iball and MacDonald, 1960) have been suggested. This type of interaction may take place to a lesser extent with nonplanar compounds such as 7,12-dimethylbenz[a]anthracene (7,12-DMBA).

More recently, some polycyclic aromatic hydrocarbons (PAH) have been shown to interact covalently with DNA following microsomal metabolic activation (Gelboin, 1969; Grover and Sims, 1968). Several suggestions have been advanced regarding the nature of the metabolically active intermediate(s) involved in the binding to DNA. One of the first suggestions was the formation of the radical cation, as a result of oxidation of the hydrocarbon (see Wilk and Girke, 1969). Another suggestion was the formation of K-region epoxides as the reactive intermediate species. Selkirk *et al.* (1971) demonstrated the formation of 5,6-epoxydibenz[a]anthracene on incubation of the parent compound with rat liver microsomes in the presence of NADPH. Similarly, the formation of 4,5-epoxide of 3,4-BP by rat liver microsomes was reported (Grover *et al.*, 1971a; Grover and Sims, 1972). Although K-region epoxides interact with DNA to a greater extent than do the parent hydrocarbons (Grover and Sims, 1970; Grover *et al.*, 1971b; Kuroki *et al.*, 1971/1972), they have very little or no carcinogenic activity in mice or rats (see E. C. Miller and Miller, 1971). It may be pointed out, however, that they are mutagenic in several systems including mammalian cells (Huberman *et al.*, 1971; Cookson *et al.*, 1971) and cause malignant transformation of cells in culture (Grover *et al.*, 1971c). The chemical nature of the products of interaction between most PAH and DNA is not known.

245

INTERAC-
TIONS OF
CARCINOGENS
WITH NUCLEIC
ACIDS

Another mode of activation has been suggested for the methylated aromatic hydrocarbons such as 7,12-DMBA, some of which are potent carcinogens (Huggins *et al.*, 1964). The first probable step involved in such activation is oxidation to hydroxymethyl derivatives (Boyland and Sims, 1965; Sims and Grover, 1968) followed by esterification of the hydroxymethyl group. Such reactions could lead to the formation of reactive carbonium ions (Dipple *et al.*, 1968; Flesher and Sydnor, 1971). Enzymatic formation of such esters, for example, a sulfate ester, has not yet been demonstrated. The model compounds 7-bromomethylbenz[*a*]anthracene and 7-bromomethyl-12-methylbenz[*a*]-anthracene, which can form carbonium ions, react *in vitro* with DNA yielding several substitution products at the 2-amino group of guanine, the 6-amino group of adenine, and to a lesser extent the 4-amino group of cytosine (Dipple *et al.*, 1971). Substitution at the C-8 position of guanine also has been demonstrated (Pochon and Michelson, 1971). It may be noted that the model bromomethyl compounds are weak carcinogens (Dipple and Slade, 1970, 1971).

Ts'o *et al.* (1969), using *in vitro* conditions, studied the nature of the binding of benzpyrenes and other polycyclic hydrocarbons to DNA. From their experiments, they have reasoned that polycyclic hydrocarbon molecules bind to DNA by hydrophobic–stacking interaction in a face-to-face mode. If the system is properly activated either by supplying radiation energy or through free radical formation, the bases of DNA and polycyclic hydrocarbons may form covalent bonds.

Photoactivation of a mixture of thymine and 3,4-BP yields a photoproduct in which 3,4-BP is joined through a single covalent bond to C-6 of thymine (Blackburn *et al.*, 1972); whether a similar reaction occurs with DNA is not known. *A priori*, there is no reason to believe that a single mechanism of activation operates in all tissues with all aromatic hydrocarbons. Broadly, one can visualize two types of interactions either separately or in combination: (1) complex formation with DNA, most probably by intercalation and particularly with planar compounds such as BP and 3-MC and to a lesser extent with nonplanar compounds such as 7,12-DMBA; and (2) covalent interaction with DNA after suitable activation *in vivo*. This pathway is probably the predominant one *in vivo*.

### 2.1.5. 4-Nitroquinoline-N-Oxide

4-Nitroquinoline-N-oxide (4NQO) and some of its derivatives are multipotent carcinogens (Nakahara *et al.*, 1957; Kawazoe *et al.*, 1969). Activated 4NQO or

246

D. S. R. SARMA,
S. RAJALAKSHMI
AND
EMMANUEL
FARBER

uncharacterized derivatives of 4NQO have been found to interact with DNA (Tada *et al.*, 1967; Matsushima *et al.*, 1967; Tada and Tada, 1971). Several probable mechanisms of interaction of 4NQO with DNA have been postulated. These include (a) reduction to the hydroxyamino derivatives, (b) conversion to a nitroso derivative, or (c) activation to a carbonium ion.

a. It is generally believed that 4NQO is reduced to 4-hydroxyaminoquinoline-*N*-oxide (4OHAQO) (Hoshino *et al.*, 1966; Kato and Takalashi, 1970). Such reduction has been shown to be mediated by the diaphorase system of both bacterial and rat liver origin (Sugimura *et al.*, 1966; Fukuda and Yamamoto, 1972). 4OHAQO by itself may not be the ultimate carcinogen, but free radicals produced from oxidation products (Nagata *et al.*, 1966*a,b*; Ishizawa and Endo, 1967; Kosuge *et al.*, 1969) or from diesters (Araki *et al.*, 1969; Enomoto *et al*, 1968) may be involved in the binding of DNA. Also, an ATP-requiring enzymatic acylation of 4OHAQO to yield the proximate carcinogen has been suggested (Tada and Tada, 1972).

b. Using a rapid-scan spectrophotometer, Matsuyama and Nagata (1972) detected the nitroso intermediate, 4-nitrosoquinoline-1-oxide. This may be an important reactive product in the carcinogenicity and the reactivity of 4NQO and 4OHAQO with DNA.

c. The formation of a carbonium ion, an active intermediate in alkylation, has been suggested (Kawazoe *et al.*, 1972). According to this proposed scheme, 4NQO may undergo replacement reactions with nucleophils, such as SH groups of proteins, with a simultaneous liberation of nitrous acid. Nitrous acid can react with primary amines *in vivo* to form diazonium ions, which on decomposition lead to the formation of carbonium ions (Kawazoe *et al.*, 1972).

### 2.1.6. Nitrofurans and Derivatives

Nitrofurans and their derivatives have been clinically used as antibacterial agents (Dodd and Stillman, 1944; Dann and Moller, 1947; Paul and Paul, 1964). They have been shown to be powerful carcinogens (Ertürk *et al.*, 1967; 1970*a,b*; 1971; Morris *et al.*, 1969). In analogy to nitroaromatic carcinogens, such as 4NQO, reduction of the nitro group to a hydroxylamino derivative appears to be a necessary metabolic activation step, either for their interaction with macromolecules or for their carcinogenic property (McCalla *et al.*, 1971; Miura and Reckendorf, 1967; Cohen *et al.*, 1973). The nature of the interaction of these derivatives with nucleic acid has yet to be determined.

### 2.1.7. Aflatoxins

The aflatoxins, a group of naturally occurring compounds, include highly potent carcinogens for liver and for other organs (Lancaster *et al.*, 1961). These compounds do not seem to be active *per se* but undergo metabolic activation prior to their reaction with DNA. Although covalent binding of aflatoxins $B_1$ and $G_1$ with DNA *in vivo* has been reported (Lijinsky *et al.*, 1970), the nature of the binding or the nature of the metabolic activation is not understood. Liver cells in

247

INTERAC-
TIONS OF
CARCINOGENS
WITH NUCLEIC
ACIDS

culture convert aflatoxin $B_1$ to a more potent cytotoxin (Scaife, 1970/1971). Garner *et al.* (1971) have reported that rat liver microsomes, in the presence of NADPH and oxygen, convert aflatoxin $B_1$ to a highly toxic product lethal to certain strains of *Salmonella typhimurium.* Their data suggest that epoxidation at the 1,2-double bond might be involved in the *in vivo* activation of this compound (Garner *et al.*, 1971). Microsomal-dependent binding of aflatoxin $B_1$ to DNA and RNA *in vitro* has been demonstrated (Garner, 1973; Swenson *et al.*, 1973). Aflatoxin $B_1$-2,3-oxide appears to be the probable reactive precursor of the RNA aflatoxin $B_1$ adduct (Swenson *et al.*, 1973).

### 2.1.8. Safrole

Safrole, a component isolated from sassafras oil, is primarily a hepatocarcinogen. It has been shown that rat and mouse liver postmitochondrial supernatant, in the presence of NADPH, oxidizes safrole to 1′-hydroxysafrole (Wislocki *et al.*, 1973). Administration of 1′-hydroxysafrole-2′, 3′-$^3$H to rats yields hepatic DNA–bound $^3$H (Wislocki *et al.*, 1973). *In vitro*, interaction of 1′-acetoxysafrole with GMP yields three products. The main one appears to be a substitution at O-6 of guanine (Borchert *et al.*, 1973).

### 2.2. Noncovalent Interactions

Noncovalent interactions can be broadly divided into two groups: (1) internal binding or intercalation, wherein the carcinogen is inserted between base pairs of the DNA duplex structure (Fig. 3), and (2) external binding, or adlineation, wherein the agent interacts with bases at sites that are not involved in base pairing. In the latter event and in contrast to intercalation, the carcinogen binds perpendicular to the planes of the bases (Arcos and Argus, 1968).

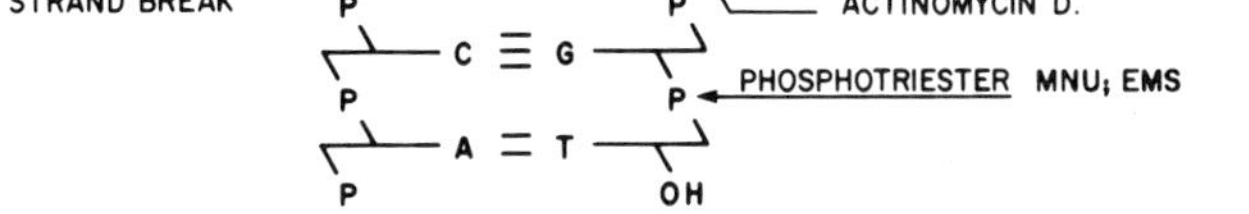

FIGURE 3. Schematic representation of chemical carcinogen–DNA interaction showing intercalation, inter- and intrastrand crosslinking, and the nature of sites liberated following strand breaks at the site of depurination.

D. S. R. SARMA,
S. RAJALAKSHMI
AND
EMMANUEL
FARBER

### 2.2.1. Intercalation

Lerman (1964) postulated the intercalation model to explain the binding of acridine to DNA and the resultant frameshift mutations. Since then, this mechanism has been suggested to explain the binding of several drugs, antibiotics, alkaloids, and some carcinogens to DNA, a detailed discussion of which is presented by Hahn (1971).

As pointed out earlier, the primary requisite for intercalation is suitable molecular geometry. Planar compounds in general intercalate most easily. Many experiments carried out to study the ability of some carcinogens such as planar polycyclic aromatic hydrocarbons, hycanthone, and actinomycin D to intercalate into DNA have been carried out *in vitro*. Caution must be used in extrapolating these data to the intact animal or organism, since intercalation depends on many variables including the state of DNA.

*In vivo* inside the nucleus, the DNA may be in a more compact or condensed form than *in vitro*, and intercalation into a compact DNA is less than in a more extended molecule (Lerman, 1971). For example, within 10–70 min following the addition of phytohemagglutinin to lymphocytes, the binding of intercalating acridine orange is about four times that obtained before phytohemagglutinin treatment (Lerman, 1971), a finding presumably due to an altered state of the DNA. Another interesting example is hycanthone, an intercalating agent that is used in the treatment of schistosomiasis. In a recent experiment, hepatic DNA from rats treated with hycanthone methanesulfonate did not show any increase in $T_m$ (Sarma *et al.*, 1973c), in contrast to its effect on DNA *in vitro* where an obvious increase in $T_m$ is observed (Weinstein and Hirschberg, 1971; Sarma *et al.*, 1973c). This intercalating drug is reported to be a carcinogen in mice with schistosomiasis (Haese *et al.*, 1973).

Intercalation has been suggested as a mechanism for the binding to DNA of planar carcinogenic polycyclic aromatic hydrocarbons such as 3,4-BP and 3-MC (Boyland, 1969; Boyland and Green, 1962; Liquori *et al.*, 1962; Nagata *et al.*, 1966a; Ts'o *et al.*, 1969). However, this postulate is controversial (Giovanella *et al.*, 1964; Van Duuren *et al.*, 1968/1969).

Actinomycin D, a weak carcinogen (Kawamata *et al.*, 1958, 1959; DiPaolo, 1960; Svoboda and Reddy, 1970), also appears to intercalate into DNA *in vitro* (Müller and Crothers, 1968; Wells, 1971). Virtually all of these studies have been carried out *in vitro*. Although a good correlation exists between frameshift mutagenicity and intercalation, a convincing correlation between carcinogenicity and extent of intercalation has yet to be established.

### 2.2.2. External Binding

External binding of several carcinogens such as 4NQO (Malkin and Zahalsky, 1966; Paul *et al.*, 1971), aflatoxins (Sporn *et al.*, 1966; Clifford and Rees, 1967; Black and Jirgensons, 1967, Schabort, 1971), and polycyclic aromatic hydrocarbons (Arcos and Argus, 1968) with DNA has been suggested. This type of binding is relatively weak compared to that of intercalation, and it is not certain at present whether such binding exists *in vivo*. Marquardt *et al.* (1971) have reported weakly bound radioactivity in rat liver DNA following the administration of $^3$H-7,12-DMBA. However, the nature of this binding remains to be clarified.

249

INTERAC-
TIONS OF
CARCINOGENS
WITH NUCLEIC
ACIDS

### 2.3. Purine-N-Oxides

The *N*-oxides of certain purines, such as adenine-1-oxide and 3-*N*-oxide derivatives of guanine and xanthine, are oncogenic and induce subcutaneous neoplasms at the site of injection and liver cancer in rats and mice (Sugiura *et al.*, 1970). The interaction of oncogenic purine-*N*-oxides with nucleic acids is not yet established. Administration of $^{14}$C-labeled 3-hydroxyxanthine does not result in any significant *in vivo* incorporation of radioactivity into adenine or guanine of RNA or DNA (Myles and Brown, 1969).

### 2.4. Carcinogenic Metals

Many inorganic metal compounds are known to be carcinogenic. However, very little is known about mechanisms by which neoplasms are induced. By virtue of being electrophilic cations, $Be^{2+}$, $Cd^{2+}$, $Co^{2+}$, $Pb^{2+}$, and $Ni^{2+}$ can interact with nucleophilic sites of macromolecules (J. A. Miller, 1970). Some of the metal ions are known to react with guanine (Shapiro, 1968) and to interact with phosphate groups of DNA (Eichhorn *et al.*, 1966). Some also interfere with the stability of the duplex structure by binding to the amino groups of the bases (Furst and Haro, 1969). Some of the carcinogenic metal ions such as $Ni^{2+}$ can depolymerize polynucleotides (Butzow and Eichhorn, 1965). The binding of some metals to the purine and pyrimidine bases can be through covalent bonds or $\pi$-electrons of the bases (Fuwa *et al.*, 1960). The nature of the *in vivo* interaction of the carcinogenic metals with nucleic acids remains to be clarified.

## 3. Interaction of Chemical Carcinogens with Mitochondrial DNA

Almost all studies with DNA and chemical carcinogens have involved total tissue or organ DNA. Since nuclear DNA represents the overwhelming mass of DNA, it is usually assumed that what is being examined in studies on cellular DNA is nuclear. Recent work by Wunderlich and associates may require a reevaluation of this assumption.

Wunderlich *et al.* (1970, 1971/1972) have observed that mitochondrial DNA in liver has 3–7 times the specific activity of nuclear DNA in rats given single injections of methyl-labeled MNU or DMN. This has led them to suggest a cytoplasmic mutation hypothesis of carcinogenesis (Wunderlich *et al.*, 1971/1972). Although interesting and provocative, these results may be in part due to the small quantity of mitochondrial DNA (1.5%; Schneider and Kuff, 1965) relative to nuclear DNA. Methylation in a highly selected portion of nuclear DNA would be

250

D. S. R. SARMA,
S. RAJALAKSHMI
AND
EMMANUEL
FARBER

greatly diluted by the large pool of poorly labeled nuclear DNA when the results are expressed as specific activity. Despite this complication, the search for selection in the type of DNA as a target for carcinogens, as is being pioneered by Wunderlich and associates, is of great potential importance in studies on chemical carcinogenesis.

## 4. Interaction of Chemical Carcinogens with RNA

### 4.1. General

Cellular ribonucleic acids play a key role as mediators in the transfer of genetic information between DNA and protein. The ultraviolet absorption–temperature curve of RNA, reaction with formaldehyde, hyperchromicity in water and at high temperature, and several other parameters, as reviewed by Kit (1960), suggest that RNA's behave hydrodynamically as homologous single chains that are coiled in such a way to permit a substantial number of intramolecular hydrogen bonds. The three-dimensional structure of tRNAs (cloverleaf model) is maintained through intramolecular hydrogen bonds at specific locations (Holley *et al.*, 1965). The heterogeneous nuclear RNA (HnRNA) of HeLa cells and Ehrlich ascites carcinoma cells has been shown to contain double-stranded regions (Jelinek and Darnell, 1972; Ryskov *et al.*, 1972). The mRNA of the same cells seems not to contain significant amounts of double-stranded regions. Thus in RNA, unlike DNA, not all nucleotides are involved in the formation of hydrogen bonds. Theoretically, one would expect more available sites for interaction of carcinogens with RNA than with DNA. In general, the interaction of RNA with chemical carcinogens has not been extensively investigated as that of DNA and of protein. Furthermore, the binding to particular species of RNA has been studied for only very few carcinogens such as 2-AAF, MNU, and ethionine. The binding of carcinogens to mRNA, HnRNA (nuclear), or "chromosomal" RNA has not been investigated to date. Such studies would appear to be very important, considering that HnRNA may serve as a precursor for cytoplasmic messenger RNA (Lindberg and Darnell, 1970; Edmonds *et al.*, 1971; Darnell *et al.*, 1971; Melli and Pemberton, 1972; Stevens and Williamson, 1972) and natural mRNA has now been found to contain methylated bases (Perry and Kelly, 1974). The existence of a unique class of RNA species which function as mediators in the initiation of DNA synthesis has been revealed by Sugino and Okazaki (1973) and Hirose *et al.* (1973). With the discovery of the presence of polyadenylate stretches associated with mRNA, it is now possible to isolate mRNA and to study carcinogen interaction with it. In the future, study of the interaction of carcinogens with these new classes of RNAs may prove to be of great value in the attempt to understand the role of altered RNA in carcinogenesis.

### 4.2. Alkylating Agents

Generally, the various sites capable of alkylation in RNA in the order of decreasing activity are N-7 of guanine > N-1 of adenine > N-3 of cytosine > N-7 of adenine > N-3 of adenine > n-3 of guanine (Shapiro, 1968, 1969). This general 251

INTERAC-
TIONS OF
CARCINOGENS
WITH NUCLEIC
ACIDS picture of activity is altered by (1) the type of alkylating agents, i.e., whether they act through an $SN_1$ or an $SN_2$ mechanism, (2) the complex environment that exists when nucleic acids are bound to proteins such as in virus particles, (3) the conformation of nucleic acids such as base stacking or hydrogen bonding, and (4) the conditions used for the alkylation reaction, i.e., whether they favor the anionic or cationic form of the heterocycles.

The interaction of DMN with cellular RNA was first demonstrated by Magee and Farber in 1962 and later by several other workers (Magee and Farber, 1962; Magee and Lee, 1963; Lee and Lijinsky, 1966; Lawley et al., 1968). The alkylation of nucleic acids of the various organs of the rat was studied by Swann and Magee (1968). DMN methylates the liver nucleic acids to a greater extent than those of other organs. MNU methylates nucleic acids of the various organs to the same extent. This differential alkylation between DMN and MNU probably results from the fact that DMN requires preliminary activation, while MNU is direct acting, and the DMN-activating enzymes are specially present in the liver. Both agents methylate RNA to a greater degree than DNA. MMS methylates the nucleic acids in several organs to the same extent as MNU, but DNA is more highly methylated than is RNA. In all these cases, the alkylated base investigated was 7-methylguanine. With respect to the formation of this major alkylated base, there seems to be no difference between DMN, MNU, MNNG, and MMS. However, Lawley and Shah (1972a) have studied the methylation of rRNA and tRNA of rabbit reticulocytes and M2 RNA of the bacteriophage using a variety of methods for the hydrolysis of methylated RNA and for the fractionation of methylated bases. The most striking difference noted by these authors (Lawley and Shah, 1972a) was the formation of O-6-methylguanine by N-alkylnitroso compounds and not by either DMS or MMS. The methylation at O-6 of guanine involves the anion form of guanine and presents an intriguing chemical problem. It is suggested (Brookes, 1971) that the intermediate alkylating species derived from the N-alkylnitroso derivatives (perhaps diazoalkanes) abstract a proton from the guanine ring rather than from the solvent, a circumstance which would favor the reaction at the O-6 atom. An alternative view is that O-6 alkylation is favored by agents reacting predominantly by the $SN_1$ mechanism. It is interesting to point out that the relative extent of methylation at the O-6 atom of guanine in RNA is about one-half that in DNA. This finding is contrary to the expectation based on the concept that involvement of the O-6 atom is hydrogen bonding of the Watson–Crick type would decrease its reactivity as found with the N-1 of adenine. The possibility that the O-6 atom of guanine in RNA is hydrogen-bonded more strongly to water if not to cytosine is worth considering. The complex environment that exists in vivo may play a vital role in the alkylation reactions in addition to the other considerations mentioned above.

The nitroso compounds are relatively more reactive at N-7 of adenine and probably N-3 of guanine but less reactive at N-1 of adenine, N-3 of cytosine, and probably N-3 of uracil as compared to either DMS or MMS. In this study, the type of RNA, i.e., whether bacteriophage RNA, ribosomal RNA, or tRNA from cells,

D. S. R. SARMA,
S. RAJALAKSHMI
AND
EMMANUEL
FARBER

had much less influence on the patterns of methylation than did the type of reagent. Studies with TMV RNA or TMV virus indicate that the methylation reaction is conformation dependent (Singer and Fraenkel-Conrat, 1969). Methylation with DMS and MMS is affected mainly by hydrogen bonding, which reduces the availability of N-1 of adenine and N-3 of cytosine. In contrast, with nitrosoguanidines, an effect in addition to that of hydrogen bonding is present, namely base stacking. With guanine and adenine, methylation is favored by base stacking, while with cytosine the opposite is found (Singer and Fraenkel-Conrat, 1969). A preferential methylation of cytosine has been noticed by these authors during the interaction of MNNG with TMV virus as compared to free TMV RNA. This is the only instance of an alkylation reaction of a group in RNA approaching in magnitude the alkylation of guanine.

Shooter et al. (1974a,b), using a RNA-containing bacteriophage R17, studied the inactivation of the phage with DMS, MMS, MNU, and MNNG. With DMS and MMS, the inactivation was mainly due to methylation at N-1 of adenine and N-3 of cytosine. However with MNU and MNNG, only about one-half of the inactivation observed could be accounted for by methylation at N-1 of adenine and N-3 of cytosine. The rest could be accounted for by methylation at O-6 of guanine and by breaks in RNA as the result of methylation of the phosphate diester group followed by hydrolysis of the unstable triester formed (Shooter et al., 1974b). In contrast to the instability of phosphotriester in RNA, the phosphotriester in DNA is relatively stable.

The ethylation of RNA by ethylating agents such as DEN, EMS, and ethylnitrosourea (ENU) has been demonstrated, and 7-ethylguanine is the major product (Magee and Lee, 1964; Swann and Magee, 1971; Magee, 1969; Singer and Fraenkel-Conrat, 1969; Ross et al., 1971; Goth and Rajewsky, 1972; Pegg, 1973). Ethylation reactions proceed more slowly than do methylations (Kriek and Emmelot, 1963) and occur to a lesser extent (Pegg, 1973).

Pegg (1973) has studied the alkylation of tRNA[fmet], tRNA[phe], tRNA[glu], and tRNA[val] by MNU and has found no significant difference in the degree of alkylation of any of the tRNA preparations examined. The major product was 7-alkylguanine, accounting for 80% of the total, but 3-methylcytosine, 6-O-methylguanine, and 1-methyl-, 3-methyl- and 7-methyladenine were also identified as products of the reactions with tRNA[fmet]. The methylated tRNA[fmet] was analyzed for preferential alkylation of certain residues by degradation with pancreatic ribonuclease and separation of oligonucleotide fragments by chromatography on DEAE-cellulose. The results revealed that the distribution of 7-alkylguanine was in agreement with that expected for a random reaction of the alkylating agent with all guanosine residues throughout the molecule. The studies were carried out under conditions where the native configuration of tRNA was maintained and hence show that the tertiary structure of the tRNA does not impart any specificity to the reaction of MNU with guanine under the conditions of study. However, the possibility that such specificity may exist for the minor products of alkylation cannot be excluded. Also, whether the same random distribution would be found with the lower levels of methylation that might be anticipated during carcinogenesis remains to be established. In this context, the work *in vitro* of Weinstein (1970) with 2-AAF and of Powers and Holley (1972) with DMS indicates that chemical interactions with tRNA need not be random but can be highly specific for even single bases in complex macromolecules when the level of interaction is low. The methylation of tRNA by MMS and DMN was reported by O'Connor *et al.* (1972). The reaction of β-propiolactone with RNA was found to yield 7-(2-carboxyethylguanine) as a major product (Roberts and Warwick, 1963).

253

INTERAC-
TIONS OF
CARCINOGENS
WITH NUCLEIC
ACIDS

### 4.2.1. Urethan

The binding of urethan to liver RNA has been studied by several workers (Boyland and Williams, 1969; Prodi *et al.*, 1970*a*; Lawson and Pound, 1971/1972, 1973*a*). The level of binding of $^3$H-urethan is higher in partially hepatectomized animals than in intact animals (Lawson and Pound, 1971/1972). However, the radioactivity declines very rapidly, a phenomenon that is apparently not due to the turnover of cellular RNAs. It is not known to which type of RNA urethan is bound or whether more than one type of RNA is involved. In mice, urethan labeled in the alkyl group and in the carbonyl carbon was found to react with nucleic acids of liver and lung. Only one radioactive spot, considered to be cytosine-5-carboxylic acid, was detected in the chromatogram (Boyland and Williams, 1969). In the rat liver, however, urethan was found to bind to all nucleotides of RNA which were obtained by alkaline and enzymatic hydrolysis (Prodi *et al.*, 1970*a*; Lawson and Pound, 1971/1972). In general, there is no agreement as to the nature of the bound molecule, i.e., whether it is an ethyl, ethoxy, or carbethoxy group. In the rat, urethan labeled only in the alkyl group was found to bind to nucleic acids (Prodi *et al.*, 1970*a*). Lawson and Pound (1973) have concluded that the bound molecule does not contain the carbonyl carbon and probably only the ethyl group.

### 4.2.2. Ethionine

The hepatic carcinogen ethionine, which is an analogue of methionine, reacts preferentially with liver tRNA *in vivo* (Farber and Magee, 1960; Stekol *et al.*, 1960; Natori, 1963; Farber *et al.*, 1967*a*; Rosen, 1968; Craddock, 1969*a*). Rosen (1968) identified $N^2$-ethyl- (23%), 7-ethyl- (10%), and $N^2,N^2$-diethyl- (2%) guanine among the ethylated purines and ribose ethylation (2′-OH of pyrimidine nucleotides). Pegg (1972) reported the presence of ethyluracil (5%), ethylcytosine (6%), $N^2$-ethyl- (25%), $N^2,N^2$-diethyl- (7%), 7-ethyl- (13%), and 1-ethyl- (2%) guanine among the ethylated bases. Similar methyl substitutions at these positions are present in the normally methylated tRNA (Craddock *et al.*, 1968; Dunn, 1959, 1963; Smith and Dunn, 1959). Since large amounts of *S*-adenosylethionine accumulate in the liver of rats administered ethionine (Farber *et al.*, 1964; Smith and Salmon, 1965; Shull *et al.*, 1966), it has been suggested that the ethylation of RNA and proteins is catalyzed by the action of enzymes that normally utilize *S*-adenosyl-L-methionine as a donor of methyl groups (Stekol, 1965; Farber,

254

D. S. R. SARMA,
S. RAJALAKSHMI
AND
EMMANUEL
FARBER

1967; Hancock, 1968). However, Ortwerth and Novelli (1969) have suggested that the ethylation of RNA *in vivo* by ethionine is not mediated through the RNA methyltransferases that can utilize S-adenosylethionine as a donor instead of S-adenosylmethionine but via a new, as yet unknown mechanisms. It is interesting to note that ethionine does not give rise to 5-ethylcytosine, although this is the major methylated base in eukaryotic DNA. It appears that there are some methyltransferases which cannot or do not use S-adenosylethionine. Ethionine has been shown to produce specific modification in the pattern of isoaccepting species for RNA$^{leu}$ (Axel *et al.*, 1967).

### 4.3. Aromatic Amines and Amides

#### 4.3.1. 2-Acetylaminofluorene and Derivatives

The binding of 2-AAF to liver tRNA and RNA *in vivo* has been reported by several workers (Henshaw and Hiatt, 1963; Marroquin and Farber, 1965; E. C. Miller, and Miller, 1969; Kriek *et al.*, 1967; Agarwal and Weinstein, 1970). The carcinogen N-acetoxy-2-AAF has been shown under certain conditions to interact preferentially with certain nucleoside residues thought to be located in exposed regions of tRNA molecules (Weinstein *et al.*, 1971; Fujimura *et al.*, 1972). This carcinogen (or its derivatives) binds to the C-8 position of guanine in nucleic acid both *in vivo* and *in vitro* (Kriek *et al.*, 1967). It was observed that the N-acetyl group is retained in the binding to RNA (Irving *et al.*, 1967) but not to DNA (Kriek, 1968). The binding of N-acetyl-2-AAF to tRNA in general (Fink *et al.*, 1970; Agarwal and Weinstein, 1970) and to tRNA$^{fmet}$ in particular (Fujimura *et al.*, 1972) has been investigated in great detail. The modified guanine is located in the single-stranded region at position 20 of the dihydrouridine loop. The cloverleaf model for tRNA$^{fmet}$ (Dube *et al.*, 1968) predicts that 18 of the 25 guanine residues present in tRNA$^{fmet}$ are in base-paired regions. Five of the remaining are presumably buried in the three-dimensional teritary structure. Two of the remaining are present in the sequence G-G-Dh of the dihydrouridine loop and would be free to react with N-acetoxy-2-AAF.

The binding of 2-AAF and its derivatives to rRNA has been demonstrated by Kriek (1968), Irving *et al.* (1967, 1969), and Agarwal and Weinstein (1970). The preferential binding of this carcinogen to rRNA during carcinogenesis has been reported by Irving and Veazey (1972).

#### 4.3.2. 2-Naphthylamine

2-Naphthylamine has been shown to be weakly carcinogenic for livers of mice when administered orally (Bonser *et al.*, 1952). Clayson reported marked differences in susceptibility to induction of tumors among different strains (Clayson, 1962). Hughes and Pilczyk (1969/1970) showed the binding of 2-naphthylamine to liver nucleic acid. The level of radioactivity bound to RNA was higher in CBA mouse liver than in C57 mouse liver. At a dose of 114 nmoles/kg, the level of binding to liver fractions was 0.0031 $\mu$mole/g liver in CBA mice and 0.0011 $\mu$mole/g liver in C57 mice (Hughes and Pilczyk, 1969/1970).

### 4.3.3. Dimethylaminoazobenzene

255

INTERAC-
TIONS OF
CARCINOGENS
WITH NUCLEIC
ACIDS

The binding of DAB to ribosomal RNA has been demonstrated by Warwick and Roberts (1967). The maximum binding to RNA was 114 nmoles/g liver (Warwick and Roberts, 1967).

### 4.3.4. Ortho-aminoazotoluene

The binding of o-AAT to liver RNA as well as DNA has been shown by Lawson (1968). Binding to DNA reached a maximum 16 h after oral administration of the chemical, whereas the peak of RNA binding occurred at an earlier time.

## 4.4. Polycyclic Aromatic Hydrocarbons

The polycyclic hydrocarbons bind firmly through covalent linkages to RNA of mouse skin *in vivo* (Brookes and Lawley, 1964; Prodi *et al.*, 1970b; Goshman and Heidelberger, 1967) and that of various cells in culture (Kuroki *et al.*, 1971/1972). In mouse embryo cells in culture, the binding index to RNA is low for the noncarcinogen dibenz[a,c]anthracene and at least 10 times higher for the carcinogenic dibenz[a,l]anthracene (Duncan *et al.*, 1969; Kuroki and Heidelberger, 1971; Duncan and Brookes, 1972). In general, it has been found that there is a greater extent of binding to nucleic acids in normal and transformable cells in cultures than in transformed tumor cells (Kuroki *et al.*, 1971/1972). The exact nature of the interactions is not clear.

## 4.5. 4-Nitroquinoline-N-Oxide

The binding of 4NQO to tRNA has been demonstrated (Andoh *et al.*, 1971; Tada and Tada, 1971). The binding sites, however, appear to be limited for each of the nucleic acids studied, tRNA, rRNA, and DNA. The binding ratios amounted to 2.6, 5.3, and 3.3 molecules of carcinogen per 10,000 nucleotide units for tRNA, rRNA, and DNA respectively. One of the suggested sites of adduct formation is between the 4-amino nitrogen of 4NQO and the C-8 of purines.

# 5. Influence of Carcinogen–Nucleic Acid Interactions on the Structure, Synthesis, and Function of DNA and RNA

## 5.1. Alterations in DNA Structure

As has been pointed out earlier, several types of chemical and physical interactions between carcinogens and DNA and RNA occur. Several alkylating carcinogens interact with groups such as O-6 and $2\text{-}NH_2$ of guanine, N-1 and $6\text{-}NH_2$ of adenine, O-4 of thymine, and N-3 and $4\text{-}NH_2$ of cytosine that are involved in hydrogen bonding. Some carcinogenic metals may interact with the amino groups

D. S. R. SARMA,
S. RAJALAKSHMI
AND
EMMANUEL
FARBER

of the DNA bases (Furst and Haro, 1969) and may lead to local denaturation. Similarly, bifunctional alkylating agents crosslink the two strands of the DNA duplex, the same strand of DNA, or two DNA duplexes. Such an interaction may interfere with the strand separation and thus affect DNA replication and transcription. Intercalation in DNA alters the helical structure of DNA (Wagner, 1971). An interaction of this kind may induce conformational changes such as from the B-form of DNA to some other form closely related to either the A-form or the helical DNA (Yang and Samejima, 1969). Such a change in conformation would involve base tilting (Wagner, 1971). Bulky molecules such as 2-AAF and its derivatives interact at C-8 of guanine and cause local denaturation of the DNA (Nelson et al., 1971). Epstein et al. (1969/1970) also have observed regions of denaturation of DNA on electron microscopic examination of DNA from livers of animals fed a regimen containing 2-AAF.

Alkylated guanines in DNA are unstable and may result in the formation of depurinated sites. Endonuclease that acts at or near the depurinated sites has been reported in rat liver (Verly et al., 1973). Van Lancker and Tomura (1972) have reported an endonuclease from rat liver that acts on ultraviolet- or X-ray-irradiated and 2-AAF-treated DNA. Such an enzymatic attack leads to DNA with single-strand breaks.

In addition to the above mentioned physical alterations in DNA structure induced in vitro by chemical carcinogens, administration of carcinogens in vivo causes single- and/or double-strand breaks in DNA. Some of the carcinogenic metals such as $Ni^{2+}$ in excess quantities can depolymerize polynucleotides (Butzow and Eichhorn, 1965).

Although the exact alterations in the hepatic DNA of urethan-treated animals are not known, the isolated DNA is resistant to hydrolysis with deoxyribonuclease and snake venom phosphodiesterase (Williams and Nery, 1971). Certain intercalating agents interfere with the processing of HnRNA (see below).

One should not overlook the physicochemical environment around nucleic acids, especially DNA, in vivo. The state or states of DNA in nature are not clear. For example, DNA in the cell is in a highly compact form, more compact than in its protein-free form. Hence any alteration of the proteins attached to DNA may alter the physical state of DNA. Alteration of the physical state of DNA during replication has been suggested (Lerman, 1971).

Furthermore, several carcinogens influence the binding of chromatin proteins to DNA in vivo (Dijkstra and Weide, 1972). Such an altered protein/DNA ratio in chromatin in vivo might be expected to have profound influences on transcription and replication. 4NQO and derivatives have been suggested to cause breaks in "linker proteins" in DNA (Andoh and Ide, 1972; Ide and Andoh, 1972), thus resulting in DNA breaks.

### 5.2. Alterations in the Synthesis and Function of DNA and RNA

Alterations in the structure of DNA and RNA as a result of carcinogen–nucleic acid interactions could have profound imfluence on the synthesis as well as the function of nucleic acids such as in transcription and translation. Furthermore, such alterations may play an important role in mutagenesis and in the initiation of carcinogenesis. Because of limitations on space, the influence of interactions of carcinogens with nucleic acids on translation and on cellular enzyme regulation is not discussed in this chapter.

257

INTERAC-
TIONS OF
CARCINOGENS
WITH NUCLEIC
ACIDS

### 5.2.1. Alterations in DNA Synthesis and Cell Cycle

Many liver carcinogens in the first few weeks of administration induce interference with cell proliferation and/or DNA synthesis in response to partial hepatectomy (Laird and Barton, 1959, 1961; Laws, 1956; Maini and Stich, 1962; Vasiliev and Guelstein, 1963; Banerjee, 1965; Simard and Daoust, 1966; Simard *et al.*, 1968; Marquardt and Philips, 1970; Rabes *et al.*, 1970; Lawson and Pound, 1971/1972; Dawson, 1972; Farber *et al.*, 1973). Jenson *et al.* (1963) also observed decreased incorporation of thymidine into DNA following administration of 7,12-DMBA. Furthermore, administration of ethionine inhibits the *in vivo* incorporation of thymidine into liver DNA (Schneider *et al.*, 1960).

Although the exact mechanism is not known, many chemical carcinogens appear not only to inhibit DNA synthesis but also to influence the cell cycle. For example, in HeLa cells damaged with MNU or with mustard gas, the replication of DNA occurs normally in the first cell cycle. However, DNA synthesis is inhibited in the second cell cycle and the cells are killed subsequently (Roberts, 1972). This type of effect of carcinogens on DNA synthesis and cell cycle appears to depend on the nature of the carcinogen and the cell type used. For example, in Chinese hamster cells, although addition of MNU during $G_1$ phase of the cell cycle inhibits the DNA synthesis in the second cell cycle, addition of half mustard gas during the $G_1$ phase inhibits the DNA synthesis in the first cell cycle itself (Roberts, 1972).

### 5.2.2. Alterations in RNA Synthesis and Function

Although several studies have been reported on the influence of carcinogens on RNA synthesis, only very few have correlated these changes with carcinogen–DNA interaction. Many of the effects are probably due to either a direct or an indirect effect of the carcinogen on the enzymes involved in the synthesis of macromolecules or due to some interference with the available pools of nucleotides.

Administration of ethionine results in the inhibition of *in vivo* hepatic RNA synthesis (Villa-Trevino *et al.*, 1966) and a decreased hepatic ATP level (Shull, 1962; Villa-Trevino *et al.*, 1963). Smuckler and Koplitz (1969) have shown that decreased RNA synthesis in ethionine-treated rats cannot be entirely due to the decreased substrate (ATP) concentration. Isolated hepatic nuclei from ethionine-treated rats are less active in synthesizing RNA even in the presence of added ATP. Smuckler and Koplitz (1969) further report that RNA synthesis using liver chromatin from ethionine-treated animals appears unaffected and suggest that ethionine treatment may inhibit the RNA polymerase activity. More recently, it

D. S. R. SARMA,
S. RAJALAKSHMI
AND
EMMANUEL
FARBER

has been observed that the decreased RNA synthesis in whole nuclei of ethionine-treated rat liver can be accounted for in an inhibition of the partially purified RNA polymerases solubilized from these nuclei (J. L. Farber *et al.*, 1974*a*). Similar to this mode of inhibition of RNA syntheses by ethionine, the inhibition of RNA syntheses following the administration of DMN (see Magee and Barnes, 1967; Stewart and Magee, 1971) is also due to a decreased activity of RNA polymerases (J. L. Farber *et al.*, 1974*b*).

A single dose of MNU (100 mg/kg) reduces the labeling by $^{14}$C-orotate of rat kidney RNA by 40% and rat liver RNA by 15–20%, the maximum effect being reached by 1.5–3 h (Kleihues, 1972). The effect in kidney appears to be due to an inhibition of uptake of $^{14}$C-orotate. The decrease in labeling by $^{14}$C-orotate of liver RNA is less marked and results from interference by MNU with the synthesis of pyrimidine nucleotides. Sublethal doses of MNU, although they depress DNA and protein synthesis, do not affect RNA synthesis in rat liver and kidney (Kleihues, 1972).

MAM-acetate has been shown to inhibit hepatic RNA synthesis *in vivo* (Zedek *et al.*, 1970). Using isolated nuclei from MAM-acetate-treated animals, Grab *et al.* (1973) reported that DNA template activity for RNA synthesis was unimpaired *in vitro* while template activity of chromatin was slightly decreased. There was a reduction in the incorporation of UTP into RNA when the "aggregate" enzyme preparation was used as the source for the template and RNA polymerase. Circular dichroism analysis revealed changes in conformation of the protein component. Inhibition of RNA synthesis following urethan in mice was observed by Lawson and Pound (1971/1972) in intact and hepatectomized animals. The rate of synthesis of labeled RNA for only 1 h was studied. Since the RNA was not fractionated, it is not known whether all or only particular species of RNA synthesis were affected.

Aflatoxin B$_1$ inhibits the synthesis of nuclear and nucleolar RNA, an effect attributed to its complexing with DNA (Edwards and Wogan, 1970; Edwards *et al.*, 1971; Floyd *et al.*, 1968; Gelboin *et al.*, 1966; Lafarge and Frayssinet, 1970; Pong and Wogan, 1970; Wagner and Drews, 1970). An active form of aflatoxin B$_1$ may be involved since no effect is observed on addition of this compound to an *in vitro* RNA polymerase system.

Chronic feeding of 2-AAF to rats results in an inhibition of hepatic RNA synthesis (Troll *et al.*, 1968). The administration of a single dose of 2-AAF was found to produce a rapid inhibition of RNA synthesis in male mouse liver. Both rRNA and tRNA in the liver were equally affected. RNA synthesis recovered by 7 h, and hydroxyurea given within 3 h following the administration of 2-AAF was found to delay the recovery of RNA synthesis (Dawson, 1972). Also, acute administration of *N*-hydroxy-2-AAF to male rats inhibited RNA synthesis. The nuclei isolated from treated rats exhibited decreased activities of both the Mg$^{2+}$- and Mn$^{2+}$-activated polymerases *in vitro* (Zieve, 1972). Using *E. coli* polymerase, Zieve (1972) observed no decrease in template activity with chromatin and DNA. Zieve concluded that inhibition of RNA synthesis by *N*-hydroxy-2-AAF is due to inactivation of polymerase. A similar conclusion was reached with hepatic nuclei

of rats treated with N-hydroxy-2-AAF, using partially purified RNA polymerases
(J. L. Farber *et al.*, 1974*a*). However, Grunberger *et al.* (1973) reported that the
inhibition of RNA synthesis after the acute administration of N-hydroxy-2-AAF
to rats is predominantly on ribosomal RNA and is due to impairment of the
nucleolar DNA template function rather than to an effect on RNA polymerase
*per se.*

259

INTERAC-
TIONS OF
CARCINOGENS
WITH NUCLEIC
ACIDS

Treatment of DNA with N-acetoxy-2-AAF *in vitro* results in a drastic reduction
in the ability of the DNA to function as a template for RNA synthesis (Zieve, 1973).
This confirms the observations of Troll *et al.* (1968) that similar treatment of DNA
with N-acetoxy-2-AAF reduces the capacity of DNA to support RNA synthesis in
the presence of RNA polymerase.

The carcinogenic metal nickel carbonyl, when administered to animals, inhibits
both *in vivo* incorporation of radioactive orotate into rat liver RNA and DNA-
dependent RNA polymerase activity (Sunderman, 1968; Sunderman, and Estahani, 1968; Beach and Sunderman, 1970). In contrast to the inhibition of RNA
synthesis by several carcinogens, administration of azo dyes results in enhanced
RNA synthesis. Nuclei from rats treated with aminoazo dyes exhibit enhanced
RNA polymerase activity. However, when exogenous polymerase such as from *E.
coli* is used for the enzyme assay, no such difference is observed. The increased
activity is considered to be the result of enhanced binding of the enzyme to the
template (Wu and Smuckler, 1971). Some carcinogens such as 3,4-BP and 3-MC
induce arylhydrocarbon hydroxylase. The increased enzyme activity is concomitant with an increase in RNA synthesis of heterogeneous type (Wiebel *et al.*, 1972).
*In vivo*, 3-MC causes an increase in the synthesis of all RNA species. The nuclei
exhibit *in vitro* an enhanced RNA polymerase activity. This increase does not
occur in adrenalectomized or hypophysectomized animals (Younger *et al.*, 1972).
3,4-BP and 7,12-DMBA cause a decrease in the rate of RNA synthesis initially,
followed by an abrupt increase well above the normal rate. It is interesting to note
that the early inhibitory effect is not observed with the noncarcinogen 1,2-BP
(Alexandrov *et al.*, 1970).

Intercalating agents appear to interfere with the processing of rRNA. Ribosomal RNA formation in mammalian cells occurs through the formation of a high
molecular weight precursor with a sedimentation coefficient of 45S. The 45S RNA
is synthesized in the nucleolus and then processed progressively in several steps to
smaller pieces, leading finally to 28S and 18S rRNA (reviewed by Darnell, 1968).
Proflavin, ethidium bromide, and ellipticine, compounds known to bind to nucleic
acid helix by intercalation, were found to inhibit the processing of 45S nucleolar
ribosomal precursor RNA in L1210 lymphoma cells (Snyder *et al.*, 1971). The
effect appears to be prompt and is not secondary to inhibition of RNA or protein
synthesis. Brinker *et al.* (1973) have reported that the intercalating dyes proflavin,
ethidium bromide, and daunomycin decrease the rate of degradation of HnRNA.
Earlier it was shown that 3% of HnRNA of HeLa cells exist in a double-stranded
structure (Jelinek and Darnell, 1972). Studies suggest that portions of at least
some HnRNA molecules serve as cytoplasmic mRNA (Lindberg and Darnell,
1970; Edmonds *et al.*, 1971; Darnell *et al.*, 1971; Melli and Pemberton, 1972;

260

D. S. R. SARMA,
S. RAJALAKSHMI
AND
EMMANUEL
FARBER

Stevens and Williamson, 1972). The double-stranded regions are believed to be destroyed during the processing of HnRNA into mRNAs (Ryskov *et al.*, 1972). The demonstration, as described above, that intercalation affects this processing raises the interesting possibility that similar effects may be exerted by carcinogens as well.

The interaction of carcinogens with mRNA is not known, although it has been suggested that such an interaction may prevent the translation of mRNA (Venitt *et al.*, 1968). The presence of poly A at the end of HnRNA and mRNA has been demonstrated (Edmonds *et al.*, 1971; Darnell *et al.*, 1971). Whether these poly A stretches can be alkylated and if so what consequences will follow are not known at present.

Although several carcinogens have been shown to interact with tRNA, very little is known regarding the effects of such interactions, either qualitative or quantitative, on protein synthesis. The binding of an AAF derivative to a residue in the valine codon GUU, the lysine codon AAG, and poly $U_3G$ completely inactivates the ability of the triplets to stimulate the binding of their respective aminoacyl tRNA (Grunberger and Weinstein, 1971; Nelson *et al.*, 1971; Grunberger *et al.*, 1970). In cases where the polymers with modified G residues are bound to ribosomes, the polypeptide chain growth is blocked when translation encounters the modified residue. Modification of poly $U_3G$ by AAF also inhibits the template function in protein synthesis. However, no miscoding is observed.

As pointed out earlier, administration of several carcinogens such as ethionine produces specific changes in the patterns of isoaccepting species for tRNAs (Axel *et al.*, 1967). Similar changes are also reported in carcinogen-induced hepatomas. The exact mechanism(s) by which such changes are induced is not clear. However, these changes could have profound influences on the qualitative and quantitative nature of the proteins synthesized.    RNA has been implicated in the initiation of DNA synthesis (Sugino and Okazaki, 1973; Hirose *et al.*, 1973). Interaction of carcinogens with such RNA remains to be investigated.

## 6. Carcinogen–DNA Interaction and Carcinogenesis

Although the existence of many carcinogen-induced alterations in DNA is now well documented with various carcinogens, as outlined above, the relationship of any of these to carcinogenesis remains speculative and problematic. Since carcinogens in general interact with proteins and RNA as well as DNA, it is possible to formulate a hypothesis in which these major cell macromolecules are the key components (e.g., Pitot and Heidelberger, 1963; Weinstein, 1970). However, these have been discussed elsewhere (Farber, 1973; Sarma *et al.*, 1974), and it does not seem appropriate in such a short discussion of carcinogens and nucleic acids to consider them further. What does seem appropriate is a brief presentation of some quantitative and qualitative aspects of carcinogen–DNA interactions and the nature and extent of the repair of the resultant alterations of

DNA. This will be followed by a discussion (Section 7) of some of the highlights and major problem areas that seem pertinent at this time to any discussion of carcinogen–nucleic acid interactions and carcinogenesis.

261

INTERAC-
TIONS OF
CARCINOGENS
WITH NUCLEIC
ACIDS

## 6.1. Carcinogen–DNA Interaction: Quantitative Analysis

As seen in Table 2, the extent of interaction of the carcinogen or its derivative with nucleic acid is relatively quite small.

The binding of carcinogen to RNA or DNA has been shown to correlate well with carcinogenesis in the case of some compounds and not in that of others. The question of the correlation of specific altered bases with carcinogenesis induced by nitrosamines and nitrosamides has been described and detailed by Magee (1972). A good correlation in regard to the variation in species specificity with 2-AAF was shown by Marroquin and Farber (1965). Roberts and Warwick (1966) reported high correlation between carcinogenic activity of DAB and its initial level of binding to rRNA. Colburn and Boutwell (1968), while studying the binding of β-propiolactone to mouse skin RNA and DNA, found a correlation with initiation of carcinogenesis. In a study using β-propiolactone and several similar alkylating agents, they concluded that binding to DNA but not to RNA or to protein correlates with tumor-initiating potency (Colburn and Boutwell, 1968). Dingman and Sporn (1967) and Brookes and Lawley (1964) also expressed similar views on the basis of their studies with a series of aminoazo dyes and polycyclic aromatic hydrocarbons, respectively.

Using K-region epoxides and other derivatives of benz[a]anthracene and dibenz[a,l]anthracene and Chinese hamster cells, Kuroki et al. (1971/1972) concluded that a good correlation was not found between the binding of the compounds to DNA and their ability to induce malignant transformation. However, in a comparative study using several hydrocarbons, Brookes (1966) pointed out that binding of these agents to RNA or protein bore no correlation to the carcinogenic potency as expressed by Iball index (1939) whereas such correlation did exist for DNA binding.

Using several derivatives of DMBA and rat liver epithelial cell lines, Schwartz (1973) has found a good correlation between the reported carcinogenicity of the derivative and its capacity to inhibit the incorporation of tritiated thymidine into acid-precipitable material.

## 6.2. Carcinogen–DNA Interaction; Qualitative Analysis

The qualitative nature of the interaction of chemical carcinogen with DNA may be of importance in the initiation of carcinogenesis (Loveless, 1969). Interaction with the groups involved in the hydrogen bonding in DNA duplex, such as O-6 of guanine, has been implicated in the carcinogenic activity of DMN in the liver (O'Connor et al., 1973; Craddock, 1973; Lawley et al., 1973). Since the groups involved in the hydrogen bonding in DNA duplex are presumably more available

262

D. S. R. SARMA,
S. RAJALAKSHMI
AND
EMMANUEL
FARBER

TABLE 2

Extent of Interaction of a Few Chemical Carcinogens with Nucleic Acids in Vivo

| Carcinogen | Dose (μmoles/kg) and route of administration | Duration of action (h) | Species and tissue | Extent of interaction (moles nucleotides/moles carcinogen) | | References |
|---|---|---|---|---|---|---|
| | | | | DNA | RNA | |
| MMS | 1090, i.p. | 4 | Rat, liver | $3.0 \times 10^3$ | | Mulivor et al. (1974) |
| DMN | 67.5, i.p. | 4 | Rat, liver | $0.2 \times 10^3$ | | Abanobi et al. (1974) |
| DEN | 2700, i.p. | 24 | Rat, liver | — | $3.8 \times 10^2$ | Magee and Lee (1964) |
| DEN | 2000, i.p. | 24 | Rat, kidney | — | $2.4 \times 10^3$ | Magee and Lee (1964) |
| Ethionine | 26, i.p. | 120 | Rat, liver | $2.7 \times 10^7$ | $5.6 \times 10^{4a}$ | Farber et al. (1967b) |
| β-Propiolactone | 97, skin | 24 | Mouse, skin | $1.3 \times 10^5$ | $6.2 \times 10^4$ | Brookes (1966) |
| Urethan | 7500, i.p. | 10 | Mouse, liver | $9.3 \times 10^3$ | $10.5 \times 10^3$ | Lawson and Pound (1973b) |
| Mustard gas | 13.3, i.p. | 0.5 | Mouse, tumor | $2.0 \times 10^4$ | $2.5 \times 10^4$ | Brookes and Lawley (1960) |
| DAB | 675, i.p. | 16 | Rat, liver | $2.3 \times 10^5$ | $2.7 \times 10^4$ | Roberts and Warwick (1966) |
| 2-AAF | 2.8, i.p. | 24 | Rat, liver | $4.0 \times 10^5$ | $1.2 \times 10^{5a}$ | Farber (1968) |
| N-Hydroxy-2-AAF | 14–15, i.p. | 24 | Rat, liver | $1.1 \times 10^5$ | $1.0 \times 10^5$ | Kriek (1969) |
| | 14–15, i.p. | 24 | Rat, liver | $1.3 \times 10^5$ | $1.0 \times 10^5$ | Kriek (1969) |
| Benzo[a]pyrene | 16, skin | 42 | Mouse, skin | $2.9 \times 10^5$ | $6.2 \times 10^4$ | Brookes and Lawley (1964) |
| 7,12-DMBA | 5.9, skin | 22 | Mouse, skin | $2.4 \times 10^5$ | $4.8 \times 10^5$ | Brookes and Lawley (1964) |

[a] Largely soluble RNA.

during DNA replication, the effect of partial hepatectomy on the qualitative and quantitative aspects of interaction of carcinogen with DNA has been studied. Available evidence pertaining to this is confusing.

263
INTERAC-
TIONS OF
CARCINOGENS
WITH NUCLEIC
ACIDS

On one hand, with urethan (Lawson and Pound, 1971/1972) or DMN (Craddock, 1973; Capps *et al.*, 1973) no differences could be found in the liver between intact animals and animals with liver regeneration. Craddock (1973) also could find no altered patterns of reaction of DMN with bases in liver DNA during liver regeneration as compared to the intact liver. Witschi *et al.* (1971) reported that the rate of loss of DNA-bound 2-AAF in regenerating and nonregenerating livers was essentially the same. On the other hand, Marquardt *et al.* (1971, 1972) have found that 7,12-DMBA shows increase binding to liver DNA during liver regeneration.

In all of these studies, replicating DNA was never isolated. Bowden and Boutwell (1973), using BrdU, attempted to separate "newly made" DNA from the parental DNA. In these experiments, the binding of the carcinogen over a period of 8 h was studied. During this long period, not only the replicating BrdU-containing DNA but also the newly made double-strand DNA might interact with the carcinogen. This could mask any differences in the differential binding of the carcinogen to replicating and nonreplicating DNA. Yuspa and Bates (1970), using cultured fetal mouse skin cells, observed that 7,12-DMBA binds to both replicated and nonreplicated DNA. In all these studies, attention was focused on the quantitative, not the qualitative, aspects of the problem, such as whether a carcinogen binds to different regions of replicating DNA as compared to nonreplicating DNA. Zeiger *et al.* (1972) have reported that 7,12-DMBA binds to both bulk and satellite DNA of mouse epidermis. Stewart and Farber (1973*a*) and Ramanathan *et al.* (1974) recently observed the nonrandom distribution of bound DMN to the DNA of rat liver chromatin.

Furthermore, some carcinogens induce single-strand breaks in liver DNA and others induce double-strand breaks (Sarma *et al.*, 1974). It is of interest to note that the apparent double-strand breaks induced by some hepatocarcinogens, such as N-nitrosodihydrouracil and 3-hydroxyxanthine, are largely repaired within 24 h. The repair of single-strand breaks in liver DNA is variable and ranges from a few hours, such as with camptothecin, MMS, 4NQO, and 4OHAQO, to weeks, such as with the hepatocarcinogens DMN, DEN, MAM, and N-hydroxy- or N-acetoxy-2-AAF. The significance of these qualitative changes with respect to carcinogenicity remains to be elucidated. Fahmy and Fahmy (1972), using several carcinogens, have observed that mainly *r* genes and tRNA genes of *Drosophila* are mutated.

### 6.3. *Repair in Vivo of DNA Damage Induced by Chemical Carcinogens*

It is apparent from the above survey that the types of interactions between chemical carcinogens and nucleic acids (DNA and RNA) are varied, and that such interactions alter both the structure and the function of nucleic acids. In order to regain normal function, the cell has devised several sophisticated processes of repair of the altered nucleic acids. Virtually nothing is known about the repair of damaged RNA. However, several aspects of DNA repair have been investigated in

D. S. R. SARMA,
S. RAJALAKSHMI
AND
EMMANUEL
FARBER

bacteria and cells in culture following exposure to ultraviolet radiation (Hanawalt, 1972; Kaplan *et al.*, 1971; Kushner *et al.*, 1971; Setlow, 1968; Howard-Flanders, 1968; Strauss, 1968), ionizing radiation (Lett *et al.*, 1967, 1970; Oremerod and Lehmann, 1971; Painter, 1970), and alkylating agents (Alexander, 1969; Roberts *et al.*, 1971; Lieberman *et al.*, 1971; Coyle and Strauss, 1969/1970; Fox and Ayad, 1971) (see also *Cold Spring Harbor Symposia on Quantitative Biology*, Vol. 33, 1968; Beers *et al.*, 1972). Very little is known about the repair of DNA induced by chemical carcinogens in an intact animal (Goodman and Potter, 1972; Cox *et al.*, 1973*a*; Damjanov *et al.*, 1973; Sarma *et al.*, 1973*a*; Rajalakshmi and Sarma, 1973; Stewart *et al.*, 1973; Stewart and Farber, 1973*b*).

Ideally, the repair of any nonphysiological alterations of the DNA molecule should result in the complete restoration of the original structure and function.

The following is a brief survey of this presumably important area in chemical carcinogenesis. The subject has been reviewed in detail by Sarma *et al.* (1974).

### 6.3.1. Removal of DNA-Bound Carcinogen or Carcinogen Metabolites

The dynamics and the mechanisms by which the cell removes the bound carcinogen (or its metabolites) are not clearly understood. In the few experiments where studied, removal of the DNA-bound carcinogen often followed multiphase kinetics and in many instances a certain percentage of bound carcinogen persisted for long periods of time.

Chemically, the simplest form of interaction between carcinogen and DNA is alkylation of one or more of the components. A few studies have been reported concerning the turnover of methyl or ethyl groups from various carcinogens. As far as is known, elimination of such alkyl groups result in the loss of the alkylated bases from the DNA.

Different methylated bases in DNA have different half-lives. For example, in *E. coli*, *O*-6-methylguanine and *N*-3-methyladenine disappear more rapidly than does 7-methylguanine (Lawley and Orr, 1970). In rat liver, the half-life of 7-methylguanine is approximately 3 days (Margison *et al.*, 1973) while that of *O*-6-methylguanine is about 13 h (O'Connor *et al.*, 1973). It is noteworthy that the half-life *in vivo* of *N*-7-methylguanine is the same whether it is derived from MMS or from DMN (Margison *et al.*, 1973). Mulivor and Sarma (1973) observed that significant amounts of depurinated sites were still present at 7 days following the administration of DMN, even though the depurinatable sites were considerably decreased at this time compared to the number at 4 h. In general, it appears that the elimination of ethylated bases from DNA is slower than the elimination of their methylated homologues (Brookes and Lawley, 1961; Lawley and Brookes, 1963).

The removal of larger carcinogens from DNA appears to have more complex kinetics. Epstein *et al.* (1969/1970) have observed that the DNA isolated from a precancerous population of rat liver cells, weeks after the termination of exposure to the dietary carcinogen 2-AAF, exhibited (1) absorption in the range of 305–310 nm, suggestive of the presence of a derivative of 2-AAF, and (2) denaturation and distortion of fibers as observed by electron microscopy. Irving and Veazey (1969) reported that approximately 10% of the radioactivity bound to rat liver DNA within 12–16 h persisted for at least 4–8 wk following the administration of 2-AAF-9-$^{14}$C. The DNA-bound carcinogen decreased in two steps. Initially the label was lost with a half-life of 10 h. Subsequently the rate of loss was slower, with a half-life of 33 h (Szafarz and Weisburger, 1969). As pointed out earlier, there appear to be at least two types of reactions of $N$-acetoxy-2-AAF with guanine in DNA. The major component (80%), $N$-(deoxyguanosine-8-yl)-2-fluorenylacetamide, has a half-life of days, while the other components (20%) remain on the DNA for periods of up to 8 wk. Warwick and Roberts (1967) have observed that after a single administration of tritiated dimethylaminoazobenzene the specific concentration of DNA-bound radioactivity decreased to approximately one-half its initial value in the first 7 days and then remained approximately constant for 3 months. Similarly, 50% of the 7,12-DMBA bound to DNA in parenchymal cells of mammary gland at 16 h was present at 14 days and 31% at 42 days following the administration of tritiated 7,12-DMBA to rats (Janss *et al.*, 1972). Persistent binding of a metabolite(s) of 2-naphthylamine to mouse liver DNA was demonstrated following a single injection of tritiated 2-naphthylamine (Hughes and Pilczyk, 1969/1970).

265

INTERAC-
TIONS OF
CARCINOGENS
WITH NUCLEIC
ACIDS

### 6.3.2. Probable Steps in the Removal of Bound Carcinogen and Subsequent Repair of the Damaged DNA

The enzymes involved in the removal of DNA-bound carcinogen *in vivo* in mammalian systems remain a challenging area for fruitful study. Removal of the bound carcinogen or its metabolite often results in depurinated DNA (King and Phillips, 1970; Mulivor and Sarma, 1973; Margison *et al.*, 1973). The enzymology of the steps involved in filling up the gaps has been clarified in bacteria, and these offer a guide to the study in mammalian systems. The several probable steps in the removal of the bound carcinogen and subsequent repair of the damaged DNA are schematically presented in Fig. 4.

*a. Recognition and Incision.* The endonuclease that acts at or near the site of carcinogen–DNA interaction has to recognize the area of attack. The recent

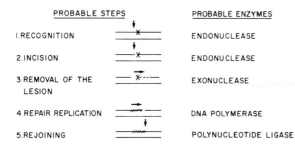

FIGURE 4. Probable steps in removal of bound carcinogen and repair of damaged DNA.

266

D. S. R. SARMA,
S. RAJALAKSHMI
AND
EMMANUEL
FARBER

observation of Van Lancker and Tomura (1972) that endonuclease purified from rat liver acts on DNA damaged either by ultraviolet light or by treatment with 2-AAF favors the possibility that the endonuclease may recognize the resultant distortion in the DNA following these treatments rather than a specific change, provided of course that the same enzyme is involved. Verly *et al.* (1973) and Verly and Paquette (1973) have reported the isolation and purification of an endonuclease from rat liver which preferentially acts on depurinated DNA. It is not known whether these two endonucleases are the same. Verly *et al.* (1973) and Verly and Paquette (1973) have claimed that their endonuclease acts at the depurinated sites. In this context, it is of importance to mention the recent observations reported by Hadi *et al.* (1973) that *E. coli* endonuclease II, which prefers alkylated DNA, acts on normal DNA as well if the assay is run at 45°C. The enzyme does not act on normal DNA at 37°C, suggesting the possibility that the enzyme recognizes local sites of denaturation that would be likely to occur at regions high in A-T at the higher temperature. The enzyme has no effect on alkylated poly dG:dC (Hadi *et al.*, 1973). Bacchetti *et al.* (1972) and Brent (1972, 1973) have studied an endonuclease in HeLa cells and in fibroblasts from normal humans and from patients with xeroderma pigmentosum which acts on ultraviolet-irradiated or γ-irradiated DNA. Whether any of these endonucleases would also recognize or act on DNA altered by chemical carcinogens is not known. The action of an endonuclease on damaged DNA should result in strand breaks.

*b. Induction of DNA Strand Breaks In Vivo by Chemical Carcinogens.* Work carried out in our laboratory (Cox *et al.*, 1973a,b; Sarma *et al.*, 1973a; Damjanov *et al.*, 1973; Stewart *et al.*, 1973; Stewart and Farber, 1973b; Rajalakshmi and Sarma, 1973) during the past 2 yr and that by Goodman and Potter (1971, 1972) indicate that administration of carcinogens to rats or mice induces hepatic DNA strand breaks *in vivo*. A wide variety of carcinogens have been tested, including methylating and ethylating nitrosamines and nitrosamides, aromatic amines,

TABLE 3
*List of Some Chemical Carcinogens That Induce Strand Breaks in Liver DNA in Vivo*

| Single-strand breaks repaired within 4–72 h | Single-strand breaks repaired slowly (72–336 h or more) |
| --- | --- |
| Methyl methanesulfonate | N-Hydroxy-2-acetylaminofluorene[a] |
| N-Methyl-N′-nitro-N-nitrosoguanidine | N-Acetoxy-2-acetylaminofluorene[a] |
| N-Nitroso-N-methylurethan | N-Nitrosopiperidine |
| 4-Nitroquinoline-N-oxide | N,N-Dinitrosopiperazine |
| 4-Hydroxyaminoquinoline-N-oxide | N-Nitrosomorpholine[a] |
| Camptothecin | N-Nitrosodimethylamine |
| Bleomycin[b] | Methylazoxymethanol acetate |
| Nitrosodihydrouracil[a] | N-Nitrosodiethylamine |
| 3-Hydroxyxanthine[a] | 2-Acetylaminofluorene |
| Hycanthone methanesulfonate[a] | |

[a] These agents in addition induce double-strand breaks.
[b] R. Cox (personal communication).

267

INTERAC-
TIONS OF
CARCINOGENS
WITH NUCLEIC
ACIDS

TABLE 4

*Hepatotoxic Compounds Inducing No Obvious Strand Breaks in Liver DNA*

| | |
|---|---|
| Cycloheximide | α-Amanitin |
| Morpholine | Isopentenyladenosine |
| Piperidine | Nitrosocitrulline |
| Piperazine | Xanthine |
| Cyclophosphamide | Sodium methanesulfonate |
| Galactosamine | Furosemide[a] |
| | Acetaminophen[a] |

[a] Parodi and Sarma (1973).

cyclic nitroso compounds, azodyes, and intercalating agents (Table 3). Although highly diverse as to structure and reactivity with DNA, they all induce single-strand breaks in liver DNA (fragmentation of the DNA seen in alkaline sucrose gradients). In addition, a few hepatocarcinogens induce double-strand breaks in liver DNA (fragmentation seen in neutral as well as alkaline sucrose gradients; Sarma *et al.*, 1973a; Stewart *et al.*, 1973). Two active hepatic carcinogens, DMN and 2-AAF, each fed under conditions that lead to liver cancer, induce liver DNA breaks (Abanobi and Sarma, 1973; Michael *et al.*, 1973). It is of interest that fragmentation of the liver DNA is progressive up to 5 wk of feeding with each carcinogen. Further feeding of DMN, even up to 14 or 15 wk, does not lead to any further fragmentation of the liver DNA. Thus there appears to be a limit to this type of damage beyond which no further significant effect is seen. It is noteworthy that several different hepatotoxic agents which are not carcinogens induce no apparent single- or double-strand breaks in liver DNA except after cell death (Table 4). Similar strand breaks induced by carcinogens have also been found in lung (Cox, personal communication), brain, kidney (Abanobi *et al.*, 1973), and intestine (Kanagalingam and Balis, personal communication). An apparently similar phenomenon has been found in certain cells in the cerebellum following X- and γ-irradiation of dogs (Wheeler and Lett, 1972). DNA breaks have been demonstrated in several different cell cultures (Andoh and Ide, 1972; Laishes and Stich, 1973; Trosko *et al.*, 1973), including cells obtained from rat liver (Michael and Williams, personal communication), following treatment with chemical carcinogens.

A good correlation appears to exist among the degree of strand break, extent of interaction of the carcinogen with DNA, and dose of the carcinogen administered. For example, there is a linear relation between the dose of administered DMN and the amount of methylated purines formed in liver DNA in the dosage range 1–30 mg/kg (Craddock, 1969b). With DNA strand breaks, there is a similar relationship in the dosage range up to 10 mg/kg. However, the strand damage reaches a maximum at this dose, while the degree of methylation of DNA appears to increase progressively with increasing dosage well beyond the 10 mg/kg dose. Thus the correlation breaks down in the higher range. Again, with DMN, one can inhibit metabolic activation by the administration of aminoacetonitrile (AAN)

268

D. S. R. SARMA,
S. RAJALAKSHMI
AND
EMMANUEL
FARBER

(Fiume *et al.*, 1970). AAN (100 mg/kg body weight), given 30 min prior to the administration of DMN (10 mg/kg body weight), inhibited almost completely the alkylation of liver RNA and DNA at 3 h following the administration of DMN. However, at 20 h following the administration of DMN, the alkylation of liver DNA and RNA reached essentially the control level (Hadjiolov, personal communication). Under similar experimental conditions, AAN markedly inhibited the liver DNA strand breaks induced by DMN at 4 h following the administration of DMN. However, by 20 h the degree of fragmentation of liver DNA was the same in both the control animals that received DMN alone and the group that received DMN plus AAN (Sarma *et al.*, 1973*b*). Therefore, in a limited number of experiments, a correlation does exist between the degree of methylation of liver DNA by DMN and the extent of strand breakage at the lower dosage range but not at the higher. The possible correlation between the type and degree of chemical interaction with DNA and strand breaks remains an important area for further study.

*c. Gap Filling.* By use of various types of cells in culture, gap filling by "unscheduled DNA synthesis" or "repair replication" has been demonstrated following treatment with chemical carcinogens (Setlow and Regan, 1972; Stich *et al.*, 1972; Roberts *et al.*, 1971; Fox and Ayad, 1971; Lieberman *et al.*, 1971; Lieberman and Forbes, 1973). Although difficulty has been experienced in observing incorporation of nucleotides except those of thymine, it is now possible to incorporate other nucleotides in some systems (Hennings, 1973; Lieberman and Poirier, 1973).

*d. Rejoining.* Rejoining, the final union of the broken strands, is presumably brought about by polynucleotide ligase, which in eukaryotic cells is an ATP-requiring enzyme. At least one ligase has been isolated from mammalian tissues including regenerating liver and hepatomas (Lindahl and Edelman, 1968; Tsukada and Ichimura, 1971; Tsukada *et al.*, 1972; Pedralinoy *et al.*, 1973).

At present, it is very difficult to correlate any particular type of carcinogen–DNA interaction with carcinogenicity. However, a working model can be developed for consideration based on the following few facts: (1) persistence of DNA-bound carcinogens or their metabolites for long periods of time, (2) persistence of depurinated sites formed as a result of loss of alkyl-guanines in liver DNA induced by several hepatocarcinogens, (3) induction of double-strand breaks in liver DNA by some hepatic carcinogens (4) occurrence of replication *in vivo* of DNA damaged with either DMN or *N*-acetoxy-2-AAF, and (5) elongation of newly made DNA strands in the presence of persisting damage in the parental DNA (Rajalakshmi and Farber, 1973; Zahner *et al.*, 1973). The last phenomenon is referred to as "bypass synthesis" and is presumably similar to that reported by Rupp and Howard-Flanders (1968) in an excision-deficient mutant of *E. coli* and by Lehmann (1972) in mouse L5178Y cells.

Replication of DNA with any damage may be deleterious. A possible miscoding lesion in the parental strand such as alkylation at O-6 and even N-7 of guanine or

269

INTERAC-
TIONS OF
CARCINOGENS
WITH NUCLEIC
ACIDS

| LESIONS IN THE PARENTAL STRAND | LESIONS IN THE NEWLY MADE STRAND |
|---|---|
| ALKYLATED BASES SUCH AS N-7-METHYLGUANINE; O-6-METHYLGUANINE OR O-4-METHYLTHYMINE | INCORRECT BASE PAIRING |
| BOUND CARCINOGEN (COVALENTLY LINKED; INTERCALATED OR CROSS LINKED) | GAP OPPOSITE TO THE DAMAGE |
| DEPURINATED REGION | GAP OPPOSITE TO THE DAMAGE |
| SINGLE STRAND BREAK OR GAP | DOUBLE STRAND BREAK |

FIGURE 5. Possible consequences of replication of damaged DNA.

O-4 of thymine may introduce errors in the newly made strand during strand replication. The noncoding lesions such as depurinated regions, single-strand breaks, or gaps are likely to become either double-strand breaks or gaps in the replicated DNA. Such damage in the newly made strand may be lethal if it is not repaired. However, the repair of these damages may be equally dangerous if nucleotides are incorporated in the absence of any available information from the complementary strand (see Fig. 5). Thus it appears that the replication of DNA with unrepaired lesions offers a mechanism by which the original damage caused by the carcinogen to the parental strand is permanently imprinted in the daughter cell. Such a permanent fixation of damage may play an important role in the initiation of carcinogenesis.

## 7. Perspectives and Conclusions

It is evident from this brief survey that any conclusions implicating altered nucleic acids in any proposed mechanism of chemical carcinogenesis must remain essentially speculative. Although there is an increasing body of information concerning various aspects of the interactions of carcinogens with nucleic acids, this factual base remains insufficient to permit anything but conjecture about how these interactions are related to carcinogenesis. Despite this inability to reach definitive conclusions, it has now become possible to begin to pinpoint areas of study that seem relevant to one or more aspects of the carcinogenic process.

   In view of the short period of exposure to a chemical carcinogen that is often sufficient to trigger the carcinogenic process, it would seem that any relevant alterations in RNA or DNA would relate to initiation. Although variations in the control of gene action almost certainly play a major role in the new patterns of cell behavior seen during the cellular evolution to cancer, the primary effects of carcinogens can be most easily related to the initial events at this time. This is most easily viewed in terms of a permanent alteration in information content, either structural or regulatory or both.

270

D. S. R. SARMA,
S. RAJALAKSHMI
AND
EMMANUEL
FARBER

What types of alterations in RNA or DNA induced by chemicals could lead to a permanent change, and how can such alterations be modified or nullified by repair processes? With respect to RNA, some of the possibilities are as follows: (1) The induction of a change in an RNA substrate for *reverse transcriptase,* resulting in a permanent transfer of misinformation to a DNA product. (2) The induction of a change in mRNA or tRNA leading to new proteins with different specificities. This could lead, in turn, to alterations either in the replication of those mac-romolecules (DNA, RNA) concerned with information storage or in the action of proteins involved in the control of DNA replication or transcription, e.g., "repressors." The repair of carcinogen-altered RNA has been essentially ignored, and yet it could be important in the study of the metabolic functions of RNA, especially as they relate to carcinogenesis.

With respect to DNA, there are many possibilities and uncertainties that relate to carcinogenesis: (1) Are interactions between carcinogens and DNA random or nonrandom? Since the location of transcribed DNA seems to vary greatly as a function of the physiological state and needs of a cell, does a carcinogen have any predilection for "available" or "unavailable" DNA? Such a selectivity could help explain the role of physiological state in the initiation of carcinogenesis. (2) What are the critical *quantitative* aspects of carcinogen–DNA interactions? One has the impression that chemical specificity of interaction decreases with increasing degrees of interaction. Thus does one pass from nonrandom to random interac-tions with increasing dosage of carcinogens? These considerations might well apply equally to various RNA's as well as DNA. (3) What are the most valid ways to measure the repair phenomena in different types of cells *in vivo* and *in vitro*? All *in vitro* culture systems involve, of necessity, cells actively proliferating or geared for active proliferation. Yet cancer *in vivo* affects many cell systems which are nonproliferating, e.g., liver, kidney, pancreas, and salivary gland. Are these differences crucial or trivial? Because of these differences, or others, can one induce a permanent change in DNA or RNA more easily in cells *in vitro* than *in vivo*, and, as a possible corollary, is repair more critical in many systems *in vivo*? What are the best indices of repair of DNA—unscheduled DNA synthesis, rejoining of broken strands, etc.? For example, in one study, by measuring unscheduled DNA synthesis in human lymphocytes exposed to the carcinogen 7-bromomethylbenzanthracene, it was found that much of the carcinogen re-mained bound to the DNA at a time when "repair" was essentially "complete" (Lieberman and Dipple, 1972). Is this a common phenomenon, and, if so, how reliable can unscheduled DNA synthesis be as a measure of DNA repair? (4) Can the role of cell proliferation in initiation be accounted for entirely as a means of converting transitory damage to DNA to permanent damage through DNA replication, or are there other considerations that are important, e.g., different receptivity of different segments of DNA or different species of RNA to interaction with carcinogen? These considerations are a few of many that seem to have possible importance in understanding any relationship of carcinogen–nucleic acid interactions to carcinogenesis. It is hoped that the clarification of these and other problem areas will lead to progressively more valid insight into the processes by which chemicals trigger the evolution to malignant neoplasia.

## ACKNOWLEDGMENTS

The authors' research included in this review was supported in part by grants from the American Cancer Society (BC-7P and Institutional Grant) and the National Institutes of Health (CA-12218, CA-12227, and AM-14882).

We wish to thank Miss Margie Tartaglione and Miss Terri Marciniszyn for their efficient secretarial assistance and patience during the preparation of this manuscript.

271

INTERAC-
TIONS OF
CARCINOGENS
WITH NUCLEIC
ACIDS

## 8. References

ABANOBI, S. E., AND SARMA, D. S. R., 1973, Unpublished observations.

ABANOBI, S. E., COX, R., DAMJANOV, I., AND SARMA, D. S. R., 1973, Unpublished observations.

ABANOBI, S. E., MULIVOR, R. A., AND SARMA, D. S. R., 1974, Unpublished observations.

AGARWAL, M. K., AND WEINSTEIN, I. B., 1970, Modifications of ribonucleic acid by chemical carcinogens. II. *In vivo* reaction of *N*-2-acetylaminofluorene with rat liver ribonucleic acid, *Biochemistry* **9**:503.

ALEXANDER, P., 1952, Interference with the formation of a nucleoprotein complex by radiomimetic compounds, *Nature (Lond.)* **169**:226.

ALEXANDER, P., 1969, Comparison of the mode of action by which some alkylating agents and ionizing radiations kill mammalian cells, *Ann. N.Y. Acad. Sci.* **163**:652.

ALEXANDROV, K., VENDRELY, C., AND VENDRELY, R., 1970, A comparative study of the action of carcinogenic substances on the RNA synthesis in mouse skin, *Cancer Res.* **30**:1192.

ANDERSON, R. A., ENOMOTO, M., MILLER, E. C., AND MILLER, J. A., 1964, Carcinogenesis and inhibition of the Walker 256 tumor in the rat by trans-4-acetylaminostilbene its *N*-hydroxy metabolite and related compounds, *Cancer Res.* **24**:128.

ANDOH, T., AND IDE, T., 1972, Strand scission and rejoining of DNA in cultured mammalian cells induced by 4-nitroquinoline 1-oxide, *Cancer Res.* **32**:1230.

ANDOH, T., KATO, K., TAKAOKA, T., AND KATSUTA, H., 1971, Carcinogenesis in tissue culture. XIII. Binding of 4-nitroquinoline-1-oxide-$^3$H to nucleic acids and proteins of L-P3 and JTC 25-P3 cells, *Int. J. Cancer* **7**:455.

ARAKI, M., KAWAZOE, Y., AND NAGATA, C., 1969, Chemical carcinogens. IX. Homolytic degradation of O,O-diacetyl-4-hydroxyaminoquinoline 1-oxide (1-acetoxy-4-acetyloxyamino-1, 4-dihydro-quinoline), *Chem. Pharm. Bull. (Tokyo)* **17**:1344.

ARCOS, J. C., AND ARGUS, M. F., 1968, Molecular geometry and carcinogenic activity of aromatic compounds: New perspectives, *Advan. Cancer Res.* **11**:305.

AXEL, R., WEINSTEIN, I. B., AND FARBER, E., 1967, Patterns of transfer RNA in normal rat liver during hepatic carcinogenesis, *Proc. Natl. Acad. Sci.* **58**:1255.

BACCHETTI, S., VAN DER PLAS, A., AND VELDHUISEN, G., 1972, A UV-specific endonucleolytic activity present in human cell, *Biochem. Biophys. Res. Commun.* **48**:662.

BANERJEE, M. R., 1965, Mitotic blockage of G2 after partial hepatectomy during 4-dimethyl-aminoazobenzene hepatocarcinogenesis, *J. Natl. Cancer Inst.* **35**:585.

BANNON, P., AND VERLY, W., 1972, Alkylation of phosphates and stability of phosphate triesters in DNA, *Europ. J. Biochem.* **31**:103.

BARTSCH, H., MILLER, J. A., AND MILLER, E. C., 1972, Activation of carcinogenic aromatic hydroxylamines by enzymatic o-acetylation, *Proc. Am. Assoc. Cancer Res.* **13**:12.

BEACH, D. J., AND SUNDERMAN, F. W., JR., 1970 Nickel carbonyl inhibition of RNA synthesis by a chromatin–RNA polymerase complex from hepatic nuclei, *Cancer Res.* **30**:48.

272

D. S. R. SARMA,
S. RAJALAKSHMI
AND
EMMANUEL
FARBER

BEERS, R. F., JR., HERRIOTT, R. M., AND TILGHMAN, R. C., eds., 1972, *Molecular and Cellular Repair Processes*, Johns Hopkins University Press, Baltimore.

BENFEY, O. T., 1970, *Introduction to Organic Reaction Mechanisms*, McGraw-Hill, New York.

BERENBLUM, I., AND TRAININ, N., 1960, Possible two-stage mechanism in experimental leukemogenesis, *Science* **132**:40.

BERGMANN, F., 1942, On the mechanism of tumor production by chemical agents, *Cancer Res.* **2**:660.

BLACK, H. S., AND JIRGENSONS, B., 1967, Interactions of aflatoxin with histones and DNA, *Plant Physiol.* **42**:731.

BLACKBURN, G. M., FENWICK, R. G., AND THOMPSON, M. W., 1972, Structure of the thymine-3,4-benzopyrene photoproduct, *Tetrahedron Letters* **7**:589.

BONSER, G. M., CLAYSON, D. B., TULL, J. W., AND PYRAH, L. N., 1952, The carcinogenic properties of 2-amino-1-naphthal hydrochloride and its parent amine 2-naphthylamine, *Brit. J. Cancer* **6**:412.

BORCHERT, P., WISLOCKI, P. G., MILLER, J. A., AND MILLER, E. C., 1973, The metabolism of the naturally occurring hepatocarcinogen safrole to 1'-acetoxy safrole and the electrophilic reactivity of 1'-acetoxy-safrole, *Cancer Res.* **33**:575.

BOUTWELL, R. K., COLBURN, N. H., AND MUCKERMAN, C. C., 1969, *In vivo* reactions of β-propiolactone, *Ann. N.Y. Acad. Sci.* **163**:751.

BOWDEN, G. T., AND BOUTWELL, R. K., 1973, The binding of 7,12-dimethylbenz(*a*)anthracene (DMBA) to replicating and non-replicating DNA *in vivo*, *Proc. Am. Assoc. Cancer Res.* **14**:28.

BOYLAND, E., 1969, The biochemistry of aromatic hydrocarbons, amines and urethane, in: *Physicochemical Mechanisms of Carcinogenesis* (E. D. Bergmann and B. Pullman, eds.), p. 25, Vol. 1 of *The Jerusalem Symposia on Quantum Chemistry and Biochemistry*, Israel Academy of Sciences and Humanities, Jerusalem.

BOYLAND, E., AND GREEN, B., 1962, The interaction of polycyclic hydrocarbons and nucleic acids, *Brit. J. Cancer* **16**:507.

BOYLAND, E., AND NERY, R., 1965, The metabolism of urethane and related compounds, *Biochem. J.* **94**:198.

BOYLAND, E., AND SIMS, P., 1965, Metabolism of polycyclic compounds: The metabolism of 7,12-dimethylbenz(*a*)anthracene by rat liver homogenates, *Biochem. J.* **95**:780.

BOYLAND, E., AND WILLIAMS, K., 1969, Reaction of urethane with nucleic acids *in vivo*, *Biochem. J.* **111**:121.

BRENT, T. P., 1972, Repair enzyme suggested by mammalian endonuclease activity specific for ultraviolet-irradiated DNA, *Nature New Biol.* **239**:172.

BRENT, T. P., 1973, A human endonuclease activity for gamma-irradiated DNA, *Biophys. J.* **13**:401.

BRINKER, J. M., MADORE, A. P., AND BELLO, L. J., 1973, Stabilization of heterogeneous nuclear RNA by intercalating drugs, *Biochem. Biophys. Res. Commun.* **52**:928.

BROOKES, P., 1966, Quantitative aspects of the reaction of some carcinogens with nucleic acids and the possible significance of such reactions in the process of carcinogenesis, *Cancer Res.* **26**:1994.

BROOKES, P., 1971, On the interaction of carcinogens with DNA, *Biochem. Pharmacol.* **20**:999.

BROOKES, P., AND LAWLEY, P. D., 1960, The reaction of mustard gas with nucleic acids *in vitro* and *in vivo*, *Biochem. J.* **77**:478.

BROOKES, P., AND LAWLEY, P. D., 1961, The reaction of mono- and di-functional alkylating agents with nucleic acids, *Biochem. J.* **80**:496.

BROOKES, P., AND LAWLEY, P. D., 1964, Evidence for the binding of polynuclear aromatic hydrocarbons to the nucleic acids of mouse skin: Relation between carcinogenic power of hydrocarbons and their binding to deoxyribonucleic acid, *Nature (Lond.)* **202**:781.

BUTZOW, J. J., AND EICHHORN, G. L., 1965, IV. Degradation of polyribonucleotides by zinc and other divalent metal ions, *Biopolymers* **3**:95.

CAPPS, M. J., O'CONNOR, P. J., AND CRAIG, A. W., 1973, The influence of liver regeneration on the stability of 7-methylguanine in rat liver DNA after treatment with *N,N*-dimethylnitrosamine, *Biochim. Biophys. Acta* **331**:33.

CLAYSON, D. B., 1962, *Chemical Carcinogenesis*, 1st ed., p. 208, Churchill, London.

CLIFFORD, J. I., AND REES, K. R., 1967, The action of aflatoxin B$_1$ on the rat liver, *Biochem. J.* **102**:65.

COHEN, S. M., ALTER, A., AND BRYAN, G. T., 1973, Distribution of radioactivity and metabolism of formic acid 2-4-(5-nitro-2-furyl)-2-$^{14}$C-2-thiazolyl hydrazide following oral administration to rats and mice, *Cancer Res.* **33**:2802.

COLBURN, N. H., AND BOUTWELL, R. K., 1968, The *in vivo* binding of β-propiolactone to mouse skin DNA, RNA and protein, *Cancer Res.* **28**:642.

273

INTERAC-
TIONS OF
CARCINOGENS
WITH NUCLEIC
ACIDS

COOKSON, M. J., SIMS, P., AND GROVER, P. L., 1971, Mutagenicity of epoxides of polycyclic hydrocarbons correlates with carcinogenicity of parent hydrocarbons, *Nature New Biol.* **234**:186.

COX, R., AND FARBER, E., 1972 Ethylation of DNA virsus: Cancer induction with ethionine, *Proc. Am. Assoc. Cancer Res.* **13**:97.

COX, R., DAMJANOV, I., ABANOBI, S., AND SARMA, D. S. R., 1973a, A method for measuring DNA damage and repair in the liver *in vivo*, *Cancer Res.* **33**:2114.

COX, R., DAMJANOV, I., AND IRVING, C. C., 1973b, Damage and repair of the hepatic DNA by ethylating carcinogens, *Proc. Am. Assoc. Cancer Res.* **14**:28.

COYLE, M. B., AND STRAUSS, B. S., 1969/1970, Characteristics of DNA synthesized by methyl methanesulfonate–treated HEp-2 cells, *Chem.-Biol. Interact.* **1**:89.

CRADDOCK, V. M., 1969a Methylation of t-RNA and ribosomal RNA in rat liver in the intact animal and the effect of carcinogens, *Biochim. Biophys. Acta* **195**:351.

CRADDOCK, V. M., 1969b, Stability of deoxyribonucleic acid methylated in the intact animal by administration of dimethylnitrosamine: Rate of breakdown *in vivo* and *in vitro* at different dosages, *Biochem. J.* **111**:497.

CRADDOCK, V. M., 1973, The pattern of methylated purines formed in DNA of intact and regenerating liver of rats treated with the carcinogen dimethylnitrosamine, *Biochim. Biophys. Acta* **312**:202.

CRADDOCK, V. M., VILLA-TREVINO, S., AND MAGEE, P. N., 1968, Occurrence of 7-methylguanine in nucleic acids of rat liver, *Biochem. J.* **107**:179.

DAMJANOV, I., COX, R., SARMA, D. S. R., AND FARBER, E., 1973, Patterns of damage and repair of liver DNA induced by carcinogenic methylating agents *in vivo*, *Cancer Res.* **33**:2122.

DANN, O., AND MOLLER, E. F., 1947, Bacteriostatically active nitro compounds of thiophene and furan, *Chem. Ber.* **80**:23.

DARNELL, J. E., 1968, Ribonucleic acids from animal cells, *Bacteriol. Rev.* **32**:262.

DARNELL, J. E., WALL, R., AND TUSHINSKI, R. J., 1971, An adenylic acid-rich sequence in messenger RNA of HeLa cells and its possible relationship to reiterated sites in DNA, *Proc. Natl. Acad. Sci.* **68**:1321.

DAWSON, K. M., 1972, Time course of the effects of AAF on mouse liver nucleic acid synthesis and its modification by inhibitors, *Chem.-Biol. Interact.* **5**:153.

DEBAUN, J. R., MILLER, E. C., AND MILLER, J. A., 1970, N-Hydroxy-2-acetylaminofluorene sulfotransferase: Its probable role in carcinogenesis and in protein (methion-S-yl) binding in rat liver, *Cancer Res.* **30**:577.

DICKENS, F., AND JONES, H. E. H., 1963, Further studies on the carcinogenic and growth-inhibitory activity of lactones and related substances, *Brit. J. Cancer* **17**:100.

DIJKSTRA, J., AND WEIDE, S. S., 1972, Changes in chromatin caused by aminoazo compounds, *Exp. Cell Res.* **72**:345.

DINGMAN, C. W., AND SPORN, M. B., 1967, The binding of metabolites of aminoazo dyes to rat liver DNA *in vivo*, *Cancer Res.* **27**:938.

DIPAOLO, J., 1960, Experimental evaluation of actinomycin D, *Ann. N.Y. Acad. Sci.* **89**:408.

DIPPLE, A., 1972, Model studies for azo dye carcinogenesis, *J. Chem. Soc. Perkin Trans.* **1**:447.

DIPPLE, A., AND SLADE, T. A., 1970, Structure and activity in chemical carcinogenesis: Reactivity and carcinogenicity of 7-bromomethylbenz(a)anthracene and 7-bromomethyl-12-methylbenz(a)anthracene, *Europ. J. Cancer* **6**:417.

DIPPLE, A., AND SLADE, T. A., 1971, Structure and activity in chemical carcinogenesis: Studies of variously substituted 7-bromomethylbenz(a)anthracenes, *Europ. J. Cancer* **7**:473.

DIPPLE, A., LAWLEY, P. D., AND BROOKES, P., 1968, Theory of tumor initiation by chemical carcinogens, dependence of activity on structure of ultimate carcinogen, *Europ. J. Cancer* **4**:493.

DIPPLE, A., BROOKES, P., MACKINTOSH, D. S., AND RAYMAN, M. P., 1971, Reaction of 7-bromomethylbenz(a)anthracene with nucleic acids, polynucleotides and nucleosides, *Biochemistry* **10**:4323.

DODD, M. E., AND STILLMAN, W. D., 1944, The *in vivo* bacteriostatic action of some simple furan derivatives, *J. Pharmacol. Exp. Ther.* **82**:11.

DRUCKREY, H., 1970, Production of colonic carcinomas by 1,2-dialkylhydrazines and azoxyalkanes in: *Carcinoma of the Colon and Antecedent Epithelium* (W. J. Burdette, ed.), p. 267, Thomas, Springfield, Ill.

DRUCKREY, H., 1972, Organospecific carcinogenesis in the digestive tract, in: *Proceedings of the Second International Symposium of the Princess Takamatsu Cancer Research Fund* (W. Nakahara, S. Takayoma, T. Sugimura, and S. Odashima, eds.), p. 73, University Park Press, Baltimore.

274

D. S. R. SARMA,
S. RAJALAKSHMI
AND
EMMANUEL
FARBER

DRUCKREY, H., PREUSSMAN, R., IVANKONIE, S., AND SCHMAHL, S., 1967a, Organotropic carcinogenic effects of 65 different N-nitroso compounds on BD-rats, Z. Krebsforsch. **69:**103.

DRUCKREY, H., PRESSMANN, R., MATZKUS, F., AND IVANKONIE, S., 1967b, Selektive Erzeugung von Darmkrebs bei Ratten durch 1,2-Dimethylhydrazin, Naturwissenschaften **54:**285.

DUBE, S. K., MARCKER, K. A., CLARK, B. F. C., AND CORY, S., 1968, Nucleotide sequence of N-formyl-methionyl-transfer RNA, Nature (Lond.) **218:**232.

DUNCAN, E. M., AND BROOKES, P., 1972, Metabolism and macromolecular binding of dibenz(a,c)anthracene and dibenz(a,h)anthracene by mouse embryo cells in culture, Int. J. Cancer **9:**349.

DUNCAN, M., BROOKES, P., AND DIPPLE, A., 1969, Metabolism and binding to cellular macromolecules of a series of hydrocarbons by mouse embryo cells in culture, Int. J. Cancer **4:**813.

DUNN, D. B., 1959, Additional components in ribonucleic acid of rat -liver fractions, Biochim. Biophys. Acta **34:**286.

DUNN, D. B., 1963, The isolation of 1-methyladenylic acid and 7-methylguanylic acid from ribonucleic acid, Biochem. J. **86:**14P.

EDMONDS, M., VAUGHAN, M. H., AND NAKAZATO, H., 1971, Polyadenylic acid sequences in the heterogeneous nuclear RNA and rapidly-labeled polyribosomal RNA of HeLa cells: Possible evidence for a precursor relationship (messenger RNA/poly(dT)-cellulose), Proc. Natl. Acad. Sci. **68:**1336.

EDWARDS, G. S., AND WOGAN, G. N., 1970, Aflatoxin inhibition of template activity of rat liver chromatin, Biochim. Biophys. Acta **224:**597.

EDWARDS, G. S., WOGAN, G. N., SPORN, M. B., AND PONG, R. S., 1971, Structure–activity relationships in DNA binding and nuclear effects of aflatoxin and analogs, Cancer Res. **31:**1943.

EICHHORN, G. L., CLARK, P., AND BECKER, E. D., 1966, Interactions of metal ions with polynucleotides and related compounds. VII. The binding of copper (II) to polynucleosides, nucleotides and deoxyribonucleic acids, Biochemistry **5:**245.

ELMORE, D. J., GULLAND, J. M., JORDAN, D. O., AND TAYLOR, H. F. W., 1948, The reaction of nucleic acids with mustard gas, Biochem. J. **42:**308.

ENOMOTO, M., SATO, K., MILLER, E. C., AND MILLER, J. A., 1968, Reactivity of the diacetyl derivative of the carcinogen 4-hydroxyaminoquinoline-1-oxide with DNA, RNA, and other nucleophiles, Life Sci. **7:**1025.

EPSTEIN, S. M., BENEDETTI, E. L., SHINOZUKA, H., BARTUS, B., AND FARBER, E., 1969/1970, Altered and distorted DNA from a premalignant liver lesion induced by 2-fluorenylacetamide, Chem.-Biol. Interact. **1:**113.

ERTÜRK, E., PRICE, J. M., MORRIS, J. E., COHEN, S. M., LEITH, R. S., VON ESCH, A. M., AND CROVETTI, A. J., 1967, The production of carcinoma of the urinary bladder in rats by feeding N-[4-(5-nitro-2-furyl)-2-thiazolyl]-formamide, Cancer Res. **27:**1998.

ERTÜRK, E., COHEN, S. M., AND BRYAN, G. T., 1970a, Induction, histogenesis and isotransplantability of renal tumors induced by formic acid 2-[4-(5-nitro-2-furyl)-2-thiazolyl]-hydrazide in rats, Cancer Res. **30:**2098.

ERTÜRK, E., MORRIS, J. E., COHEN, S. M., PRICE, J. M., AND BRYAN, G. T., 1970b, Transplantable rat mammary tumors induced by 5-nitro-2-furyldehyde semicarbazone and by formic acid 2-[4-(5-nitro-2-furyl)-2-thiazolyl]-hydrazide, Cancer Res. **30:**1409.

ERTÜRK, E., MORRIS, J. E., COHEN, S. M., VON ESCH, A. M., CROVETTI, A. J., PRICE, J. M., AND BRYAN, G. T., 1971, Comparative carcinogenicity of formic acid 2-[4-(5-nitro 2-furyl)-2-thiazolyl]-hydrazide and related chemicals in the rat, J. Natl. Cancer Inst. **47:**437.

FAHMY, O. G., AND FAHMY, M. J., 1972, Mutagenic selectivity for the RNA-forming genes in relation to the carcinogenicity of alkylating and polycyclic aromatics, Cancer Res. **32:**550.

FARBER, E., 1963, Ethionine carcinogenesis, Advan. Cancer Res. **7:**383.

FARBER, E., 1967, Ethionine fatty liver, Advan. Lipid Res. **5:**119.

FARBER, E., 1968, Biochemistry of carcinogenesis, Cancer Res. **28:**1859.

FARBER, E., 1973, Carcinogenesis, cellular evolution as a unifying thread: Presidential address, Cancer Res. **33:**2537.

FARBER, E., AND MAGEE, P. N., 1960, The probable alkylation of liver ribonucleic acid by the hepatic carcinogens dimethylnitrosamine and ethionine, Biochem. J. **76:**58P.

FARBER, E., SHULL, K. H., VILLA-TREVINO, S., LOMBARDI, B., AND THOMAS, M., 1964, Biochemical pathology of acute hepatic adenosinetriphosphate deficiency, Nature (Lond.) **203:**34.

FARBER, E., McCONOMY, J., FRANZEN, B., MARROQUIN, F., STEWART, G. A., AND MAGEE, P. N., 1967a, Interaction between ethionine and rat liver ribonucleic acid and protein in vivo, Cancer Res. **27:**1761.

FARBER, E., McCONOMY, J., AND FRUMANSKI, B., 1967b, Relative degrees of labeling of liver DNA and RNA with ethionine, *Proc. Am. Assoc. Cancer Res.* **8**:16.

FARBER, E., PARKER, S., AND GRUENSTEIN, M., 1973, Unpublished observations.

FARBER, J. L., SHINOZUKA, H., SERRONI, A., AND FARMER, R., 1974a, Reversal of the ethionine-induced inhibition of rat liver RNA polymerases *In vivo* by adenine, *Lab. Invest.* (in press).

FARBER, J. L., AND HERZOG, J., 1974b, Unpublished observations.

FARBER, J. L., HERZOG, J., SERRONI, A., AND BRIESMEISTER, B., 1974c, Unpublished observations.

FINK, L. M., NISHIMURA, S., AND WEINSTEIN, I. B., 1970, Modifications of ribonucleic acid by chemical carcinogens I. *In vitro* modification of transfer ribonucleic acid by N-acetoxy-2-acetylaminofluorene, *Biochemistry* **9**:496.

FIUME, L., CAMPADELLI-FIUME, G., MAGEE, P. N., AND HOLSMAN, J., 1970, Cellular injury and carcinogenesis: Inhibition of metabolism of dimethylnitrosamine by aminoacetonitrile, *Biochem. J.* **120**:601.

FLESHER, J. W., AND SYDNOR, K. L., 1971, Carcinogenicity of derivatives of 7,12-dimethylbenz(a)anthracene, *Cancer Res.* **31**:1951.

FLOYD, L. R., UNUMA, T., AND BUSCH, H., 1968, Effects of aflatoxin $B_1$ and other carcinogens upon nucleolar RNA of various tissues in the rat, *Exp. Cell Res.* **51**:423.

FOX, M., AND AYAD, S. R., 1971, Characteristics of repair synthesis in P388 cells treated with methylmethanesulphonate, *Chem.-Biol. Interact.* **3**:193.

FUJIMURA, S., GRUNBERGER, D., CARVAJAL, G., AND WEINSTEIN, I. B., 1972, Modification of RNA by chemical carcinogen: Modification of E. Coli formylmethionine tRNA with N-acetoxy-2-acetylaminofluorene, *Biochemistry* **11**:3629.

FUKUDA, S., AND YAMAMOTO, N., 1972, Detection of activating enzymes for-nitroquinoline 1-oxide activation with a microbial assay system, *Cancer Res.* **32**:435.

FURST, A., AND HARO, R. T., 1969, Possible mechanisms of metal ion carcinogenesis, in: *Physicochemical Mechanisms of Carcinogenesis* (E. D. Bergmann and B. Pullman, eds.), p. 310, Vol. 1 of *The Jerusalem Symposia on Quantum Chemistry and Biochemistry*, Israel Academy of Sciences and Humanities, Jerusalem.

FUWA, K., WARREN, W. E. C., DRUYAN, R., BARTHOLOMAY, A., AND VALEE, B. L., 1960, Nucleic acids and metals. II. Transition metals as determinants of the Conformation of ribonucleic acids, *Proc. Natl. Acad. Sci.* **46**:1298.

GARNER, R. C., 1973, Microsomal-dependent binding of aflatoxin-$B_1$ to DNA, RNA, polynucleotides and protein *in vitro*, *Chem.-Biol. Interact.* **6**:125.

GARNER, R. C., MILLER, E. C., MILLER, J. A., GARNER, J. V., AND HANSON, R. S., 1971, Formation of a factor lethal for S. typhimurium TA1530 and TA1531 on incubation of aflatoxin $B_1$ with rat liver microsomes, *Biochem. Biophys. Res. Commun.* **45**:774.

GELBOIN, H. V., 1969, A microsome-dependent binding of benzo(a)pyrene to DNA, *Cancer Res.* **29**:1272.

GELBOIN, H. V., WIRLHAM, J. S., WILSON, R. G., FRIEDMAN, M., AND WOGAN, G. N., 1966, Rapid and marked inhibition of rat liver RNA polymerase by aflatoxin $B_1$, *Science* **154**:1205.

GIOVANELLA, B. C., McKINNEY, L. E., AND HEIDELBERGER, C., 1964, On the reported solubilization of carcinogenic hydrocarbons in aqueous solutions of DNA, *J. Mol. Biol.* **8**:20.

GOODMAN, J. I., AND POTTER, V. R., 1971, Early effects of 3'-methyl-4-dimethylaminoazobenzene (MeDAB) administration: Evidence of an increased turnover of hepatic DNA, *Proc. Am. Assoc. Cancer Res.* **12**:36.

GOODMAN, J. I., AND POTTER, V. R., 1972, Evidence for DNA repair synthesis and turnover in rat liver following ingestion of 3'-methyl-4-dimethylaminoazobenzene, *Cancer Res.* **32**:766.

GOSHMAN, L. M., AND HEIDELBERGER, C., 1967, Binding of tritium-labeled polycyclic hydrocarbons to DNA of mouse skin, *Cancer Res.* **27**:1678.

GOTH, R., AND RAJEWSKY, M. F., 1972, Ethylation of nucleic acid by ethylnitrosourea-1-$C^{14}$ in the fetal and adult liver, *Cancer Res.* **32**:1501.

GRAB, D. J., ZEDECK, M. S., SURSTOCKI, N. I., AND SONENBERG, M., 1973, *In vitro* synthesis of RNA with "aggregate" enzyme, chromatin and DNA from liver of methylazoxymethanol acetate-treated rats, *Chem.-Biol. Interact.* **6**:259.

GROVER, P. L., AND SIMS, P., 1968, Enzyme-catalysed reactions of polycyclic hydrocarbons with deoxyribonucleic acids and protein *in vitro*, *Biochem. J.* **110**:159.

GROVER, P. L., AND SIMS, P., 1970, Interactions of the k-region epoxides of phenanthrene and dibenz(a,h)anthracene with nucleic acids and histone, *Biochem. Pharmacol.* **19**:2251.

275

INTERAC-
TIONS OF
CARCINOGENS
WITH NUCLEIC
ACIDS

276

D. S. R. SARMA,
S. RAJALAKSHMI
AND
EMMANUEL
FARBER

GROVER, P. L., AND SIMS, P., 1972, Metabolic formation of a k-region epoxide of benzo(a)pyrene, Proc. Am. Assoc. Cancer Res. 13:25.

GROVER, P. L., HEWER, A., AND SIMS, P., 1971a, Epoxides as microsomal metabolites of polycyclic hydrocarbons, FEBS Letters 18:76.

GROVER, P. L., FORRESTER, J. A., AND SIMS, P., 1971b, Reactivity of the k-region epoxides of some polycyclic hydrocarbons towards the nucleic acids and proteins of BHK 21 cells, Biochem. Pharmacol. 20:1297.

GROVER, P. L., SIMS, P., HUBERMAN, E., MARQUARDT, H., KUROKI, T., AND HEIDELBERGER, C., 1971c, In vitro transformation of rodent cells by K-region derivatives of polycyclic hydrocarbons, Proc. Natl. Acad. Sci. 68:1098.

GRUNBERGER, D., AND WEINSTEIN, I. B., 1971, Modifications of ribonucleic acid by chemical carcinogens. III. Template activity of polynucleotides modified by N-acetoxy-2-acetylaminofluorene, J. Biol. Chem. 246:1123.

GRUNBERGER, D., NELSON, J., CANTOR, R. C., AND WEINSTEIN, I. B., 1970, Coding and conformational properties of oligonucleotides modified with the carcinogens N-2-acetylaminofluorene, Proc. Natl. Acad. Sci. 66:488.

GRUNBERGER, G., YU, F. L., GRUNBERGER, D., AND FEIGELSON, P., 1973, Mechanism of N-hydroxy-2-acetylaminofluorene inhibition of rat hepatic ribonucleic acid synthesis, J. Biol. Chem. 248:6278.

HADI, I. S. M., KIRTIKAR, D., AND GOLDTHWAIT, D. A., 1973, Endonuclease II of Excherichia coli degradation of double- and single-stranded deoxyribonucleic acid, Biochemistry 12:2747.

HAESE, W. H., SMITH, D. L., AND BUEDING, E., 1973, Hycanthone-induced hepatic changes in mice infected with Schistosoma mansoni, J. Pharmacol. Exp. Ther. 186:430.

HAHN, F. E., 1971, Progress in Molecular and Subcellular Biology, Vol. 2, Springer, New York.

HANAWALT, P. C., 1972, Repair of genetic material in living cells, Endeavour 31:83.

HANCOCK, R. L., 1968, Soluble RNA ethylase activity of normal and neoplastic mouse tissues, Cancer Res. 28:1223.

HAWKS, A., SWANN, P. F., AND MAGEE, P. N., 1972, Probable methylation of nucleic acids of mouse colon by 1,2-dimethylhydrazine in vivo, Biochem. Pharmacal. 21:432.

HEATH, D. F., 1961, Mechanism of the hepatotoxic action of dialkylnitrosamine, Nature (Lond.) 192:170.

HENNINGS, H., 1973, DNA repair after treatment of mouse skin cell cultures with β-propiolactone (BPL), Proc. Am. Assoc. Cancer Res. 14:70.

HENSHAW, E. C., AND HIATT, H. H., 1963, Binding of fluorenylacetamide to rat liver RNA in vivo, Proc. Am. Assoc. Cancer Res. 4:27.

HIROSE, S., OKAZAKI, R., AND TAMANOI, F., 1973, Mechanism of DNA chain growth. XI. Structure of RNA-linked DNA fragments of Escherichia coli, J. Mol. Biol. 77:501.

HOLLEY, R. W., APGAR, J., EVERETT, G. A., MADISON, J. T., MARQUISEE, M., MERRILL, S. H., PENSWICK, J. R., AND ZAMIR, A., 1965, Structure of a ribonucleic acid Science 147:1462.

HOSHINO, H., FUMIKO, F., OKABE, K., AND SUGIMURA, T., 1966, Metabolism of 4-nitroquinoline 1-oxide. II. In vivo conversion of subcutanously injected 4-nitroquinoline 1-oxide to 4-aminoquinoline 1-oxide and 4-hydroxyaminoquinoline 1-oxide in rats, Gann 57:71.

HOWARD-FLANDERS, P., 1968, DNA repair, Ann. Rev. Biochem. 37:175.

HUBERMAN, E., ASPIRAS, L., HEIDELBERGER, C., GROVER, P. L., AND SIMS, P., 1971, Mutagenicity to mammalian cells of epoxides and other derivatives of polycyclic hydrocarbons, Proc. Natl. Acad. Sci. 68:3195.

HUGGINS, C., GRAND, L., AND FUKUNISHI, R., 1964, Aromatic influences on the yields of mammary cancers following administration of 7,12-dimethylbenz(a)anthracene, Proc. Natl. Acad. Sci. 51:737.

HUGHES, P. E., AND PILCZYK, R., 1969/1970, The in vivo binding of metabolites of 2-naphthylamine to mouse-liver DNA, RNA and protein, Chem.-Biol. Interact. 1:307.

IBALL, J., 1939, The relative potency of carcinogenic compounds, Am. J. Cancer 35:188.

IBALL, J., AND MACDONALD, S. G. G., 1960, The crystal structure of 20-methylcholanthrene, Z. Kristallog. 114:439.

IDE, T., AND ANDOH, T., 1972, Scissions of proteins linking DNA in cultured mammalian cells induced by 4-nitroquinoline-1-oxide and their repair, Cancer Res. 32:1236.

INGOLD, C. K., 1970, Structure and Mechanism in Organic chemistry, 2nd ed., pp. 421–555, G. Bell and Sons, Edinburgh.

IRVING, C. C., 1970, in: Metabolic Conjugation and Metabolic Hydrolysis, Vol. 1 (W. H. Fishman, ed.), p. 53, Academic Press, New York.

IRVING, C. C., 1971, Metabolic activation of N-hydroxy compounds by conjugation, *Xenobiotica* 1:387.

IRVING, C. C., 1973, Interaction of chemical carcinogens with DNA, in: *Methods in Cancer Research*, Vol VII (H. Busch, ed.), p. 189, Academic Press, New York.

IRVING, C. C., AND RUSSELL, L. T., 1970, Synthesis of the O-glucuronide of N-2-fluorenylhydroxylamine: Reaction with nucleic acids and the guanosine 5'-monophosphate, *Biochemistry* 9:2471.

IRVING, C. C., AND VEAZEY, R. Z., 1969, Persistent binding of 2-acetylaminofluorene to rat liver DNA *in vivo* and consideration of the mechanism of binding of N-hydroxy-2-acetylaminofluorene to rat liver nucleic acids, *Cancer Res.* 27:1779.

IRVING, C. C., AND VEAZEY, R. A., 1972, Preferential binding of 2-acetylaminofluorene to rat liver rRNA during early stages of hepatocarcinogenesis, *Biochem. Biophys. Res. Commun.* 47:1159.

IRVING, C. C., VEAZEY, R. A., AND WILLARD, R. F., 1967, The significance and mechanism of the binding of 2-acetylaminofluorene and N-hydroxy-2-acetylaminofluorene to rat liver ribonucleic acid *in vivo*, *Cancer Res.* 27:720.

IRVING, C. C., VEAZEY, R. A., AND HILL, G. T., 1969, Reaction of the glucuronide of the carcinogen N-hydroxy-2-acetylaminofluorene with nucleic acids, *Biochim. Biophys. Acta* 179:189.

IRVING, C. C., JANSS, D. H., AND RUSSELL, L. T., 1971, Lack of N-hydroxy-2-acetylaminofluorene sulfotransferase activity in the mammary gland and Zymbal's gland of the rat, *Cancer Res.* 31:387.

ISHIZAWA, M., AND ENDO, H., 1967, On the mode of action of a potent carcinogen, 4-hydroxylaminoquinoline 1-oxide, on bacteriophage $T_4$, *Biochem. Pharmacol.* 16:637.

JANSS, D. H., MOON, R. C., AND IRVING, C. C., 1972, The binding of 7,12-dimethylbenz(a)anthracene to mammary parenchymal DNA and protein *in vivo*, *Cancer Res.* 32:254.

JELINEK, W., AND DARNELL, J. E., 1972, Double-stranded regions in heterogeneous nuclear RNA from HeLa cells, *Proc. Natl. Acad. Sci.* 69:2537.

JENSON, E. V., FORD, E., AND HUGGINS, C., 1963, Depressed incorporation of thymidine-$^3$H into deoxyribonucleic acid following administration of 7,12-dimethylbenzanthracene, *Proc. Natl. Acad. Sci.* 50:454.

KAPLAN, J. C., KUSHNER, S. R., AND GROSSMAN, L., 1971, Enzymatic repair of DNA. III. Properties of the UV-endonuclease and UV-exonuclease, *Biochemistry* 10:3315.

KATO, M., AND TAKALASHI, A., 1970, Characteristics of nitro reduction of the carcinogenic agent, 4-nitroquinoline N-oxide, *Biochem. Pharmacol.* 19:45.

KAWAMATA, J., NAKABAYASHI, N., KAWAI, A., AND USHIDA, T., 1958, Experimental production of sarcoma in mice with actinomycin, *Med. J. Osaka Univ.* 8:753.

KAWAMATA, J., NAKABAYASHI, N., KAWAI, A., FUJITA, H., IMANISHI, M., AND IKEGAMI, R., 1959, Studies on the carcinogenic effect of actinomycin, *Biken's J.* 2:105.

KAWAMOTO, S., IDA, N., KIRSCHBAUM, A., AND TAYLOR, G., 1958, Urethan and leukemogenesis in mice, *Cancer Res.* 18:725.

KAWAZOE, Y., ARAKI, M., AOKI, K., AND NAKAHARA, W., 1969, Structure–carcinogenicity relationship among derivatives of 4-nitro- and 4-hydroxyaminoquinoline-1-oxide, *Biochem. Pharmacol.* 16:631.

KAWAZOE, Y., ARAKI, M., AND HUANG, G. F., 1972, Chemical aspects of carcinogenesis by 4-nitroquinoline 1-oxide, : *Proceedings of the Second International Symposium of the Princess Takamatsu Cancer Research Fund* (W. Nakahara, S. Takayama, T. Sugimura, and S. Odashima, eds.), p. 1, University Park Press, Baltimore.

KING, C. M., AND KRIEK, E., 1965, The differential reactivity of the oxidation products of O-aminophenols towards proteins and nucleic acid, *Biochim. Biophys. Acta* 111:147.

KING, C. M., AND PHILLIPS, B., 1970, Instability of fluorenylamine-substituted polynucleotides: Loss of carcinogen and production of an altered nucleic acid, *Chem.-Biol. Interact.* 2:267.

KING, C. M., AND PHILLIPS. B., 1972, Mechanism of introduction of fluorenylamine (FA) substituents into nucleic acid by rat liver, *Proc. Am. Assoc. Cancer Res.* 13:43.

KIT, S., 1960, Studies on structure, composition, metabolism of tumour RNA, in: *Cell Physiology of New Phases: Fourteenth Annual Symposium on Fundamental Cancer Research*, p. 337, University of Texas M. D. Anderson Hospital and Tumor Institute, University of Texas Press, Austin.

KLEIHUES, P., 1972, N-Methyl-N-nitrosourea induced changes in the labeling by ($^{14}$C) orotate of RNA and acid-soluble fractions in rat kidney and liver, *Chem.-Biol. Interact.* 5:309.

KOSUGE, T., ZENDA, H., YOKOTA, M., SAWANISHI, H., AND SUZUKI, Y., 1969, Further evidence for formation of 4-nitrosoquinoline-1-oxide, *Chem. Pharm. Bull. (Tokyo)* 17:2181.

KRIEK, E., 1968, Difference in binding of 2-acetylaminofluorene to rat liver deoxyribonucleic acid and ribosomal ribonucleic acid *in vivo*, *Biochim. Biophys, Acta* 161:273.

277

INTERAC-
TIONS OF
CARCINOGENS
WITH NUCLEIC
ACIDS

278

D. S. R. SARMA,
S. RAJALAKSHMI
AND
EMMANUEL
FARBER

KRIEK, E., 1969, On the mechanism of action of aromatic amines *in vivo:* Differences in binding to ribosomal RNA and DNA, in:*Physico-chemical Mechanisms of Carcinogenesis* (E. D. Bergman and B. Pullman, eds.), p. 136,Vol. 1 of *The Jerusalem Symphosia on Quantum Chemistry and Biochemistry,* Israel Academy of Sciences and Humanities, Jerusalem.

KRIEK, E., 1972, Persistent binding of a new product of the carcinogen N-hydroxy-N-2-acetylaminofluorene with guanine in rat liver DNA *in vivo, Cancer Res.* **32:**2042.

KRIEK, E., AND EMMELOT, P., 1963, Methylation and breakdown of microsomal and soluble ribonucleic acid from rat liver by diazomethane, *Biochemistry* **2;**733.

KRIEK, E., MILLER, J. A., JUHL, V., AND MILLER, E. C., 1967, 8-(N-2-Fluorenylacetamide)guanosine, an arylamidation reaction product of guanosine and the carcinogen N-acetoxy-N-2-fluorenylacetamide in neutral solution, *Biochem. J.* **6:**177.

KRÜGER, F. W., 1972, New Aspects in metabolism of carcinogenic nitrosamine, in: *Proceedings of the Second International Symposium of the Princess Takamatsu Cancer Research Fund* (W. Nakahara, S. Takayama, T. Sugimura, and S. Odashima, eds.), p. 213, University Park Press, Baltimore.

KRÜGER, F. W., 1973, Metabolism of nitrosamines *in vivo.* II. On the methylation of nucleic acids by aliphatic di-n-alkyl-nitrosamines *in vivo,* caused by $\beta$-oxidation: The increased formation of 7-methylguanine after application of $\beta$-hydroxypropyl-propyl-nitrosamine compared to that after application of di-n-propyl-nitrosamine, *Z. Krebsforsch.* **79:**90.

KRÜGER, F. W., AND BERTRAM, B., 1973, Metabolism of nitrosamines *in vivo.* III. On the methylation of nucleic acids by aliphatic di-n-alkyl-nitrosamines *in vivo* resulting from $\beta$-oxidation: The formation of 7-methylguanine after application of 2-oxo-propyl-propyl-nitrosamine and methyl-propyl-nitrosamine, *Z. Krebsforsch.* **80:**189.

KUROKI, T., AND HEIDELBERGER, C., 1971, The binding of polycyclic aromatic hydrocarbons to the DNA, RNA and proteins of transformable cells in culture, *Cancer Res.* **31:**2168.

KUROKI, T., HUBERMAN, E., MARQUARDT, H., SELKIRK, J. K., HEIDELBERGER, C., GROVER, P. L., AND SIMS, P., 1971/1972, Binding of k-region epoxides and other derivatives of benz(a)anthracene and dibenz(a,h)anthracene to DNA, RNA, and proteins of transformable cells, *Chem.-Biol. Interact.* **4:**389.

KUSHNER, S. R., KAPLAN, J. C., ONO, H., AND GROSSMAN, L., 1971, Enzymatic repair of deoxyribonucleic acid. IV. Mechanism of photoproduct excision, *Biochemistry* **10:**3325.

LAFARGE, C., AND FRAYSSINET, C., 1970, The reversibility of inhibition of RNA and DNA synthesis induced by aflatoxin in rat liver, a tentative explanation for carcinogenic mechanism, *Int. J. Cancer* **6:**74.

LAIRD, A. K., AND BARTON, A. D., 1959, Cell growth and the development of tumours, *Nature (Lond.)* **183:**1655.

LAIRD, A. K., AND BARTON, A. D., 1961, Cell proliferation in precancerous liver: Relation to presence and dose of carcinogen, *J. Natl. Cancer Inst.* **27:**827.

LAISHES, B. A., AND STICH, H. F., 1973, Repair synthesis and sedimentation analysis of DNA of human cells exposed to dimethylnitrosamine and activated dimethylnitrosamine, *Biochem. Biophys. Res. Commun.* **52:**827.

LANCASTER, M. C., JENKINS, F. P., AND PHILIP, J. M., 1961, Toxicity associated with certain samples of dry nuts, *Nature (Lond.)* **192:**1095.

LAQUEUR, G. L., AND SPATZ, M., 1968, Toxicology of cycasin, *Cancer Res.* **28:**2262.

LAWLEY, P. D., 1966, Effects of some chemical mutagens and carcinogens on nucleic acids, *Prog. Nucl. Acid Res. Mol. Biol.* **5:**89.

LAWLEY, P. D., 1972a, Some aspects of the cellular response to chemical modifications of nucleic acid purines, in: *Purines, Theory and Experiment The Jerusalem Symposia on Quantum Chemistry and Biochemistry,* (E. D. Bergmann and P. Pullman, eds.), pp. 579–591, Vol. 4 of Israel Academy of Sciences and Humanities, Jerusalem.

LAWLEY, P. D., 1972b, The action of alkylating mutagens and carcinogens on nucleic acids: N-Methyl-N-nitroso compounds as methylating agents, in: *Proceedings of the Second International Symposium of the Princess Takamatsu Cancer Research Fund* (W. Nakahara, S. Takayama, T. Sugimura, and S. Odashima, eds.), p. 237, University Park Press, Baltimore.

LAWLEY, P. D., 1973, Reaction of N-methyl-N-nitrosourea (MNUA) with ³²P labeled DNA: Evidence for formation of phosphotriesters, *Chem.-Biol. Interact.* **7:**127.

LAWLEY, P. D., AND BROOKES, P., 1963, Further studies on the alkylation of nucleic acids and their constituent nucleotides, *Biochem. J.* **89:**127.

LAWLEY, P. D., AND ORR, D. J., 1970, Specific excision of methylation products from DNA of *Escherichia coli* treated with N-methyl-N'-nitro-N-nitrosoguanidine, *Chem.-Biol. Interact.* **2:**154.

LAWLEY, P. D., AND SHAH, S. A., 1972a, Methylation of ribonucleic acid by the carcinogens dimethyl-sulfate N-methyl-N-nitrosourea and N-methyl-N'-nitro-N-nitrosoguanidine, comparisons of chemical analysis at the nucleoside and base levels, *Biochem. J.* **128**:117.

LAWLEY, P. D., AND SHAH, S. A., 1972b, Reaction of alkylating mutagens and carcinogens with nucleic acids: Detection and estimation of a small extent of methylation at O-6 of guanine in DNA by methylmethanesulfonate *in vivo, Chem.-Biol. Interact.* **5**:286.

LAWLEY, P. D., AND SHAH, S. A., 1973, Methylation of DNA by $^3$H-$^{14}$C-methyl-labeled N-methyl-N-nitrosourea—evidence for transfer of the intact methyl group, *Chem.-Biol. Interact.* **7**:115.

LAWLEY, P. D., AND THATCHER, C. J., 1970, Methylation of deoxyribonucleic acid in cultured mammalian cells by N-methyl-N'-nitro-N-nitrosoguanidine: The influence of cellular thiol concentrations on the extent of methylation and the 6-oxygen atom of guanine as a site of methylation, *Biochem. J.* **116**:693.

LAWLEY, P. D., BROOKES, P., MAGEE, P. N., CRADDOCK, V. M., AND SWANN, P. F., 1968, Methylated bases in liver nucleic acids from rats treated with dimethylnitrosamine, *Biochim. Biophys. Acta* **157**:646.

LAWLEY, P. D., ORR, D. J., AND SHAH, S. A., 1971/1972, Reaction of alkylating mutagens and carcinogens with nucleic acids: N-3 of guanine as a site of alkylation by N-methyl-N-nitrosourea and dimethylsulfate, *Chem.-Biol. Interact.* **4**:431.

LAWLEY, P. D., ORR, D. J., SHAH, S. A., FARMER, P. B., AND JARMAN, M., 1973, Reaction products from N-methyl-N-nitrosourea and deoxyribonucleic acid containing thymidine residues: Synthesis and identification of a new methylation product $O^4$-methylthymidine, *Biochem. J.* **135**:193.

LAWS, J. O., 1959, Tissue regeneration and tumour development, *Brit. J. Cancer* **13**:669.

LAWSON, T. A., 1968, The binding of O-aminoazotoluene to deoxyribonucleic acid, ribonucleic acid and protein in the C57 mouse, *Biochem. J.* **109**:917.

LAWSON, T. A., AND CLAYSON, D. B., 1969, Differences in binding of orthoaminoazotoluene to macromolecules of female and male C57 mouse liver, in: *Physico-chemical Mechanisms of Carcinogenesis* (E. D. Bergmann and B. Pullman, eds.), p. 226, Vol. 1 of *The Jerusalem Symposia on Quantum Chemistry and Biochemistry,* Israel Academy of Sciences and Humanities, Jerusalem.

LAWSON, T. A., AND POUND, A. W., 1971, Reaction of urethane with mouse liver nucleic acids *in vivo,* Pathology **3**:223.

LAWSON, T. A., AND POUND, A. W., 1971/1972, The interaction of ($^3$H) ethyl carbamate with nucleic acids of regenerating mouse liver, *Chem.-Biol. Interact.* **4**:329.

LAWSON, T. A., AND POUND, A. W., 1973a, The interaction of carbon-12-labeled alkyl carbomates, labeled in the alkyl- and carbonyl-positions, with DNA *in vivo, Chem.-Biol. Interact.* **6**:99.

LAWSON, T. A., AND POUND, A. W., 1973b, The prolonged binding of ethyl carbamate-($^{14}$C) to DNA in regenerating and intact mouse liver, *Europ. J. Cancer* **9**:491.

LEE, K. Y., AND LIJINSKY, W., 1966, Alkylation of rat liver RNA by cyclic N-nitrosamines *in vivo, J. Natl. Cancer Inst.* **37**:401.

LEHMANN, A. R., 1972, Postreplication repair of DNA in ultraviolet-irradiated mammalian cells, *J. Mol. Biol.* **66**:319.

LERMAN, L. S., 1964, Acridine mutagens and DNA structure, *J. Cell. Comp. Physiol.* **64**:1 (Suppl. 1).

LERMAN, L. S., 1971, Intercalability, the "y" transition, and the state of DNA in nature, in: *Progress in Molecular and Subcellular Biology,* Vol. 2 (F. E. Hahn, ed.), p. 382, Springer, New York.

LETT, J. T., PARKINS, G. M., AND ALEXANDER, P., 1962, Physiochemical changes produced in DNA after alkylation, *Arch. Biochem. Biophys.* **97**:80.

LETT, J. T., CALDWELL, I., DEAN, C. J., AND ALEXANDER, P., 1967, Rejoining of x-ray induced breaks in the DNA of leukemia cells, *Nature (Lond.)* **214**:790.

LETT, J. T., KLUCIS, E. S., AND SUN, C., 1970, On the size of the DNA in the mammalian chromosome substructural sununits, *Biophys. J.* **10**:277.

LIEBERMAN, M. W., AND DIPPLE, A., 1972, Removal of bound carcinogen during DNA repair in non-dividing human lymphocytes, *Cancer Res.* **32**:1855.

LIEBERMAN, M. W., AND FORBES, P. D., 1973, Demonstration of DNA repair in normal and neoplastic tissues after treatment with proximate chemical carcinogens and ultraviolet radiation, *Nature New Biol.* **241**:199.

LIEBERMAN, M. W., AND POIRIER, M. C., 1973, Deoxyribonucleoside incorporation during DNA repair of carcinogen-induced damage in human diploid fibroblasts, *Cancer Res.* **33**:2097.

LIEBERMAN, M. W., BANEY, R. N., LEE, R. E., SELL, S., AND FARBER, E., 1971, Studies on DNA repair in human lymphocytes treated with proximate carcinogens and alkylating agents, *Cancer Res.* **31**:1297.

LIJINSKY, W., LOO, J., AND ROSS, A. E., 1968, Mechanism of alkylation of nucleic acids by nitrosodimethylamine, *Nature (Lond.)* **218**:1174.

279

INTERAC-
TIONS OF
CARCINOGENS
WITH NUCLEIC
ACIDS

280

D. S. R. SARMA,
S. RAJALAKSHMI
AND
EMMANUEL
FARBER

LIJINSKY, W., LEE, K. Y., AND JALLAGHER, C. H., 1970, Interaction of aflatoxins B₁ and G₁ with tissues of the rat, *Cancer Res.* **30:**2280.

LINDAHL, T., AND EDELMAN, G. M., 1968, Polynucleotide ligase from myeloid and lymphoid tissues, *Proc. Natl. Acad. Sci.* **61:**680.

LINDBERG, U., AND DARNELL, J. E., 1970, SV40-specific RNA in the nucleus and polyribosomes of transformed cells, *Proc. Natl. Acad. Sci.* **65:**1089.

LINGENS, F., HAERLIN, F., AND SUSSMUTH, R., 1971, Mechanisms of mutagenesis by *N*-methyl-*N'*-nitro-*N*-nitrosoguanidine (MNNG): Methylation of nucleic acids by *N*-trideuteriomethyl-*N'*-nitro-*N*-nitrosoguanidine (D₃-MNNG) in the presence of cysteine and in cells of *Escherichia coli*, *FEBS Letters* **13:**241.

LIQUORI, A. M., DELERMA, B., ASCOLI, F., BOTRÉ, C., AND TRASCITTI, M., 1962, Interaction between DNA and polycyclic aromatic hydrocarbons, *J. Mol. Biol.* **5:**521.

LOTLIKAR, P. D., AND LUHA, L., 1971a, Enzymatic *N*-acetylation of *N*-hydroxy-2-aminofluorene by liver cytosol from various species, *Biochem. J.* **123:**287.

LOTLIKAR, P. D., AND LUHA, L., 1971b, Acylation of carcinogenic hydroxamic acids by carbamoylphosphate to form reactive esters, *Biochem. J.* **124:**69.

LOVELESS, A., 1969, Possible relevance of *O*-6 alkylation of deoxyguanosine to the mutagenicity and carcinogenicity of nitrosamines and nitrosamides, *Nature (Lond.)* **223:**206.

MAGEE, P. N., 1969, Interactions of carcinogens *in vivo*, in: *Physico-chemical Mechanisms of Carcinogenesis* Vol. 1 of i *The Jerusalem Symposia on Quantum Chemistry and Biochemistry*, (E. D. Bergmann and B. Pullman, eds.), pp. 298–304, Israel Academy of Science and Humanities, Jerusalem.

MAGEE, P. N., 1972, Possible mechanisms of carcinogenesis and mutagenesis by nitrosamines, in: *Proceedings of the Second International Symposium of the Princess Takamatsu Cancer Research Fund* (W. Nakahara, S. Takayama, T. Sugimura, and S. Odashima, eds.), p. 259, University Park Press, Baltimore.

MAGEE, P. N., AND BARNES, J. M., 1967, Carcinogenic nitroso compounds, *Advan. Cancer Res.* **10:**163.

MAGEE, P. N., AND FARBER, E., 1962, Methylation of rat liver nucleic acids by dimethylnitrosamine *in vivo*, *Biochem. J.* **83:**114.

MAGEE, P. N., AND HULTIN, T., 1962, Toxic liver injury and carcinogenesis: Methylation of rat liver slices by dimethylnitrosamine *in vitro*, *Biochem. J.* **83:**106.

MAGEE, P. N., AND LEE, K. Y., 1963, Experimental toxic liver injury by some nitrosamines, *Ann. N.Y. Acad. Sci.* **104:**916.

MAGEE, P. N., AND LEE, K. Y., 1964, Cellular injury and carcinogenesis: Alkylation of ribonucleic acid of rat liver by diethylnitrosamine and *n*-butylmethylnitrosamine *in vivo*, *Biochem. J.* **91:**35.

MAGEE, P. N., AND SCHOENTAL, R., 1964, Carcinogenesis by nitroso compounds, *Brit. Med. Bull.* **20:**102.

MAINI, M. M., AND STICH, H. F., 1962, Chromosomes of tumor cells III. Unresponsiveness of precancerous hepatic tissues and hepatomas to a mitotic stimulus, *J. Natl. Cancer Inst.* **28:**753.

MALKIN, M. F., AND ZAHALSKY, A. C., 1966, Interaction of the water-soluble carcinogen 4-nitroquinoline *N*-oxide with DNA, *Science* **154:**1665.

MARGISON, G. P., CAPPS, M. J., O'CONNOR, P. J., AND CRAIG, A. W., 1973, Loss of 7-methylguanine from rat liver DNA after methylation *in vivo* with methylmethanesulfonate or dimethylnitrosamine, *Chem.-Biol. Interact.* **6:**119.

MARQUARDT, H., AND PHILIPS, F. S., 1970, The effects of 7,12-dimethylbenz(a)anthracene on the synthesis of nucleic acids in rapidly dividing hepatic cells in rats, *Cancer Res.* **30:**2000.

MARQUARDT, H., BENDICH, A., PHILIPS, F. S., AND HOFFMANN, D., 1971, Binding of G-³H-7,12-dimethylbenz(a)anthracene to DNA of normal and rapidly dividing hepatic cells of rats, *Chem.-Biol. Interact.* **3:**1.

MARQUARDT, H., PHILIPS, F. S., AND BENDICH, A., 1972, DNA binding and inhibition of DNA synthesis after 7,12-dimethylbenz(a)anthracene administered during the early prereplicative phase in regenerating rat liver, *Cancer Res.* **32:**1810.

MARROQUIN, F., AND FARBER, E., 1965, The binding of 2-acetylaminofluorene to rat liver ribonucleic acid *in vivo*, *Cancer Res.* **25:**1262.

MATSUMOTO, H., AND HIGA, H. H., 1966, Studies on methylazoxymethanol, the aglycone of cycasin: Methylation of nucleic acids *in vitro*, *Biochem. J.* **98:**20C.

MATSUSHIMA, T., KOBUNA, I., AND SUGIMURA, T., 1967, *In vivo* interaction of 4-nitroquinoline 1-oxide and derivatives with DNA, *Nature (Lond.)* **216:**508.

281

INTERAC-
TIONS OF
CARCINOGENS
WITH NUCLEIC
ACIDS

MATSUYAMA, A., AND NAGATA, C., 1972, Detection of the unstable intermediate 4-nitrosoquinoline 1-oxide, in: *Proceedings of the Second International Symposium of the Princess Takamatsu Cancer Research Fund* (W. Nakahara, S. Takayama, T. Sugimura, and S. Odashima, eds.), p. 35, University Park Press, Baltimore.

MCCALLA, D. R., REUVERS, A., AND KITAI, R., 1968, Inactivation of biologically active N-methyl-N-nitroso compounds in aqueous solution: Effect of various conditions of pH and illumination, *Canad. J. Biochem.* **46**:807.

MCCALLA, D. R., REUVERS, A., AND KAISER, C., 1971, Activation of nitrofurazone in animal tissues, *Biochem. Pharmacol.* **20**:3532.

MELLI, M., AND PEMBERTON, R. E., 1972, New method of studying the precursor–product relationship between high molecular weight RNA and messenger RNA, *Nature New Biol.* **236**:172.

MICHAEL, R. O., SARMA, D. S. R., DAMJANOV, I., COX, R., AND FARBER, E., 1973, Unpublished observations.

MILLER, E. C., AND MILLER, J. A., 1969, Studies on the mechanism of activation of aromatic amine and amide carcinogens to ultimate carcinogenic electrophilic reactants, *Ann. N.Y. Acad. Sci.* **163**:731.

MILLER, E. C., AND MILLER, J. A., 1971, The mutagenicity of chemical carcinogens: Correlations, problems, and interpretations, in: *Chemical Mutagens: Principles and Methods for Their Detection*, Vol. 1 (A. Hollander, ed.), p. 83, Plenum Press, New York.

MILLER, E. C., SMITH, J. Y., AND MILLER, J. A., 1970, Lack of correlation between the formation of the glucouronide of N-hydroxy-2-acetyl aminofluorene (N-GLO-AAF) and susceptibility to hepatic carcinogenesis, *Proc. Am. Assoc. Cancer Res.* **11**:56.

MILLER, J. A., 1970, Carcinogenesis by chemicals: An overview—G. H. A., Clowes memorial lecture, *Cancer Res.* **30**:559.

MILLER, J. A., AND MILLER, E. C., 1969, Metabolic activation of carcinogenic aromatic amines and amides via N-hydroxylation and N-hydroxy-esterification and its relationship to ultimate carcinogens as electrophilic reactants, in: *Physico-chemical Mechanisms of Carcinogenesis* (E. D. Bergmann and B. Pullman, eds.), p. 237, Vol. 1 of *The Jerusalem Symposia on Quantum Chemistry and Biochemistry*, Israel Academy of Sciences and Humanities, Jerusalem.

MILLER, J. A., LIN, J.-K., AND MILLER, E. C., 1970, N-(Guanosin-8-yl) and N-(deoxyguanosin-8-yl) N'-methyl-4-aminoazobenzene: Degradation products of hepatic RNA and DNA in rats administered N'-methyl-4-aminoazobenzene, *Proc. Am. Assoc. Cancer Res.* **11**:56.

MIRVISH, S. S., 1968, The carcinogenic action and metabolism of urethane and N-hydroxyurethane, *Advan. Cancer Res.* **11**:1.

MIURA, K., AND RECKENDORF, H. K., 1967, The nitrofurans, *Prog. Med. Chem.* **5**:320.

MORRIS, J. E., PRICE, J. M., LALICH, J. J., AND STEIN, R. J., 1969, The carcinogenic activity of some 5-nitrofuran derivatives in the rat, *Cancer Res.* **29**:2145.

MULIVOR, R. A., AND SARMA, D. S. R., 1973, Unpublished observations.

MULIVOR, R. A., ABANOBI, S. E., AND SARMA, D. S. R., 1974, Unpublished observations.

MÜLLER, W., AND CROTHERS, D. M., 1968, Studies on the binding of actinomycin and related compounds to DNA, *J. Mol. Biol.* **35**:251.

MURAMATSU, M., AND BUSCH, H., 1967, Isolation, composition and function of nucleoli of tumors and other tissues, *Meth. Cancer Res.* **2**:303.

MYLES, A., AND BROWN, G. B., 1969, Purine N-oxides. XXX. Biochemical studies of the oncogen 3-hydroxyxanthine, *J. Biol. Chem.* **244**:4072.

NAGASAWA, H. T., SHIROTA, F. N., AND MATSUMOTO, H., 1972, Decomposition of methylazoxymethanol, the aglycone of cycasin, in $D_2O$, *Nature (Lond.)* **236**:234.

NAGATA, C., KODAMA, M., TAGASHIRA, Y., AND IMAMURA, A., 1966a, Interaction of polynuclear aromatic hydrocarbons, 4-nitro-quinoline-1-oxides, and various dyes with DNA, *Biopolymers* **4**:409.

NAGATA, C., KATAOKA, N., IMAMURA, A., KAWAZOF, Y., AND CHIHARA, G., 1966b, Electronic spin resonance study on the free radicals produced from 4-hydroxyaminoquinoline-1-oxide and its significance in carcinogenesis, *Gann* **57**:323.

NAGATA, Y., AND MATSUMOTO, H., 1969, Studies on methylazoxymethanol: Methylation of nucleic acids in the fetal rat brain, *Proc. Soc. Exp. Biol. Med.* **132**:383.

NAKAHARA, W., FUKUOKA, F., AND SUGIMURA, T., 1957, Carcinogenic action of 4-nitroquinoline 1-oxide, *Gann* **48**:129.

NATORI, Y., 1963, VI. Sex-dependent behaviour of methionine and ethionine in rats, *J. Biol. Chem.* **238**:2075.

282

D. S. R. SARMA,
S. RAJALAKSHMI
AND
EMMANUEL
FARBER

NELSON, J. H., GRUNBERGER, D., CANTOR, C. R., AND WEINSTEIN, I. B., 1971, Modification of ribonucleic acid by chemical carcinogen. IV. Circular dichroism and proton magnetic resonance studies of oligonucleotides modified with N-2-acetylaminofluorene, J. Mol. Biol. 62;331.

NERY, R., 1968, Some aspects of the metabolism of urethane and N-hydroxy urethane in rodents, Biochem. J. 106:1.

NERY, R., 1969, Acylation of cytosine by ethyl N-hydrocarbamate and its acyl derivatives and the binding of these agents to nucleic acids and proteins, J. Chem. Soc. Section E 1860.

O'CONNOR, P. J., CAPPS, M. J., CRAIG, A. W., LAWLEY, P. D., AND SHAH, S. A., 1972, Differences in the patterns of methylation in rat liver ribosomal ribonucleic acid after reaction in vivo with methyl methanesulfonate and N,N-dimethylnitrosamine, Biochem. J. 129:519.

O'CONNOR, P. J., CAPPS, M. J., AND CRAIG, A. W., 1973, Comparative studies of the hepatocarcinogen N,N-dimethylnitrosamine in vivo: Reaction sites in rat liver DNA and the significance of their relative stabilities, Brit. J. Cancer 27:153.

OREMEROD, M. G., AND LEHMANN, A. R., 1971, Artifacts arising from the sedimentation of high molecular weight DNA on sucrose gradients, Biochim. Biophys. Acta 247:369.

ORTWERTH, B. J., AND NOVELLI, D. G., 1969, Studies on the incorporation of L-ethionine-ethyl-1-$^{14}$C into the transfer RNA of rat liver, Cancer Res. 29:380.

PAINTER, R. B., 1970, Repair of DNA in mammalian cells, Curr. Topics Radiation Res. 7:45.

PARODI, S., AND SARMA, D. S. R., 1973, Unpublished observations.

PAUL, H. E., AND PAUL, M. F., 1964, The nitrofurans—chemotherapeutic properties, in: Experimental Chemotherapy, Vol. II (R. J. Schnitzer and F. Hawkins, eds.), p. 307, Academic Press, New York.

PAUL, J. S., MONTGOMERY, P. O'B., JR., AND LOUIS, J. B., 1971, A proposed model of the interaction of 4-nitroquinoline 1-oxide with DNA, Cancer Res. 31:413.

PAULING, L., 1970, General Chemistry, Freeman, San Fransisco.

PEDRALINOY, G. C. F., SPADARI, S., CIARROCCHI, G., PEDRINI, A. M., AND FALASCHI, A., 1973, Two forms of the DNA ligase of human cells, Europ. J. Biochem. 39:343.

PEGG, A. E., 1972, Ethylation of rat liver t-RNA after administration of L-ethionine, Biochem. J. 128:59.

PEGG, A. E., 1973, Alkylation of transfer RNA by N-methyl-N-nitrosourea and N-ethyl-N-nitrosourea, Chem.-Biol. Interact. 6:393.

PERRY, R. P., AND KELLY, D. E., 1974, Existence of methylated messenger RNA in mouse L cells, Cell 1:37.

PITOT, H. C., AND HEIDELBERGER, C., 1963, Metabolic regulatory circuits and carcinogenesis, Cancer Res. 23:1694.

POCHON, F., AND MICHELSON, A. M., 1971, Action of the carcinogen 7-bromomethylbenz(a)anthracene on synthetic polynucleotides, Europ. J. Biochem. 21:144.

POIRIER, L. A., MILLER, J. A., MILLER, E. C., AND SATO, K., 1967, N-Benzoyloxy-N-methyl-4-aminoazobenzene: Its carcinogenic activity in the rat and its reactions with proteins, nucleic acids and their constituents in vitro, Cancer Res. 27:1600.

PONG, R. S., AND WOGAN, G. N., 1970, Time course and dose–response characteristics of aflatoxin B$_1$ effects on rat liver RNA polymerase and ultrastructure, Cancer Res. 30:294.

POWERS, D. M., AND HOLLEY, R. W., 1972, Selective chemical methylation of yeast alanine transfer RNA, Biochim. Biophys. Acta 287:456.

PREUSSMANN, R., DRUCKREY, H., IVANKOVIC, S., AND HODENBERG, A. V., 1967, Chemical structure and carcinogenicity of aliphatic hydrazo, azo, and azoxy compounds and of triazenes, potential in vivo alkylating agents, Ann. N.Y. Acad. Sci. 163:697.

PRODI, G., ROCCHI, P., AND GRILLI, S., 1970a, In vivo interaction of urethan with nucleic acids and proteins, Cancer Res. 30:2887.

PRODI, G., ROCCHI, P., AND GRILLI, S., 1970b, Binding of 7,12-dimethylbenz(a)anthracene and benzopyrene to nucleic acids and proteins of organs in rats, Cancer Res. 30:1020.

PULLMAN, B., AND PULLMAN, A., 1959, The electronic structure of the purine pyrimidine pairs of DNA, Biochim. Biophys. Acta 36:343.

RABES, H., HARTENSTEIN, R., AND SCHOLZE, P., 1970, Specific stages of cellular response to homeostatic control during diethylnitrosamine-induced carcinogenesis, Experientia 26:1356.

RAJALAKSHMI, S., AND FARBER, E., 1973, DNA synthesis in liver of rats treated with DMN, Fed. Proc. 32:833.

RAJALAKSHMI, S., AND SARMA, D. S. R., 1973, Rapid repair of hepatic DNA damage induced by camptothecin in the intact rat, Biochem. Biophys. Res. Commun. 53:1268.

RAMANATHAN, R., SARMA, D. S. R., RAJALAKSHMI, S., AND FARBER, E., 1974, Unpublished observations.

REINER, B., AND ZAMENHOF, 1957, Studies on the chemically reactive groups of deoxyribonucleic acids, *J. Biol. Chem.* **228**:475.

RHAESE, H. J., AND FREESE, E., 1969, Chemical analysis of DNA alteration. IV. Reaction of oligodeoxynucleotides with monofunctional alkylating agents leading to backbone breakage, *Biochim. Biophys. Acta* **190**:418.

ROBERTS, J. J., 1969, The binding of metabolites of 4-dimethylaminoazobenzene and 2-methyl-4-dimethylaminoazobenzene to hooded rat macromolecules during chronic feeding, in: *Physico-chemical Mechanisms of Carcinogenesis* (E. Bergmann and B. Pullman, eds.), p. 229, Vol. 1 of *The Jerusalem Symposia on Quantum Chemistry and Biochemistry*, Israel Academy of Sciences and Humanities, Jerusalem.

ROBERTS, J. J., 1972, Repair of alkylated DNA in mammalian cells, in: *Molecular and Cellular Repair Processes* (R. F. Beers, R. M. Herriott, and R. C. Tilghman, eds.), p. 226, Johns Hopkins University Press, Baltimore.

ROBERTS, J. J., AND WARWICK, G. P., 1961, Reaction of $^3$H-labelled butter yellow *in vivo* and N-hydroxy-methylaminoazobenzene *in vitro*, *Biochem. J.* **93**:1897.

ROBERTS, J. J., AND WARWICK, G. P., 1963, The reaction of β-propiolactone with guanosine, deoxyguanylic acid and RNA, *Biochem. Pharmacol.* **12**:1441.

ROBERTS, J. J., AND WARWICK, G. P., 1966, The covalent binding of metabolites of di-methylaminoazobenzene, β-naphthylamine and aniline to nucleic acids *in vivo*, *Int. J. Cancer* **1**:179.

ROBERTS, J. J., PASCOE, J. M., SMITH, B. A., AND CRATHRON, A. R., 1971, Quantitative aspects of the repair of alkylated DNA in cultured mammalian cells. II. Non-semiconservative DNA synthesis ("repair synthesis") in HeLa and Chinese hamster cells following treatment with alkylating agents, *Chem.-Biol. Interact.* **3**:49.

ROSEN, L., 1968, Ethylation *in vivo* of purines in rat liver t-RNA by L-ethionine, *Biochem. Biophys. Res. Commun.* **33**:546.

ROSS, A. E., KEEFER, L., AND LIJINSKY, W., 1971, Alkylation of nucleic acids of rat liver and lung by deuterated N-nitrosodiethylamine *in vivo*, *J. Natl. Cancer Inst.* **47**:789.

RUPP, W. P., AND HOWARD-FLANDERS, P., 1968, Discontinuities in the DNA synthesized in an excision-defective strain of *Escherichia coli* following ultraviolet irradiation, *J. Mol. Biol.* **31**:291.

RYSKOV, A. P., FARASHYAN, V. R., AND GEORGIEV, G. P., 1972, Ribonuclease-stable base sequences specific exclusively for giant dRNA, *Biochim. Biophys. Acta* **262**:568.

SARMA, D. S. R., MICHAEL, R. O., STEWART, B. W., COX, R., AND DAMJANOV, I., 1973a, Patterns of damage and repair of rat liver DNA induced by chemical carcinogens *in vivo*, *Fed. Proc.* **32**:833.

SARMA, D. S. R., RAJALAKSHMI, S., AND HADJILOV, D., 1973b, Unpublished observations.

SARMA, D. S. R., ZUBROFF, J., AND RAJALAKSHMI, S., 1973c, Unpublished observations.

SARMA, D. S. R., RAJALAKSHMI, S., AND FARBER, 1974, DNA repair in chemical carcinogenesis, *Biochim. Biophys. Acta. Cancer Rev.*, in press.

SASAKI, T., AND YOSHIDA, T., 1935, Production of carcinoma of the liver by feeding O-aminoazotoluene, *Arch. Pathol. Anat.* **295**:175.

SCAIFE, J. F., 1970/1971, Aflatoxin B$_1$: Cytotoxic mode of action evaluated by mammalian cell cultures, *FEBS Letters* **12**:143.

SCHABORT, J. C., 1971, The differential interaction of aflatoxin B$_2$ with deoxyribonucleic acids from different sources and with purines and purine nucleosides, *Chem.-Biol.Interact.* **3**:371.

SCHNEIDER, J. H., CASSIR, R., AND CHORDIKON, F., 1960, Inhibition of incorporation of thymidine into DNA by amino acid antagonists *in vivo*, *J. Biol. Chem.* **235**:1437.

SCHNEIDER, W. C., AND KUFF, E. L., 1965, The isolation and some properties of rat liver mitochondrial deoxyribonucleic acid, *Proc. Natl. Acad. Sci.* **54**:1650.

SCHULZ, U., AND McCALLA, D. R., 1969, Reactions of cysteine with N-methyl-N-nitroso-P-toluene sulfonamide and N-methyl-N'-nitro-N-nitrosoguanidine, *Canad. J. Biochem.* **47**:2021.

SCHWARTZ, A. G., 1973, The protective effect of estradiol-17β against polycyclic hydrocarbon cytotoxicity, *Cancer Res.* **33**:2431.

SELKIRK, J. K., HUBERMAN, E., AND HEIDELBERGER, C., 1971, An epoxide is an intermediate in the microsomal metabolism of the chemical carcinogen, dibenz(a,h)anthracene, *Biochem. Biophys. Res. Commun.* **43**:1010.

SETLOW, R. B., 1968, The photochemistry, photobiology and repair of polynucleotides, *Prog. Nucl. Acid Res. Mol. Biol.* **8**:257.

SETLOW, R. B., AND REGAN, J. D., 1972, Defective repair of N-acetoxy-2-acetylaminofluorene-induced lesions in the DNA of xeroderma pigmentosum, *Biochem. Biophys. Res. Commun.* **46**:1019.

283

INTERAC-
TIONS OF
CARCINOGENS
WITH NUCLEIC
ACIDS

284

D. S. R. SARMA,
S. RAJALAKSHMI
AND
EMMANUEL
FARBER

SHANK, R. C., AND MAGEE, P. N., 1967, Similarities between the biochemical actions of cycasin and dimethylnitrosamine, *Biochem. J.* **105**:521.

SHAPIRO, R., 1968, Chemistry of guanine and its biologically significant derivatives, *Prog. Nucl. Acid Res. Mol. Biol.* **8**:73.

SHAPIRO, R., 1969, Reactions with purines and pyrimidines, *Ann. N.Y. Acad. Sci.* **163**:624.

SHOOTER, K. V., HOUSE, R., AND MERRIFIELD, K., 1974a, Biological effects of phosphotriester formation, *Biochem. J.* **137**:313.

SHOOTER, K. V., HOUSE, R., SHAH, S. A., AND LAWLEY, P. O., 1974b, The molecular basis for biological interaction of nucleic acid: The activity of methylating agents on the RNA containing bacteriophage R-17, *Biochem. J.* **137**:303.

SHULL, K. H., 1962, Hepatic phosphorylase and adenosine triphosphate levels in ethionine treated rats, *J. Biol. Chem.* **237**:P.C.1734.

SHULL, K. H., McCONOMY, J., VOGT, M., CASTILLO, A., AND FARBER, E., 1966, On the mechanism of induction of hepatic adenosine triphosphate deficiency by ethionine, *J. Biol. Chem.* **241**:5060.

SIMARD, A., AND DAOUST, R., 1966, DNA synthesis and neoplastic transformation in rat liver parenchyma, *Cancer Res.* **26**:1665.

SIMARD, A., COUSINEAU, G., AND DAOUST, R., 1968, Variations in the cell cycle during azo dye hepatocarcinogenesis, *J. Natl. Cancer Inst.* **41**:1257.

SIMS, P., AND GROVER, P. L., 1968, Quantitative aspects of the metabolism of 7,12-dimethylbenz(a)anthracene by liver homogenates from animals of different age, sex and species, *Biochem. Pharmacol.* **17**:1751.

SINGER, S., AND FRAENKEL-CONRAT, H., 1969, Chemical modification of viral ribonucleic acid. VIII. The chemical and biological effects of methylating agents and nitrosoguanidine on tobacco mosaic virus, *Biochemistry* **8**:3266.

SMITH, J. D., AND DUNN, D. B., 1959, The occurrence of methylated guanines in ribonucleic acids from several sources, *Biochem. J.* **72**:294.

SMITH, R. C., AND SALMON, W. D., 1965, Formation of S-adenosylethionine by ethionine-treated rats, *Arch. Biochem. Biophys.* **111**:191.

SMUCKLER, E. A., AND KOPLITZ, M., 1969, The effects of carbon tetrachloride and ethionine on RNA synthesis *in vivo* and in isolated rat liver nuclei, *Arch. Biochem. Biophys.* **132**:62.

SNYDER, A. L., KANN, H. E., JR., AND KOHN, K. W., 1971, Inhibition of the processing of ribosomal precursor RNA by intercalating agents, *J. Mol. Biol.* **5**:555.

SPATZ, M., AND LAQUEUR, G. L., 1967, Transplacental induction of tumours in Sprague-Dawley rats with crude cycad material, *J. Natl. Cancer Inst.* **38**:233.

SPORN, M. B., DINGMAN, C. W., PHELPS, H. L., AND WOGAN, G. N., 1966, Aflatoxin $B_1$: Binding to DNA *in vitro* and alteration of RNA metabolism *in vivo*, *Science* **151**:1539.

STACEY, K. A., COFF, M., COUSENS, S. F., AND ALEXANDER, P., 1957/1958, The reactions of the "radiomimetic" alkylating agents with macromolecules *in vitro*, *Ann. N.Y. Acad. Sci.* **68**:682.

STEKOL, J. A., 1965, in: *Transmethylation and Methionine Biosynthesis* (S. K. Shapiro and F. Schiewk, eds.), p. 231, University of Chicago Press, Chicago.

STEKOL, J. A., MODY, U., AND PERRY, J., 1960, The incorporation of the carbon of the ethyl group of ethionine into liver nucleic acids and the effect of ethionine feeding on the content of nucleic acids in rat liver, *J. Biol. Chem.* **235**:P.C.54.

STEVENS, R. H., AND WILLIAMSON, A. R., 1972, Specific IgG mRNA molecules from myeloma cells in heterogeneous nuclear and cytoplasmic RNA containing poly-A, *Nature (Lond.)* **239**:143.

STEWART, B. W., AND FARBER, E., 1973a, Unpublished observations.

STEWART, B. W., AND FARBER, E., 1973b, Strand breakage in rat liver DNA and its repair following administration of cyclic nitrosamines, *Cancer Res.* **33**:3209.

STEWART, B. W., AND MAGEE, P. N., 1971, Effect of single dose of dimethylnitrosamine on biosynthesis of nucleic acid and protein in rat liver and kidney, *Biochem. J.* **125**:943.

STEWART, B. W., AND MAGEE, P. N., 1972, Metabolism and some biochemical effects of N-nitrosomorpholine, *Biochem. J.* **126**:21P.

STEWART, B. W., FARBER, E., AND MIRVISH, S. S., 1973, Induction by an hepatic carcinogen, 1-nitroso-5,6-dihydrouracil, of single and double strand breaks of liver DNA with rapid repair, *Biochem. Biophys. Res. Commun.* **53**:773.

STICH, H. F., SAN, R. H., MILLER, J. A., AND MILLER, E. C., 1972, Various levels of DNA repair synthesis in xeroderma pigmentosum cells exposed to the carcinogens N-hydroxy- and N-acetoxy-2-acetylaminofluorene, *Nature New Biol.* **238**:9.

285

INTERAC-
TIONS OF
CARCINOGENS
WITH NUCLEIC
ACIDS

STRAUSS, B. S., 1968, DNA repair mechanisms and their relation to mutation and recombination, *Cur. Topics Microbiol. Immunol.* **44**:1.

SUGIMURA, T., OKABE, K., AND NAGAO, M., 1966, The metabolism of 4-nitroquinoline-1-oxide, a carcinogen. III. An enzyme catalysing the conversion of 4-nitroquinoline-1-oxide to 4-hydroxyaminoquinoline-1-oxide in rat liver and hepatomas, *Cancer Res.* **26**:1717.

SUGINO, A., AND OKAZAKI, R., 1973, RNA-linked DNA fragments *in vitro, Proc. Natl. Acad. Sci.* **70**:88.

SUGIURA, K., TELLER, M. N., PARHAM, J. C., AND BROWN, G. B., 1970, A comparison of the oncogenicities of 3-hydroxyxanthine, guanine-3-*N*-oxide and some related compounds, *Cancer Res.* **30**:184.

SUNDERMAN, F. W., JR., 1968, Nickel carcinogenesis, *Dis. Chest* **54**:41.

SUNDERMAN, F. W., JR., AND ESTAHANI, M., 1968, Nickel carbonyl inhibition of RNA polymerase activity in hepatic nuclei, *Cancer Res.* **28**:2565.

SVOBODA, D., AND REDDY, J., 1970, Invasive tumors induced in rats with actinomycin D, *Cancer Res.* **30**:2771.

SWAN, P. F., AND MAGEE, P. N., 1968, Nitrosamine-induced carcinogenesis: the alkylation of nucleic acids of the rat by *N*-methyl-*N*-nitrosourea, dimethylnitrosamine, dimethyl sulfate and methyl-methanesulphonate. *Biochem. J.* **110**:39.

SWAN, P. F., AND MAGEE, P. N., 1971, The alkylation of N-7 of guanine of nucleic acids of the rat by diethylnitrosamine, *N*-ethyl-*N*-nitrosourea and ethylmethane-suphonate. *Biochem. J.* **125**:841.

SWANN, P. F., PEGG, A. E., HAWKS, A., FARBER, E., AND MAGEE, P. N., 1971, Evidence for ethylation of rat liver deoxyribonucleic acid after administration of ethionine, *Biochem. J.* **123**:175.

SWENSON, D. H., MILLER, J. A., AND MILLER, E. C., 1973, 2,3-Dihydro-2,3-dihydroxy-aflatoxin B$_1$: An acid hydrolysis product of an RNA–aflatoxin B$_1$ adduct formed by hamster and rat liver microsomes *in vitro, Biochem. Biophys. Res. Commun.* **53**:1260.

SZAFARZ, D., AND WEISBURGER, J. H., 1969, Stability of binding of label from *N*-hydroxy-*N*-2-fluorenylacetamide to intracellular targets, particularly deoxyribonucleic acid in rat, *Cancer Res.* **29**:962.

TADA, M., AND TADA, M., 1971, Interaction of a carcinogen, 4-nitroquinoline-1-oxide, with nucleic acids: Chemical degradation of the adducts, *Chem.-Biol. Interact.* **3**:225.

TADA, M., AND TADA, M., 1972, Enzymatic activation of the carcinogen 4-hydroxyaminoquinoline-1-oxide and its interaction with cellular macromolecules, *Biochem. Biophys. Res. Commun.* **46**:1025.

TADA, M., TADA, M., AND TAKADASHI, T., 1967, Interaction of a carcinogen, 4-hydroxy-aminoquinoline 1-oxide with nucleic acids, *Biochem. Biophys. Res. Commun.* **29**:469.

TROLL, W., BELMAN, S., AND LEVINE, E., 1963, The effects of metabolites of 2-naphthylamines and the mutagen hydroxylamine on the thermal stability of DNA and polyribonucleotides, *Cancer Res.* **23**:841.

TROLL, W., BELMAN, S., BERKOWITZ, E., CHIEMLEWICZ, Z. F., AMBRUS, J. L., AND BARDOS, T. J., 1968, Differential responses of DNA and RNA polymerase to modifications of the template rat liver DNA caused by action of the carcinogen acetylaminofluorene *in vivo* and *in vitro, Biochim. Biophys. Acta* **157**:16.

TROLL, W., RINDE, E., AND DAY, P., 1969, Effect on N-7 and C-8 substitution of guanine in DNA on $T_m$, buoyant density and RNA polymerase priming, *Biochim. Biophys. Acta* **174**:211.

TROSKO, J. E., FRANK, P., CHU, E. H. Y., AND BECKER, J. E., 1973, Caffeine inhibition of post-replication repair of *N*-acetoxy-2-acetylaminofluorene damaged DNA in Chinese hamster cells, *Cancer Res.* **33**:2444.

TS'O, P. O. P., LESKO, S. A., AND UMANS, R. S., 1969, The physical binding and the chemical linkage of benzpyrene to nucleotides, nucleic-acids and nucleohistones, in: *Physico-chemical Mechanisms of Carcinogenesis* (E. D. Bergmann and B. Pullman, eds.), p. 106, Vol. 1 of *The Jerusalem Symposia on Quantum Chemistry and Biochemistry*, Israel Academy of Sciences and Humanities, Jerusalem.

TSUKADA, K., AND ICHIMURA, M., 1971, Polynucleotide ligase from rat liver after partial hepatectomy, *Biochem. Biophys. Res. Commun.* **42**:1156.

TSUKADA, K., HOKARI, S., HAYASAKI, N., AND ITO, N., 1972, Increased activity of polynucleotide ligase from rat hepatoma induced by *N*-2-fluorenylacetamide, *Cancer Res.* **32**:886.

VAN DUUREN, B. L., GOLDSCHMIDT, B. M., AND SELTZMAN, H. H., 1968/1969, The interaction of mutagenic and carcinogenic agents with nucleic acids, *Ann. N.Y. Acad. Sci.* **153**:744.

VAN LANCKER, J. L., AND TOMURA, T., 1972, A mammalian DNA repair endonuclease, *Proc. Am. Assoc. Cancer Res.* **13**:122.

286

D. S. R. SARMA,
S. RAJALAKSHMI
AND
EMMANUEL
FARBER

VASILIEV, J. M., AND GUELSTEIN, V. I., 1963, Sensitivity of normal and neoplastic cells to the damaging action of carcinogenic substances: A review, *J. Natl. Cancer Inst.* **31:**1123.

VENITT, S., BROOKES, P., AND LAWLEY, P. D., 1968, Effects of alkylating agents on the induced synthesis of β-galactosidase by *Escherichia coli* B$_{s-1}$, *Biochim. Biophys. Acta* **155:**521.

VERLY, W. G., AND PAQUETTE, Y., 1973, An endonuclease for depurinated DNA in rat liver, *Canad. J. Biochem.* **51:**1003.

VERLY, W. G., PAQUETTE, Y., AND THIBODEAU, L., 1973, Nuclease for DNA apurinic sites may be involved in the maintenance of DNA in normal cells, *Nature New Biol.* **244:**67.

VILLA-TREVINO, S., SHULL, K. H., AND FARBER, E., 1963, The role of adenosine triphosphate deficiency in ethionine-induced inhibition of protein synthesis, *J. Biol. Chem.* **238:**1757.

VILLA-TREVINO, S., SHULL, K. H., AND FARBER, E., 1966, The inhibition of liver ribonucleic acid synthesis by ethionine, *J. Biol. Chem.* **241:**4670.

WAGNER, L., AND DREWS, J., 1970, The effect of aflatoxin B$_1$ on RNA synthesis and breakdown in normal and regenerating rat liver, *Europ. J. Cancer* **6:**465.

WAGNER, T. A., 1971, Physical studies on the interaction of lysergic acid diethylamide and trypanocidal dyes with DNA and DNA-containing genetic material, in: *Progress in Molecular and Subcellular Biology*, Vol. 2 (F. E. Hahn, ed.), p. 152, Springer, New York.

WALKER, I. G., AND EWART, D. F., 1973, The nature of single strand breaks in DNA following treatment of L-cells with methylating agents, *Mutation Res.* **19:**331.

WALPOLE, A. L., ROBERTS, D. C., ROSE, F. L., HENDRY, J. A., AND HOMER, R. F., 1954, Cytotoxic agents. IV. The carcinogenic actions of some monofunctional ethyleneimine derivatives, *Brit. J. Pharmacol. Chemother.* **9:**306.

WARWICK, G. P., 1967, The covalent binding of metabolites of tritiated 2-methyl-4-dimethylaminoazobenzene to rat liver nucleic acids and proteins and the carcinogenicity of the unlabelled compound in partially hepatectomized rats, *Europ. J. Cancer* **3:**227.

WARWICK, G. P., 1969, The covalent-binding of metabolites of 4-dimethylaminoazobenzene to liver nucleic acids *in vivo*: The possible role of cell proliferation in cancer initiation, in: *Physico-chemical mechanisms of Carcinogenesis* (E. Bergmann and B. Pullman, eds.), p. 218, Vol. 1 of *The Jerusalem Symposia on Quantum Chemistry and Biochemistry*, Israel Academy of Sciences and Humanities, Jerusalem.

WARWICK, G. P., AND ROBERTS, J. J., 1967, Persistent binding of butter yellow metabolites to rat liver DNA, *Nature (Lond.)* **213:**1206.

WEINSTEIN, I. B., 1970, Modifications in transfer RNA during chemical carcinogenesis, in: *Genetic concepts and Neoplasia*, p. 380, University of Texas M. D. Anderson Hospital and Tumor Institute, Williams and Wilkins, Baltimore.

WEINSTEIN, I. B., AND HERSCHBERG, E., 1971, Mode of action of miracil D, in: *Progress in Molecular and Subcellular Biology*, Vol. 2 (F. E. Hahn, ed.), p. 232, Springer, New York.

WEINSTEIN, I. B., GRUNBERGER, D., FUJIMURA, S., AND FINK, L. M., 1971, Chemical carcinogens and RNA, *Cancer Res.* **31:**651.

WEISBURGER, J. H., AND WEISBURGER, E. K., 1973, Biochemical formation and pharmacological, toxicological, and pathological properties of hydroxylamines and hydroxamic acids, *Pharmacol. Rev.* **25:**1.

WEISBURGER, J. H., YAMAMOTO, R. S., WILLIAMS, G. M., GRANTHAM, P. H., MATSUSHIMA, T., AND WEISBURGER, E. K., 1972, On the sulfate ester of *N*-hydroxy-*N*-2-fluorenylaceamide as a key ultimate hepatocarcinogen in the rat, *Cancer Res.* **32:**491.

WELLS, R. D., 1971, The binding of actinomycin D to DNA, in: *Progress in Molecular and Subcellular Biology*, Vol. 2 (F. E. Hahn, ed.), p. 21, Springer, New York.

WHEELER, K. T., AND LETT, J. T., 1972, Formation and rejoining of DNA strand breaks in irradiated neurons: *In vivo, Radiation Res.* **52:**59.

WIEBEL, F. J., MATTHEWS, E. G., AND GELBOIN, H. V., 1972, Ribonucleic acid synthesis-dependent induction of aryl hydrocarbon hydroxylase in the absence of ribosomal ribonucleic acid synthesis and transfer, *J. Biol. Chem.* **242:**4711.

WILK, M., AND GIRKE, W., 1969, Radical cation of carcinogenesis alternant hydrocarbons, amines, and azodyes and their reactions with nucleobases, in: *Physico-chemical Mechanisms of Carcinogenesis* (E. D. Bergmann and B. Pullman, eds.), p. 91, Vol. 1 of *The Jerusalem Symposia on Quantum Chemistry and Biochemistry*, Israel Academy of Sciences and Humanities, Jerusalem.

WILLIAMS, K., AND NERY, R., 1971, Aspects of the mechanism of urethane carcinogenesis, *Xenobiotica* **1:**545.

287
INTERAC-
TIONS OF
CARCINOGENS
WITH NUCLEIC
ACIDS

WISLOCKI, P. G., BORCHERT, P., MILLER, E. C., AND MILLER, J. A., 1973, Further studies on the metabolism and carcinogenicity of safrole, *Proc. Am. Assoc. Cancer Res.* **14:**19.

WITSCHI, H., EPSTEIN, S. M., AND FARBER, E., 1971, Influence of liver regeneration on the loss of fluorenylacetamide derivative bound to liver DNA, *Cancer Res.* **31:**270.

WU, Y. S., AND SMUCKLER, A. E., 1971, The acute effect of aminoazobenzene and some of its derivatives on RNA polymerase activity in isolated rat liver nuclei, *Cancer Res.* **31:**239.

WUNDERLICH, V., SCHÜTT, M., BÖTTGER, M., AND GRAFFI, A., 1970, Preferential alkylation of mitochondrial deoxyribonucleic acid by $N$-methyl-$N$-nitrosourea, *Biochem. J.* **118:**99.

WUNDERLICH, V., TEZLAFF, I., AND GRAFFI, A., 1971/1972, Studies on nitrosodimethylamine: Preferential methylation of mitochondrial DNA in rats and hamsters, *Chem.-Biol. Interact.* **4:**81.

YANG, J. T., AND SAMEJIMA, T., 1969, Optical rotary dispersion and circular dichroism of nucleic acids, in: *Progress in Nucleic Acid Research and Molecular Biology*, Vol. 9, p. 224, Academic Press, New York.

YOUNGER, L. R., SALMON, R., WILSON, R. W., PEACOCK, A. C., AND GELBOIN, H. V., 1972, Effects of polycyclic hydrocarbons on ribonucleic acid synthesis in rat liver nuclei and hamster embryo cells, *Mol. Pharmacol.* **8:**452.

YUSPA, S. H., AND BATES, R. R., 1970, The binding of benz($a$)anthracene to replicating and non-replicating DNA in cell culture, *Proc. Soc. Exp. Biol. Med.* **135:**732.

ZAHNER, A., RAJALAKSHMI, S., AND SARMA, D. S. R., 1973, Unpublished observations.

ZEDEK, M. S., STEINBERG, S. S., POYNTER, R. N., AND MCGOWAN, J., 1970, Biochemical and pathological effects of methylazoxymethanol-acetate—A potent carcinogen, *Cancer Res.* **30:**801.

ZEIGER, R. S., SALOMON, R., KINOSHITA, N., AND PEACOCK, A. C., 1972, The binding of 9,10-dimethyl-1,2-benzanthracene to mouse epidermal satelite DNA *in vivo*, *Cancer Res.* **32:**643.

ZIEVE, F. J., 1972, Inhibition of rat liver ribonucleic acid polymerase by the carcinogen $N$-hydroxy-2-fluorenylacetamide, *J. Biol. Chem.* **247:**5987.

ZIEVE, F. J., 1973, Effects of the carcinogen $N$-acetoxy-2-fluorenylacetamide on the template properties of deoxyribonucleic acid, *Mol. Pharmacol.* **9:**658.

# 9

# Some Effects of Chemical Carcinogens on Cell Organelles

DONALD SVOBODA AND JANARDAN REDDY

## 1. Introduction

There is no single ultrastructural feature that distinguishes the malignant cell from its normal counterpart, and, with some exceptions, the premalignant state, although conceptually useful, has not been identifiable morphologically. Nevertheless, ultrastructural studies of tissues and cells from animals given chemical carcinogens have disclosed many early, intermediate, and late alterations in cell structure that have helped to clarify the biological interaction between a carcinogen or its metabolite and specific organelles. In addition, such studies have made possible comparisons between the cellular responses to carcinogenic injury and other forms of cell damage, thereby placing the problem of carcinogenesis in an appropriately larger biological perspective. Although morphological description of the responses of cells to carcinogens cannot substitute for biochemical analysis of the significance of such responses, nonetheless descriptive morphology serves as a useful step preliminary to other forms of investigation.

Investigations dealing with the effects of several carcinogens on the ultrastructure of rat liver have been reviewed in some detail previously (Svoboda and Higginson, 1968). These investigations, made prior to 1968, will be summarized briefly in this chapter. In addition, more recent studies of ultrastructural responses to carcinogens, those published since 1968, will be discussed, with

DONALD SVOBODA AND JANARDAN REDDY ● Department of Pathology, University of Kansas Medical Center, Kansas City, Kansas.

TABLE 1

*Design of Study of Acute Effects of Selected Chemical Carcinogens on Rat Liver Cells*

| Agent | Dose and route | Time of liver biopsy and sacrifice (hours) |
|---|---|---|
| Aflatoxin $B_1$ | 0.45 mg/kg (p.o.) | 24, 48, 72* |
| Diethylnitrosamine | 140 mg/kg (i.p.) | 24, 48, 72 |
| Dimethylnitrosamine | 22.5 mg/kg (i.p.) | 24, 48, 72 |
| Ethionine | 1 mg/g (i.p.) | 12, 24 |
| Lasiocarpine | 80 mg/kg (i.p.) | 1, 4, 6, 8, 12, 24, 48, 72 |
| 3'-Methyl-4-dimethylaminoazobenzene | 300 mg/kg (o.o.) | 24, 48 |
| Tannic acid | 700 mg/kg (s.c.) | 1, 3, 6, 12, 18, 24, 48, 72, 120 |
| Thioacetamide | 60 mg/kg (i.p.) | 18, 24, 48 |

* Two animals were studied at each interval with every agent.

emphasis on familiar chemical carcinogens and their effects on rat liver since this is the system that has been most used in the authors' laboratories as well as by others. For convenience and brevity, routes and doses as well as intervals of sacrifice are given in Table 1, while comparisons of morphological effects of the respective carcinogens are included in Tables 2, 3, and 4.

## 2. The Carcinogens

The carcinogens, dosages, routes of administration, and intervals of sacrifice for acute experiments that are used in our laboratories are given in Table 1. The most conspicuous and consistent light microscopic changes are listed in Table 2.

The early histological changes were found to include nuclear enlargement with dimethylnitrosamine (DMN) and thioacetamide and increase in number of nucleoli with ethionine. Decreased basophilia of centrilobular parenchymal cells and of the peripheral zone was apparent with tannic acid and aflatoxin $B_1$, respectively, while cells with increased acidophilia were present after thioacetamide and diethylnitrosamine (DEN). Lysosomes were conspicuous as PAS-positive cytoplasmic globules following lasiocarpine, while cytoplasmic swelling followed 3'-methyldimethylaminoazobenzene (3'-Me-DAB). Most of the carcinogens caused slight to moderate necrosis and a variable degree of inflammatory cellular infiltrate.

The acute ultrastructural changes in rat liver cells following administration of the respective carcinogens are summarized in Table 3. All carcinogens used caused increase in smooth endoplasmic reticulum (ER) and detachment of ribosomes from the rough ER (Figs. 1 and 2), resulting in increased numbers of ribosomes free in the hyaloplasm (Fig. 3). Similarly, there was zonal or diffuse loss of glycogen and a variable increase in cytoplasmic fat with all of the carcinogens. The number of lysosomes appeared only slightly increased with most carcinogens. Mitochondria underwent variable degrees of swelling, and with thioacetamide and aflatoxin $B_1$ there were dense matrix granules resembling calcium in some

291

SOME EFFECTS
OF CHEMICAL
CARCINOGENS
ON CELL
ORGANELLES

TABLE 2

Light Microscopic Changes in Rat Liver after Acute Doses of Carcinogens

| Agent | Number of hours | Nucleus | Cytoplasm | Glycogen | Necrosis | Oval cell and bile duct proliferation | Fat | Cell infiltration |
|---|---|---|---|---|---|---|---|---|
| Aflatoxin B$_1$ | 24–72 | | Decreased basophilia (P) | Decreased (P & M) | + (P) | ± | | Neutrophils and mononuclear (P) |
| Diethylnitrosamine | 24–72 | | Acidophilic cells (F) | Decreased (C) | Hemorrhagic ++ (C) | | | Macrophages, neutrophils (C) |
| Dimethylnitrosamine | 24–72 | Enlarged | Vacuoles (M & P) | Decreased (C) | ++ (C) | | | Neutrophils (C) |
| Ethionine | 24 | Increased numbers of nucleoli | Slight diffuse vacuolization | | | | | |
| Lasiocarpine | 24 | | Periodic acid-Schiff globules; swelling | Decreased | + (C) | | | |
| 3'-Methyldimethyl-aminoazobenzene | 24–28 | | Swelling | Decreased | | | | Mononuclear (C) |
| Tannic acid | 12–72 | | Decreased basophilia (C) | Decreased | + (C & F) | | + | Neutrophils (C) |
| Thioacetamide | 24–48 | Enlarged | Acidophilic cells (C) | Decreased | + (C) | ± | | |

P = peripheral zone; M = midzone; C = central zone; F = focal.

TABLE 3

*Early Ultrastructural Changes in Liver Cells Produced by Hepatocarcinogens (up to 72 h)*

| Carcinogen | Nucleolus | Nucleoplasm | Rough endoplasmic reticulum | Smooth endoplasmic reticulum | Golgi |
|---|---|---|---|---|---|
| Aflatoxin B₁ | Macrosegregation | Increased inter-chromatin granules | Detachment of ribosomes | Increase ++ Concentric association with glycogen | |
| Diethylnitro-samine | | | Detachment of ribosomes | Increase + | |
| Dimethyl-nitrosamine | Microsegregation | | Detachment of ribosomes | Increase + | |
| Ethionine | Microsegregation | Increased inter-chromatin granules | Detachment of ribosomes | Increase + | |
| Lasiocarpine | Macro- and micro-segregation | Increased interchromatin granules "Satellite" granules | Detachment of ribosomes; Extensive dilatation | Increase ++ | Dilated; numerous small, dense deposits |
| 3'-Methyldimethyl-aminoazobenzene | Macrosegregation | | Detachment of ribosomes | Increase ++ | |
| Tannic acid | Macrosegregation | Increased interchromatin granules; Iron containing inclusions | Detachment of ribosomes | Increase ++ | Slight dilatation |
| Thioacetamide | Increased granular component ++; microsegregation | Increased interchromatin granules | Detachment of ribosomes; polysomes conspicuous | Increase ++ | |

**293**

SOME EFFECTS
OF CHEMICAL
CARCINOGENS
ON CELL
ORGANELLES

| Mitochondria | Lysosomes | Microbodies | Glycogen | Fat | Remarks |
|---|---|---|---|---|---|
| Swelling + (centrolobular) Dense deposits (? calcium) Decrease or loss of matrix granules | Increase ++ | | Lost throughout most of lobule; slight centrolobular preservation | Medium to large globules ++ | |
| | Increase + | | Sharply demarcated centrolobular loss | Increase + | "Coated" vesicles++ |
| | | Moderate increase in number | Sharply demarcated centrolobular and periportal loss; retained in midzonal areas | Increase + | "Coated" vesicles++ interruptions in plasma membranes |
| Irregular swelling; not uniform in any single cell or from to cell | Increase +++ | | Uniform loss throughout all zones | Increase ++ | Nuclear changes throughout lobules; cytoplasmic changes primarily centrolobular |
| Focal mitochondrial swelling | Increase + | | Uniform decrease throughout all zones | Increase + | "Coated" vesicles |
| Slight swelling + | Increase + | | General loss at 6 h, restoration in periportal areas by 12 h | Increase ++ | Focal cytoplasmic necrosis most prominent in centrolobular zones |
| Dense deposits (? calcium) in occasional cells | Increase + | Moderate increase in number | Generally lost throughout lobule except for scattered midzonal cells | Increase + | |

TABLE 4

*Chronic Ultrastructural Changes Produced in Liver Cells by Hepatocarcinogens*

| Carcinogen | Nucleolus | Nucleoplasm | Rough endoplasmic reticulum | Smooth endoplasmic reticulum | Golgi |
|---|---|---|---|---|---|
| Aflatoxin $B_1$ | Microsegregation; slight | | Slight dilatation; detachment of ribosomes | Increased ++ | |
| Diethylnitrosamine | | | Detachment of ribosomes; polysomes conspicuous | Increased ++ | Dilated, empty vesicles |
| Dimethylnitrosamine | Multiple clumped and cord-like condensations of fibrillar component; microsegregation | Increased interchromatin granules + | Slight detachment of ribosomes | Small aggregates of vesicles ++ | Dilated, empty vesicles |
| Ethionine | Enlarged; involved both fibrillar and granular components Occasional nucleoli surrounded by a membrane | Marked increase in interchromatin granules ++ Cytoplasmic invaginations + Increased perichromatin granules + | Prominent detachment of ribosomes | Increased ++ | Dilated vesicles with dense droplets ++ |
| Lasiocarpine | Microsegregation in megalocytes | Increased interchromatin granules + Cytoplasmic invaginations | Dilatation; detachment of ribosomes | Increased ++ | Dilated vesicles |
| 3'-Methyldimethyl-aminoazobenzene | Occasional nucleoli with condensations of fibrillar component | Ribosomes | Detachment of close association | Increased ++; vacuoles; with glycogen; | Dilated, empty |
| Tannic acid | Enlargement (rare) | Increased interchromatin granules Iron-containing inclusions | Dilatation + detachment of ribosomes | Increased + | |
| Thioacetamide | Increased size; granular component; prominent "cavities" in nucleoli | Increased extent of interchromatic spaces | Detachment of ribisomes | Increased ++ | Dilated, empty vesicles |

| Mitochondria | Lysosomes | Microbodies | Glycogen | Fat | Remarks |
|---|---|---|---|---|---|
| Marked elongation of occasional profiles | + | | Patchy loss in scattered foci of enlarged, vacuolated cells | + | Occasional dilated bile canaliculi |
| Swollen (slight) | + | | Centrolobular loss | + | |
| Swollen: occasionally ruptured; decreased number and length of cristae, abnormal disposition of cristae; bizarre forms; paucity of matrix granules; interlocking protrusion and evaginations (all changes most marked in periportal zones) | + | Increased in some cells + | Patchy loss | ++ | |
| Matrix granules reduced or absent | + | | Moderate centrolobular loss | ++ | |
| Large circular dense deposits in matrix | | | | | |
| Variation in size and shape; scalloping of margins | ++ | | Decreased | + | |
| | + | | Decreased | Large vacuoles in close association with mitochondria | |
| | + | | Decreased | + | |
| Decreased number of matrix granules | + | Increased in some cells + | Centrolobular loss; cells lacking glycogen coincided with those having greatest degree of nucleolar enlargement | ++ | Annulate lamellae in many cells |

DONALD
SVOBODA
AND JANARDAN
REDDY

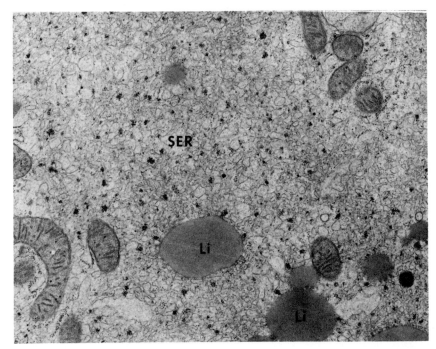

FIGURE 1. Portion of hepatocyte cytoplasm of a rat, following treatment with diethylnitrosamine. Marked proliferation of smooth endoplasmic reticulum (SER) is evident. Li, Lipid droplets. ×22,000.

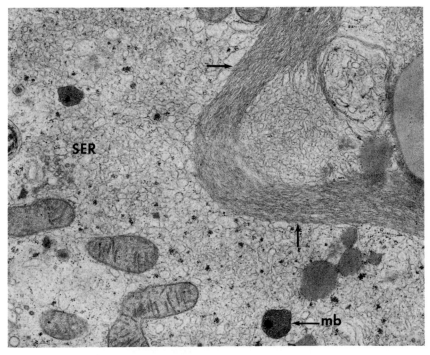

FIGURE 2. Diethylnitrosamine treatment. In several cells, the increase in SER is associated with the occurrence of myelin figures (arrows). mb, Microbody. ×22,000.

297

SOME EFFECTS
OF CHEMICAL
CARCINOGENS
ON CELL
ORGANELLES

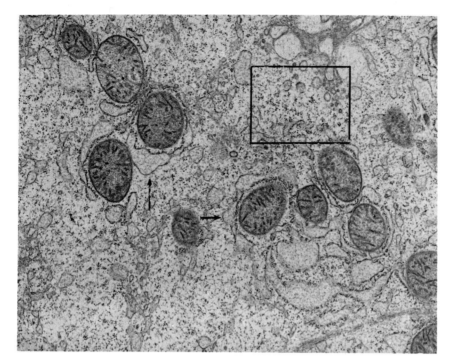

FIGURE 3. At 2 h following lasiocarpine administration, marked disaggregation of ribosomes occurs in liver cells. Free ribosomes are abundant in the area outlined. Rough endoplasmic reticulum channels are dilated and reveal areas devoid of ribosomes (arrows). ×15,000.

cells. The most uniform ultrastructural changes in the nucleus consisted of redistribution and rearrangement and/or quantitative differences in the fibrillar and granular components of the nucleolus (Figs. 4–9). For purposes of comparison, we have used the terms "macrosegregation," "microsegregation," and "nucleolar enlargement" to categorize and describe the nucleolar abnormalities in rat liver cells after administration of carcinogens. It should be pointed out that these terms need not imply qualitative or functional differences nor need they be mutually exclusive after administration of a single carcinogen.

Macrosegregation has also been termed "nucleolar capping." In this category, separation of granules and fibrils tended to occur in large, distinct, and relatively pure zones. Such changes were typical with aflatoxin $B_1$, lasiocarpine, 3'-Me-DAB, and tannic acid (Figs. 6–9). In most instances, the nucleolar diameter was smaller than normal. Microsegregation, on the other hand, designates a condition in which there were definite, compact condensations of the fibrillar component of the nucleolus. The condensations were multiple and irregular in size and shape, and tended to occur in interrupted or continuous plaquelike configurations either within or at the periphery of a dispersed nucleolus. Microsegregation was conspicuous with DMN (Fig. 10) at 6 days and with lasiocarpine at 1 h (prior to macrosegregation). It was also present in some cells 18 h after administration of tannic acid. Simple nucleolar enlargement was the typical response to

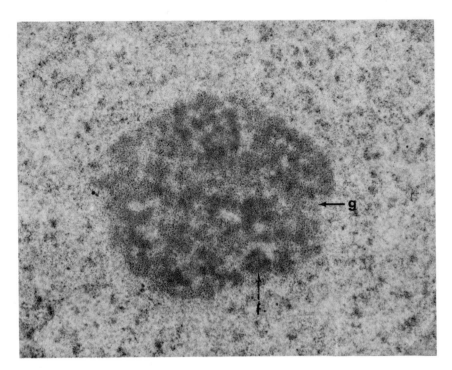

FIGURE 4. Nucleolus of normal rat liver cell in which the granular (g) and fibrillar (f) components are closely intermingled. ×37,000.

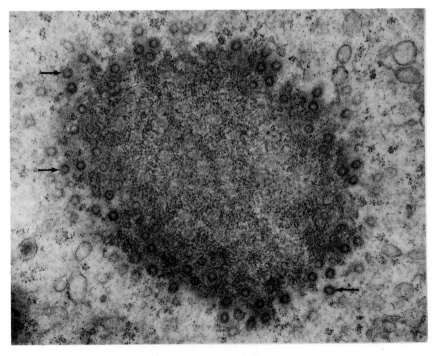

FIGURE 5. Tangential section of the normal nucleus revealing numerous pores (arrows) in the nuclear membranes. ×66,000.

299

SOME EFFECTS
OF CHEMICAL
CARCINOGENS
ON CELL
ORGANELLES

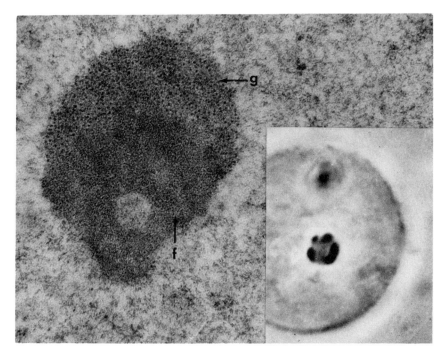

FIGURE 6. Aflatoxin B$_1$, 24 h. The granular (g) and fibrillar (f) components of the rat liver cell nucleolus are segregated to form two distinct areas. This type of change is known as macrosegregation. The nucleolar abnormalities (caps) can be recognized if isolated nuclei are examined with a phase contrast microscope (inset). ×39,000.

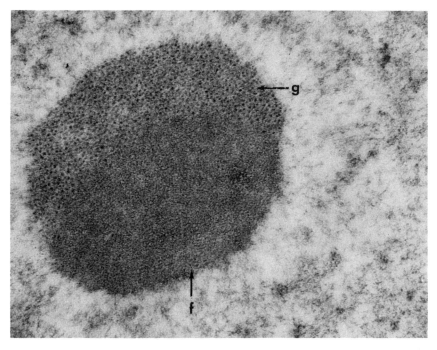

FIGURE 7. Lasiocarpine, 12 h. The nucleolus shows macrosegregation with separation of granular (g) and fibrillar (f) components. ×41,000.

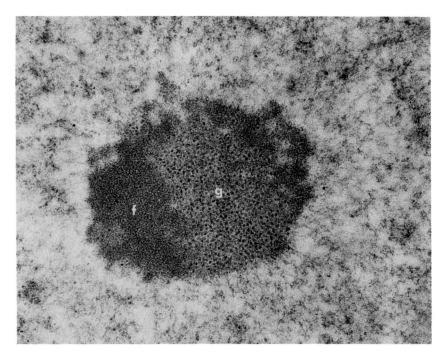

FIGURE 8. 3′-Methyldimethylaminoazobenzene, 24 h. Distinct separation of granules (g) and fibrils (f) resulting in macrosegregation. ×33,000.

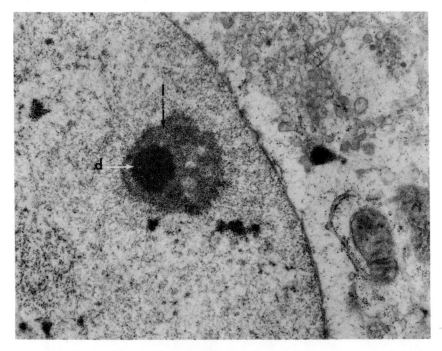

FIGURE 9. Tannic acid, 6 h. The nucleolar alteration produced by this agent is highly characteristic. One or more dark zones (d) composed of densely packed ribonucleoprotein granules are located in the nucleolus. These are surrounded by light areas (l) containing a mixture of granules and fibrils. ×21,800.

301

SOME EFFECTS
OF CHEMICAL
CARCINOGENS
ON CELL
ORGANELLES

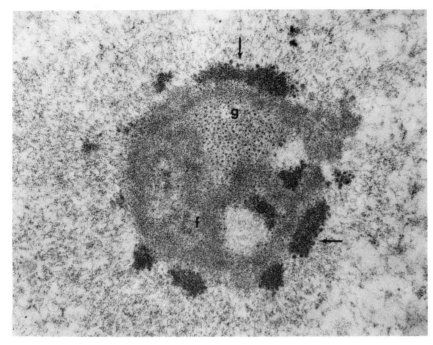

FIGURE 10. Dimethylnitrosamine, 36 h. Granules (g) and fibrils (f) are irregularly separated. Dense condensations (arrows) are seen at the periphery. This change is known as microsegregation. ×49,000.

thioacetamide and ethionine (Figs. 11 and 12). With thioacetamide the enlargement was due predominantly to increase in the granular component, while with ethionine there was increase in both the fibrillar and granular components.

While it might be argued that the terms "macrosegregation" and "microsegregation" are imprecise or arbitrary, or that they do not reflect functional consequences of the nucleolar alterations, they are intended only to be descriptive of morphological rearrangement of nucleolar constituents without implying a single or consistent biochemical equivalent. They may merely represent different degrees of severity or different stages of a spectrum of related changes. Moreover, the terms have been generally accepted and used in the literature, suggesting that they are useful in arriving at a common terminology.

The chronic ultrastructural changes in rat liver cells due to aflatoxin $B_1$, DEN, DMN, ethionine, lasiocarpine, 3'-Me-DAB, tannic acid, and thioacetamide are summarized in detail in Table 4 (for additional related references, see Svoboda and Higginson, 1968). Most carcinogens caused alterations in either the proportion or the ultrastructural configuration of the nucleolar constituents—increase in interchromatin granules or perichromatin granules (ethionine) or enlargement of the interchromatinic spaces (thioacetamide). The most consistent cytoplasmic changes were increased smooth ER and detachment of ribosomes from ergastoplasmic membranes; these changes probably persisted from the acute intervals.

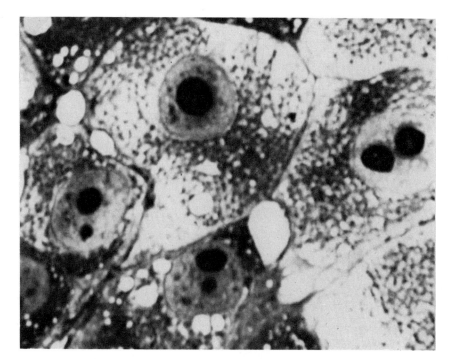

FIGURE 11. Thioacetamide, daily for 9 days. Megalocytosis of liver cells is evident in 0.5-μm-thick sections of Epon-embedded tissue. The nuclei and nucleoli are markedly enlarged. ×800.

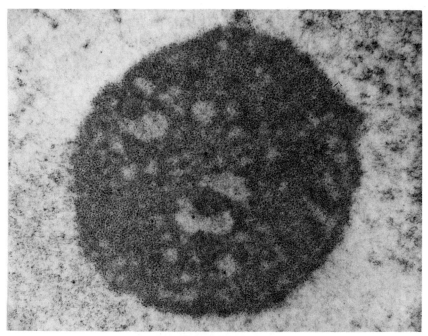

FIGURE 12. Thioacetamide, daily for 9 days. The nucleolus is enlarged significantly and is composed predominantly of granular component. The fibrillar component is significantly diminished. ×19,000.

DMN caused the most severe mitochondrial alterations, consisting of marked enlargement and bizarre-shaped profiles with decrease in length and number of cristae—changes most conspicuous in the periportal zones. Golgi areas were usually dilated but with empty vesicles and vacuoles, while the number of lysosomes appeared slightly increased in number with all carcinogens. The number of microbodies appeared to be focally increased only with thioacetamide and DMN. Glycogen was variably decreased, occasionally in a zonal pattern, while cytoplasmic lipid was increased.

None of the carcinogens caused specific changes in either acute or chronic stages that were sufficiently characteristic to identify the carcinogen by the ultrastructural responses it evoked.

303

SOME EFFECTS
OF CHEMICAL
CARCINOGENS
ON CELL
ORGANELLES

## 2.1. Aflatoxins

Aflatoxin $B_1$, a metabolite of *Aspergillus flavus*, a mold that grows on several cereals and legume crops, is the most potent hepatocarcinogen so far identified. For a comprehensive review, the reader is referred to the book by Goldblatt (1969) and the review by Wogan (1965).

The main histological changes in acute experiments with aflatoxin $B_1$ were slight periportal necrosis, peripheral and midzonal loss of glycogen, and decreased basophilia in the peripheral zones. In chronic experiments, there were several small foci of hyperbasophilic cells as well as aggregates of large pale cells lacking glycogen. Even at the time of appearance of hepatomas, the remaining nontumor liver was not cirrhotic nor did it show cholangiofibrosis or proliferation of oval cells or of bile ducts. Newberne and Wogan (1968) noted a similar distinction between basophilic cells which they believed progressed to poorly differentiated carcinomas and larger, pale eosinophilic cells which developed into well-differentiated carcinomas. By electron microscopy, the early changes due to aflatoxin $B_1$ were macrosegregation of the nucleolus and an increase in interchromatin granules. Similar nucleolar changes were described by Butler (1966) and by Bernhard *et al.* (1965). In chronic experiments, there was microsegregation of the nucleolus. Detachment of ribosomes was conspicuous in both acute and chronic experiments.

Butler reported that a maximum concentration of aflatoxin in the liver was reached approximately 1 h after oral administration; by 6 h most had gone, and at 24 h, when histological changes were identifiable, only a trace of the toxin was discernible. The earliest ultrastructural change seen by Butler was at 1 h and consisted of dilatation of ER cisterns and detachment of fibrosomes. By 6 h, there were mitochondrial and nucleolar changes. Butler (1966) concluded that there was a correlation between disruption of rough ER and inhibition of protein synthesis but that neither was related to the nucleolar abnormalities. Svoboda *et al.* (1966) illustrated marked separation of the fibrillar and granular elements of the nucleolus in a rhesus monkey 48 h after a dose of 2.6 mg/kg body weight of pure aflatoxin $B_1$. In addition, in rhesus monkeys given 0.45–2.6 mg/kg of pure aflatoxin $B_1$, the livers showed histological changes that were distinctly different from those occurring in rats and ducklings. Instead of periportal necrosis, the histological changes in the liver of a rhesus monkey given 2.6 mg/kg of pure aflatoxin consisted of individual cell necrosis and eosinophilic Councilman-like bodies, the overall pattern resembling the changes seen in viral hepatitis in man.

The changes induced in the fine structure of rat liver cells by synthetic aflatoxins $M_1$ and $B_1$ at a dose of 1 mg/kg were indistinguishable from those caused by the natural toxins at approximately half the dose. The main alterations were macrosegregation of nucleolar constituents, proliferation of smooth ER, and detachment of ribosomes from ergastoplasmic membranes. Synthetic aflatoxins $M_1$ and $B_1$ caused qualitatively similar acute effects in the rat liver and appeared to be approximately equal in potency.

In a comparative study of the effects of aflatoxin $B_1$ on the nucleoli of Morris hepatomas and adult and embryonic rat liver, Unuma et al. (1967) found that although acute treatment produced marked changes in nucleolar structure, continued treatment with the same dose caused little change other than nucleolar enlargement. In hamsters given a mixture of aflatoxins by intraperitoneal injection, it was found that, at their death 7 months later, they had hemorrhagic necrosis and megalocytosis (marked enlargement of hepatic parenchymal cells) usually at the periphery of the lobule, suggesting that the megalocytes represent a regenerative response to preexistent periportal necrosis caused by aflatoxin. In this species, aflatoxins caused marked enlargement of proximal tubular epithelium. The increase in size involved both nucleus and cytoplasm; nucleoli were prominent and often multiple. In the jejunum and ileum of hamsters, the toxins caused decrease in height and increase in width of the villi with reduction in mucosal thickness and villous atrophy (Herrold, 1969).

Aflatoxin $B_1$ in addition to being a hepatocarcinogen in trout, was shown by ammoniacal silver stain after one 400 $\mu$g/kg dose to cause a 41% loss of chromatin stainability with 65% loss of histone and acidic proteins relative to DNA. Losses of chromatin protein were restored within 48 h (Childs et al., 1972). Busch et al. (1963) suggested that any substance which inhibits rapidly sedimenting nucleolar RNA also produces segregation of nucleolar, granular, and fibrillar elements. In a study which included careful temporal comparisons between nucleolar changes and alterations in enzyme activity, Pong and Wogan (1970) showed that over a 36-h period after administration of aflatoxin there was close correlation between changes in liver cell nucleoli and RNA polymerase activity. RNA polymerase activity was maximally inhibited at 15 min (60%) but returned to normal at 36 h. Macrosegregation of nucleoli was apparent at 1 h and persisted until 12 h, but was essentially recovered by 36 h. The nucleolar changes were apparent after a dose of 0.2 mg/kg of aflatoxin $B_1$ but not after 0.1 mg/kg, a dose capable of causing only 5% inhibition of RNA polymerase activity. Although enzyme inhibition was maximal within 15 min after dosing, the most extensive nucleolar changes did not occur until 1 h, indicating that macrosegregation is not a prerequisite for maximum enzyme inhibition.

*2.2. Azo Dyes*

305
SOME EFFECTS
OF CHEMICAL
CARCINOGENS
ON CELL
ORGANELLES

The sequence of light microscopic changes in livers of rats given carcinogenic azo dyes has been well documented previously (Firminger and Mulay, 1952; Opie, 1944).

In experiments in our laboratories dealing principally with 3'-Me-DAB, the typical hyperplastic nodules with bile duct proliferation were apparent by 14 wk. During the first 48 h, the most pronounced changes were swelling of the cytoplasm with a decrease in the amount of glycogen and centrilobular infiltration of mononuclear cells. By electron microscopy, both microsegregation and macrosegregation (Fig. 8) of the nucleolus, detachment of ribosomes with an increase in the amount of smooth ER, and focal mitochondrial swelling with slight increase in lysosomes were apparent. There was uniform decrease in glycogen throughout the entire lobule with a slight increase in fat. "Coated" vesicles were also apparent. Studies reported from other laboratories (Porter and Bruni, 1959; Timme and Fowle, 1963) dealing with ultrastructural effects of azo dyes should also be consulted.

In chronic experiments using 3'-Me-DAB, occasional nucleoli showed condensations of the fibrillar component, while, in the cytoplasm, detachment of ribosomes, increased amounts of smooth ER in close association with glycogen, and dilated empty Golgi vacuoles were prominent. In addition, there were fat vacuoles in close association with mitochondria.

The earliest studies of the ultrastructural effect of 3'-Me-DAB were those of Porter and Bruni (1959) and Nigam (1965). Both studies showed similar reduction of glycogen with increase in smooth ER and detachment of ribosomes due to 3'-Me-DAB.

There is a close parallel between the biochemical and morphological abnormalities that follow injury induced in liver cells by administration of DAB. Ketterer *et al.* (1967) showed that the earliest change in liver cells after one dose of DAB was detachment of polyribosomes with disorganization and vesiculation of cisterns of granular ER followed by disaggregation of the polyribosomes and impaired microsomal amino acid incorporation which reached a maximum at 24 h.

Hyperbasophilic areas appear with some regularity in the liver of rats given carcinogenic azo dyes and have been studied intensively by Simard and Daoust (1966), who demonstrated that these hyperbasophilic foci were sites of accelerated synthesis of DNA in preneoplastic liver. Karasaki (1969) showed that the hyperbasophilic foci contained proliferating cells which were poorly differentiated but had several morphological features characteristic of DAB-induced tumors (Svoboda, 1964) and suggested that the hyperbasophilic foci represented sites of dedifferentiated liver cells having accelerated rates of proliferation leading to growth of liver tumors.

A study of LaFontaine and Allard (1964) showed that ultrastructural changes produced in rat liver cells by a noncarcinogenic azo dye duplicated most of the ultrastructural changes produced by the closely related and potent carcinogen

3'-Me-DAB. These nonspecific changes included disorganization and fragmentation of cisterns of the rough ER, with large cytoplasmic aggregates of tubules and vesicles resulting from hypertrophy of both smooth and granular ER. In addition, 2-Me-DAB apparently caused an increase in the number of mitochondria per cell. Perhaps the most important interpretation that can be made from this study is that noncarcinogenic chemicals closely related structurally to their carcinogenic counterparts are capable of causing remarkably similar ultrastructural alterations in the parenchymal liver cells of rats.

In an interesting study of the functional capacities and ultrastructural properties of hyperbasophilic foci, Karasaki (1969) showed by radioautography that only those cells which were proliferating, as determined by thymidine uptake into the nuclei, were poorly differentiated. These labeled cells had a high nucleocytoplasmic ratio, and the cytoplasm had almost completely lost the specialized elements that characterize hepatocytes. There were prominent nucleoli, increased numbers of free ribosomes, and absence of smooth ER, microbodies, bile canaliculi, and glycogen granules. The author concluded that hyperbasophilic foci represented sites of marked dedifferentiation of liver cells followed by rapid cellular proliferation leading to neoplasms. Lantos *et al.* (1973) showed that with vitamin E deficiency alone there was marked variation in size and shape of the mitochondria, often with abnormal cristae that showed no relation with the inner mitochondrial membrane.

## 2.3. Ethionine

For a complete and authoritative discussion on the role of ethionine in hepatic carcinogenesis, the reader should consult the review by Farber (1963). Of the early light microscopic changes occurring within 24 h after a dose of 1 ml/kg of DL-ethionine to inbred male F344 rats, the most conspicuous was an increase in the numbers of nucleoli with only slight diffuse vacuolization of the cytoplasm. By 2 wk, rats given 0.25% ethionine showed slight fat accumulation and large, often multiple eosinophilic nucleoli; at 14 wk, these were accompanied by slight oval cell proliferation. By electron microscopy, the acute change (up to 72 h) after administration of ethionine was microsegregation of the nucleolus with marked increase in the number of interchromatin granules. The most prominent cytoplasmic changes were detachment of ribosomes and slight increase in the amount of smooth ER. In chronic experiments, nucleoli were markedly enlarged because of an increase in both the granular and the fibrillar components, but no form of separation of these components was present. There was a marked increase in the amount of interchromatin granules, which commonly formed complex branching patterns. This change became noticeably more severe after 12 wk on the carcinogen and was accompanied by an increase in the number of perichromatin granules. Between 6 and 12 wk, cytoplasmic invaginations into nuclei were common and occasionally nucleoli surrounded by a membrane were noted. A few small areas of focal cytoplasmic necrosis were present, and electron-dense droplets were present in the Golgi vesicles. The normal dense granules that occur in the mitochondrial matrix were reduced or totally absent in various organelles. Smooth ER remained increased. Both nuclear and cytoplasmic changes persisted at 18 wk.

307
SOME EFFECTS
OF CHEMICAL
CARCINOGENS
ON CELL
ORGANELLES

The ultrastructure of interphase nuclei of rat liver cells in ethionine intoxication was described extensively by Miyai and Steiner (1965). With subacute ethionine intoxication, the authors described a number of interesting nuclear changes including reduction in the amount of peripheral chromatin and the number of chromatin centers as well as reduction in nucleolus-associated chromatin. The perichromatin granules were normal, and occasionally the interchromatin granules formed large aggregates. The nucleolus in some instances was enlarged, with clear, prominent vacuoles. The authors also described occasional nucleoli surrounded by membrane as well as membranous condensation of the interchromatin substance and invaginations of cytoplasmic blebs into the nucleus. They concluded that the nuclear changes were attributable to the toxic action of ethionine either through competition with methionine, alterations in energy balance, production of ethylated metabolites, incorporation of ethionine into protein, or production of abnormal nucleic acids or through a combination of some or all of these processes.

In addition to the other cytoplasmic changes that occur in chronic ethionine intoxication of rat liver cells, Steiner et al. (1964) described complex concentric circular arrays of membranes associated with glycogen granules and indicated that liver cells of hyperplastic nodules had resumed glycogen storage and considered it likely that neoplasms arose from such cells. Similarly, Epstein et al. (1967) showed that nodules induced with ethionine retained glycogen despite a period of fasting or administration of glucagon. Also, ethionine-induced nodules showed decrease in activity of glucose-6-phosphatase and glycogen phosphorylase.

It was Farber (1963) who initially suggested that the nucleolar lesions were related to a fall in hepatic ATP concentration. In a study relating ATP levels and capacity for enzyme induction, Meldolesi et al. (1967) showed that in ethionine-treated rats the ATP level and induction of enzymes with phenobarbital were reduced but partially restored when adenine was also given. There was significant correlation between ATP level and capacity for enzyme induction. With respect to ultrastructural changes, Meldolesi et al. (1967) felt that some of the ethionine-induced alterations such as cytoplasmic fat, mitochondrial swelling, dilatation of the endoplasmic reticulum, and reduction of free and attached ribosomes were correlated with the decrease of ATP. In contrast, they suggested that hyperplasia of smooth ER and the formation of myelin figures were probably independent of ATP deficiency.

Shinozuka et al. (1968) confirmed earlier findings that at about $1\frac{1}{2}$ h after ethionine injection in rats electron-dense masses appeared in the nucleolonema. By 6–8 h, the nucleoli showed partial fragmentation into small dense masses and enlarged aggregates of interchromatin granules occurred. By 12 h, there was almost complete fragmentation of nucleoli, but if adenine was given previously it prevented the development of these nucleolar changes. If adenine was given 8 h after ethionine, it reversed the nucleolar lesion by 12 h. Methionine given at 8 h also caused earlier partial recovery of thionine-induced nucleolar changes. The authors, like Farber, suggested that the nucleolar changes are consequence of ATP deficiency induced by ethionine and suggested that the nucleolar alterations caused by ethionine differ from those induced by actinomycin and other drugs that combine directly with DNA. They also suggested that nucleolar disassociation and segregation produced by actinomycin are not the consequence of inhibition of RNA synthesis as such, but instead are due to molecular interactions which lead to such inhibition. In a later but closely related study, Shinozuka and Farber (1969) showed that the nucleolar fragmentation was reversible if the animal was given ATP precursors such as adenine or ethionine. The data suggest that synthesis of new protein is not essential for recovery of nucleolar structure and that such recovery probably represents reaggregation and restoration of preexistent nucleolar fragments. In a study comparing the time sequence of recovery of the nucleolus and the cytoplasm following acute ethionine intoxication, Shinozuka *et al.* (1970) showed that, between 20 and 24 h after administration of ethionine, nucleoli began to recover their structure and hepatic ATP levels and RNA synthesis began to show signs of recovery, although protein synthesis remained inhibited and lipid accumulation and disaggregation of polyribosomes were maintained. Between 36 and 48 h, many nucleoli were normal although the cytoplasm still showed persistent lipid droplets and numerous concentric lamellar collections. Polyribosomes began to appear by 36 h and protein synthesis was returned to 50% of control values while ATP levels were at 60% of normal. This study and related references from this group present evidence that reformation of nucleoli takes place in the absence of significant protein synthesis but not in the absence of RNA synthesis. Both suggest that ethionine-induced nucleolar lesions are probably related to ATP deficiency induced by ethionine. Following administration of ethionine, the decrease in nuclear ATP is considerably less than the decrease in cytoplasmic ATP (Okazaki *et al.*, 1968). The lesser degree of ATP inhibition in the nucleus may allow earlier recovery of nucleolar structure than of the changes in cytoplasm. Natural recovery of nucleolar ultrastructure after ethionine was also reported by Miyai and Ritchie (1970). They showed that 1 mg/g body weight of DL-ethionine given by intraperitoneal injection to female rats caused fragmentation of the nucleolus as well as fragmentation and dilatation of cisterns of rough ER. Both membrane-bound and free ribosomes were dispersed and did not form coiled aggregates. The smooth ER had begun to proliferate and flipid droplets had accumulated. By 36 h, many nucleoli formed ropelike configurations and smooth ER was abundant. By 48 h, the ultrastructure of the nucleolus was normal and some ribosomes had reaggregated. Between 84 and 96 h, the ultrastructure of the cytoplasm was almost completely recovered.

Merkow *et al.* (1971) showed that the ultrastructural alterations in hyperplastic nodules induced by ethionine and 2-FAA were similar. In fasted animals, but not in fed ones, the cells in the hyperplastic nodules showed a marked clustering of smooth ER with some diminution or decrease of rough ER. Annulate lamellae in continuity with the endoplasmic reticulum were noted rarely. Mitochondria within the nodules showed a close association with either smooth or rough ER. According to these authors, all changes occurred only in hyperplastic nodules, not in the adjacent liver. In a related study, Merkow et al. (1972) showed that, in hyperplastic liver nodules induced by ethionine, ultrastructural characteristics were similar within cells of the same or different nodules, while among hepatocellular carcinoma cells there was a great deal of heterogeneity. Similar comparisons were true when the carcinogen was 2-FAA. The hyperplastic nodules induced by either chemical had a number of fine structural similarities to hepatoma cells associated with the same carcinogen. These similarities included increased amounts and clustering of smooth ER, presence of annulate lamellae, decreased parallel arrays of rough ER, and tendency for rough ER to surround the mitochondria.

## 2.4. Nitrosamines

For detailed reports of the histological changes, the biochemical and carcinogenic effects, and the metabolism of N-nitroso compounds, the reader is referred to the review by Magee (1963) and the more recent one by Magee and Barnes (1967).

### 2.4.1. Morphology

In acute experiments, the light microscopic alterations following DEN (Diethylnitrosamine) and DMN (dimethylnitrosamine) were not strikingly different. Both caused centrilobular hemorrhagic necrosis and loss of glycogen. Moderate nuclear enlargement was apparent with DMN. In chronic experiments, DEN caused irregularity in size of liver cells followed by irregular nodular hyperplasia. DMN also caused acidophilic degeneration of centrilobular cells, and occasionally large hyperchromatic nuclei were apparent. The early light microscopic changes with both DEN and DMN (24–72 h) consisted of enlargement of the nucleus with focal acidophilic cells and decreased amount of glycogen in central zones along with centrilobular hemorrhagic necrosis and infiltration by macrophages and neutrophils in these central areas.

By electron microscopy, an early ultrastructural change induced by DMN was microsegregation (Fig. 10), while both DMN and DEN caused detachment of ribosomes and increase in the amount of smooth ER. It appeared that DMN caused a moderate increase in the number of microbodies, although this is questionable. DEN caused a sharply demarcated centrilobular loss of glycogen, while DMN caused sharply demarcated centrilobular and periportal loss; both agents caused slight increase in fat and "coated" vesicles having interruptions in the plasma membranes were noted with both.

### 2.4.2. Dimethylnitrosamine

In early studies of the effects of DMN on liver cells, Emmelot and Benedetti (1961) showed that a single dose caused breakdown of the characteristic lamellar organization of the endoplasmic reticulum and marked increase in the number of free ribosomes. Geil *et al.* (1968) showed that in the liver cells of female rats given DMN the only persistent cytoplasmic abnormalities in late stages of the experiment were moderately reduced stores of glycogen and hypertrophy of smooth ER. There were focal condensations of the fibrillar component of the nucleolus first appearing after 170 days of treatment, condensations which persisted throughout the experiment in some cells. Tumor cells also showed large nucleoli with focal condensations of fibrillar components.

Williams and Hulton (1973) found that administration of DMN to mice for 2 h resulted in 60% inhibition of hepatic protein synthesis accompanied by disaggregation of both free and membrane-bound polysomes.

Hard and Butler (1971*b*) stated that, among other evidence, the fact that adenocarcinomas induced in the rat kidney by DMN contained microbodies indicated their derivation from proximal tubular epithelial cells. However, the microbodies in this study were not clearly illustrated. A related study (Hard and Butler, 1971*a*) demonstrated that DMN-induced kidney tumors originated from interstitial cells having the morphology of fibroblasts in the vicinity of the glomerular hilus. Abnormal interstitial cells could be recognized as early as 3 wk, and by 6 wk some of the cell forms characteristic of tumors were present.

### 2.4.3. Diethylnitrosamine and Other Nitrosamines

An exceedingly detailed study of the light and electron microscopic changes in rat liver following the administration of nitrosomorpholine has been reported by Bannasch (1968). Although comprehensive, the descriptions were limited to the cytoplasm and did not include the nucleus. Several of the acute changes were nonspecific and included dilatation of cisterns with loss of ribosomes accompanied by assorted mitochondrial changes. Many of the latter appeared to be minor and were probably nonspecific. Bannasch described cells with prominent accumulations of glycogen associated with membranes resembling the complexes described by Steiner *et al.* (1964). Bannasch termed these "lamellar cistern complexes," but the addition of another term for a finding adequately described previously is probably superfluous. Like Steiner *et al.* (1964), Bannasch considered that hepatomas induced with nitrosomorpholine developed from those parenchymal cells that showed enhanced glycogen storage. He suggested that enhanced glycogen storage in peripheral cells indicates a precancerous reaction, while loss of glycogen in the central cells is simply a sign of cell injury. He also suggested that mitochondrial partitions do not indicate mitochondrial division since he did not observe such a partition lead to complete transection. Considering the plasticity of the wide variety of configurational changes in mitochondria as viewed by phase microscopy, mitochondrial partitions need not indicate division. Difficulty in interpretation of mitochondrial partitions could be solved by examination of serial sections.

Bruni (1973) showed that an early abnormality caused by DEN was an increase in the smooth ER of some liver cells in the form of tubules and vesicles. Between 49 and 70 days, however, small foci of liver cells were found that differed from the others because they had little or no smooth ER, and this system was also lacking in the tumors that occurred later. The scarcity of smooth ER, in Bruni's opinion, caused the neoplastic liver cells to resemble fetal liver cells. The author concluded that the few cells free of smooth ER between 49 and 70 days might represent the initial stage in tumor formation and that the fine structure of these cells expressed permanently arrested differentiation. It is clear from these studies that various authors feel that changes in glycogen and decrease in smooth ER may be important in the carcinogenic process. From a broader perspective, it would appear that neither of these changes is sufficiently specific or consistent in the process of malignant transformation.

311
SOME EFFECTS
OF CHEMICAL
CARCINOGENS
ON CELL
ORGANELLES

## 2.5. Pyrrolizidine Alkaloids

The pyrrolizidine alkaloids constitute a large group of naturally occurring environmental toxins derived from several families of plants distributed in various parts of the world (Kingsbury, 1964). Their chemistry and metabolism and the pathological alterations resulting from both acute and chronic alkaloid poisoning in animals have been reviewed comprehensively by McLean (1970). In acute doses, several of these alkaloids cause centrilobular hemorrhagic necrosis of the liver, segregation of the nucleolus, and disaggregation of polyribosomes associated with rapid inhibition of RNA polymerase activity and of RNA synthesis. Chronic administration results in progressive enlargement of liver parenchymal cells (megalocytosis), focal periportal fibrosis, bile duct proliferation, and, occasionally, cirrhosis of the liver. An early report by Reddy and Svoboda (1968) pointed out that abnormalities in nucleolar ultrastructure and disaggregation of polyribosomes in liver cells were associated with simultaneous inhibition of hepatic RNA and protein synthesis.

The first study of the effects of the pyrrolizidine alkaloids lasiocarpine and monocrotaline on the fine structure of rat liver cells was reported by Svoboda and Soga (1966). Related studies are those by Cook *et al.* (1950), Schoental and Magee (1959), Schoental and Head (1955, 1957), and Schoental (1963).

The pyrrolizidine alkaloids, esters of a basic alcohol containing a pyrrolizidine group, are toxic to man and animals and differ from most hepatotoxic and carcinogenic substances in that they are capable of causing severe chronic and progressive liver disease after a single dose. In addition, some of these alkaloids cause a number of cellular changes which differ from those induced by the more familiar and widely used hepatotoxic agents. These differences include the formation of cellular aggregates on the lumen surface of central veins, often causing total occlusion of the vessels, atypical regenerative response manifested by formation of liver cells 3–4 times the normal size (termed "megalocytosis"), and the presence of prominent cytoplasmic globules, probably lysosomes, in the acute stage of poisoning. It has been suggested that the alkaloids act as alkylating agents and possess mutagenic and carcinogenic properties which may be related to their effect on genetic material of cells. In humans, these agents have been incriminated in venoocclusive disease, cirrhosis, and Chiari's syndrome in those parts of the world where they are given as a medicinal tonic or consumed in flour contaminated with alkaloid-containing seeds.

The early electron microscopic study by Svoboda and Soga (1966) indicated that after the administration of lasiocarpine or an extract of *Crotalaria* microsegregation occurred in 30 min, along with macrosegregation and increase in interchromatin granules, prominent between 2 and 8 h (Fig. 7). The nucleolar changes returned to normal by 72 h but were accompanied by a decrease in hepatic RNA and protein content. Nuclear alterations were followed by formation of focal cytoplasmic necrosis and aggregations of cells resembling macrophages on the lumen surface of central veins.

In a later comparative study (Svoboda and Higginson, 1968), the early (24 h) changes in the liver of male rats following lasiocarpine consisted of formation of numerous lysosomes, decrease in glycogen, and centrilobular necrosis. By electron microscopy, there was macro- and microsegregation of the nucleolus with increased interchromatin granules and electron-dense satellite granules. In the cytoplasm, there was detachment of ribosomes with extensive dilatation of the rough ER, increase in smooth ER, and numerous small dense droplets in the Golgi areas. Mitochondria showed irregular swelling which was not consistent from cell to cell. There was uniform loss of glycogen throughout all of the zones of the liver with moderate increase in fat. The nuclear changes were present throughout the lobule, while those of the cytoplasm were most conspicuous in the centrilobular areas. In chronic experiments, the most obvious change in parenchymal cells was the formation of megalocytes. These showed microsegregation of their nucleoli. The increase in interchromatin granules persisted, and there were numerous invaginations of cytoplasm into the nucleus. In the cytoplasm, there was dilatation of the rough ER with detachment of ribosomes and increase in the amount of smooth ER. Mitochondria showed some variation in size and shape with scalloping of margins, and there was a moderate increase in lysosomes with decrease in glycogen and slight increase in fat.

Monneron (1969) found that within 10 min after injection of lasiocarpine or aflatoxin to intact or partially hepatectomized rats numerous helical polysomes occurred. They recovered by 24 h; some attached to the endoplasmic reticulum and others located close to the nuclear membrane. They appeared prior to the nucleolar changes due to these two agents, and their occurrence was not prevented by previous administration of actinomycin D. The sudden and early occurrence of these polysomes may be related to the production of a special type of transient messenger RNA (Monneron *et al.*, 1971). It is important to note that this author also found the same unusual configuration of polysomes in the cytoplasm of Kupffer cells.

## 2.6. Thioacetamide

The acute histological changes within 24–48 h after administration of thioacetamide were enlargement of nuclei and occasional acidophilic cells in the centrilobular zone. Glycogen was decreased, and there was slight centrilobular necrosis. By electron microscopy, there was nucleolar enlargement due to increase in the granular component (Fig. 12). In addition, there was increase in interchromatin granules. In the cytoplasm, as with all of the other carcinogens, there were detachment of ribosomes and increase in smooth endoplasmic reticulum. Polysomes were conspicuous, as were dense deposits, possibly calcium, in occasional mitochondria. Lysomes increased slightly, and there was a moderate increase in the number of microbodies. There was general decrease in glycogen throughout the lobules except for scattered midzonal cells. Fat was slightly increased. In chronic experiments, the most notable change was increase in size of the nucleolus, again principally due to increase in the granular component; in addition, there were prominent electron-lucent cavities in nucleoli. The extent of interchromatinic spaces was increased. Detachment of ribosomes and increase in smooth endoplasmic reticulum persisted, while the Golgi vesicles were dilated but empty and the mitochondria showed a decreased number of the normal electron-dense matrix granules. Lysosomes were only slightly increased and microbodies appeared to continue to be increased in some cells. There was centrilobular loss of glycogen in those cells having the greatest degree of nucleolar enlargement. Fat was increased and annulate lamellae were prominent in many cells. Two weeks after withdrawal of the carcinogen, only a few enlarged nucleoli remained. Some oval cells and small amounts of ceroid were present until 8 wk, when cytoplasmic basophilia was uniformly restored and most nucleoli recovered their normal structure.

Kendrey (1968) reported that the principal effect of thioacetamide, studied up to 101 days, was nuclear and nucleolar enlargement with increase in smooth ER and decrease in rough ER. He also reported a decrease in the number of free ribosomes, which is rather questionable. Animals given thioacetamide for 5 months showed a marked increase in nuclear water as well as in dry mass (Malvaldi, 1969). Smith *et al.* (1968) reported that nuclei of liver cells of mice fed thioacetamide contained lipid cysts in the nucleus by 3 days and were more frequent after 9 days. Such cysts were found as well in nuclei of mouse hepatomas transplanted subcutaneously.

Koshiba *et al.* (1971) found that the nucleoli of thioacetamide-treated rat liver exhibited two major differences from the normal. First, there was a marked increase in the relative number of RNP particles so that the overall appearance of the nucleoli was far more granular, an observation which has been confirmed in the authors' laboratories; second, the size of the RNP particles was greater than normal. Extraction produced a thirtyfold increase in the yield of nucleolar RNP particles per 100 g of liver.

## 3. Organelles

In considering the response of cell organelles to the effects of carcinogens, it is important to bear in mind the severe sampling limitations imposed by current techniques of transmission electron microscopy in assessing the normal cell ultrastructure. Similarly, it is important to be aware of ultrastructural alterations that might occur in liver cells simply as a result of the nutritional status of experimental animals. It has been shown, for example, that simple prolonged protein deficiency in rats caused marked loss of granular endoplasmic reticulum with enlargement of mitochondria which contained large cavities in their matrix as well as defects in their limiting membranes. There was prominent dilatation of endoplasmic reticulum progressing to the formation of large cytoplasmic "lakes." In addition to the cytoplasmic changes, there was nucleolar enlargement with pronounced segregation of the granular and fibrillar components. The nuclei of several cells contained irregular branching cleftlike defects. Nair *et al.* (1970) showed that there was a diurnal rhythm of enzyme activity in rat liver cells accompanied by proliferation of smooth ER. At the time when enzyme activity was maximum, the amount of smooth ER was also maximum and *vice versa*. When the rhythm of the enzyme activity was abolished, as in blinded rats, the diurnal rhythm in endoplasmic reticulum was also abolished. These studies show that, even under normal circumstances, there may be quantitative increases or decreases in cytoplasmic structures and that before such changes can be attributed to carcinogens or toxic chemicals the normal baseline information must be available. Loud (1968) studied the fractional volumes in cytoplasm of liver cells occupied by mitochondria, peroxisomes, lysosomes, lipid, and glycogen as well as the surface density of smooth and rough ER and mitochondrial envelope and cristae. The results provide a basis at the ultrastructural level for reasonably accurate quantitative comparison of normal and pathologically altered liver cells by morphological means. The authors showed that parenchymal cells in normal rat liver are at least 80% homogeneous with respect of those structural parameters measured. Where significant intralobular differences in ultrastructure do exist, they are most pronounced in the two or three layers of cells surrounding the central vein. Weibel *et al.* (1969) showed that 1 ml of normal rat liver contains $169 \times 10^6$ nuclei and $90 \times 10^6$ nuclei of other cells as well as $280 \times 10^9$ mitochondria. Hepatocyte cytoplasm accounts for 77% of liver volume and the mitochondria for 18%. The surface area of the endoplasmic reticulum membranes in 1 ml of liver has been measured at 11 m$^2$, two-thirds of that in the rough form. The surface area of mitochondrial cristae in 1 ml of liver has been estimated at 6 m$^2$. One hepatocyte contains about 370 microbodies, which contribute only 1.5% of the cytoplasmic volume. Although somewhat laborious, this type of morphometric analysis allows one to consider the normal liver cell in a somewhat different light than by mere examination of electron micrographs for subjective impressions. The paper of Weibel *et al.* (1969) should be consulted for quantitation of organelles in liver cells expressed in several different terms. The authors also point out the problems that arise in quantitative estimation of cell organelles and the artifacts that may originate from homogenization and preparation of cell fractions for biochemical analysis.

## 3.1. Endoplasmic Reticulum

For a general review of the functions of endoplasmic reticulum and a comprehensive discussion of functional and morphological modifications in this organelle due to chemical injury and other pathological states, the reader is referred to the review by Stenger (1970). In the authors' laboratories, all the carcinogens listed in Table 1 caused some increase in smooth endoplasmic reticulum and detachment of ribosomes in both acute and chronic stages. These changes persisted with aflatoxin $B_1$, thioacetamide, DMN, and DEN, but with ethionine and 3'-Me-DAB the ribosome–ergastoplasm complex was virtually normal in most cells by 6 wk after withdrawal. Detachment of polysomes and their disaggregation along with proliferation of smooth ER have been recorded with several carcinogens (Baglio and Farber, 1965), including aflatoxin (Villa-Trevino and Leaver, 1968), 4-dimethylaminoazobenzene (Ketterer *et al.*, 1967), lasiocarpine, and others (Harris *et al.*, 1969; Ashworth *et al.*, 1965; Benedetti and Emmelot, 1966; Butler, 1966; Mikata and Luse, 1964; Popper *et al.*, 1960; Porter and Bruni, 1959; Svoboda *et al.*, 1966; Mukherjee *et al.*, 1963; Reddy *et al.*, 1970).

It must be emphasized, however, that detachment of ribosomes and proliferation of smooth ER occur with several noncarcinogens (Fouts and Rogers, 1965; Herdson *et al.*, 1965; Hruban *et al.*, 1965; Orrenius and Ericsson, 1966). Rubin *et al.* (1968) showed that ethanol causes proliferation of smooth endoplasmic reticulum and associated drug-metabolizing enzymes.

In conclusion, it is clear that few irreversible or specific changes in cytoplasmic membranes or in other cell organelles are demonstrable at the ultrastructural level as solely due to carcinogens. Although various degrees of increase in smooth ER and detachment of ribosomes persisted throughout acute and chronic experiments, the former may only represent detoxification by induced enzymes and the latter may reflect toxic injury. An interesting study by LaFontaine and Allard (1964) showed that all of the cytoplasmic changes produced by the potent carcinogen 3'-Me-DAB were also induced by the noncarcinogenic analogue 2-Me-DAB.

## 3.2. Plasma Membrane

In the acute experiments with the carcinogens listed in Table 1, the only consistent change in plasma membranes was the formation of coated vesicles, which appeared to originate from plasma membranes but were occasionally located deep in the cytoplasm. They were present during the acute experiments after administration of DEN, DMN, and 3'-Me-DAB. In chronic experiments, they were not present. Coated vesicles have been noted in several cell types, and Novikoff and Shin (1964) suggested that these vesicles transport material from the endoplasmic reticulum. Friend and Farquhar (1967) suggested that the coated vesicles could reflect accelerated transport of material through specialized portions of the plasma membrane. For additional references to coated vesicles, the reader is referred to the article by Svoboda and Higginson (1968).

## 3.3. Mitochondria, Lysosomes, Microbodies

The most unusual and consistent abnormalities in ultrastructure of mitochondria were those following DMN; they did not occur with other carcinogens. The abnormal form of mitochondria included marked enlargement, occasional rupture of limiting membranes, and many bizarre shapes with an abnormal number and distribution of cristae. Many adjacent profiles showed interlocking protrusions and invaginations of their membrane. These abnormal forms apparently occurred in too few cells to be reflected in alterations in P:O ratios. Emmelot and Benedetti (1961) found that mitochondria isolated from rat livers 3 h after *in vivo* administration of 10 mg of DMN behaved normally, but by 24 h after a dose of 20 mg there was some degree of respiratory inhibition and diminished oxidative phosphorylation. In these studies, although there was swelling of some mitochondria, most retained normal ultrastructure. Compared to the carcinogens we have studied in our laboratories, the mitochondrial changes due to DMN were relatively severe in their morphological manifestations and have not been reported previously. Mukherjee *et al.* (1963) showed that liver tissue does not react uniformly to dimethylnitrosamine, and this could cause some variation in electron microscopic and biochemical observations following administration of this carcinogen. In our experiments, for example, it was clear by both light and electron microscopic examination that the enlarged and bizarre forms of mitochondria following DMN were confined to a small number of cells in the immediate periportal area. If these morphological changes had any biochemical consequences, they were diluted by the presence of unaltered mitochondria in midzonal and centrilobular areas.

In the experiments in these authors' laboratories, there was a slight to moderate increase in the number of lysosomes in both acute and chronic experiments as well as in the final tumor cell. In our initial observations, we felt that responses of hepatic lysosomes to chemical carcinogens were comparatively inconspicuous and probably were a result of toxicity. In addition, we have observed lysosomes in fetal rat liver cells, where, presumably, injury is minimal and considerably less than that occurring in the postnatal animal. Because of the great morphological variety of lysosomes in many pathological conditions, it is difficult to formulate any persuasive conclusions regarding their relationship to neoplasia. We are inclined to reiterate our previous opinion (Svoboda and Reddy, 1970) that responses of lysosomes after the administration of carcinogens are, like changes in the Golgi apparatus, fat, and glycogen, quite variable and nonspecific.

Important studies by Allison and Mallucci (1964) showed that the carcinogens dimethylbenzanthracene, methylcholanthrene, 1,2,5,6-dibenzanthracene, and 3,4-benzpyrene (studied in monkey kidney cells, HeLa cells, macrophages, and chick embryo cells as well as *in vivo* in mice given subcutaneous injections of DMBA) concentrated in the lysosomes and appeared to decrease the stability of the lysosome membrane so that high concentrations could bring about release of lysosome enzymes into the cytoplasm. The same phenomena were reported following x-irradiation (Brandes *et al.*, 1967).

In experiments dealing more directly with experimental chemical carcinogenesis, Kampschmidt and Wells (1969) showed that both free and latent activities of several lysosomal enzymes increased after 4 wk of feeding 3'-Me-DBA. Several enzymes, with the exception of acid phosphatase, increased significantly, but both free and total activities declined when the rats were returned to a regular diet at 12 wk.

317

SOME EFFECTS
OF CHEMICAL
CARCINOGENS
ON CELL
ORGANELLES

The role of microbodies in tumors has not been studied extensively, and, in fact, comparatively little is known about the biological role of microbodies, although it is now apparent that they are present in a wide variety of tissues and cells. The occurrences, distributions, and possible roles of microbodies (peroxisomes) have been reviewed by Svoboda and Reddy (1973). In previous studies (Svoboda and Higginson, 1968), it was found that microbodies were slightly increased in number after administration of DMN or thioacetamide in both acute and chronic stages but tumor cells contained fewer microbodies than did normal cells. Afzelius and Schoental (1967) described a decrease in number of microbodies within megalocytes induced with pyrolizidine alkaloids; however, this was merely a visual estimate and was not strictly quantitative.

## 3.4. Nucleolus

The most comprehensive review of the biology of the nucleolus in tumor cells, especially liver nucleoli, and the effects of drugs on nucleoli is the book by Busch and Smetana (1970). Yasuzumi et al. (1970) compared nucleolar changes occurring after administration of 3'-Me-DAB, 2-fluorenylacetamide, and DL-ethionine and found that the changes in nuclei were similar in all instances and consisted of nucleolar enlargement. The increase in size of nuclei was due principally to an increase in the granular component. The authors also described a decrease in number of perichromatin granules, but such estimates made from inspection of electron micrographs may not be entirely reliable. Paul et al. (1971) showed that carcinogenic derivatives of 4-nitroquinoline-N-oxide resulted in a preponderance of Chang cell nucleoli showing macrosegregation, while weakly carcinogenic ones resulted primarily in microsegregation. Thus there may be a relationship between nucleolar segregation and carcinogenicity among the 4-nitroquinoline oxides; however, it may be valid only for this group of carcinogens. Reddy and Svoboda (1968) showed that 3'-Me-DAB, lasiocarpine, DMN, and tannic acid all inhibited the in vivo corporation of radioactive uridine into nuclear and ribosomal RNA at a time when nucleolar segregation was most pronounced. Further, Specific activity of nuclear and ribosomal RNA in rats treated with the hepatocarcinogens was significantly lower than that of controls. In addition to inhibition of RNA synthesis, the RNA polymerase activity in segregated nuclei was decreased. RNA synthesis returned to normal when nucleolar morphology recovered. It should not be construed, however, that structural or biochemical modifications in nuclear behavior represent necessary or specific events in the carcinogenic process, and, in fact, reports of nucleolar capping with noncarcinogenic agents in rat liver suggest the contrary. Many of the nucleolar changes recovered or did not even occur when carcinogens were given in low chronic doses to induce tumors. Harris et al. (1968) showed that after the administration of lasiocarpine, actinomycin D, or tannic acid the isolated nucleoli from rat liver maintained a form closely resembling their morphology in situ, suggesting that metabolic studies on isolated nucleoli after experimentally induced morphological abnormalities may be reasonably representative of the abnormality that exists *in vivo*.

In general, it would appear that although some degree of redistribution of fibrillar and granular nucleolar constituents occurs with several carcinogens, the importance of such changes is questionable, since with aflatoxin $B_1$, lasiocarpine, and 3'-Me-DAB similar nucleolar alterations are present in Kupffer cells. Moreover, although hypophysectomy inhibits induction of hepatic tumors by azo dyes (Lee and Goodall, 1968) in rats given 3'-Me-DAB 24 h prior to sacrifice and in rats given lasiocarpine, characteristic nucleolar changes occur.

It appears that many ultrastructural changes in nucleoli of rat liver cells are nonspecific and are related to a variety of biochemical alterations in addition to changes in RNA synthesis.

Although there is evidence to support the principal importance of the nucleus, particularly DNA, in the carcinogenic process, the morphological changes that occur in the nucleolus appear to be as nonspecific as those occurring in the cytoplasm.

## 4. Comment

With the carcinogens listed in Table 1, most of the ultrastructural changes in nontumor cells recovered in 4–8 wk after withdrawal. No specific nuclear or cytoplasmic alterations could be related with certainty to a single carcinogen but instead appeared to be associated with most carcinogens or with the state of toxicity. Increased smooth ER, dilatation of the smooth ER, focal cytoplasmic degradation, and occasional increase in interchromatin granules were the only changes persisting 4–8 wk after withdrawal of the carcinogen. The cytoplasmic changes following administration of carcinogens appear to be nonspecific reactions of toxicity or manifestations of enzyme induction. The changes in nuclei and nucleoli also appear to be nonspecific with respect to carcinogenesis even though the ultrastructural alterations in the nucleus may represent fundamental disturbances that occur prior to those in the cytoplasm. Many of the ultrastructural nuclear changes described either recover or do not occur when the carcinogens are given in low chronic doses sufficient to induce tumors. Accordingly, nucleolar segregation and simultaneous inhibition of RNA synthesis may be manifestations only of acute toxicity of the chemicals independent of their carcinogenic potential. Similarly, there is serious question whether the nucleolar alterations have been studied sufficiently to subclassify the patterns of change. At present, it appears that many of the ultrastructural changes are nonspecific and are related to a variety of biochemical alterations in addition to changes in RNA synthesis.

To summarize the ultrastructural features of tumors induced by the carcinogens in Table 1 and on the basis of available literature regarding experimental liver tumors, it is apparent that tumor cells contain less granular endoplasmic reticulum, increased numbers of free ribosomes, generally fewer and smaller mitochondria, and enlarged nucleoli. In the preneoplastic intervals, prior to the induction of frank tumors, nucleolar enlargement and increased numbers of free

319
SOME EFFECTS
OF CHEMICAL
CARCINOGENS
ON CELL
ORGANELLES

ribosomes are also frequent; therefore, the transitions between normal cells, preneoplastic cells, and malignant cells are not marked by any constant changes in ultrastructure at present levels of resolution. No carcinogen produced a tumor with sufficiently characteristic ultrastructure that could serve to identify which chemical it was. Virus particles were not found in any of tumors induced in our laboratories. We have not observed any characteristic or uniform ultrastructural abnormality in the nontumor cells of rats bearing chemically induced primary hepatomas.

Newer techniques may permit fruitful investigation of the carcinogenic process from a morphological point of view. For example, freeze-etching and freeze-cleavage might be useful for study of the nuclear membrane. Such techniques should confirm or deny the report of Miyai and Steiner (1965) regarding changes in nuclear pores during subacute ethionine intoxication. Similarly, the advent of scanning electron microscopy, if used with proper experimental hypotheses, might very well reveal important surface membrane changes in several types of tissues and cells which have been exposed to carcinogens.

ACKNOWLEDGMENTS

The work from the authors' laboratories was supported in part by Grants CA-5680, ESO-0629 and GM-15956 from the United States Public Health Service. We wish to thank the editors and publishers of *Cancer Research* and *Laboratory Investigation* for permission to republish tabular material published previously in those journals. Technical assistance was given by Faye Brady, Diane Knox and Lynne Schmutz. We thank Juanita Stika for her cooperation in preparation of the manuscript.

## 5. *References*

AFZELIUS, B., AND SCHOENTAL, R., 1967, The ultrastructure of the enlarged hepatocytes induced in rats with a single oral dose of retrorsine, a pyrrolizidine (*Senecio*) alkaloid, *J. Ultrastruct. Res.* **20**:328.

ALLISON, A., AND MALLUCCI, L., 1964, Lysosomes in dividing cells, with special reference to lymphocytes, *Lancet* **2**:1371.

ASHWORTH, C., WERNER, D., GLASS, M., AND ARNOLD, N., 1965, Spectrum of fine structural changes in hepatocellular injury due to thioacetamide, *Am. J. Pathol.* **47**:917.

BAGLIO, C., AND FARBER, E., 1965, Correspondence between ribosome aggregation patterns in rat liver homogenates and in electron micrographs following administration of ethionine, *J. Mol. Biol.* **12**:466.

BANNASCH, P., 1968, The cytoplasm of hepatocytes during carcinogenesis: Electron- and light-microscopical investigations of the nitrosomorpholine-intoxicated rat liver, in: *Recent Results in Cancer Research*, Vol. 19, Springer New York.

BENEDETTI, E., AND EMMELOT, P., Effect of dimethylnitrosamine on the endoplasmic reticulum of rat liver cells, *Lab. Invest.* **15**:209.

BERNHARD, W., FRAYSSINET, C., LAFARGE, C., AND LE BRETON, E., 1965, Lesions nucleolaires precoces provoquees par l'aflatoxine dans les cellules hepatiques du rat, *Compt. Rend. Acad. Sci.* **261**:1785.

BRANDES, D., SLOAN, K., ANTON, E., AND BLOEDORN, F., 1967, The effect of X-irradiation on the lysosomes of mouse mammary gland carcinoma, *Cancer Res.* **27**:731.

BRUNI, C., 1973, Distinctive cells similar to fetal hepatocytes associated with liver carcinogenesis by diethylnitrosamine: Electron microscopic study, *J. Natl. Cancer Inst.* **50:**1513.

BUSCH, H., AND SMETANA, K., *The Nucleolus*, 1970, Academic Press, New York.

BUSCH, H., BYVOET, P., AND SMETANA, K., 1963, The nucleolus of the cancer cell: A review, *Cancer Res.* **23:**313.

BUTLER, W. H., 1966, Early hepatic parenchymal changes induced in the rat by aflatoxin $B_1$, *Am. J. Pathol.* **49:**113.

CHILDS, E., AYRES, J., AND KOEHLER, P., 1972, Aflatoxin $B_1$—Effects on rainbow trout liver chromatin, *Biochem. Pharmacol.* **21:**3053.

COOK, J., DUFFY, E., AND SCHOENTAL, R., 1950, Primary liver tumours in rats following feeding with alkaloids of *Senecio jacobaea*, *Brit. J. Cancer* **4:**405.

EMMELOT, P., AND BENEDETTI, E., 1961, Some observations on the effect of liver carcinogens on the fine structure and function of the endoplasmic reticulum of rat liver, in: *Protein Biosynthesis* (R. Harris, ed.), pp. 99–123, Academic Press, London and New York.

EMMELOT, P., AND BENEDETTI, E., 1966, On the possible involvement of the plasma membrane in the carcinogenic process, in: *Carcinogenesis: A Broad Critique*, pp. 471–533, M. D. Anderson Hospital and Tumor Institute, University of Taxas, Houston, Williams and Wilkins, Baltimore.

EPSTEIN, S., ITO, N., MERKOW, L., AND FARBER, E., 1967, Cellular analysis of liver carcinogenesis: The induction of large hyperplastic nodules in the liver with 2-fluorenylacetamide of ethionine and some aspects of their morphology and glycogen metabolism, *Cancer Res.* **27:**1702.

FARBER, E., 1963, Ethionine carcinogenesis, *Advan. Cancer Res.* **7:**383.

FIRMINGER, H., AND MULAY, A., 1952, Histochemical and morphologic differentiation of induced tumors of the liver in rats, *J. Natl. Cancer Inst.* **13:**19.

FOUTS, J., AND ROGERS, L., 1965, Morphological changes in the liver accompanying stimulation of microsomal drug metabolizing enzyme activity by phenobarbital, chlordane, benzpyrene or methylcholanthrene in rats, *J. Pharmacol. Exp. Ther.* **147:**112.

FRIEND, D., AND FARQUHAR, M., 1967, Functions of coated vesicles during protein absorption in the rat vas deferens, *J. Cell Biol.* **35:**357.

GEIL, J., STENGER, R., BEHKI, R., AND MORGAN, W., 1968, Hepatotoxic and carcinogenic effects of dimethylnitrosamine in low dosage: Light and electron microscopic study, *J. Natl. Cancer Inst.* **40:**713.

GOLDBLATT, L. A., 1969, *"Aflatoxin": Scientific Background, Control, and Implications* (L. Goldblatt, ed.), Academic Press, New York and London.

HARD, G., AND BUTLER, W., 1971a, Ultrastructural study of the development of interstitial lesions leading to mesenchymal neoplasia induced in the rat renal cortex by dimethylnitrosamine, *Cancer Res.* **31:**337.

HARD, G., AND BUTLER, W., 1971b, Ultrastructural aspects of renal adenocarcinoma induced in the rat by dimethylnitrosamine, *Cancer Res.* **31:**366.

HARRIS, C., REDDY, J., AND SVOBODA, D., 1968, Isolation and ultrastructure of nucleoli altered *in vivo*, *Exp. Cell Res.* **51:**268.

HARRIS, C., REDDY, J., CHIGA, M., AND SVOBODA, D., 1969, Polysome disaggregation in rat liver by lasiocarpine, *Biochim. Biophys. Acta* **182:**587.

HERDSON, P., GARVIN, P., AND JENNINGS, R., 1964, Reversible biological and fine structural changes produced in rat liver by a thiohydantoin compound, *Lab. Invest.* **13:**1014.

HERROLD, K., 1969, Aflatoxin induced lesions in Syrian hamsters, *Brit. J. Cancer* **23:**655.

HRUBAN, Z., SWIFT, H., DUNN, F., AND LEWIS, D., 1965, Effect of $\beta$-3-furylalanine on the ultrastructure of the hepatocytes and pancreatic acinar cells, *Lab. Invest.* **14:**70.

KAMPSCHMIDT, R., AND WELLS, D., 1969, Acid hydrolase activity during the induction and transplantation of hepatomas in the rat, *Cancer Res.* **29:**1028.

KARASAKI, S., 1969, The fine structure of proliferating cells in preneoplastic rat livers during azo-dye carcinogenesis, *J. Cell Biol.* **40:**322.

KENDREY, G., 1968, Fine structural changes in rat liver cells in response to prolonged thioacetamide, *Pathol. Europ.* **3:**96.

KETTERER, B., HOLT, S., AND ROSS-MANSELL, P., 1967, The effect of a single intraperitoneal dose of the Hepatocarcinogen 4-dimethylaminoazobenzene on the rough-surfaced endoplasmic reticulum of the liver of the rat, *Biochem. J.* **103:**692.

KINGSBURY, J., 1964, *Poisonous Plants of the U.S. and Canada*, pp. 425–435, Prentice-Hall, Englewood Cliffs, N.J.

321

SOME EFFECTS
OF CHEMICAL
CARCINOGENS
ON CELL
ORGANELLES

KOSHIBA, K., THIRUMALACHARY, C., DASKAL, Y., AND BUSCH, H., 1971, Ultrastructural and biochemical studies on ribonucleoprotein particles from isolated nucleoli of thioacetamide-treated rat liver, *Exp. Cell. Res.* **68**:235.

LAFONTAINE, J., AND ALLARD, C., 1964, A light and electron microscope study of the morphological changes induced in rat liver cells by the azo dye 2-Me-DAB, *J. Cell Biol.* **22**:143.

LANTOS, P., KETTERER, B., AND HOLT, S., 1973, The ultrastructure of the hepatocyte of the vitamin E deficient rat and the effect of a single intraperitoneal dose of N,N-dimethyl-4-aminoazobenzene on the stability of its fractionated polysomes, *Exp. Mol. Pathol.* **18**:68.

LEE, K., AND GOODALL, C., 1968, Methylation of ribonucleic acid and deoxyribonucleic acid and tumour induction in livers of hypophysectomized rats treated with dimethylnitrosamine, *Biochem. j.* **106**:767.

LOUD, A., 1968, A quantitative stereological description of the ultrastructure of normal rat liver parenchymal cells, *J. Cell Biol.* **37**:27.

MAGEE, P., 1963, Cellular injury and chemical carcinogenesis by N-nitroso compounds, in: *Cancer Progress, Volume 1963* (R. Raven, ed.), pp. 56–66, Butterworths, London.

MAGEE, P., AND BARNES, J., 1967, Carcinogenic nitro compounds, *Advan. Cancer Res.* **10**:163–246.

MALVALDI, G., 1969, Changes in dry mass of rat liver nuclei in chronic thioacetamide poisoning, *Experientia* **25**:955.

MCLEAN, E., 1970, The toxic actions of Pyrrolizidine (*Senecio*) alkaloids, *Pharmacol. Rev.* **22**:429.

MELDOLESI, J., CLEMENTI, F., CHIESARA, E., CONTI, F., AND FANTI, A., 1967, Cytoplasmic changes in rat liver after prolonged treatment with low doses of ethionine and adenine, *Lab. Invest.* **17**:265.

MERKOW, L., EPSTEIN, S., SLIFKIN, M., FARBER, E., AND PARDO, M., 1971, Ultrastructural alterations within hyperplastic liver nodules induced by ethionine, *Cancer Res.* **31**:174.

MERKOW, L., EPSTEIN, S., SLIFKIN, M., FARBER, E., AND PARDO, M., 1972, The cellular analysis of liver carcinogenesis. V. Ultrastructural alterations within hepatocellular carcinoma induced by ethionine, *Lab. Invest.* **26**:300.

MIKATA, A., AND LUSE, S., 1964, Ultrastructural changes in the rat liver produced by N-2-fluorenyldiacetamide, *Am. J. Pathol.* **44**:455.

MIYAI, K., AND RITCHIE, A., 1970, Natural resolution of hepatic ultrastructural changes induced by DL-ethionine, *Am. J. Pathol.* **61**:211.

MIYAI, K., AND STEINER, J., 1965, Fine structure of interphase liver cell nuclei in subacute ethionine intoxication, *Exp. Mol. Pathol.* **4**:525.

MONNERON, A., 1969, Experimental induction of helical polysomes in adult rat liver, *Lab. Invest.* **20**:178.

MONNERON, A., LIEW, C., AND ALLFREY, V., 1971, Isolation and biological activity of mammalian helical polyribosomes, *J. Mol. Biol.* **57**:335.

MUKHERJEE, T., GUSTAFSSON, R., AFZELIUS, B., AND ARRHENIUS, E., 1963, Effects of carcinogenic amines on amino acid incorporation by liver systems. II. A morphological and biochemical study on the effect of dimethylnitrosamine, *Cancer Res.* **23**:944.

NAIR, V., CASPER, R., SIEGEL, S., AND BAU, D., 1970, Regulation of the diurnal rhythm in hepatic drug metabolism, *Fed. Proc.* **29**:804 (abst.).

NEWBERNE, P., AND WOGAN, G., 1968, Sequential morphologic changes in aflatoxin $B_1$ carcinogenesis in the rat, *Cancer Res.* **28**:770.

NIGAM, V., 1965, Glycogen metabolism in liver during DAB carcinogenesis, *Brit. J. Cancer* **19**:912.

NOVIKOFF, A., AND SHIN, W., 1964, The endoplasmic reticulum in the Golgi zone and its relation to microbodies, Golgi apparatus and autophagic vacuoles in rat liver cells, *J. Micros.* **3**:187.

OKAZAKI, K., SHULL, K., AND FARBER, E., 1968, Effects of ethionine on adenosine triphosphate levels and ionic composition of liver cell nuclei, *J. Biol. Chem.* **243**:4661.

OPIE, E. L., 1944, The pathogenesis of tumors of the liver produced by butter yellow, *J. Exp. Med.* **80**:231.

ORRENIUS, S., AND ERICSSON, J., 1966, On the relationship of liver glucose-6-phosphatase to the proliferation of endoplasmic reticulum in phenobarbital induction, *J. Cell Biol.* **31**:243.

PAUL, J., ROSS, W., AND MONTGOMERY, P., JR., 1971, Ultrastructural nucleolar segregation and carcinogenicity among the 4-nitroquinoline-1-oxides, *J. Natl. Cancer Inst.* **47**:367.

PONG, R., AND WOGAN, G., 1970, Time course and dose–response characteristics of aflatoxin $B_1$ effects on rat liver polymerase and ultrastructure, *Cancer Res.* **30**:294.

POPPER, H., STERNBERG, S., OSER, B., AND OSER, M., 1960, The carcinogenic effect of aramite in rats, *Cancer* **13**:1035.

PORTER, K., AND BRUNI, C., 1959, An electron microscope study of the early effects of 3'-Me-DAB on rat liver cells, *Cancer Res.* **19**:997.

REDDY, J., AND SVOBODA. D., 1968, The relationship of nucleolar segregation to ribonucleic acid synthesis following the administration of selected hepatocarcinogens, *Lab. Invest.* **19**:132.

REDDY, J., CHIGA, M., HARRIS, C., AND SVOBODA, D., 1970, Polyribosomal disaggregation in rat liver following administration of tannic acid, *Cancer Res.* **30**:58.

RUBIN, E., HUTTERER, F., AND LIEBER, C., 1968, Ethanol increase hepatic smooth endoplasmic reticulum and drug-metabolizing enzymes, *Science (N.Y.)* **159**:1469.

SCHOENTAL, R., 1963, Pyrrolizidine (*Senecio*) alkaloids and their hepatotoxic action, *Biochem. J.* **88**:57p.

SCHOENTAL, R., AND HEAD, M., 1955, Pathological changes in rats as a result of treatment with monocrotaline, *Brit. J. Cancer* **9**:229.

SCHOENTAL, R., AND HEAD, M., 1957, Progression of liver lesions in rats by temporary treatment in pyrrolizidine (*Senecio*) alkaloids, and the effects of betaine and high casein diet, *Brit. J. Cancer* **11**:535.

SCHOENTAL, R., AND MAGEE, P., 1959, Further observations on the subacute and chronic liver changes in rats after a single dose of various pyrrolizidine (*Senecio*) alkaloids, *J. Pathol. Bacteriol.* **78**:471.

SHINOZUKA, H., AND FARBER, E., 1969, Reformation of nucleoli after ethionine-induced fragmentation in the absence of significant protein synthesis, *J. Cell Biol.* **41**:280.

SHINOZUKA, H., GOLDBLATT, P., AND FARBER, E., 1968, The disorganization of hepatic cell nucleoli induced by ethionine and its reversal by adenine, *J. Cell Biol.* **36**:313.

SHINOZUKA, H., REID, I., SHULL, K., LIANG, H., AND FARBER, E., 1970, Dynamics of liver cell injury and repair. I. Spontaneous reformation of the nucleolus and polyribosomes in the presence of extensive cytoplasmic damage induced by ethionine, *Lab. Invest.* **23**:253.

SIMARD, A., AND DAOUST, R., 1966, DNA synthesis and neoplastic transformation in rat liver parenchyma, *Cancer Res.* **26**:1665.

SMITH, E., NOSANCHUK, J., SCHNITZER, B., AND SWARM, R., 1968, Fatty inclusions and microcysts, *arch. Pathol.* **85**:175.

STEINER, J., MIYAI, K., AND PHILLIPS, M., 1964, Electron microscopy of membrane-particle arrays in liver cells of ethionine-intoxicated rats, *Am. J. Pathol.* **44**:169.

STENGER, R., 1970, Organelle pathology of the liver: The endoplasmic reticulum, *Gastroenterology* **58**:554.

SVOBODA, D., 1964, Fine structure of hepatomas induced in rats with *p*-dimethylaminoazobenzene, *J. Natl. Cancer Inst.* **33**:315.

SVOBODA, D., AND HIGGINSON, J., 1968, A comparison of ultrastructural changes in rat liver due to chemical carcinogens, *Cancer Res.* **28**:1703.

SVOBODA, D., AND REDDY, J., 1970, Some effects of carcinogens on the structure and activity of liver cells, in: *Metabolic Aspects of Food Safety* (F. Roe, ed.), Chap. 19, pp. 533–567, Blackwell, Oxford and Edinburgh.

SVOBODA, D., AND REDDY, J., 1973, Some biological properties of microbodies (peroxisomes), in: *Pathobiology Annual* (H. Ioachin, ed.), Appleton-Century-Crofts, New York.

SVOBODA, D., AND SOGA, J., 1966, Early effects of pyrrolizidine alkaloids on the fine structure of rat liver cells, *Am. J. Pathol.* **48**:347.

SVOBODA, D., GRADY, H., AND HIGGINSON, J., 1966, Aflatoxin $B_1$ injury in rat and monkey liver, *Am. J. Pathol.* **49**:1023.

TIMME, A., AND FOWLE, L., 1963, Effects of *p*-dimethylaminoazobenzene on the fine structure of rat liver cells, *Nature (Lond.)* **200**:694.

UNUMA, T., MORRIS, H., AND BUSCH, H., 1967, Comparative studies of the nucleoli of Morris hepatomas, embryonic liver, and aflatoxin $B_1$–treated liver of rats, *Cancer Res.* **27**:2221.

VILLA-TREVINO, S., AND LEAVER, D., 1968, Effects of the hepatotoxic agents retrorsine and aflatoxin $B_1$ on hepatic protein synthesis in the rat, *Biochem. J.* **109**:87.

WEIBEL, E., STAUBLI, W., GNAGI, R., AND HESS, F., 1969, Correlated morphometric and biochemical studies on the liver cell. I. Morphometric model, stereologic methods, and normal morphometric data for rat liver, *J. Cell Biol.* **42**:68.

WILLIAMS, G., AND HULTIN, T., 1973, Ribosomes of mouse liver following administration of dimethylnitrosamine, *Cancer Res.* **33**:1796.

WOGAN, G., 1965, *Mycotoxins in Foodstuffs* (G. Wogan, ed.), pp. 153–273, Proceedings of a Symposium held at Massachusetts Institute of Technology, 1964, M.I.T. Press, Cambridge, Mass.

YASUZUMI, G., SUGIHARA, R., ITO, N., KONISHI, Y., AND HIASA, Y., 1970, Fine structure of nuclei as revealed by electron microscopy. VII. Hyperplastic liver nodules in rat induced by 3'-methyl-4-dimethylaminoazobenzene, 2-fluorenylacetamide and DL-ethionine, *Exp. Cell Res.* **63**:83.

# 10

# Sequential Aspects of Chemical Carcinogenesis: Skin

Isaac Berenblum

## 1. Origin of the Concept of Sequential Stages of Skin Carcinogenesis

The existence of sequential stages of carcinogenesis first became apparent in connection with skin response, by the convergence of two independent lines of inquiry: The primary aim in the one case was to try to explain why experimentally induced papillomas in rabbit skin tended so often to regress, but also to answer the more basic question of whether such apparently unstable growths were indeed truly neoplastic (Rous and Kidd, 1941; MacKenzie and Rous, 1941; see also Friedewald and Rous, 1944a,b, 1950). The aim in the other case was to study the nature of the newly discovered cocarcinogenic action of croton oil in mouse skin, and at a more fundamental level to try to understand—in functional rather than morphological terms—the nature of the changes in skin during the long latent period of carcinogenesis (Berenblum, 1941a,b; see also Berenblum and Shubik, 1947a,b, 1949a,b).

In the rabbit experiments referred to above, it was possible to show that papillomas that had apparently regressed completely could be made to reappear at the identical sites by means of nonspecific stimuli (e.g., by punching holes in the ear or by applications of substances such as turpentine and chloroform). This led Rous and his associates to conclude (1) that foci of tumor cells, no longer visible to the naked eye, remained in a "latent" or dormant state, capable of being "reawakened," and (2) that the induction process on the one hand and the

Isaac Berenblum ● The Weizmann Institute of Science, Rehovot, Israel.

subsequent growth process on the other depended on different kinds of stimuli and therefore involved independent mechanisms—referred to as "initiation" and "promotion."

In the mouse experiments, the cocarcinogenic agent, croton oil, was found capable of enhancing tumor induction when it was applied after a subeffective dose of carcinogenic hydrocarbon, but not when applied beforehand. This was taken to mean that the starting of the carcinogenic process and its completion involved separate mechanisms—referred to at the time as "precarcinogenic" and "epicarcinogenic," respectively (with yet a third stage, called "metacarcinogenic," responsible for the subsequent transformation of benign papillomas into malignant tumors). (Other terms, introduced by workers such as Mottram, 1944a,b, and Tannenbaum, 1944b, soon disappeared from the literature.)

Although the rabbit experiments and the mouse experiments just referred to were apparently related in the interpretative sense, they did differ in two important respects:

1. In the rabbit experiments, the primary action (initiation) was continued for a long enough time to cause tumors to appear, while the secondary action (promotion) caused those once regressed to reappear. In the mouse experiments, the primary action (precarcinogenic) was insufficient to produce tumors, while the secondary action (epicarcinogenic) caused visible tumors to appear for the first time.

2. In the rabbit experiments, the secondary action was nonspecific; in the mouse experiments, a definitely specific kind of action (e.g., by croton oil) was required, many other skin irritants proving ineffective (see Shubik, 1950a; Saffiotti and Shubik, 1963).

Nevertheless, in the interest of conformity, and in order to avoid confusion, one single terminology—of initiation and promotion, as proposed by Rous and colleagues—became accepted by everyone for both kinds of effects.

The early studies on sequential stages of skin carcinogenesis briefly outlined above have been extensively reviewed in the past (e.g., see Berenblum, 1944, 1947, 1954a,b, 1960; Salaman, 1958; Salaman and Roe, 1964; Wolstenholme and O'Connor, 1959; Saffiotti amd Shubik, 1963; Boutwell, 1964). They need not therefore be discussed again in great detail here. Attention will be paid only to some of the more crucial and controversial features of these early studies, as an introduction to contemporary work in the field. (For reviews of more recent developments, see Van Duuren, 1969; Berenblum, 1969, 1974; Hecker, 1971a.)

## 2. The Search for Other Initiators and Promoters of Skin Carcinogenesis

One of the limitations of the original two-stage technique for mouse skin carcinogenesis was that the initiating action had to depend on the use of a complete carcinogen (acting for a very brief period, so that the potential promoting action did not have a chance of expressing itself). This complication was ultimately eliminated by the discovery that urethan could act cocarcinogeni-

cally with croton oil on mouse skin when the two were applied concurrently (Graffi 325
SEQUENTIAL
ASPECTS OF
CHEMICAL
CAR-
CINOGENESIS:
SKIN *et al.*, 1953) and as a pure initiator when applied first, with croton oil treatment given later (e.g., Salaman and Roe, 1953). The initiating action of urethan on the skin could as well be demonstrated by administering the compound systemically, with croton oil applied locally to the skin (Haran and Berenblum, 1956; Ritchie, 1957), as was similarly known to be the case with 2-acetylaminofluorene (Ritchie and Saffiotti, 1955) and with various carcinogenic hydrocarbons (Graffi *et al.*, 1955: Berenblum and Haran-Ghera, 1957*b*). (For confirmation of systemic initiating action of carcinogenic hydrocarbons on mouse skin using the active principle of croton oil as promoter for bocal application, see Hecker and Paul 1968.)

Other initiators for skin carcinogenesis (which were themselves either noncarcinogenic or only weakly carcinogenic) included β-radiation (Shubik *et al.*, 1953*b*); benz[*a*]anthracene, β-propiolactone, triethylene melamine (TEM), and 4-*N,N*-di(2-chloroethyl)butyric acid (Roe and Salaman, 1955; Roe and Glendenning, 1956); some esters of methanesulfonic acid (Roe, 1957); *N*-phenylcarbamate, an analogue of urethan (Van Esch *et al.*, 1958); and dibenz[*a,c*]anthracene (Van Duuren, 1969). On the other hand, negative results were obtained with anthracene and borderline results with phenanthrene, pyrene, and a number of other compounds (see Salaman and Roe, 1956*c*). Negative results were also obtained with acridine orange, acridine yellow, and certain antimetabolites of nucleic acid synthesis (Trainin *et al.*, 1964).

For promoting action, apart from that of croton oil, the following were found to possess some activity for mouse skin: iodoacetic acid and chloracetophenone (Gwynn and Salaman, 1953); phenol and some of its analogues (Rusch *et al.*, 1955), including anthranil (1,8,9-trihydroxyanthracene) (Bock and Burns, 1963) and related compounds (Segal *et al.*, 1971); certain straight-chain hydrocarbons, such as *n*-dodecane (Shubik *et al.*, 1956; Saffiotti and Shubik, 1956) and some other alkanes and 1-alkanols (Sicé, 1966); cantharidin (Hennings and Boutwell, 1970); citrus oils (Roe and Peirce, 1960); *Euphorbia* lattices (Roe and Peirce, 1961), the active constituents of which are related to those of croton oil (see Hecker, 1971*b*); and cigarette condensates (Gelhorn, 1958; Wynder and Hoffman, 1961; Van Duuren *et al.*, 1966*a*; Roe and Walters, 1965). (For skin irritants lacking promoting action for mouse skin, see Shubik, 1950*a*, and Saffiotti and Shubik, 1963: these included turpentine, acridine, fluorene, phenanthrene, castor oil, ricinoleic acid, oleic acid, and silver nitrate.)

Much interest was shown, at one time, in the promoting properties of certain surface-acting lipophilic–hydrophilic substances belonging to the "Tween" and "Span" group of detergents (Setälä *et al.*, 1954; see Setälä, 1960). These substances required very high concentrations to be effective as promoting agents for the skin and also possessed considerable carcinogenic activity of their own (Della Porta *et al.*, 1960).

Since none of the newer promoting agents possessed any clear advantages over croton oil, most of them being more weakly acting and some having undesirable side-effects, it became all the more pressing to isolate and identify the active principle(s) of croton oil itself. After many unsuccessful (or partially successful) attempts in various laboratories, Hecker and his associates (see reviews by Hecker, 1968, 1971a; but see also Van Duuren, 1969) succeeded in isolating and characterizing a number of phorbol diesters with specific fatty acid chains in particular positions in the phorbol molecule (see Fig. 1), the most active derivative, TPA, possessing pronounced promoting activity in high dilution for mouse skin. Unesterified phorbol proved to be entirely inactive as a promoter for skin carcinogenesis, although it was later shown to be active systemically for certain other tissues (see Section 7).

## 3. Quantitative Analysis of the Two-Stage Mechanism

The initiation–promotion hypothesis, as proposed for mouse skin, with croton oil as promoting agent, lent itself to quantitative analysis as a basis for judging its validity. If tumor induction consisted of an initial transformation of a normal cell into a dormant tumor cell, and if the "dormancy" of the latter had to be overcome by a different kind of action, then the following premises could be formulated and submitted to experimental testing:

1. Initiating action—presumably a mutation-like process—should be completed very rapidly, most of the long latent period of carcinogenesis being taken up with the promoting phase.
2. The total tumor incidence should theoretically be determined by the potency of the initiating stimulus, while the speed of action (i.e., the actual latent period) should depend on the efficiency and persistence of action of the promoting agent.
3. If the conversion, by initiating action, of a normal cell into a dormant tumor cell is essentially an irreversible process—a valid assumption if it represents a mutational change in the genome—then a delay in the interval between completion of initiating action and the start of promoting action should not seriously affect the incidence of tumors but merely cause a corresponding delay in their time of appearance.
4. Since promoting action could only operate on cells already transformed by initiating action, reversal of the procedure—i.e., applying the promoting agent before the initiating agent—should be ineffective in producing tumors.
5. Artificial inhibitors of carcinogenesis (Anticarcinogenic agents) might be expected to operate more readily on the promoting phase than on the initiating phase.

At first, the model for the detailed study of the initiating–promoting system involved 8 weekly applications of a carcinogenic hydrocarbon, followed by twice weekly applications of croton oil for several months. Mottram (1944a,b) then introduced a useful simplification by demonstrating that a single application of the carcinogen was sufficient for initiating action. Quantitative analysis of the results thus became easier to interpret. (The use of urethan as a "pure" initiator for skin carcinogenesis, with phorbol esters as promoter—see Section 2—provided further refinements of the technique in later experiments.)

Early attempts to determine the time required for initiating action involved removal of the hydrocarbon with appropriate solvents after brief intervals (followed by standard croton oil treatment). Even as short a time as 15 min proved adequate for effective initiating action (Ball and McCarter, 1960). But since appreciable amounts of the hydrocarbon had by then already penetrated the cells (and thus were no longer extractable), the true time of action by the initiator might have been longer than 15 min.

A different approach to the problem was to use actinomycin D as an inhibitor of the initiating phase of skin carcinogenesis and to determine its optimal effect in relation to the time of application of the initiator (Gelboin *et al.*, 1965). The results (although conflicting with those of others; see Section 6) led Gelboin and colleagues to conclude that the process of initiation—the actual transformation into a dormant tumor cell—involved metabolic changes during one mitotic cycle, which took about a day for completion.

Although none of the results so far available provide sufficiently accurate data as to the exact speed of initiating action, there seems little doubt that the time is of the order of hours rather than weeks or months. This is compatible with the concept of a mutational change in the genome of the cell (see Section 8).

In contrast to this, promoting action is undoubtedly a very slow process, occupying the greater part of the latent period of carcinogenesis. This is supported by the need for long-continued treatment with croton oil in order for tumors to develop by the two-stage technique. Promotion can also be arrested by the application of anticarcinogenic agents (see reviews by Crabtree, 1947; Van Duuren and Melchione, 1969).

It should be noted, however, that under certain favorable conditions a single application of a carcinogen to the mouse's skin, without supplementary (promoting) action, can sometimes cause tumors to develop (Mider and Morton, 1939; Law, 1941; Cramer and Stowell, 1943; Terracini *et al.*, 1960). Tumors are particularly likely to occur when the application is made during the "resting phase" of the hair cycle (see Andreasen and Engelbreth-Holm, 1953; Borum, 1954). This can be attributed to the fact that during the "resting phase" the hydrocarbon remains for at least a week dissolved in the sebum in the hair follicles, and thus has time to act as promoter as well as initiator, in contrast to what happens during the "growth phase" of the hair cycle, when there is active sebum secretion, causing the hydrocarbon to be "washed out" within a day or two (Berenblum *et al.*, 1958).

The second of the abovementioned five premises—that the final tumor yield by the two-stage technique should be quantitatively related to the dose of initiating agent—was experimentally confirmed using different known concentrations of carcinogenic hydrocarbon applied locally (Berenblum and Shubik, 1949a; McCarter *et al.*, 1956) or using urethan applied locally (Roe and Salaman, 1954) or administered systematically (Berenblum and Haran-Ghera, 1957a), and followed in each case by standard croton oil treatment.

The irreversible nature of initiating action (the third of the five premises) was likewise confirmed, in this case by testing the two-stage process with varying intervals between the initiating action and the start of the promoting action. No falling off in tumor yield resulted, in most cases, from lengthening the interval between initiation and promotion, whether the initiator was a carcinogenic hydrocarbon applied locally (Berenblum and Shubik, 1947b, 1949b; Van Duuren, 1969) or urethan administered systemically (Berenblum and Haran-Ghera, 1957a). (For an apparent exception, see Section 6.)

Evidence in support of the fourth premise—that tumors should fail to appear when the sequence of initiating action and promoting action is reversed—was quoted at the very outset (see Section 1) as the basis of the two-stage mechanism in skin. It has since been confirmed under more stringent conditions (see Berenblum and Haran, 1955; Roe, 1959).

As for the fifth premise—that anticarcinogenic agents should operate more readily on the promoting phase (which can in any case be interrupted by discontinuing the croton oil treatment) than on the initiating phase (which is generally assumed to be essentially an irreversible process)—evidence in support of this goes back to the time of the original discovery of anticarcinogenic action (see Berenblum, 1929), when it was shown that sulfur mustard could seriously interfere with tar carcinogenesis in the skin, even when applied quite late. Another early example, this time operating systemically, was the observation by Tannenbaum (1944a) that the inhibiting effect of caloric restriction of the diet operated during the promoting phase of skin carcinogenesis. (For further details, see Section 6.)

## 4. Critique of the Two-Stage Hypothesis

The experimental data presented so far deal with evidence in support of the initiation–promotion theory of skin carcinogenesis. However, the theory has been subjected to criticism from time to time. This called, in turn, for further tests to try, if possible, to meet the objections raised.

The earliest criticism, which actually questioned the very concept inherent in the initiation–promotion theory, was regarding the existence of "dormant tumor cells" as precursors of visibly growing tumors. The doubts arose from some early experiments by Orr (1934, 1935, 1937) indicating that vascular and fibrocytic changes in the chorium rather than specific, irreversible changes in the covering epithelium determined the development of skin tumors (however, see Ritchie, 1952a,b). The criticism seemed to receive strong support from subsequent experiments involving reciprocal grafting of carcinogen-treated "initiated" skin to normal sites and of normal skin to "initiated" sites, followed in both cases by croton oil treatment (Billingham et al., 1951; Marchant and Orr, 1953, 1955). Tumors should theoretically have developed preferentially in the skin grafts that had received initiating action prior to transplantation, whereas in fact they arose more frequently at the sites where "initiated" skin had been excised and normal skin grafted in its place. This was interpreted by Orr (1958) to conflict with the notion of dormant tumor cells (although he had admitted, in an earlier publication, the possibility that such postulated dormant tumor cells might have remained behind in the skin appendages, thus accounting for the anomalous results). Later, using genetic markers to determine the origin of induced tumors in skin, Lappé (1968, 1969) and Steinmuller (1971) were able to establish that skin tumors were indeed derived from dormant tumor cells carried over in grafts.

329

SEQUENTIAL
ASPECTS OF
CHEMICAL
CAR-
CINOGENESIS:
SKIN

The fact that the papillomas in mouse skin produced by the two-stage process tended to regress more commonly than those produced by repeated applications of a carcinogenic hydrocarbon (Shubik, 1950b; Saffiotti and Shubik, 1956; Frei and Kingsley, 1968) raised some doubts as to whether the former method of induction was truly comparable to conventional carcinogenesis. Van Duuren et al. (1966b), while confirming the high regression rate when using crude croton oil as promoter, failed to observe it when using one of the semipurified active constituents of croton oil—thus suggesting that some unknown anticarcinogen might be present in the crude croton oil, largely responsible for the regression.

Another somewhat disturbing feature of the two-stage technique was that croton oil possessed some carcinogenic activity of its own—usually producing no more than an occasional papilloma per group of control mice (Roe, 1956b), although in some strains the incidence could be very high (see Boutwell et al., 1957). There is always the theoretical possibility that, in these cases, croton oil acted as a promoting agent with respect to dormant tumor cells that arose spontaneously rather than as a complete carcinogen. Such an eventuality would make it impossible ever to prove the noncarcinogenicity of a "pure" promoter. Actually, in practice, the background carcinogenicity of croton oil rarely interferes with the interpretation of results using the two-stage technique.

There is, finally, the "irreversibility" of the initiating phase to be considered—as demonstrated by the maintenance of the same tumor yield, however long the interval between the initiating action and the start of promoting action (in one experiment as long as 43 weeks; see Berenblum and Shubik, 1949b).

While these results have been repeatedly confirmed under various conditions (see Graffi, 1953; Berenblum and Haran-Ghera, 1957a; Van Duuren, 1969) and partly confirmed (i.e., with some falling off only) under conditions of poor health of the animals (Roe and Salaman, 1954), a discordant result has been reported by Roe et al. (1972), with a striking falling off in incidence when the interval between initiating action (by DMBA) and promoting action (by TPA, one of the active principles of croton oil) was 50 wk. The authors themselves conclude that "this finding is not necessarily at variance with the postulate of irreversibility of the formation of 'latent tumour cells'" and suggest, as an alternative explanation, the possibility of regression of induced tumors, at a very early stage, resulting from immunosurveillance.

In summary, the initiation–promotion hypothesis seems to have stood up reasonably well since its original formulation more than 30 yr ago, although calling for (1) minor modifications and elaboration of the initial scheme (see Section 5), (2) consideration of factors capable of influencing initiation or promotion (see Section 6), (3) extension of the scheme to systems other than skin carcinogenesis (see Section 7), and (4) attempts to explain the nature of initiation and promotion in functional terms and also, if possible, in biochemical terms (see Section 8).

## 5. Extensions of the Two-Stage System

It already seemed apparent from one of the early experiments (Berenblum, 1941b) that in addition to promoting action, croton oil was capable of encouraging induced papillomas to become malignant ("metacarcinogenic" action; see Section 1). This aspect of the problem has since been followed up under more varying conditions (see Shubik, 1950b; Shubik et al., 1953a; Roe, 1956a,b; Salaman and Roe, 1956a,b; Boutwell et al., 1957; Van Duuren et al., 1966b). (The phenomenon is, strictly speaking, an aspect of tumor progression—see Foulds, 1954—and therefore "postcarcinogenic" rather than part of the process of carcinogenesis per se.) The results of these subsequent studies may be summarized as follows:

1. The transition from a benign papilloma to a malignant tumor represents at least one, and possibly several, irreversible steps (Shubik, 1950b; Shubik et al., 1953a).
2. These changes usually occur spontaneously—e.g., even after a single application of a carcinogen, without subsequent treatment of any kind (e.g., see Mider and Morton, 1939; Shubik et al., 1953a; Roe, 1956a).
3. Since the rate and extent of progression to malignancy vary greatly from one papilloma to another in the same animal, the process is not under systemic control, but determined within the benign tumor cell.
4. However, progression to malignancy can be artificially stimulated by additional croton oil treatment (Berenblum, 1941b), as confirmed by Roe (1956a), more so with the use of the active constituents of croton oil (Van Duuren et al., 1966b), and even more effectively by repeated applications of a carcinogenic hydrocarbon or by supplementary hydrocarbon treatment after the two-stage hydrocarbon–croton oil technique (Shubik, 1950b).

As for the initiation–promotion process itself, further divisions have been proposed, based on evidence suggesting (1) that there is a pre-initiating phase (Pound and Bell, 1962; Pound and Withers, 1963) and (2) that the promoting phase is itself made up of two separate stages (Boutwell, 1964).

The evidence for a pre-initiating phase arose from the observation that with urethan as initiator and croton oil as promoter an enhanced tumor response could be elicited when the skin was, in addition, prepainted with croton oil (Pound and Bell, 1962). This did not negate the earlier claims that reversal of the initiation promotion process failed to cause tumors to appear, since subsequent croton oil treatment was still essential and since the augmentation also occurred as a result of pretreatment with such nonspecific stimuli as acetic acid, trichloracetic acid, xylene, turpentine, or cantharidin (itself an anticarcinogenic agent when applied during the promoting phase), or even by scarification (Pound and Withers, 1963). Furthermore, the need for such pretreatment was observed only in relation to urethan as initiator, not with DMBA (7,12-dimethylbenz[a]anthracene) and only slightly so with β-propiolactone as initiator (Hennings *et al.*, 1969). The most plausible explanation of the phenomenon is that initiating action requires the cells to be in a state of mitotic division (*cf.* Gelboin *et al.*, 1965)—a process which is stimulated by all skin irritants, including carcinogenic hydrocarbons (acting at the same time as initiator), but not by urethan, which therefore calls for additional "preinitiation stimulation" for optimal effects.

331
SEQUENTIAL
ASPECTS OF
CHEMICAL
CAR-
CINOGENESIS:
SKIN

The proposal for two separate stages of promotion rested on the fact that when DMBA as initiator was followed by croton oil for 5 wk and then by turpentine for a further 5 wk, the tumor yield was significantly higher than when the DMBA was followed by turpentine first and by croton oil afterward under otherwise identical conditions (Boutwell, 1964). The mechanism of this complex situation is not yet understood.

## 6. Factors Influencing Initiation and Promotion

There are many factors capable of influencing the outcome of carcinogenic action—both positively (cocarcinogenic) and negatively (anticarcinogenic). These may be further subdivided according to whether the influence is on the scope of action of the carcinogen or on the response of the animal. (For a detailed classification of the various types of cocarcinogenic action, see Berenblum, 1969. It should be noted that promoting action represents only one special kind of cocarcinogenic action, connected with tissue response.)

The advantages of studying cocarcinogenic and anticarcinogenic action *vis-à-vis* the separate stages of initiation and promotion are twofold: (1) the mechanisms of action of cocarcinogenic and anticarcinogenic agents might thus become better understood, and (2) cocarcinogenic and anticarcinogenic agents (especially the latter) could serve as experimental tools for more detailed study of the mechanisms of initiation and promotion.

Cocarcinogenic and anticarcinogenic factors that operate by influencing the scope of action of carcinogens do so by affecting their rates of absorption in the body, their penetration into the target cells, their metabolic fate, their detoxification and rate of excretion from the body, etc. Such influences can, of course, also be involved in carcinogenesis by the two-stage process, especially in connection with initiating action (which depends on a single, brief action of a relatively small dose of initiator), and perhaps less so in connection with promoting action (which involves oversaturation of the tissues by the promoting agent for long periods).

An interesting example of interference with the scope of action of an initiator was the inhibition of tumor induction when phenanthrene was added to DMBA at the initiating phase (Huh and McCarter, 1960). This could not be attributed to competitive absorption into, or action on, the target cells—as generally suspected when reduction of tumor yield results from repeated applications of a strong and weak carcinogen at the same time (Riegel *et al.*, 1951; see also Falk *et al.*, 1964)—since in the present case the phenanthrene was shown actually to increase the amount of DMBA absorbed. But neither was it likely to alter the responsiveness of the target cell. Hydrocarbons are known, however, to stimulate the action of hydrolases, capable of detoxifying carcinogens, not only in the liver (Conney *et al.*, 1957; Arcos *et al.*, 1961) but also in the skin (Gelboin and Blackburn, 1964), and phenanthrene might conceivably have acted in this way.

Much more is known about the influence of cocarcinogenic and anticarcinogenic factors affecting tissue response at the two respective stages of skin carcinogenesis.

There is, first, the genetic angle to be considered. The promoting action of croton oil is species specific—i.e., effective for the skin of the mouse but not of the rat, guinea pig, or rabbit (Shubik, 1950a). Even its efficiency for mouse skin varies greatly according to strain (unpublished data by the author), and by selective breeding it is possible to obtain relatively susceptible and relatively resistant strains to skin tumor induction by the two-stage technique (Boutwell, 1964). There is, unfortunately, practically no information about the action of other skin promoters tested in species and strains that are resistant to croton oil promoting action.

With regard to specific modifiers of initiation or promotion, inhibitors (anticarcinogenic agents) proved, on the whole, to be more useful as analytical tools than stimulators (cocarcinogenic agents).

The earliest example of a potent anticarcinogenic agent for mouse skin, shown to operate during the promoting phase (actually demonstrated long before the concept of initiation and promotion was formulated), was sulfur mustard ($\beta\beta'$-dichlorethylsulfide), which caused inhibition of tumor induction even when it was applied quite late during the course of tar carcinogenesis (Berenblum, 1929). Many subsequent examples of anticarcinogenic agents for mouse skin were investigated in relation to total carcinogenesis rather than to the separate stages (see Crabtree, 1947), and do not therefore concern us here. (For a recent review of the subject, connected more specifically with initiation and promotion, see Van Duuren and Melchionne, 1969.)

An interesting early example of systemic anticarcinogenic action on mouse skin carcinogenesis—resulting from caloric restriction of the diet—was, once again, shown to operate during the promoting phase, being more effective during the late stages than during the first 10 wk of benzpyrene skin carcinogenesis (Tannenbaum, 1944a). In fact, Boutwell and Rusch (1951) were able definitely to exclude any influence of caloric restriction on the initiating phase.

Studies of hormonal influences on carcinogenesis in general (see Bielschowsky and Horning, 1958) include some inquiries in relation to skin response, although only in a few instances were these designed to determine the response of the separate phases of initiation and promotion.

Meites (1958) found that thyroxine (by mouth) caused pronounced inhibition of tumor induction, and thiouracil caused some augmentation, when tested in connection with the DMBA–croton oil two-stage technique. The evidence pointed strongly to the effect being on the promoting phase. (There were, unfortunately, no separate groups in which the feeding was confined to the initiating phase.)

333
SEQUENTIAL
ASPECTS OF
CHEMICAL
CAR-
CINOGENESIS:
SKIN

Ritchie *et al.* (1953) studied the effect of cortisone on the hyperplasia-producing action of croton oil on mouse skin and observed little influence except for a slight increase in the mitotic rate. When tested in relation to DMBA–croton oil two-stage treatment, no demonstrable effect of cortisone could be detected. Engelbreth-Holm and Asboe-Hansen (1953) claimed, however, that cortisone administered together with continued DMBA treatment caused some inhibition but did not prevent the development of papillomas; subsequently, Boutwell (1964) demonstrated definite inhibition of the promoting phase of skin carcinogenesis when cortisone was applied to the skin or administered orally.

In a critical study of the role of adrenal imbalance in skin carcinogenesis, Trainin (1963) administered hydrocortisone during the initiating and promoting phases for excessive adrenal action and performed adrenalectomy (with subsequent reimplantation of isologous adrenal tissue at the end of the required periods) for deficient action. The initiating phase remained unchanged by either form of added treatment, but the promoting phase was strongly inhibited by the hydrocortisone feeding and greatly enhanced by adrenalectomy. (See also Belman and Troll, 1971 for the influence of other steroid hormones.)

The choice of possible inhibitors of skin carcinogenesis as potential tools for study of the mechanism of initiation and promotion has, in recent years, been dictated more by biochemical considerations—based on existing knowledge of their metabolic effects on cell replication, etc. Actinomycin D is a case in point, being known to interfere with DNA-dependent RNA synthesis in the cell (Bates *et al.*, 1968) although possessing many toxic side-effects as well.

The effect of actinomycin D on the two-stage system of skin carcinogenesis as originally tested by Gelboin *et al.* (1965; see also Bates *et al.*, 1968) pointed to specific inhibition of the initiating phase: the inhibition was pronounced when the actinomycin D was applied on day 0 or 1 relative to the application of the initiator, weak when applied 7 days before or 4 days after, and absent when applied on day 7 or later. When administered systemically, instead of being applied locally on the skin, actinomycin had no effect at all. The conclusions drawn from these results were (1) that initiation took place during the mitotic cycle of the cell affected, (2) that this involved metabolic changes requiring 1 day for completion, and (3) that actinomycin D interfered with this specific metabolic pathway.

Both the results and the conclusions derived from them were questioned by others (see Hennings and Boutwell, 1967; Van Duuren, 1969), whose results (under somewhat different conditions of dosage, etc.) pointed rather to an effect on the promoting phase, inhibition occurring when the actinomycin D was applied as late as 30 days after the initiator (Van Duuren, 1969). Some of the effects observed by Gelboin *et al.* (1965) might well have been due to nonspecific, toxic action, causing death of some of the initiated cells, although this was partly answered by later quantitative studies (Bates *et al.*, 1968) using lower doses than in the original experiments.

A similar lack of agreement occurred with the use of poly I/C (a synthetic double-stranded RNA) as inhibitor, Gelboin and his associates (Gelboin and Levy, 1970; Gelboin et al., 1972) observing inhibition of the promoting phase, while Kreibich et al. (1970) found the inhibition confined to the initiating phase. (Poly I/C has many interesting biological properties, including the stimulation of cells to synthesize interferon, development of resistance to virus replication, and stimulation of cellular and humoral immunity.)

Troll et al. (1970) tested three inhibitors of proteases (tosyl lysine chloromethyl ketone, tosyl phenylalanine chloromethyl ketone, and tosyl arginine chloromethyl ketone) for effects on the two-stage skin carcinogenesis, and found all to inhibit the promoting phase. Another inhibitor of the promoting phase was the fungal antibiotic griseofulvin (Vesselinovitch and Mihailovich, 1968). Similarly, aflatoxin $B_1$ proved to be an inhibitor of the promoting phase, while dl-diepoxybutane and acridine orange inhibited the initiating phase (Van Duuren et al., 1969).

In view of the interest taken nowadays in the possibility of "immunosurveillance" as a controlling factor in carcinogenesis (Miller et al., 1963; Grant et al., 1966), it is interesting to note that depression of the immune response by injection of antithymocyte serum (ATS), at either the initiating phase or the promoting phase of skin carcinogenesis, did not affect the tumor yield or average latent period (Haran-Ghera and Lurie, 1971), although progression from benign tumors to malignancy was enhanced in the ATS-treated groups.

In summary, while no consistent pattern has yet emerged from the studies involving interference with the separate components of the two-stage process of skin carcinogenesis, there seems little doubt that the method of approach is a sound one, likely to throw light eventually on the mechanism of initiation and promotion.

## 7. Promoting Action in Other Tissues

The subject of sequential stages of carcinogenesis in tissues other than skin will be dealt with elsewhere in this volume. Here, we are concerned with only one aspect of the problem—with skin initiators and promoters (or compounds closely related to them) which act as promoters for other tissues. Two compounds come up for special consideration: (1) urethan, a pure initiator for skin, and (2) unesterified phorbol, itself inactive as a skin promoter, although some of its fatty acid derivatives (see Fig. 1) constitute the active constituents of croton oil.

Urethan was already known to be a complete carcinogen for the lung (Nettleship et al., 1943) and for a number of other tissues (see Tannenbaum and Silverstone, 1958; Mirvish, 1968) long before the discovery that, for mouse skin, it acted only as a cocarcinogen in association with croton oil when the two were applied concurrently (Graffi et al., 1953) but acted as a pure initiator when applied first and croton oil later (Salaman and Roe, 1953; Haran and Berenblum, 1956). It was all the more unexpected to find that urethan also possessed promoting action in relation to radiation leukemogenesis (Berenblum and Trainin, 1960). (Its

335

SEQUENTIAL
ASPECTS OF
CHEMICAL
CAR-
CINOGENESIS:
SKIN

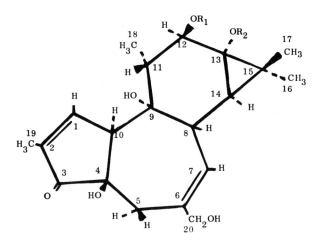

| COMPOUND | SUBSTITUENTS (positions) | | PROMOTING ACTIVITY on Mouse Skin |
|---|---|---|---|
| | 12 ($R_1$) | 13 ($R_2$) | |
| Phorbol | H | H | — |
| TP | $CO-(CH_2)_{12}-CH_3$ | H | — |
| PT | H | $CO-(CH_2)_{12}-CH_3$ | + + |
| TPA | $CO-(CH_2)_{12}-CH_3$ | $COCH_3$ | + + + + |
| 4$\alpha$-PDD | $CO-(CH_2)_8-CH_3$ | $CO-(CH_2)_8-CH_3$ | — |

FIGURE 1. Phorbol and some of its derivatives.

cocarcinogenic action, when administered concurrently with X-irradiation, had previously been demonstrated by Kawamoto *et al.*, 1958.)

Urethan thus remains as quite a unique compound—having initiating action for one tissue (mouse skin) and promoting action for another (hematopoietic tissue), and being a complete carcinogen for the lung and several other tissues.

A particularly intriguing feature of the chemical–biological relationship among the isolated and identified constituents of croton oil (see Fig. 1) responsible for promoting action in skin carcinogenesis was that activity depended on the lengths of the two fatty acid chains and their positions of attachment (12 and 13) to the phorbol nucleus, while unesterified phorbol itself was found to be completely inactive as a promoter for the skin (see Hecker, 1971a).

One possible explanation was that unesterified phorbol, being more water soluble than the diesters, was unable to penetrate the skin when applied topically. This was tested by administering phorbol systemically after an initial application of DMBA to the skin (Berenblum and Lonai, 1970). The results were negative as far as skin response was concerned, but as high percentage of the phorbol-treated mice (with or without prior DMBA treatment) developed leukemia. Unesterified phorbol could thus no longer be considered biologically inactive. (The skin test calls for repetition, with considerably higher doses of phorbol than were available for the abovementioned experiment.)

That unesterified phorbol did possess systemic promoting action for tissues other than skin was demonstrated in mice (Armuth and Berenblum, 1972), for the liver and lungs, using a subeffective dose of dimethylnitrosamine as initiator, and also in rats for mammary carcinogenesis, using a subeffective oral dose of DMBA as initiator (Armuth and Berenblum, 1974).

Both naturally occurring and semisynthetic compounds closely or somewhat remotely related to phorbol and its derivatives are now available (see Hecker, 1971*b*). These should provide useful material for tests of the kind described above as a means of elucidating the mechanism of promoting action in skin carcinogenesis. (For other biological and biochemical properties of phorbol esters, see Hecker and Paul, 1968, Van Duuren and Sivak, 1968, Sivak *et al.*, 1969, Paul and Hecker, 1969, Kreibich and Hecker, 1971, Bach and Goerttler, 1971, Kreibich *et al.*, 1971, Gaudin *et al.*, 1971, 1972.)

## 8. The Mechanism of the Two-Stage Process

The earlier efforts to explain, in biological terms, how the two-stage initiation–promotion process operated were largely based on speculative considerations (see Berenblum, 1954*b*), and the few attempts made to submit these to experimental verification (e.g., by Trainin *et al.*, 1964; see below) did not prove too successful. The application of biochemical methods provided more reliable means of interpreting the earlier biological results and offered a working hypothesis of carcinogenic action.

That neoplasia might depend on a mutation in the genome of a somatic cell is a very old idea (see Bauer, 1928)—generally referred to as the "somatic cell mutation" theory of cancer. The theory did have the merit of accounting for (1) the irreversibility of neoplasia (i.e., the fact that the newly acquired properties were passed on to the daughter cells on cell division), (2) the almost infinite variety of tumors, and (3) the fact that each individual tumor tended to "breed true to type." The apparent objection to the theory was that a mutation is, by definition, virtually an instantaneous process, whereas carcinogenesis is one of the slowest biological processes known. With the introduction of the two-stage hypothesis, however, this criticism disappeared, since one could now postulate that only the initiating phase was mutational.

(Attempts have been made, from time to time, to account for the long latent period of carcinogenesis on the basis of a series of random mutations—e.g., see Charles and Luce-Clausen, 1942; Iversen and Arley, 1950; Fisher and Hollomon, 1951; Nordling, 1953—thus implying that promoting action is also mutational. The idea becomes untenable when one considers, for instance, the fact that initiating action and promoting action fail to operate in reverse order.)

To test the "modified" mutation theory, mice were painted with acridine orange, and a number of other known mutagens, for possible initiating action, followed by standard croton oil treatment (Trainin *et al.*, 1964). The results were disappointingly negative. (The fact that some of the mutagens are known to act by intercalation between base pairs in the nucleic acid chain, rather than by covalent binding with the nucleic acid as in the case of true initiators or carcinogens in general—see below—renders these negative results less disturbing than might appear at first sight.)

As for the biological approach to explain the mode of action of promoting agents, the crucial issue seemed to be the following: Why should promoting action be necessary at all, once a normal cell is converted into a (dormant) tumor cell by initiating action? Should not the normal tendency for periodic mitotic division be sufficient to make the dormant tumor cell develop into a progressively growing mass?

The answer, based on fundamental principles of cell kinetics, was that cell division in a tissue such as skin epithelium leads to a state of growth equilibrium, with 50% of the progeny (whether of normal cells or of dormant tumor cells) remaining stem cells and 50% maturing and eventually dying to produce surface keratin. The essential feature of promoting action, it was suggested (Berenblum, 1954*b*), was to cause a disequilibrium in this kinetic cell equation, resulting in a clone of tumor cells which would thereafter grow continuously without further stimulation. Although seemingly satisfactory as a hypothetical model, it did not in fact explain how promoting action operates.

We come next to an important new phase in carcinogenesis, in which biochemical studies of the binding capacities of carcinogens (or their active metabolites) with specific receptors in the cell began to provide valuable information about the mode of action of carcinogens.

The capacity of aminoazo dye carcinogens to bind covalently with specific proteins in the liver (Miller and Miller, 1947, 1966) was found to apply to polycyclic aromatic hydrocarbons as well, in the case of skin (Wiest and Heidelberger, 1953; Heidelberger and Moldenhauer, 1956; Abell and Heidelberger, 1962), and, in fact, to all the known complete carcinogens (see Magee and Farber, 1962; Mirvish, 1969; Grover and Sims, 1970; Prodi *et al.*, 1970).

At the same time, evidence began to accumulate that of carcinogens had the capacity to bind covalently with nucleic acids (e.g., Brookes and Lawley, 1964; Goshman and Heidelberger, 1967; Warwick, 1969) and that such binding was generally restricted to those tissues that responded carcinogenically to these compounds (see Magee and Farber, 1962; Mirvish, 1969; Prodi *et al.*, 1970).

While the consistent evidence of nucleic acid binding provided strong support for the "somatic mutation" theory—at least with respect to the initiating phase—the equally consistent evidence of protein binding was thought, for a time, to represent an alternative explanation of carcinogenesis—e.g., by acting on the genetic control mechanism (Pitot and Heidelberger, 1963)—as an extension of the theory of Jacob and Monod (1961) for normal genetic control.

Recent metabolic studies, especially in the field of skin carcinogenesis, suggest, however, that nucleic acid binding and protein binding are stages, rather than alternative mechanisms, of carcinogenic action, the former responsible for initiating action and the latter for promoting action (see Scribner and Boutwell, 1972; Berenblum, 1974). This is supported by data on the binding capacities of "incomplete" carcinogens:

1. The binding capacity of urethan with nucleic acids is most pronounced in skin (Prodi *et al.*, 1970)—the tissue for which it acts as a pure initiator.

2. Certain noncarcinogenic hydrocarbons which nevertheless possess cocarcinogenic properties—e.g., dibenz[*a,c*]anthracene and 5,6-dimethoxydibenz[*a,h*]anthracene—bind strongly with skin proteins (Oliverio and Heidelberger, 1958; Abell and Heidelberger, 1962; Heidelberger and Moldenhauer, 1956), although, according to Van Duuren (1969), the former compound is an initiator and binds with nucleic acids in the skin.

3. The highly potent promoter TPA (the active constituent of croton oil) binds weakly with skin proteins (Traut *et al.*, 1971; Scribner and Boutwell, 1972), while other inflammation-producing substances do not possess this property. There appears, however, to be a strange anomaly here in that an analogue of TPA, 4α-PDD (see Fig. 1), which lacks promoting action, also binds weakly with skin proteins (Traut *et al.*, 1971).

Further details are presented in the author's review (Berenblum, 1974), in which various possibilities are discussed as to the way in which protein binding might account for the promoting phase of carcinogenesis.

## 9. References

ABELL, C. W., AND HEIDELBERGER, C., 1962, Interaction of carcinogenic hydrocarbons with tissues. VIII. Binding of tritium-labeled hydrocarbons to the soluble proteins of mouse skin, *Cancer Res.* **22:**931.

ANDREASEN, E., AND ENGELBRETH-HOLM, J., 1953, On the significance of the mouse hair cycle in experimental carcinogenesis, *Acta Pathol. Microbiol. Scand.* **32:**165.

ARCOS, J. C., CONNEY, A. H., AND BUU-HOI, N. P., 1961, Induction of microsomal enzyme synthesis by polycyclic aromatic hydrocarbons of different molecular sizes, *J. Biol. Chem.* **236:**1291.

ARMUTH, V., AND BERENBLUM, I., 1972, Systemic promoting action of phorbol in liver and lung carcinogenesis in AKR mice, *Cancer Res.* **32:**2259.

ARMUTH, V., AND BERENBLUM, I., 1974, Promotion of mammary carcinogenesis and leukemogenic action by phorbol in virgin female Wistar rats, *Cancer Res.* **34:** (in press).

BACH, H., AND GOERTTLER, K., 1971, Morphologische Untersuchungen zur hyperplasiogenen Wirkung des biologisch aktiven Phorbolesters A₁, *Virchows Arch. Abt. B Zellpathol.* **8:**196.

BALL, J. K., AND MCCARTER, J. A., 1960, A study of dose and effect in initiation of skin tumours by a carcinogenic hydrocarbon, *Brit. J. Cancer* **14:**577.

BATES, R. R., WORTHAM, J. S., COUNTS, W. B., DINGMAN, C. W., AND GELBOIN, H. V., 1968, Inhibition by actinomycin D of DNA synthesis and skin tumorigenesis induced by 7,12-dimethylbenz(a)anthracene, *Cancer Res.* **28:**27.

BAUER, K. H., 1928, *Mutationstheorie der Geschwülst-Entstehung*, Julius Springer, Berlin.

BELMAN, S., AND TROLL, W., 1971, The inhibition of croton oil-promoted mouse skin tumorigenesis by steroid hormones, *Cancer Res.* **32:**450.

BERENBLUM, I., 1929, The modifying influence of dichloroethyl sulphide on the induction of tumours in mice by tar, *J. Pathol. Bacteriol.* **32:**425.

BERENBLUM, I., 1941a, The cocarcinogenic action of croton resin, *Cancer Res.* **1:**44.

BERENBLUM, I., 1941b, The mechanism of carcinogenesis: A study of the significance of cocarcinogenic action and related phenomena, *Cancer Res.* **1**:807.

BERENBLUM, I., 1944, Irritation and carcinogenesis, *Arch. Pathol.* **38**:233.

BERENBLUM, I., 1947, Cocarcinogenesis, *Brit. Med. Bull.* **4**:343.

BERENBLUM, I., 1954a, Carcinogenesis and tumor pathogenesis, *Advan. Cancer Res.* **2**:129.

BERENBLUM, I., 1954b, A speculative review: The probable nature of promoting action and its significance in the understanding of the mechanism of carcinogenesis, *Cancer Res.* **14**:471.

BERENBLUM, I., 1960, Carcinogenesis in relation to skin cancer, *Med. J. Austral.* **2**:721.

BERENBLUM, I., 1969, A re-evaluation of the concept of cocarcinogenesis, *Prog. Exp. Tumor Res.* **11**:21.

BERENBLUM, I., 1974, The two-stage mechanism of carcinogenesis in biochemical terms, in: *The Physiopathology of Cancer*, 3rd ed., Vol. 1, p. 393, S. Karger, Basel.

BERENBLUM, I., AND HARAN, N., 1955, The significance of the sequence of initiating and promoting actions in the process of skin carcinogenesis in the mouse, *Brit. J. Cancer* **9**:268.

BERENBLUM, I., AND HARAN-GHERA, N., 1957a, A quantitative study of the systemic initiating action of urethane (ethyl carbamate) in mouse skin carcinogenesis, *Brit. J. Cancer* **11**:77.

BERENBLUM, I., AND HARAN-GHERA, N., 1957b, The induction of the initiating phase of skin carcinogenesis in the mouse by oral administration of 9:10-dimethyl-1:2-benzanthracene, 20-methylcholanthrene, 3:4-benzpyrene, and 1:2:5:6-dibenzanthracene, *Brit. J. Cancer* **11**:85.

BERENBLUM, I., AND LONAI, V., 1970, The leukemogenic action of phorbol, *Cancer Res.* **30**:2744.

BERENBLUM, I., AND SHUBIK, P., 1947a, The role of croton oil applications, associated with a single painting of a carcinogen, in tumor induction in the mouse's skin, *Brit. J. Cancer* **1**:379.

BERENBLUM, I., AND SHUBIK, P., 1947b, A new, quantitative, approach to the study of the stages of chemical carcinogenesis in the mouse's skin, *Brit. J. Cancer* **1**:383.

BERENBLUM, I., AND SHUBIK, P., 1949a, An experimental study of the initiating stage of carcinogenesis, and a re-evaluation of the somatic cell mutation theory of cancer, *Brit. J. Cancer* **3**:109.

BERENBLUM. I., AND SHUBIK, P., 1949b, The persistence of latent tumour cells induced in the mouse's skin by a single application of 9:10-dimethyl-1:2-benzanthracene, *Brit. J. Cancer* **3**:384.

BERENBLUM, I., AND TRAININ, N., 1960, Possible two-stage mechanism in experimental leukemogenesis, *Science* **132**:40.

BERENBLUM, I., HARAN-GHERA, N., AND TRAININ, N., 1958, An experimental analysis of the "hair cycle effect" in mouse skin carcinogenesis, *Brit. J. Cancer* **12**:402.

BIELSCHOWSKY, F., AND HORNING, E. S., 1958, Aspects of endocrine carcinogenesis, *Brit. Med. Bull.* **14**:106.

BILLINGHAM, R. E., ORR, J. W., AND WOODHOUSE, D. L., 1951, Transplantation of skin components during chemical carcinogenesis with 20-methylcholanthrene, *Brit. J. Cancer* **5**:417.

BOCK, F. C., AND BURNS, R., 1963, Tumor-promoting properties of anthranil (1,8,9-anthratriol), *J. Natl. Cancer Inst.* **30**:393.

BORUM, K., 1954, The role of the mouse hair cycle in epidermal carcinogenesis, *Acta Pathol., Microbiol. Scand.* **34**:542.

BOUTWELL, R. K., 1964, Some biological aspects of skin carcinogenesis, *Prog. Exp. Tumor Res.* **4**:207.

BOUTWELL, R. K., AND RUSCH, H. P., 1951, The absence of an inhibiting effect of caloric restriction on papilloma formation, *Cancer Res.* **11**:238.

BOUTWELL R. K., BOSCH, D., AND RUSCH, H. P., 1957, On the role of croton oil in tumor formation, *Cancer Res.* **17**:71.

BROOKES, P., AND LAWLEY, P. D., 1964, Alkylating agents, *Brit. Med. Bull.* **20**:91.

CHARLES, D. R., ANS LUCE-CLAUSEN, E. M., 1942, The kinetics of papilloma formation in benzpyrene-treated mice, *Cancer Res.* **2**:261.

CONNEY, A. H., MILLER, E. C., AND MILLER, J. A., 1957, Substrate-induced synthesis and other properties of benzpyrene hydroxylase in rat liver, *J. Biol. Chem.* **228**:753.

CRABTREE, H. G., 1947, Anti-carcinogenesis, *Brit. Med. Bull.* **4**:345.

CRAMER, W., AND STOWELL, R. E., 1943, Skin carcinogenesis by a single application of 20-methylcholanthrene, *Cancer Res.* **3**:36.

DELLA PORTA, G., SHUBIK, P., DAMMERT, K., AND TERACINI, B., 1960, Role of polyoxyethylene sorbitan monostearate in skin carcinogenesis in mice, *J. Natl. Cancer Inst.* **25**:607.

ENGELBRETH-HOLM, J., AND ASBOE-HANSEN, G., 1953, Effect of cortisone on skin carcinogenesis in mice, *Acta Pathol. Microbiol. Scand.* **32**:560.

FALK, H. L., KOTIN, P., AND THOMPSON, S., 1964, Inhibition of carcinogenesis, *Arch. Environ. Health* **9**:169.

FISHER, J. C., AND HOLLOMON, J. H., 1951, A hypothesis for the origin of cancer foci, *Cancer* **4**:916.

FOULDS, L., 1954, The experimental study of tumor progression, *Cancer Res.* **14**:327.

FREI, J. V., AND KINGSLEY, W. F., 1968, Observations on chemically induced regressing tumors of mouse epidermis, *J. Natl. Cancer Inst.* **41**:1307.

FRIEDEWALD, W. F., AND ROUS, P., 1944a, The initiating and promoting elements in tumor production: An analysis of the effects of tar, benzpyrene, and methylcholanthrene on rabbit skin, *J. Exp. Med.* **80**:101.

FRIEDEWALD, W. F., AND ROUS, P., 1944b, The determining influence of tar, benzpyrene, and methylcholanthrene on the character of the benign tumors induced therewith in rabbit skin, *J. Exp. Med.* **80**:127.

FRIEDEWALD, W. F., AND ROUS, P., 1950, The pathogenesis of deferred cancer: A study of the after-effects of methylcholanthrene upon rabbit skin, *J. Exp. Med.* **91**:459.

GAUDIN, D., GREGG, R. S., AND YIELDING, K. L., 1971, DNA repair inhibition: A possible mechanism of action of co-carcinogens, *Biochem. Biophys. Res. Commun.* **45**:630.

GAUDIN, D., GREGG, R. S., AND YIELDING, K. L., 1972, Inhibition of DNA repair by cocarcinogens, *Biochem. Biophys. Res. Commun.* **48**:945.

GELBOIN, H. V., AND BLACKBURN, N. R., 1964, The stimulatory effect of 3-methylcholanthrene on benzpyrene hydroxylase activity in several rat tissues: Inhibition by actinomycin D and puromycin, *Cancer Res.* **24**:356.

GELBOIN, H. V., AND LEVY, H. B., 1970, Polyinosinic-polycytidylic acid inhibits chemically induced tumorigenesis in mouse skin, *Science* **167**:205.

GELBOIN, H. V., KLEIN, M., AND BATES, R. R., 1965, Inhibition of mouse skin tumorigenesis by actinomycin D, *Proc. Natl. Acad. Sci.* **53**:1353.

GELBOIN, H. V., KINOSHITA, N., AND WIEBEL, F. J., 1972, Microsomal hydrolases: Studies on the mechanism of induction and their role in polycyclic hydrocarbon action, in: *Environment and Cancer*, 24th Annual Symposium on Fundamental Cancer Research, M. D. Anderson Hospital and Tumor Institutes, Houston, Williams and Wilkins, Baltimore, p. 214.

GELHORN, A., 1958, The cocarcinogenic activity of cigarette tobacco tar, *Cancer Res* **18**:510.

GOSHMAN, L. M., AND HEIDELBERGER, C., 1967, Binding of tritium-labeled polycyclic hydrocarbons to DNA of mouse skin, *Cancer Res.* **27**:1678.

GRAFFI, A., 1953, Untersuchungen über den Mechanismus der Cancerogenese und die Wirkungsweise cancerogener Reize, *Abh. Deutsch. Akad. Wiss. Berl. Klasse Med. Wiss.* **1**:1 (quoted by Roe et al., 1972).

GRAFFI, A., VLAMYNCK, E., HOFFMANN, F., AND SCHULZ, I., 1953, Untersuchungen über die geschwülstlösende Wirkung verschiedener chemischer Stoffe in der Kombination mit Crotonöl, *Arch. Geschwulstforsch.* **5**:110.

GRAFFI, A., SCHARSACH, F., AND HEYER, E., 1955, Zur Frage der Initialwirkung cancerogener Kohlenwasserstoffe auf die Mäusehaut nach intravenöser, intraperitonealer und oraler Applikation, *Naturwissenschaften* **42**:184.

GRANT, G. A., ROE, F. J. C., AND PIKE, M. C., 1966, Effect of neonatal thymectomy on the induction of papillomata and carcinomata by 3,4-benzopyrene in mice, *Nature (Lond.)* **210**:603.

GROVER, P. L., AND SIMS, P., 1970, Interactions of K-region epoxides of phenanthrene and dibenz(a,h)anthracene with nucleic acids and histones, *Biochem. Pharmacol.* **19**:2251.

GWYNN, R. H., AND SALAMAN, M. H., 1953, Studies on co-carcinogenesis: SH-reactors and other substances tested for co-carcinogenic action in mouse skin, *Brit. J. Cancer* **7**:482.

HARAN, N., AND BERENBLUM, I., 1956, The induction of the initiating phase of carcinogenesis in the mouse by oral administration of urethane (ethyl carbamate), *Brit. J. Cancer* **10**:57.

HARAN-GHERA, N., AND LURIE, M., 1971, Effect of heterologous antithymocyte serum on mouse skin tumorigenesis, *J. Natl. Cancer Inst.* **46**:103.

HECKER, E., 1968, Cocarcinogenic principles from the seed oil of *Croton tiglium* and from other Euphorbiaceae, *Cancer Res.* **28**:2338.

HECKER, E., 1971a, Isolation and characterization of the cocarcinogenic principles from croton oil, in: *Methods in Cancer Research*, Vol. 6 (H. Busch, ed.), p. 439.

HECKER, E., 1971b, New phorbol esters and related cocarcinogens, in: *Proceedings of the Xth International Cancer Congress, Houston, Texas*, Vol. 5, p. 213, Year Book Medical Publishers, Chicago.

HECKER, E., AND PAUL, D., 1968, Zum biochemischen Mechanismus der Tumorgenese der Maushaut. I. Verteilung und Stoffwechsel intragastral verfütterten 9-10-Dimethyl-(1,2)-benzanthracens in der Maus, *Z. Krebsforsch.* **71**:153.

HEIDELBERGER, C., AND MOLDENHAUER, M. G., 1956, The interaction of carcinogenic hydrocarbons with tissue constituents. IV. A quantitative study of the binding to skin proteins of several C$^{14}$-labeled hydrocarbons, *Cancer Res.* **16**:442.

HENNINGS, H., AND BOUTWELL, R. K., 1967, On the mechanism of inhibition of benign and malignant skin tumors by actinomycin D., *Life Sci.* **6**:173.

HENNINGS, H., AND BOUTWELL, R. K., 1970, Studies on the mechanism of skin tumor promotion, *Cancer Res.* **30**:312.

HENNINGS, H., BOWDEN, G. T., AND BOUTWELL, R. K., 1969, The effect of croton oil pretreatment on skin tumor initiation in mice, *Cancer Res.* **29**:1773.

HUH, T.-Y., AND McCARTER, J. A., 1960, Phenanthrene as an anti-initiating agent, *Brit. J. Cancer* **14**:591.

IVERSEN, S., AND ARLEY, N., 1950, On the mechanism of experimental carcinogenesis, *Acta Pathol. Microbiol. Scand.* **27**:773.

JACOB, F., AND MONOD, J., 1961. On the regulation of gene activity, *Cold Spring Harbor Symp. Quant. Biol.* **26**:193.

KAWAMOTO, S., IDA, N., KIRSCHBAUM, A., AND TAYLOR, G., 1958, Urethan and leukemogenesis in mice, *Cancer Res.* **18**:725.

KREIBICH, G., AND HECKER, E., 1971, Phorbol ester stimulates choline incorporation, *Naturwissenschaften* **58**:323.

KREIBICH, G., SÜSS, R., KINZEL, V., AND HECKER, E., 1970, On the biochemical mechanism of tumorigenesis in mouse skin. III. Decrease of tumor yields by poly I/C administered during initiation of skin by an intragastric dose of 7,12-dimethyl-benz(a)anthracene, *Z. Krebsforsch.* **74**:383.

KREIBICH, G., WITTE, I., AND HECKER, E., 1971, On the biochemical mechanism of tumorigenesis in mouse skin. IV. Methods for determination of fate and distribution of phorbolester TPA, *Z. Krebsforsch.* **76**:113.

LAPPÉ, M. A., 1968, Evidence for the antigenicity of papillomas induced by 3-methylcholanthrene, *J. Natl. Cancer Inst.* **40**:823.

LAPPÉ, M. A., 1969, Tumour specific transplantation antigens: Possible origin in premalignant lesions, *Nature (Lond.)* **223**:82.

LAW, L. W., 1941, Multiple skin tumors in mice following a single painting with 9:10-dimethyl-1:2-benzanthracene, *Am. J. Pathol.* **17**:827.

MACKENZIE, I., AND ROUS, P., 1941, The environmental disclosure of latent neoplastic changes in tarred skin, *J. Exp. Med.* **73**:391.

MAGEE, P. N., AND FARBER, E., 1962, Toxic liver injury and carcinogenesis: Methylation of rat-liver nucleic acids by dimethylnitrosamine *in vivo*, *Biochem. J.* **83**:114.

MARCHANT, J., AND ORR, J. W., 1953, Further attempts to analyse the roles of epidermis and deeper tissues in experimental chemical carcinogenesis by transplantation and other methods, *Brit. J. Cancer* **7**:329.

MARCHANT, J., AND ORR, J. W., 1955, A further investigation of the role of skin components in chemical carcinogenesis, *Brit. J. Cancer* **9**:128.

McCARTER, J. A., SZERB, J. C., AND THOMPSON, G. E., 1956, The influence of area of skin exposed, duration of exposure, and concentration in determining tumor yield in the skin of the mouse after a single application of a carcinogenic hydrocarbon, *J. Natl. Cancer Inst.* **17**:405.

MEITES, J., 1958, Effects of thyroxine and thiouracil on induction of tumors in mice by 9,10-dimethyl-1,2-benzanthracene and croton oil, *Cancer Res.* **18**:176.

MIDER, G. B., AND MORTON, J. J., 1939, Skin tumors following a single application of methylcholanthrene in C57 brown mice, *Am. J. Pathol.* **15**:299.

MILLER, E. C., AND MILLER, J. A., 1947, The presence and significance of bound aminoazo dyes in the livers of rats fed *p*-dimethylaminoazobenzene, *Cancer Res.* **7**:468.

MILLER, E. C., AND MILLER, J. A., 1966, Mechanism of chemical carcinogenesis: Nature of proximate carcinogens and interactions with macromolecules, *Pharmacol. Rev.* **18**:805.

MILLER, J. F. A. P., GRANT, G. A., AND ROE, F. J. C., 1963, Effect of thymectomy on the induction of skin tumours by 3,4-benzopyrene, *Nature (Lond.)* **199**:920.

MIRVISH, S. S., 1968, The carcinogenic action and metabolism of urethan and N-hydroxyurethan, *Advan. Cancer Res.* **11**:1.

MIRVISH, S. S., 1969, *In vivo* binding of tritium-labelled dimethyl-and diethyl-nitrosamine to the nucleic acids and proteins of rat liver, in: *Physico-chemical Mechanism of Carcinogenesis*, Vol. 1, 305. Israel Academy of Sciences and Humanities, Jerusalem.

MOTTRAM, J. C., 1944a, A developing factor in experimental blastogenesis, *J. Pathol. Bacteriol.* **56**:181.

MOTTRAM, J. C., 1944b, A sensitizing factor in experimental blastogenesis, *J. Pathol. Bacteriol.* **56**:391.

NETTLESHIP, A., HENSHAW, P. S., AND MEYER, H. L., 1943, Induction of pulmonary tumors in mice with ethyl carbamate (urethane), *J. Natl. Cancer Inst.* **4**:309.

NORDLING, C. O., 1953, A new theory on the cancer-inducing mechanism, *Brit. J. Cancer* **7**:68.

OLIVERIO, V. T., AND HEIDELBERGER, C., 1958, The interaction of carcinogenic hydrocarbons with tissues. V. Some structural requirements for binding of 1,2,5,6-dibenzanthracene, *Cancer Res.* **18**:1094.

ORR, J. W., 1934, The influence of ischaemia on the development of tumours, *Brit. J. Exp. Pathol.* **15**:73.

ORR, J. W., 1935, The effect of interference with the vascular supply on the induction of dibenzanthracene tumours, *Brit. J. Exp. Pathol.* **16**:121.

ORR, J. W., 1937, The results of vital staining with phenol red during the progress of carcinogenesis in mice treated with tar, dibenzanthracene and benzpyrene, *J. Pathol. Bacteriol.* **44**:19.

ORR, J. W., 1958, The mechanism of chemical carcinogenesis, with particular reference to the time of development of irreversible changes in the epithelial cells, *Brit. Med., Bull.* **14**:99.

PAUL, D., AND HECKER, E., 1969, On the biochemical mechanism of tumorigenesis in mouse skin. II. Early effects on the biosynthesis of nucleic acids induced by initiating doses of DMBA and by promoting doses of phorbol–12.13-diester TPA, *Z. Krebsforsch.* **73**:149.

PITOT, H. C., AND HEIDELBERGER, 1963, Metabolic regulatory circuits and carcinogenesis, *Cancer Res.* **23**:1694.

POUND, A. W., AND BELL, J. R., 1962, The influence of croton oil stimulation on tumour initiation by urethane in mice, *Brit. J. Cancer* **16**:690.

POUND, A. W., AND WITHERS, H. R., 1963, The influence of some irritant chemicals and scarification on tumour initiation by urethane in mice, *Brit. J. Cancer* **17**:460.

PRODI, G., ROCHI, P., AND GRILLI, S., 1970, *In vivo* interaction of urethan with nucleic acids and protein, *Cancer Res.* **30**:2887.

RIEGEL, B., WARTMAN, W. B., HILL, W. T., REEB, B. B., SHUBIK, P., AND STANGER, D. W., 1951, Delay of methylcholanthrene skin carcinogenesis in mice by 1,2,5,6-dibenzfluorene, *Cancer Res.* **11**:301.

RITCHIE, A. C., 1952a, The effect of local injections of adrenalin on epidermal carcinogenesis in the mouse, *J. Natl. Cancer Inst.* **12**:839.

RITCHIE, A. C., 1952b, The effect of arterial occlusion on epidermal carcinogenesis in the rabbit, *J. Natl. Cancer Inst.* **12**:847.

RITCHIE, A. C., 1957, Epidermal carcinogenesis in the mouse by intraperitoneally administered urethane followed by repeated applications of croton oil, *Brit. J. Cancer* **11**:206.

RITCHIE, A. C., AND SAFFIOTTI, U., 1955, Orally administered 2-acetylaminofluorene as an initiator and as a promoter of epidermal carcinogenesis in the mouse, *Cancer Res.* **15**:84.

RITCHIE, A. C., SHUBIK, P., AND LEROY, E. P., 1953, The effect of cortisone on the hyperplasia produced in mouse skin by croton oil, *Cancer Res.* **13**:45.

ROE, F. J. C., 1956a, The development of malignant tumours of mouse skin after "initiating" and "promoting" stimuli. I. The effect of a single application of 9,10-dimethyl-1,2-benzanthracene (DMBA), with and without subsequent treatment with croton oil, *Brit. J. Cancer* **10**:61.

ROE, F. J. C., 1956b, The development of malignant tumours of mouse skin after "initiating" and "promoting" stimuli. III. The carcinogenic action of croton oil, *Brit. J. Cancer* **10**:72.

ROE, F. J. C., 1957, Tumor initiation in mouse skin by certain esters of methanesulfonic acid, *Cancer Res.* **17**:64.

ROE, F. J. C., 1959, The effect of applying croton oil before a single application of 9,10-dimethyl-1,2-benzanthracene (DMBA), *Brit. J. Cancer* **13**:87.

ROE, F. J. C., AND GLENDENNING, O. M., 1956, The carcinogenicity of β-propiolactone for mouse-skin, *Brit. J. Cancer* **10**:357.

ROE, F. J. C., AND PEIRCE, W. E. H., 1960, Tumor promotion by citrus oils: Tumors of the skin and urethral orifice in mice, *J. Natl. Cancer Inst.* **24**:1389.

ROE, F. J. C., AND PEIRCE, W. E. H., 1961, Tumor promotion by euphorbia lattices, *Cancer Res.* **21**:338.

ROE, F. J. C., AND SALAMAN, M. H., 1954, A quantitative study of the power and persistence of the tumour-initiating effect of ethyl carbamate (urethane) on mouse skin, *Brit. J. Cancer* **8**:666.

ROE, F. J. C., AND SALAMAN, M. H., 1955, Further studies on incomplete carcinogenesis: Triethylene melamine (T.E.M.) 1,2-benzanthracene, and β-propiolactone, as initiators of skin tumour formation in the mouse, *Brit. J. Cancer* **9**:177.

343

SEQUENTIAL
ASPECTS OF
CHEMICAL
CAR-
CINOGENESIS:
SKIN

ROE, F. J. C., AND WALTERS, M. A., 1965, Some unsolved problems in lung cancer etiology, *Prog. Exp. Tumor Res.* **6:**126.

ROE, F. J. C., CARTER, R. L., MITCHLEY, B. C. V., PETO, R., AND HECKER, .E., 1972, On the persistence of tumour initiation and the acceleration of tumour progression in mouse skin tumorigenesis, *Int. J. Cancer* **9:**264.

ROUS, P., AND KIDD, J. G., 1941, Conditional neoplasms and subthreshold neoplastic states, *J. Exp. Med.* **73:**365.

RUSCH, H. P., BOSCH, D., AND BOUTWELL, R. K., 1955, The influence of irritants on mitotic activity and tumor formation in mouse epidermis, *Acta Unio Int. Contra. Cancrum* **11:**699.

SAFFIOTTI, U., AND SHUBIK, P., 1956, The effects of low concentrations in epidermal carcinogenesis: A comparison with promoting agents, *J. Natl. Cancer Inst.* **16:**961.

SAFFIOTTI, U., AND SHUBIK, P., 1963, Studies on promoting action in skin carcinogenesis, *Natl. Cancer Inst. Monogr.* **10:**489.

SALAMAN, M. H., 1958, Cocarcinogenesis, *Brit. Med. Bull.* **14:**116.

SALAMAN, M. H., AND ROE, F. J. C., 1953, Incomplete carcinogens: Ethyl carbamate (urethane) as an initiator of skin tumour formation in the mouse, *Brit. J. Cancer* **7:**472.

SALAMAN, M. H., AND ROE, F. J. C., 1956a, The development of malignant tumours of mouse skin after "initiating" and "promoting" stimuli. II. The influence of alternate applications of croton oil on malignant tumour-production by repeated applications of dilute 9,10-dimethyl-1,2-benzanthracene (DMBA), *Brit. J. Cancer* **10:**70.

SALAMAN, M. H., AND ROE, F. J. C., 1956b, The development of malignant tumours of mouse skin after "initiating" and "promoting" stimuli. IV. Comparison of the effects of single and divided doses of 9,10-dimethyl-1,2-benzanthracene (DMBA), *Brit. J. Cancer* **10:**79.

SALAMAN, M. H., AND ROE, F. J. C., 1956c, Further tests for tumour-initiating activity: N,N-Di-(20-chloroethyl)-p-aminophenylbutyric acid (CB1348) as an initiator of skin tumour formation in the mouse, *Brit. J. Cancer* **10:**363.

SALAMAN, M. H., ROE, F. J. C., 1964, Cocarcinogenesis, *Brit. Med. Bull,* **20:**139.

SCRIBNER, J. D., AND BOUTWELL, R. K., 1972, Inflammation and tumor promotion: Selective protein induction in mouse by tumor promoters, *Europ. J. Cancer* **8:**617.

SEGAL, A., KATZ, C., AND VAN DUUREN, B. L., 1971, Structure and tumor-promoting activity of anthranil (1,8-dihydroxy-9-anthrone) and related compounds *J. med. Chem.* **14:**1152.

SETÄLÄ, K., 1960, Progress in carcinogenesis, tumor-enhancing factors: A bio-assay of skin tumor formation, *Prog. Exp. Tumor Res.* **1:**225.

SETÄLÄ, K., SETÄLÄ, H., AND HOLSTI, P., 1954, A new physicochemically well-defined group of tumor-promoting (cocarcinogenic) agents for mouse skin, *Science* **120:**1075.

SHUBIK, P., 1950a, Studies on the promoting phase in the stages of carcinogenesis in mice, rats, rabbits, and guinea pigs, *Cancer Res.* **10:**13.

SHUBIK, P., 1950b, The growth potentialities of induced skin tumors in mice: The effect of different methods of chemical carcinogenesis, *Cancer Res.* **10:**713.

SHUBIK, P., BASERGA, R., AND RITCHIE, A. C., 1953a, The life and progression of induced skin tumors in mice, *Brit. J. Cancer* **7:**342.

SHUBIK, P., GOLDFARB, A. R., RITCHIE, A. C., AND LISCO, H., 1953b, Latent carcinogenic action of beta-irradiation on mouse epidermis, *Nature (Lond.)* **171:**934.

SHUBIK, P., SAFFIOTTI, U., FELDMAN, R., AND RITCHIE, A. C., 1956, Studies on promoting action in skin carcinogenesis, *Proc. Am. Assoc. Cancer Res.* **2:**146.

SICÉ, J., 1966, Tumor-promoting activity of n-alkanes and 1-alkanols, *Toxicol. Appl. Pharmacol.* **9:**70.

SIVAK, A., RAY, F., AND VAN DUUREN, B. L., 1969, Phorbol ester tumor-promoting agents and membrane stability, *Cancer Res.* **29:**624.

STEINMULLER, D., 1971, A reinvestigation of epidermal transplantation during chemical carcinogenesis, *Cancer Res.* **31:**2080.

TANNENBAUM, A., 1944a, The dependence of the genesis of induced skin tumors on the caloric intake during different stages of carcinogenesis, *Cancer Res.* **4:**673.

TANNENBAUM, A., 1944b, The importance of differential considerations of the stages of carcinogenesis in the evaluation of cocarcinogenic and anticarcinogenic effects, *Cancer Res.* **4:**678.

TANNENBAUM, A., AND SILVERSTONE, H., 1958, Urethan (ethyl carbamate) as a multipotential carcinogen, *Cancer Res.* **18:**1225.

TERRACINI, B., SHUBIK, P., AND DELLA PORTA, G., 1960, A study of skin carcinogenesis in the mouse with single applications of 9,10-dimethyl-1,2-benzanthracene of different dosages, *Cancer Res.* **20:**1538.

TRAININ, N., 1963, Adrenal imbalance in mouse skin carcinogenesis, *Cancer Res.* **23**:415.

TRAININ, N., KAYE, A. M., AND BERENBLUM, I., 1964, Influence of mutagens on the initiation of skin carcinogenesis, *Biochem. Pharmacol.* **13**:263.

TRAUT, M., KREIBICH, G., AND HECKER, E., 1971, Über die Proteinbildung carcinogener Kohlwasserstoffe und cocarcinogener Phorbolester, in: *Aktuelle Probleme aus dem Gebiet der Cancerologie*, Vol. 3, p. 91, Springer, Berlin.

TROLL, W., KLASSEN, A., AND JANOFF, A., 1970, Tumorigenesis in mouse skin: Inhibition by synthetic inhibitors of proteases, *Science* **169**:1211.

VAN DUUREN, B. L., 1969, Tumor-promoting agents in two-stage carcinogenesis, *Prog. Exp. Tumor Res.* **11**:31.

VAN DUUREN, B. L., AND MELCHIONNE, S., 1969, Inhibition of tumorigenesis, *Prog. Exp. Tumor Res.* **12**:55.

VAN DUUREN, B. L., AND SIVAK, A., 1968 Tumor-promoting agents from *Croton tiglium* L. and their mode of action, *Cancer Res.* **28**:2349.

VAN DUUREN, B. L. SIVAK, A., SEGAL, A., ORRIS, L., AND LANGESETH, L., 1966a, The tumor-promoting agents of tobacco leaf and tobacco smoke condensate, *J. Natl. Cancer Inst.* **37**:519.

VAN DUUREN, B. L., LANGSETH, L., SIVAK, A., AND ORRIS, L., 1966b, The tumor-enhancing principles of *Croton tiglium* L. II. A comparative study, *Cancer Res.* **26**:1729.

VAN DUUREN, B. L., SIVAK, A., KATZ, C., AND MELCHIONNE, S., 1969, Inhibition of tumor induction in two-stage carcinogenesis on mouse skin, *Cancer Res.* **29**:947.

VAN ESCH, G. J., VAN GENDEREN, H., AND VINK, H. H., 1958, The production of skin tumours in mice by oral treatment with urethane, isopropyl-*n*-phenyl carbamate or isopropyl-*N*-chlorophenyl carbamate in combination with skin-painting with croton oil and Tween 60, *Brit. J. Cancer* **12**:355.

VESSELINOVITCH, S. D., AND MIHAILOVICH, N., 1968, The inhibitory effect of griseofulvin on the "promotion" of skin carcinogenesis, *Cancer Res.* **28**:2463.

WARWICK, .G. P., 1969, The covalent binding of metabolites of 4-dimethylaminoazobenzene to liver nucleic acids *in vivo*, in *Physico-chemical Mechanisms of Carcinogenesis*, Vol. 1, p. 218, Israel Academy of Sciences and Humanities, Jerusalem.

WIEST, W. G., AND HEIDELBERGER, C., 1953, The interaction of carcinogenic hydrocarbons with tissue constituents. II. 1,2,5,6-Dibenzanthracene-9,10-$C^{14}$ in skin, *Cancer Res.* **13**:250.

WOLSTENHOLME, G. E., AND O'CONNOR, M., eds., 1959, *Carcinogenesis: Mechanisms of Action*, Ciba Foundation Symposium, Churchill, London.

WYNDER, E. L., AND HOFFMAN, D., 1961, A study of tobacco carcinogenesis. VIII. The role of the acidic fractions as promoters, *Cancer* **14**:1306.

# 11

# Sequential Aspects of Liver Carcinogenesis

GEORGE TEEBOR

## 1. Introduction

The widespread use of precancerous tissue in research is predicated on the hope that changes manifested by such tissue will reveal critical aspects of the neoplastic transformation. The investigator must first decide which parameters of cell function he will measure in the preneoplastic period. Such decisions are generally influenced by current research trends in cell biology in the hope that a perturbation of a particular cell function is essential to malignancy. Once this decision has been made, the technical problems are essentially two. First is the differentiation of toxic effects of the carcinogen from those related to malignancy, and second is the identification and isolation of the true preneoplastic population.

In the case of the first problem, it is clear that such experimental parameters as species, strain, sex, age, dose regimen, and the nature of the carcinogen itself can all affect the interpretation of results. Time and frequency of measurements of the particular cell property under investigation are critical since animals adapt to the carcinogen and many acute changes subside during the course of the regimen.

The second problem is even more critical. Since the appearance of tumors is generally focal, characterization of the preneoplastic population is of the utmost importance. If such identification is not made, then changes measured may well be the reflection of a heterogeneous response and pertinent changes will probably be masked.

GEORGE TEEBOR ● Department of Pathology, New York University School of Medicine, New York, New York.

For these reasons, an understanding of sequential events in a particular carcinogenic system is necessary for a rational evaluation of data. The use of the liver in experimental oncogenesis is widespread, and for good reason. Hepatocellular carcinomas can be induced by virtually every class of carcinogen, the carcinogen can be administered orally with the daily diet, dosage schedules can be varied, the organ can be visualized by laparotomy during the course of the regimen, and relatively large amounts of tissue are available for experimental work. What changes are common to all classes of carcinogens? It is now generally agreed that prior to the appearance of carcinoma, areas of hepatocellular proliferation appear throughout the parenchyma. These are first discernible microscopically, and as carcinogen administration progresses they become grossly apparent. Their relationship to malignancy is still not certain in that there is no definitive evidence showing that carcinomas arise only from these hyperplastic populations. There have been reports which have described atypical cells within these areas of hyperplasia and concluded that these cells represent the earliest evidence of malignancy (Epstein *et al.*, 1967). Becker and Klein (1971), utilizing the mitotic inhibitor L-asparaginase, reported that within such nodules there were populations of cells whose mitotic activity was not suppressed while that of the vast majority of the cells was. In this respect, these apparent subpopulations were similar to autonomous neoplasms rather than hyperplastic normal parenchyma. The hyperplastic nodule can be induced under a wide variety of regimens, but the most successful employ either ethionine or N-2-fluorenylacetamide (FAA). The use of the nodule as an example of premalignant tissue has been amply reviewed by Farber (1973a), who has also stressed the evolutionary nature of carcinogenesis.

The nature of changes which precede the appearance of nodules is less well characterized. Furthermore, the development of nodules is generally accompanied by cirrhosis. The relationship of this reparative process to carcinogenesis is also not clearly defined.

It seems that all changes which develop are, to a great extent, dose dependent. The higher the dose of carcinogen employed, the greater the yield of tumors and the more malignant the tumors generally are. Furthermore, both the early and late changes in the hepatic parenchyma are more pronounced as the dose of carcinogen increases.

Early toxic changes are more pronounced in the central portion of the hepatic lobule. Changes include glycogen depletion, disruption of internal membranes, deformation of mitochondria, nuclear abnormalities, and actual necrosis (Bannasch, 1968). These changes are increasingly severe with increasing doses of carcinogen, and vary with the type of carcinogen used. In order to induce carcinomas, some carcinogens have to be employed at doses which lead to widespread necrosis, while others induce much less damage (Magee and Barnes, 1956). Alkyl-amine hepatocarcinogenesis is characterized by widespread necrosis, while tumors may be induced by FAA with relatively little evidence of cell death

(Teebor and Seidman, 1970). Unfortunately, no insight into the nature of the critical carcinogenic target is discernible from these differences.

The toxicity of carcinogens has been confirmed by a variety of experimental results. The best known deal with inhibition of the mitotic response to partial hepatectomy in rats. A single oral dose of FAA inhibits mitosis (Becker and Klein, 1971). Similar results have been reported with N,N-dimethyl-4-aminoazobenzene DAB and in mice after short-term administration of o-aminoazotoluene (AAT) (Vasiliev and Guelstein, 1963).

Functional changes in membranes have been indirectly demonstrated by results which showed profound alterations in the labilization of glucose-6-phosphatase by detergent from isolated membranes of livers of animals fed FAA for short periods of time (Teebor and Seidman, 1970). Instead of the usual 50% or so increase in activity associated with enzyme detergent activation, three- to fourfold increase in activity was found in membranes from rats fed carcinogen for a few weeks. The toxic nature of this phenomenon was evident since these results occurred in both male rats, which are susceptible to FAA tumorigenesis, and females, which are not. The phenomenon of altered enzyme induction was also described, and it was reported that a wide variety of enzymes of amino acid catabolism were not inducible by dietary or hormonal administration (Poirier and Pitot, 1969). Such changes appeared long before morphological evidence of hyperplasia or cirrhosis.

There is little doubt that most of these effects are the result of the direct interaction of cellular constituents with the carcinogen. Binding to all compartments has been demonstrated, and this results in abnormal function in all of them. Binding of carcinogen to nucleic acids has profound effects on parameters of DNA synthesis and RNA synthesis. Carcinogens such as aflatoxin, FAA, 7,12-dimethylbenzanthracene DMBA, and nitroquinoline oxide have all inhibited RNA polymerase activity and decreased the activity of the DNA as a template for exogenous RNA polymerase. This subject has been well reviewed by Irving (1973). Short-term administration of carcinogens has also resulted in the appearance of breaks in the DNA of hepatocytes. Both double- and single-strand breaks have been reported as present, and carcinogenic substances have been classified by their ability to cause either single- or double-strand breaks in rat liver DNA (Farber, 1973b). The former may be reparable by cellular mechanisms, such as have been demonstrated in cell culture systems. Double-strand breaks are presumably irreparable and probably lead to permanent damage to the genome.

All of these interesting studies are corroborative of the hypothesis that the interaction of chemical carcinogens with cellular constituents can have profound, measurable effects on hepatic cellular function. However, it is also evident that these toxic events occur after doses that are far beneath the threshold necessary for the induction of carcinoma. This would not preclude a relationship to malignancy, but what renders these changes suspect as fundamental is their disappearance from the preneoplastic hyperplastic population. Hyperplastic cells, in contrast to acutely intoxicated liver, respond with a vigorous mitotic activity after partial hepatectomy, indicating both that they are functionally capable of cell division and that the stimulus to cell division is still effective in these hyperplastic resistant populations. Such data have been reported in rats administered FAA (Becker and Klein, 1971) and in mice fed AAT (Vasiliev and Guelstein, 1963). These nodules also manifest a far more normal pattern of enzyme induction than do cells of acutely intoxicated liver. The responses to dietary and hormonal inducers have been shown to be near normal, and the severe aberrations of activity of glucose-6-phosphatase, after detergent labilization, are not evident in hyperplastic tissue (Teebor and Seidman, 1970). It must be stated, however, that a definite alteration in carbohydrate metabolism does take place since starvation does not deplete the nodules of glycogen to the extent of normal tissue (Epstein *et al.*, 1967). The relationship of this perturbation in carbohydrate metabolism to neoplasia is as yet not evident.

The data of most studies indicate that under continuing carcinogen administration a population of proliferating cells appear which are considerably less susceptible to the toxic effects of the carcinogen than the original population. This loss of sensitivity is associated with a moderate degree of metabolic abnormalities, but if the carcinogen is withdrawn soon after the appearance of these cells the hyperplastic lesions regress (Teebor and Becker, 1971). This indicates that their existence represents a response to the continuing presence of carcinogen and is indeed dependent on it.

This mechanism of increased resistance, and the origin of this population of cells, is not well understood. Bannasch (1968) has gone to great lengths to document the hypothesis that the central portion of the liver lobule is susceptible to the toxic effects of the carcinogen, leading to necrosis, fibrosis, and cirrhosis, while the peripheral portion of the lobule gives rise to glycogen-rich cells which are presumably malignant precursors. The differences between the two populations may be due to differences in the metabolism of the carcinogen continuously administered to the animal. The toxic component may be a metabolic product mediated by the cell enzyme machinery, and this may differ within the lobule. Hence one population of cells proliferates at the expense of the other, and this proliferating population is at increased risk for malignant transformation. This hypothesis is, in principle, supported by a variety of reports which indicate normal functional heterogeneity in the liver lobule. Glycogen, acid phosphatase, and pentose-shunt enzymes have all been described as being concentrated peripherally, while mitochondria, lysosomes, and peroxisomes are more numerous in central protions. Several workers have shown that after partial hepatectomy the mitotic response is predominantly periportal, a finding in keeping with the demonstration that the hyperplastic lesions of carcinogenesis arise peripherally. Heterogeneity has been also well demonstrated by the finding that the greatest induction of smooth endoplasmic reticulum is in the central portion of the lobule after phenobarbital administration (Becker and Lane, 1968).

### 3. Methods of Determining the Sequence of Events in Hepatocarcinogenesis

All of these observations suggest that the carcinogenic process involves a complex series of interactions between the chemical and cellular constituents which are not uniform throughout the lobule. Such a hypothesis is obviously consistent with dose–effect relationships. The more toxically suppressed the vulnerable population, the more the secondary hyperplastic population becomes manifest. Hence, the higher the dosage, the larger the nodules which appear in a given time, and the more likely tumors are to appear in this expanding susceptible population.

349
SEQUENTIAL
ASPECTS OF
LIVER
CAR-
CINOGENESIS

How can this hypothesis be corroborated experimentally? The critical question seems to be related to metabolism of the carcinogen and its distribution within the liver cells. One would like to know whether there is increased or decreased binding to portions of the cells in vulnerable and resistant populations. Were such differences manifest, they might differentiate the potential carcinogenic target from nonspecific toxic ones. The difficulties in pursuing this line of investigation are many. Studies of this type demand the maintenance of large populations of experimental animals under continuing carcinogen administration. Such a population is vulnerable to infections, and a continuing high mortality rate persists.

Selection of tissue for study involves dissection of proliferating areas from nonproliferating areas. In order to insure high yields of hyperplastic tissue, the dose administered must be on the high side; otherwise, the experiments are not feasible. The most effective way to examine carcinogenic distribution is through the use of radioactively labeled carcinogen. If metabolism of the carcinogen is essential to the process, then the labeled compound should be administered in the same fashion as that given during the regimen. This necessitates intubation if the daily diet contains the carcinogens, and large amounts must be given. The selection of the label is critical since metabolism may remove it or exchange of a nonspecific type may take place. The pitfalls in such experimentation are best illustrated by an example of data using FAA labeled with carbon-14 in the aromatic moiety and with tritium in the acetyl moiety (Irving *et al.*, 1970). When administered to male and female rats, the proportion of $^{14}C$ bound to nucleic acids was identical in both groups. However, the male rats retained 7 times as much of the $^{3}H$ label in the nucleic acids as did females. Since the male rats develop tumors and the females do not, this suggests that the retention of the acetyl moiety is related to carcinogenicity. Such experiments have not been performed within male rat liver to determine whether binding to DNA of hyperplastic resistant areas is different than in toxically suppressed areas. The cost of labeled carcinogen is high, the specific activity is extremely low, administration is uncertain if orally given, and, in practice, each animal to be given such a tracer dose should first undergo laparotomy to determine that hyperplastic areas are well developed to insure an adequate yield of tissue. All such experiments, of course, are predicated on the assumption that covalent binding is essential to carcinogenicity. If other interactions such as ionic bonding are critical, then the standard procedure of isolating tissue macromolecules will disrupt such bonds and labeled carcinogen will be lost.

The effects of the carcinogen can also be assessed indirectly by determining the continuing vulnerability of the cellular DNA to breaks which are carcinogen induced. Differential repair may be going on in the various populations, which may lead to expression of certain properties. This area of investigation is still very poorly developed in animal tissue since the usual parameters for measuring repair used in cell culture are not directly applicable. A few reports have indicated enzyme activity in rat liver which was able to endonucleolytically incise both ultraviolet-irradiated DNA (Van Lancker and Tomura, 1972) and apurinic sites on DNA (Verly et al., 1973), but this work is still in its preliminary stages.*

It may also be possible to test whether differential metabolism of carcinogen in hyperplastic areas is occurring. Ames et al. (1974) have shown that incubation of most carcinogens with phenobarbital-induced hepatic microsomes leads to the formation of products mutagenic for bacteria. It would be of considerable interest to determine whether such activity was present in the microsomal fraction of hyperplastic tissue, and to determine whether differences were manifested between such fractions and those of nonhyperplastic tissue.

Such experiments will be illuminating only if binding of chemical carcinogens to cell components is essential for the carcinogenic processes. If the carcinogen simply establishes a suitable toxic field for ultimate viral transformation, then these data will shed little light on the relationship of carcinogen interactions and the ultimate malignant transformation. It must be noted that the appearance of RNA virus in a wide series of primarily induced hepatomas (FAA) has been reported by Weinstein et al. (1972). To date, they have not reported such virus in preneoplastic tissue, but further experiments may reveal this to be so.

## 4. References

AMES, B. N., DURSTON, W. E., YAMASAKI, E., AND LEE, F. D., 1973, Carcinogens are mutagens: A single test system combining liver homogenates for activation and bacteria for detection, *Proc. Natl. Acad. Sci.* **70:**2281.

BANNASCH, P., 1968, The cytoplasm of hepatocytes during carcinogenesis, in: *Recent Results in Cancer Research*, Vol. 19, Springer, New York.

BECKER, F. F., AND LANE, N. P., 1968, Regeneration of the mammalian liver. VI. Retention of phenobarbital–induced cytoplasmic alterations in dividing hepatocytes, *Am. J. Pathol.* **52:**211.

BECKER, F. F., AND KLEIN, K. M., 1971, The effect of L-asparaginase on mitotic activity during N-fluorenylacetamide hepatocarcinogenesis: Sub-populations of nodule cells, *Cancer Res.* **31:**169.

EPSTEIN, S. M., ITO, N., MERKOW, L., AND FARBER, E., 1967, Cellular analysis of liver carcinogenesis: The induction of large hyperplastic nodules in the liver with 2-fluorenylacetamide or ethionine and some aspects of their morphology and glycogen metabolism, *Cancer Res.* **27:**1702.

FARBER, E., 1973a, Hyperplastic liver nodules, in: *Methods in Cancer Research*, Vol. VII (H. Busch, ed.), Academic Press, New York and London.

FARBER, E., 1973b, Carcinogenesis—Cellular evolution as a unifying thread: Presidential address, *Cancer Res.* **33:**2537.

IRVING, C. C., 1973, Interaction of chemical carcinogens with DNA, in: *Methods in Cancer Research*, Vol. VII (H. Busch, ed.), Academic Press, New York and London.

IRVING, C. C., VEAZEY, R. A., AND PEELER, V. A., 1970, Differences in binding of 2-acetylaminofluorene (AAF) and its N-hydroxy metabolite to liver nucleic acids of male and female rats, *Proc. Am. Assoc. Cancer Res.* **11:**39.

MAGEE, P. N., AND BARNES, J. M., 1956, The production of malignant primary hepatic tumours in the rat by feeding dimethylnitrosamine, *Brit. J. Cancer* **10:**114.

*Note Added in Proof: Purification of an endonuclease from rat liver which causes single-strand nicks in ultraviolet irradiated and FAA-bound double-stranded DNA has been reported. Van Lancker, J. L., and Tomura, T., 1974, *Biochim. Biophys. Acta* **353:**99.

Poirier, L. A., and Pitot, H. C., 1969, Dietary induction of some enzymes of amino acid metabolism during 2-acetylaminofluorene feeding, *Cancer Res.* **29:**464.

Teebor, G. W., and Seidman, I., 1970, Retention of metabolic regulation in the hyperplastic hepatic nodule induced by N-2-fluorenylacetamide, *Cancer Res.* **30:**1095.

Teebor, G. W., and Becker, F. F., Regression and persistence of hyperplastic hepatic nodules induced by N-2-fluorenylacetamide and their relationship to hepatocarcinogenesis, *Cancer Res.* **31:**1.

Van Lancker, J. L., and Tomura, T., 1972, Mammalian DNA repair endonuclease, *Proceedings of the American Association for Cancer Research,* Abstract 487.

Vasiliev, J. M., and Guelstein, V. I., 1963, Sensitivity of normal and neoplastic cells to the damaging actions of carcinogenic substances: A review, *J. Natl. Cancer Inst.* **31:**1123.

Verly, W. G., Paquette, Y., and Thibodeau, L., 1973, Nuclease for DNA apurinic sites may be involved in the maintenance of DNA in normal cells, *Nature New Biol.* **244:**67.

Weinstein, I. B., Gebert, R., Stadler, U. C., Orenstein, J. M., and Axel, R., 1972, Type C virus from cell cultures of chemically induced rat hepatomas, *Science* **178:**1098.

351

SEQUENTIAL
ASPECTS OF
LIVER
CAR-
CINOGENESIS

# Neoantigen Expression in Chemical Carcinogenesis

ROBERT W. BALDWIN AND MICHAEL R. PRICE

## 1. Introduction

Neoplastic transformation induced by chemical carcinogens results in the expression in transformed cells of antigens which are not present in their normal counterparts, at least in the adult host. In the early studies with chemically induced tumors (Foley, 1953; Baldwin, 1955; Prehn and Main, 1957), neoantigens were defined by their capacity to elicit immunity to transplanted tumor and were termed "tumor-specific transplantation antigens." It is now evident that immune responses are elicited against these antigens in the autochthonous host, and they must be viewed as a limiting (or enhancing) component of chemical carcinogenesis. It is therefore now appropriate to refer to these neoantigens, which are also viewed as components of the tumor cell surface membrane, as "tumor-associated rejection antigens." Following the development of transplanted tumor models in syngeneic hosts for studying tumor immune mechanisms, *in vitro* methods have been introduced for detecting cellular and humoral responses to tumor-associated antigens. Techniques such as membrane immunofluorescence staining of viable tumor cells in suspension and *in vitro* assays of serum antibody and lymphocyte cytotoxicity against cultured tumor cells almost certainly are detecting antigens expressed at the cell surface. Moreover, the specificities of these reactions are often identical to those of the tumor rejection antigens. Even so, it is preferable to refer to the neoantigens detected by these *in vitro* techniques as "tumor-associated surface antigens," since their identity to rejection antigens in most cases is not proven.

ROBERT W. BALDWIN and MICHAEL R. PRICE ● Cancer Research Campaign Laboratories, University of Nottingham, Nottingham, England.

354

ROBERT W.
BALDWIN
AND
MICHAEL R.
PRICE

During the past few years, it has been realized that chemically induced tumors may express a diversity of neoantigens in addition to the classical tumor rejection antigens. These include reexpressed embryonic antigens ("tumor-associated embryonic antigens,") which may in some cases function as rejection antigens. Also, proteins modified by interaction with carcinogen metabolites may be present for a limited period of time. Almost all of these antigens are immunogenic in the autochthonous host, so they may elicit immune reactions which modify tumor growth to some extent. Even though some of these tumor-associated antigens are not highly functional as targets for immunosurveillance reactions, they may be viewed as essential markers of transformed cells and so be invaluable for studying transformation and metabolic events during carcinogenesis.

## 2. Neoantigens on Chemically Induced Tumors

### 2.1. Tumor-Associated Neoantigens

Considerable effort in the past 20 yr has been devoted to characterizing tumor-associated rejection antigens (TARA) expressed at the cell surface of chemically induced tumors which operate to promote reactions leading to the control of progressive neoplastic growth and possibly to the ultimate destruction of tumor

TABLE 1
*Expression of Tumor-Associated Neoantigens on Chemically Induced Tumors*

| Carcinogen | Tumor type | Species | Neoantigen detected | | |
|---|---|---|---|---|---|
| | | | Tumor-associated rejection antigen (TARA) | Tumor-associated surface antigen (TASA) | Tumor-associated embryonic antigen (TAEA) |
| Polycyclic hydrocarbons | | | | | |
| 3-methyl-cholanthrene (MCA) | Sarcoma | Mouse | + | + | + |
| | | Rat | + | + | + |
| | | Guinea pig | + | + | |
| | Mammary carcinoma | Mouse | + | | |
| | | Rat | + | | |
| | Lymphoma | Mouse | + | | |
| | Skin papilloma/ carcinoma | Mouse | + | | |
| | Bladder papilloma/ carcinoma | Mouse | + | + | |
| | | Rat | + | + | |
| | *In vitro* transformed prostate cells | Mouse | + | + | |
| | 3T3 cells transformed *in vitro*, maintained *in vivo* | Mouse | + | | |
| | Normal fibroblasts, transformed and maintained *in vitro* and *in vivo* | Mouse | + | | |

TABLE 1 (*cont.*)

355

NEOANTIGEN
EXPRESSION
IN CHEMICAL
CAR-
CINOGENESIS

| Carcinogen | Tumor type | Species | Neoantigen detected | | |
|---|---|---|---|---|---|
| | | | Tumor-associated rejection antigen (TARA) | Tumor-associated surface antigen (TASA) | Tumor-associated embryonic antigen (TAEA) |
| Dibenz[*a,h*]anthracene | Sarcoma | Mouse | + | | |
| | | Guinea pig | + | | |
| 7,12-Dimethylbenz[*a*] anthracene (DMBA) | Sarcoma | Mouse | + | + | + |
| | | Guinea pig | + | + | |
| | Epithelioma | Mouse | + | | |
| Benzo[*a*]pyrene | Sarcoma | Mouse | + | | + |
| | | Rat | + | | + |
| Dibenzo[*a,i*]pyrene | Sarcoma | Mouse | + | | |
| Aminoazo dyes | | | | | |
| 4-Dimethylaminoazo-benzene (DAB) | Hepatoma | Rat | + | + | + |
| 3'-Methyl-DAB | Hepatoma | Rat | + | | |
| *o*-Aminoazotoluene | Hepatoma | Mouse | + | | |
| 5-[[*l*-(Dimethylamino)-phenyl]azo]-quinoline | Hepatoma | Rat | + | + | |
| Aromatic amines | | | | | |
| N-2-Fluorenyl-acetamide (FAA) | Mammary carcinoma | Rat | + | + | + |
| | Hepatoma | Rat | + | + | |
| | Ear duct carcinoma | Rat | + | + | + |
| Alkylnitrosamines | | | | | |
| Diethylnitrosamine (DENA) | Hepatoma | Rat | + | + | |
| | | Guinea pig | + | + | |
| Nitrosoguanidine | *In vitro* transformed prostate cells | Mouse | | + | |
| Miscellaneous | | | | | |
| Urethan | Pulmonary adenoma | Mouse | + | + | |
| Mineral oil | Plasma cell tumor | Mouse | + | + | |
| Plastic film | Sarcoma | Mouse | + | + | |

cells (Table 1). It has been possible to evaluate the contribution of these components to tumor immunity only by detailed examination of a range of chemically induced tumors and by design of highly controlled experimental procedures using syngeneic hosts for transplantation tests. The expression of tumor-associated surface antigens (TASA) in several tumor systems has also been characterized both by phenomena which they evoke *in vivo* and by the *in vitro* analyses of cell-mediated and humoral immune reactions in tumor-immune hosts. In a number of instances, these antigenic components have been isolated as cell-free preparations, and it is now feasible to critically define not only their expression and involvement in tumor immunity but also their characteristics as membrane-associated products.

ROBERT W.
BALDWIN
AND
MICHAEL R.
PRICE

## 2.1.1. Polycyclic Hydrocarbons

Early studies by Foley (1953), Baldwin (1955), and Prehn and Main (1957) using transplanted 3-methylcholanthrene (MCA) induced sarcomas in the rat or mouse showed that by appropriate manipulation of the progressively growing tumor (surgical excision or ligation of tumor blood supply), the treated animals were subsequently resistant to challenge inocula of viable cells of the same tumor. Comparably, animals treated with tumor cells attenuated by irradiation (Révész, 1960; Klein et al., 1960) or cytotoxic drugs (Apffel et al., 1966) developed the capacity to reject cells of the immunizing MCA-induced sarcoma. In these investigations, the state of immunity conferred exhibited a high degree of specificity, and protection was generally evident only against the transplanted tumor to which the animal had previously been exposed. The specificity of these tumor rejection reactions has in the past been a point of some controversy, although as a result of studies on a variety of chemically induced tumor systems in the mouse, rat, and guinea pig using both transplantation techniques and in vitro assays of cell-mediated and humoral immunity, this question has been at least partially resolved and the expression of tumor rejection antigens defined. For example, sarcomas induced by polycyclic hydrocarbons, and in particular MCA, which has been used extensively in these studies, are considered to be strongly immunogenic, and immunized animals are frequently protected against large numbers of cells of the immunizing sarcoma but not cells of other sarcomas induced by the same carcinogen (reviewed by Baldwin, 1973). Among the many workers who have confirmed these findings, Reiner and Southam (1967, 1969) also reported that immunization with a pool of several MCA-induced murine sarcomas in some instances produced protection against other sarcomas not included in the immunizing pool. While this may indicate that these tumors share a weakly expressed common rejection antigen(s) as well as a distinct tumor-specific component, it was concluded by Basombrío (1970) that this is not the case, and as a result of extensive studies, cross-resistance was found to be a nonreproducible event.

Cross-reacting tumor rejection antigens have also been reported in MCA-induced sarcomas maintained by transplantation in strain 2 guinea pigs (Holmes et al., 1971). This, however, may be accounted for by viral contamination since viral particles were detected by electron microscopy in some of the sarcomas studied and this strain is known to be susceptible to virus-associated leukemia. Conversely, MCA-induced guinea pig sarcomas in strain 13 animals display individually distinct tumor rejection antigens (Morton et al., 1965; Oettgen et al., 1968).

While rejection antigens associated with MCA-induced sarcomas are generally considered to display individual specificity, bladder carcinomas and papillomas induced by this carcinogen in the mouse and rat show an "organ-type" specificity, and it has been reported that immunization with tumor cells significantly inhibited bladder papilloma formation induced by MCA (Taranger et al., 1972a,b). This, however, represents a unique system requiring more comprehensive analysis, since cross-reactivity in rejection tests has not generally been found in tumors induced by MCA at other tissue sites (e.g., mammary carcinomas studied by Prehn, 1962, and Kim, 1970, and the well-established sarcoma system already discussed). Moreover, the rejection antigens demonstrable on tumors induced by a range of other polycyclic hydrocarbons show the characteristic high degree of specificity. These latter systems include squamous cell carcinomas (Pasternak *et al.*, 1964; Tuffrey and Batchelor, 1964) and sarcomas (Pasternak, 1963; Oettgen *et al.*, 1968) induced by 7,12-dimethylbenz[*a*]anthracene, together with sarcomas induced by dibenz[*a,h*]anthracene (Prehn, 1960; Morton *et al.*, 1965), benzo[*a*]pyrene (Delorme and Alexander, 1964; Globerson and Feldman, 1964), and dibenzo[*a,i*]pyrene (Old *et al.*, 1962).

357
NEOANTIGEN
EXPRESSION
IN CHEMICAL
CAR-
CINOGENESIS

While sarcomas induced by MCA are in most cases consistently immunogenic, there is a species variability with respect to the number of viable cells which treated animals are able to reject. Thus challenge inocula with up to 6 g of viable tumor tissue may be rejected by guinea pigs immunized by implantation of X-irradiated sarcoma tissue (Oettgen *et al.*, 1968), whereas transplantation resistance in the rat or mouse may be overcome by much smaller challenges with between $10^6$ and $10^8$ viable sarcoma cells (Baldwin, 1955; Klein *et al.*, 1960). The immunogenicity of MCA-induced sarcomas within a single species is also subject to variability (Baldwin, 1955; Old *et al.*, 1962; Johnson, 1968; Takeda, 1969; Bartlett, 1972), and an inverse relationship between latency period of induction and immunogenic potential has been reported in some studies (Old *et al.*, 1962; Johnson, 1968). In an extensive analysis of this phenomenon, Bartlett (1972) determined that early arising murine sarcomas showed a wide range of immunogenicities, whereas with progressively increasing latency periods of induction the proportion of highly immunogenic tumors in the population decreased. Thus, while host immunoselection leading to antigen loss may be a contributory factor modifying the immunogenicity of tumors with long latent periods of induction, it is evident that antigenic variability is a real effect in chemical carcinogenesis.

A well-developed cellular immune response to tumor-associated antigens is viewed to be necessary for tumor rejection responses to be effective. This has been clearly exemplified in studies showing that sensitized lymphocytes have the capacity to adoptively transfer tumor immunity to normal syngeneic hosts (K. E. Hellström and Hellström, 1969). Also, the specific cytotoxic effect of lymphoid cells from immune donors has been detected in neutralization tests in which inhibition of growth of MCA-induced murine sarcomas was achieved by immunization of normal recipients with mixtures of tumor cells and sensitized lymph node cells (Klein *et al.*, 1960; Borberg *et al.*, 1972) or peritoneal exudate cells (Old *et al.*, 1962).

Comprehensive analyses of cell-mediated immune reactions to antigens expressed on MCA-induced sarcomas have been performed using *in vitro* cytotoxicity assays. The validity of these techniques has been substantiated in transplanted tumor systems, and their potential for exploring immune responses in the autochthonous host has yet to be fully realized. The occurrence and specificity of the cell-mediated immune reaction to MCA-induced sarcomas in

358

ROBERT W.
BALDWIN
AND
MICHAEL R.
PRICE

several species has been defined using both colony inhibition and microcytotoxicity tests (Hellström *et al.*, 1968, 1970; Baldwin and Moore, 1971; Cohen *et al.*, 1972). The individual specificity of the surface antigens associated with these tumors was revealed since lymphoid cell cytotoxicity was specifically directed against cells of the immunizing sarcoma. One exception to this general rule has been reported by Taranger *et al.* (1972*a,b*), who found that lymph node cells from mice sensitized against (or bearing) MCA-induced bladder carcinomas were cytotoxic for cells of the immunizing tumor as well as other MCA-induced bladder carcinomas. Furthermore, it was established that peripheral blood lymphocytes from rats sensitized to MCA-induced papillomas or carcinomas were cross-reactive. It was also shown that papillomas and carcinomas induced in a number of ways, including bladder implantation of MCA in paraffin, paraffin pellets alone, or cholesterol or silastic pellets, expressed common neoantigens (I. Hellström and Hellström, 1972; Taranger *et al.*, 1972*b*). These results have been interpreted as showing that chemically induced bladder tumors express organ-specific neoantigens comparable to those demonstrable on human bladder tumors (Bubenik *et al.*, 1970*a,b*; O'Toole *et al.*, 1972*a,b*, 1973), and in support of this argument it was established that lymphoid cells from bladder tumor-bearing rats and mice were not cytotoxic for sarcomas induced by either polyoma or MCA. The characteristics of the neoantigens on these bladder tumors require further evaluation, however, since antigens showing comparable specificities have been demonstrated on N-2-fluorenylacetamide-induced, and spontaneously developing, rat mammary carcinomas which are probably tumor-associated embryonic antigens (Baldwin and Embleton, 1974).

Delayed hypersensitivity reactions elicited by tumor cells or cell extracts have proved most useful in characterizing antigens expressed on guinea pig sarcomas induced by MCA or other polycyclic hydrocarbons (Oettgen *et al.*, 1968; Suter *et al.*, 1972). Complementary to these *in vivo* investigations has been the use of tests involving detection of the inhibition of migration of sensitized macrophages by tumor cells or cell extracts in order to evaluate the tumor-specific immune reactions to MCA-induced sarcomas in both guinea pigs (Bloom *et al.*, 1969; Suter *et al.*, 1972) and mice (Halliday and Webb, 1969; Halliday, 1971).

Further evidence demonstrating the occurrence and confirming the individual specificity of surface antigens expressed on MCA-induced sarcomas in the mouse and rat comes from analyses of humoral antibody reactions to these tumors. While sarcoma cells are not susceptible to cytotoxic antibody in short-term cytotoxicity assays (Old and Boyse, 1965), colony inhibition techniques allow the detection of complement-dependent cytotoxic antibody in sera from immune animals. In this way, serum either from mice immunized by surgical excision of tumor (Hellström *et al.*, 1968) or from rats treated with γ-irradiated tumor grafts (Baldwin and Moore, 1971) inhibited the capacity of cultured sarcoma cells to form colonies. Conversely, tumor cell growth was not inhibited by normal control serum or by serum from animals immunized against other sarcomas. Comparable effects have also been obtained in tests employing the microcytotoxicity assay of Takasugi and Klein (1970) to detect cytotoxic antibody in the serum of mice immunized against transplanted MCA-induced sarcomas (Bloom, 1970; Bloom and Hildemann, 1970).

In addition to the complement-dependent cytotoxic antibody demonstrable in serum of rats immunized against transplanted MCA-induced sarcomas Baldwin and Moore, 1971), we have identified specific I$\gamma$G antibody reacting with the tumor cell surface as assessed by indirect membrane immunofluorescence techniques (Baldwin *et al.*, 1971*a,c*, 1972*a*). Using eight transplanted sarcomas and a panel of 26 tumor-immune sera, we found that in only one of 122 cross-tests did a serum react to give positive membrane immunofluorescence staining with viable cells of a different sarcoma. Furthermore, except in this one case, absorption of tumor-specific antibody could be accomplished only with cells of the immunizing sarcoma, even though absorptions were carried out with 100 times the number of cells of the immunizing tumor required to effect antibody neutralization. It was therefore concluded that weak common antigens were not expressed at the cell surface.

Less extensive studies have been performed using MCA-induced murine sarcomas. In an early study by Lejneva *et al.* (1965), positive membrane immunofluorescence reactions were observed when sarcoma cells were reacted with serum from mice immune to the corresponding tumor. The specificity of this effect was not fully established in cross-tests with other transplanted sarcomas. Attempts have also been made with MCA-induced murine sarcomas to develop radioimmunoassay techniques for the demonstration of cell surface antigens. These methods are often difficult to adequately control because of the nonspecific uptake of the radiolabel by nonviable cells in the population, although Harder and McKhann (1968) were able to demonstrate cell surface antigens on single cell suspensions using radioiodinated antibody preparations. This indirect isotopic antiglobulin assay procedure has recently been adapted by Burdick *et al.* (1973) for use on a microscale with cell monolayers in culture in the wells of Microtest II plates. In this way, antibody directed against tumor-associated antigens was detected with sensitivity, and the technique was considered suitable for evaluating possible cross-reactivity between different MCA-induced sarcomas.

### 2.1.2. Aminoazo Dyes

Tumor-associated rejection antigens expressed on aminoazo dye–induced hepatomas in mice (Müller, 1968) and rats (Gordon, 1965; Baldwin and Barker, 1967*a*) were initially demonstrated by the induction of immunity to transplanted tumor cells in syngeneic animals. Two major features displayed by rat hepatomas induced by 4-dimethylaminoazobenzene (DAB) are that the tumors are consistently immunogenic so that immunized animals are able to reject up to $5 \times 10^5$ to $10^6$ viable cells and that each tumor expresses an individually distinct tumor rejection antigen (reviewed by Baldwin, 1973). A direct parallel is thus evident between these hepatomas and many of the MCA-induced sarcoma systems already discussed.

The cellular and humoral immune responses to tumor-associated surface antigens on DAB-induced rat hepatomas have been analyzed using a variety of *in*

359

NEOANTIGEN
EXPRESSION
IN CHEMICAL
CAR-
CINOGENESIS

360

ROBERT W.
BALDWIN
AND
MICHAEL R.
PRICE

TABLE 2

*Demonstration of Immune Responses to Tumor-Associated Neoantigens in Rats Immunized Against Transplanted DAB-Induced Hepatomas*

| Immune response | Method of detection | Antigen detected | Reference |
|---|---|---|---|
| Transplantation immunity [a,b,c] | Rejection of transplanted hepatoma cells | TARA | Baldwin and Barker (1967a) |
| Cytotoxic lymph node cells [a,b] | Colony inhibition test | TASA | Baldwin and Embleton (1971a) |
| | Microcytotoxicity test | TASA | Baldwin *et al.* (1973c) |
| Complement-dependent cytotoxic antibody [a,b] | Colony inhibition test | TASA | Baldwin and Embleton (1971a) |
| | Microcytotoxicity test | TASA | Baldwin *et al.* (1973c) |
| Humoral antibody | Membrane immuno-fluorescence test | TASA | Baldwin and Barker (1967b) Baldwin *et al.* (1971a,c 1972a) |

[a] Immune response induced by implantation of γ-irradiated (15,000 R) hepatoma grafts.
[b] Immune response induced by excision of progressively growing hepatoma grafts.
[c] Immune response induced by administration of viable hepatoma cells in admixture with peritoneal exudate cells from rats immunized by implantation of γ-irradiated (15,000 R) hepatoma grafts.

*vivo* and *in vitro* techniques, as shown in Table 2. In these investigations, the immune reactions demonstrated were, in each case, directed only against the tumor-specific component and no cross-reactions between individual hepatomas were observed. For example, lymph node cells and serum (in the presence of added complement) from rats immunized against transplanted hepatomas are cytotoxic only against plated cells of the immunizing tumor (Baldwin and Embleton, 1971a; Baldwin *et al.*, 1973c). Similarly serum from immune animals will react in membrane immunofluorescence tests only with surface antigens of cells from the immunizing hepatoma (Baldwin and Barker, 1967b; Baldwin *et al.*, 1971a,c, 1972a). In Table 2, a distinction between the antigens associated with these hepatomas (i.e., TARA or TASA) has been made. However, the individual specificity of the immune response to hepatoma neoantigens as measured by a variety of *in vivo* or *in vitro* techniques (Table 2) would suggest that in this system the cell surface–expressed antigen and rejection antigen are the same component of the cell membrane. This well-characterized model system has subsequently been used to evaluate the contribution of cellular and humoral immune responses in both the actively immunized and the tumor-bearing individual (Baldwin *et al.*, 1973c,e).

### 2.1.3. Aromatic Amines

Although aromatic amines constitute a major class of chemical carcinogens, only the immunological properties of rat tumors induced by N-2-fluorenylacetamide (FAA) have been analyzed in detail. These tumors appear deficient in tumor-associated rejection antigens since they do not display consistent or marked immunogenicity in transplant rejection tests. For example, by excision of growing tumor or by implantation of irradiated tumor grafts, only two of 11 mammary carcinomas showed resistance to further challenge with viable tumor cells (Baldwin and Embleton, 1969a). Comparably, tumor transplantation resistance could be induced only against three of ten FAA-induced rat hepatomas and one of three ear duct carcinomas (Baldwin and Embleton, 1971*b*). Compared to the MCA-induced rat sarcomas or DAB-induced rat hepatomas, the degree of resistance elicited in these experiments was low, as reflected by the maximum number of tumor cells ($10^3$ to $10^5$) rejected by immunized rats (Baldwin and Embleton, 1969*a*, and 1971*b*).

361
NEOANTIGEN
EXPRESSION
IN CHEMICAL
CAR-
CINOGENESIS

Variability in the expression of tumor rejection antigens on FAA-induced tumors is clearly demonstrated in these studies, and this is in accord with the studies of Bartlett (1972) showing similar variability of immunogenicity in MCA-induced murine sarcomas. None of these tumor rejection studies can establish whether some tumors are totally deficient in tumor rejection antigens, and it may be possible to conduct more precise studies using sensitive assays of cell-mediated and humoral immune reactions. In this respect, however, tumor-specific antibody was detected by membrane immunofluorescence tests in sera from rats immunized against the few weakly immunogenic FAA-induced tumors (Baldwin and Embleton, 1971*b*). These immune sera reacted only with the surface of cells of the immunizing tumor, showing a close correlation with tumor immunogenicity. Furthermore, sera taken from rats similarly treated with cells of tumors displaying no significant tumor rejection reactions did not react positively in membrane immunofluoresence reactions. In contrast, it has been established that lymph node cells taken from rats bearing FAA-induced mammary carcinomas were cytotoxic *in vitro* for cells of the corresponding tumor, even though in some cases the tumor lacked significant immunogenicity as evaluated by tumor transplant rejection tests (Baldwin and Embleton, 1974). These tumor-bearer lymph node cells were also cytotoxic for cells of other tumors (FAA-induced or spontaneously arising) of the same histological type, whereas reactivity with other tumor types was observed only infrequently. The nature of the neoantigens eliciting these reactions has not yet been defined, although they appear to differ from the well-characterized individual tumor antigens. Since it can be shown that the cytotoxicity of FAA-tumor-bearer lymph node cells can be abrogated by pretreatment of target tumor cells with multiparous rat serum, it is likely that tumor-associated embryonic antigens are being detected (see Section 2.2). This demonstrates an inherent difficulty in that the *in vitro* assays of tumor immune reactions may not be detecting the same neoantigens which are functional as tumor rejection antigens (Klein, 1973).

### 2.1.4. Alkylnitrosamines

Diethylnitrosamine (DENA) induced hepatomas in strain 2 guinea pigs are significantly immunogenic, immunity to syngeneic transplanted tumor being induced by excision of tumor grafts or by intradermal or intramuscular injection of subthreshold cell doses such that progressive growth is prevented (Zbar *et al.*, 1969). These tumors have been studied by Rapp and his associates as models for immunotherapy (Zbar *et al.*, 1971, 1972*a*,*b*; Bartlett and Zbar, 1972) since tumor growth can be suppressed by injecting hepatoma cells in admixture with Bacillus

362

ROBERT W.
BALDWIN
AND
MICHAEL R.
PRICE

Calmette Guérin (BCG). Regression of hepatoma–BCG mixed inocula leads to suppression of tumor implanted simultaneously at another site, and, furthermore, direct intratumoral injection of BCG into an established tumor graft suppresses its development and limits metastatic spread to the draining lymph nodes.

The adoptive transfer of immunity by peritoneal exudate cells from guinea pigs immunized with DENA-induced hepatomas results in a marked cell-mediated immune response, this being detected either by suppression of tumor growth or by the production of delayed hypersensitivity reactions (Kronman *et al.*, 1969; Wepsic *et al.*, 1970; Zbar *et al.*, 1970). The specificity of these reactions has indicated that the rejection antigens expressed by DENA-induced guinea pig hepatomas are individually distinct, and heterologous antisera prepared against intact tumor cells have, after appropriate absorption, been rendered monospecific, reacting in complement fixation tests only with homologous tumor cells (Leonard *et al.*, 1972). Using these antisera in membrane immunofluorescence studies, Leonard (1973) demonstrated that cell surface–expressed tumor antigens were mobile within the membrane plane and that after apparent removal (by extrusion) of surface antigen–antibody complexes, resynthesis of tumor antigen occurred. These findings were interpreted to reflect the manner in which soluble tumor antigen or antigen–antibody complexes could be continuously released from the tumor *in vivo*.

Rat hepatomas induced by DENA are also immunogenic, and syngeneic animals treated with $\gamma$-irradiated tumor grafts are resistant to challenge with cells of the immunizing tumor (Baldwin and Embleton, 1971*b*). No extensive analyses of cell-mediated and humoral immune response to these tumors are as yet available, although serum from rats immunized against one hepatoma has been found to contain antibody reacting weakly in membrane immunofluorescence tests with cells of the homologous tumor (Baldwin and Embleton, 1971*b*). Comparably, tumor-associated surface antigens have been demonstrated on one line of mouse prostate cells transformed *in vitro* by nitrosoguanidine, these findings being compatible with the antigenicity of cells of the same line transformed by MCA (Embleton and Heidelberger, 1972). DENA-induced murine pulmonary adenocarcinomas do not, however, exhibit significant immunogenicity, and protection against challenge with as few as $2 \times 10^4$ tumor cells was not induced in mice immunized by irradiated tumor grafts (Pasternak *et al.*, 1966).

### 2.1.5. Isolation and Characterization of Tumor-Associated Antigens

Considerable attention has recently been directed toward the isolation of tumor-associated rejection antigens and tumor-associated surface antigens with a view to defining their physicochemical characteristics and molecular expression at the cell surface, and elucidating their contribution to cellular and humoral immune reactions in the tumor-bearing or tumor-immune host. It is evident from Table 3 that in the chemically induced tumor systems already examined, tumor-associated antigens display a variability either in their cellular localization or in the degree to which they are associated with tumor cell membranes as exemplified by the diverse extraction procedures employed to liberate water-soluble antigen fractions. For example, with polycyclic hydrocarbon–induced guinea pig sarcomas, tumor rejection antigens are released into the soluble cytoplasmic fraction following homogenization in isotonic saline (Oettgen *et al.*, 1968; Bloom *et al.*, 1969; Suter *et al.*, 1972) or exposure of cells to low-intensity ultrasound (Holmes *et al.*, 1970). These soluble preparations retain the capacity to evoke transplantation resistance to viable tumor cell challenge and to induce delayed hypersensitivity reactions as measured by skin tests and by the inhibition of migration of sensitized peritoneal macrophages. However, with DAB-induced rat hepatomas (Baldwin and Glaves, 1972; Baldwin *et al.*, 1972*d*, 1973*d*; Harris *et al.*, 1973), MCA-induced rat sarcomas (Thomson and Alexander, 1973), and DENA-induced guinea pig hepatomas (Meltzer *et al.*, 1971, 1972; Leonard *et al.*, 1972), more vigorous treatments of cells or cell membrane fractions are necessary to release water-soluble antigenic components, implying that these determinants represent more integrated structures of the tumor cell membrane. In this respect, perhaps the most effective procedures currently available for antigen solubilization involve limited papain digestion of cell membranes or salt extraction (3.0–3.5 M KCl) of tumor cells or cell homogenates. With the latter technique, it was originally proposed that antigen solubilization was accomplished by a reduction of ordered structure of water molecules intimately associated with membrane protein, thus allowing hydrophobic regions of the protein to become detached from their lipid environment and dispersing membrane molecules in the aqueous media (Reisfeld and Kahan, 1970, 1972). However, Mann (1972) has suggested that products arising from 3 M KCl solubilization of whole cells may in fact be released by the action of soluble intracellular and possibly membrane-bound proteolytic enzymes. This would imply that membrane-associated antigens solubilized by either limited proteolysis with papain or salt extraction might represent similar macromolecular fragments. Indeed, this is supported by the findings of Thomson and Alexander (1973) demonstrating that antigenic activity liberated from MCA-induced rat sarcomas by papain or 3 M KCl was associated with material having an apparent molecular weight range of 40,000–50,000.

As already mentioned, tumor rejection antigens atypically can be isolated from polycyclic hydrocarbon-induced guinea pig sarcomas following tumor cell rupture. This might be taken to indicate that these determinants are associated with soluble intracellular moieties. However, in order to elicit rejection reactions, these antigens must almost certainly show expression at the cell surface either to participate in humoral reactions with antibody or to operate in cell–cell interactions. Hence the anomalous properties of polycyclic hydrocarbon-induced guinea pig sarcoma antigens may either reflect an inherent lability of the tumor cell membrane or indicate that the components isolated are immunologically active soluble precursors of the antigens inserted into the plasma membrane.

The cell surface localization of tumor rejection antigens associated with DAB-induced rat hepatomas is now well established (Baldwin, 1973). The indirect

TABLE 3

*Isolation and Characterization of Tumor-Associated Antigens from Chemically Induced Tumors*

| Tumor system | Preparation of antigenic fraction | Nature of antigenic fraction | Antigen detected by assay of | Reference |
|---|---|---|---|---|
| **Polycyclic hydrocarbon-induced tumors** | | | | |
| MCA-induced murine sarcomas | 7000g supernatant of tissue homogenates | Cell membranes and soluble cytoplasmic protein | Tumor rejection | Pilch (1968) |
| | Fluorocarbon extract of 7000g supernatant of tissue homogenates | Dispersed membrane lipoprotein and soluble cytoplasmic protein | Tumor rejection | Pilch (1968) |
| | EDTA–borate extraction of ascites cells | Cell "ghost" membranes | Tumor rejection | McCollester (1970) |
| MCA-induced rat sarcomas | 3.5 M KCl extraction of tissue homogenates | Soluble component, mol wt 40,000–50,000 (protein or glycoprotein) | Antibody inhibition[a] | Thomson and Alexander (1973) |
| | Papain digestion of cell membranes | Soluble component(s), mol wt <100,000 | Antibody inhibition | Thomson et al. (1973) |
| | Membrane ultrafiltration of tumor-bearer serum | Cell membrane fraction | Antibody inhibition[b] | Baldwin and Pimm (unpublished findings) |
| | Nitrogen cavitation of cells | | Antibody formation | Baldwin, Price, and Pimm (unpublished findings) |
| | Papain digestion of cell membranes | Soluble component(s) (protein or glycoprotein) | Antibody inhibition | |
| MCA-induced guinea pig sarcomas | 100,000g supernatant of tissue homogenate | Soluble cytoplasmic protein | Delayed hypersensitivity | Oettgen et al. (1968) |
| | | | Tumor rejection | Bloom et al. (1969) |
| | Exposure of cells to low-intensity ultrasound | Soluble component(s) | Tumor rejection | Holmes et al. (1970) |
| | Isotonic saline extraction of tissue fragments | Soluble component(s): smallest component, mol wt ~50,000; largest component, mol wt >10⁶ | Macrophage migration inhibition | Suter et al. (1972) |
| DMBA-induced murine lymphomas | Zonal centrifugation of cell homogenate fractions | Cell "ghost" membranes | Tumor rejection | Wolf and Avis (1970) |
| DMBA-induced guinea pig sarcomas | 100,000g supernatant of tissue homogenates | Soluble cytoplasmic protein | Delayed hypersensitivity | Oettgen et al. (1968) |
| | | | Tumor rejection | Bloom et al. (1969) |
| | | | Macrophage migration inhibition | |
| | Isotonic saline extraction of tissue fragments | Soluble components: smallest component, mol wt 50,000; largest component; mol wt >10⁶ | Macrophage migration inhibition | Suter et al. (1972) |

| Tumor | Method of preparation | Nature of antigen | Assay | Reference |
|---|---|---|---|---|
| **Aminoazo dye-induced tumors** | | | | |
| 4-Dimethylaminoazobenzene-induced rat hepatomas | Hypotonic salt elution of cells | Particulate membrane lipoprotein | Antibody inhibition | Baldwin and Moore (1968) |
| | Nitrogen cavitation of cells | Fragmented and vesicular cell membranes | Antibody inhibition | Baldwin and Moore (1969) |
| | Zonal centrifugation of cell homogenate fractions | Fragmented and vesicular plasma membrane fractions | Antibody formation<br>Antibody inhibition<br>Antibody formation | Baldwin et al. (1973b)<br>Baldwin et al. (1971b)<br>Baldwin and Price (unpublished findings) |
| | Papain digestion of cell membranes | Soluble component(s) (protein or glycoprotein)<br>Soluble protein or glycoprotein components: major component, mol wt ~ 55,000 | Antibody inhibition<br>Antibody formation<br>Antibody inhibition<br>Lymph node cell cytotoxicity inhibition[c] | Baldwin and Glaves (1972)<br>Baldwin et al. (1972d, 1973d)<br>Baldwin et al. (1973f) |
| | EDTA extraction of cell membranes | Soluble component(s) (protein or glycoprotein) | Antibody inhibition | Harris et al. (1973) |
| | β-Glucosidase extraction of cell membranes | Soluble components: major component, mol wt ~ 50,000–60,000 | Antibody inhibition<br>Antibody formation | Baldwin, Bowen, and Price (unpublished findings) |
| | Gel filtration of tumor-bearer serum | Soluble component(s), mol wt <150,000 | Antibody inhibition<br>Antibody formation | Baldwin et al. (1973a) |
| **Alkylnitrosamine-induced tumors** | | | | |
| DENA-induced guinea pig hepatomas | 3 M KCl extraction of cells | Soluble component, mol wt 75,000–150,000 (protein or glycoprotein) | Delayed hypersensitivity | Meltzer et al. (1971) |
| | | | Delayed hypersensitivity<br>Tumor rejection | Leonard et al. (1972) |
| | | | Delayed hypersensitivity<br>Macrophage migration inhibition<br>Lymphocyte transformation | Meltzer et al. (1972) |

[a] Antigen detected by its capacity to inhibit the interaction of antitumor antibody with the surface of tumor cells (e.g., as measured by membrane immunofluoresence).
[b] Antigen detected by its capacity to elicit antibody syngeneic animals.
[c] Antigen detected by its capacity to inhibit the in vitro cytotoxicity of sensitized lymph node cells for cultured tumor cells.

366
ROBERT W.
BALDWIN
AND
MICHAEL R.
PRICE

membrane immunofluorescence technique employed in several studies to evaluate the unique specificity of these antigens (Baldwin and Barker, 1967b; Baldwin et al., 1971a,c) by definition detects antigen–antibody interactions occurring at the cell surface. Also, on tumor cell rupture, antigenic activity is retained by membrane fractions of cell homogenates, and only these fractions have the capacity to absorb antibody from the serum of rats positively immunized against transplanted tumor cells (Baldwin and Moore, 1968, 1969; Baldwin and Price, unpublished findings). Although hepatoma membrane fractions have been found not to induce transplantation resistance, they retain the capacity to elicit the formation of antibody reacting with cells of the homologous tumor (Baldwin et al., 1973b). Comparably, antigen fractions solubilized from hepatoma cell membranes by proteolysis also evoke humoral antibody production (Baldwin and Glaves, 1972). These preparations have been partially purified to yield a major soluble antigenic protein or glycoprotein fraction displaying a molecular weight of approximately 55,000, together with a range of larger antigenic components, these being most probably macromolecular aggregates of the smaller antigenic moiety (Baldwin et al., 1973d). These findings are essentially comparable with those of Suter et al. (1972), who have shown that extraction of guinea pig sarcomas with isotonic saline liberates soluble tumor-specific antigen separable into two distinct fractions, one having a molecular weight of 50,000 and the other being in excess of $10^6$.

In all of the studies discussed, the origin of material for antigen extraction has been tumor cells or cell homogenates. However, recent findings suggest alternative sources of antigen in a soluble form which is highly suitable for further purification. With rats bearing either large intraperitoneal implants of a DAB-induced hepatoma (Baldwin et al., 1973a) or subcutaneous grafts of an MCA-induced rat sarcoma (Thomson et al., 1973), it has been determined that the serum from these animals contains soluble tumor-associated antigen both in a free form and complexed with specific antibody. The immune complexes have been dissociated relatively easily by acid or salt treatment of serum, allowing antigen to be separated from antibody on a molecular size basis, since the former displays an apparent molecular weight of significantly less than 100,000–150,000. On a practical level, these results indicate that it is possible to obtain antigenically active material not only from the tumor cell but also from body fluids of the tumor-bearing individual.

As a direct consequence of the studies outlined and by consideration of the more comprehensive summary of investigations in Table 3, it is evident that in a number of chemically induced tumor systems, tumor-associated antigens may now be prepared as subcellular membrane-expressed and soluble components. Without doubt, this latter finding is of great significance since the ability to obtain soluble antigen fractions indicates that it is further possible to apply classical separative and analytical biochemical techniques to define these components which under appropriate conditions may initiate rejection responses in the tumor-bearing animal.

## 2.2. Tumor-Associated Embryonic Antigens

367

NEOANTIGEN
EXPRESSION
IN CHEMICAL
CAR-
CINOGENESIS

Reexpressed embryonic antigens have been detected on a variety of chemically induced tumors. These neoantigens are expressed during specific stages of embryogenesis, although they are apparently not present on normal adult tissues. Current interest in these antigens has stemmed largely from the early work of Abelev *et al.* (1963), who reported that fetal protein (termed "$\alpha$-fetoprotein") present in the serum of newborn but not adult mice was also secreted into the circulation by *o*-aminoazotoluene-induced mouse hepatomas (reviewed by Abelev, 1971). The recurrence of $\alpha$-fetoproteins in serum from animals bearing aminoazo dye–induced hepatomas is now a well-documented phenomenon (Stanislawski-Birencwajg *et al.*, 1967; Watabe *et al.*, 1972; Kitagawa *et al.*, 1972; Kroes *et al.*, 1972), and it has been possible to detect $\alpha$-fetoprotein in early stages of hepatocarcinogenesis before overt tumors are apparent (Hull *et al.*, 1969; Kitagawa *et al.*, 1972; Kroes *et al.*, 1972; 1973; De Néchaud and Uriel, 1973). In this respect, however, Uriel *et al.* (1973) have found that the cell type producing $\alpha$-fetoprotein is not, in fact, the hepatoma cell but rather a "transitional liver cell" which is distinct from both normal neoplastic hepatocytes and is present in hepatocellular carcinomas as well as in fetal and neonatal liver. The origin of this cell type is not known, although this finding may explain the lack of correlation between serum levels of $\alpha$-fetoprotein and the size and/or morphological type of the tumors and also the presence of $\alpha$-fetoprotein in pathological situations other than primary liver cancer.

$\alpha$-Fetoproteins are usually detected by reaction with xenogeneic antisera, although their immunogenicity in the tumor-bearing host is less well established. There are, however, other embryonic antigens expressed on chemically induced tumors which are immunogenic in the autochthonous host, and these have been demonstrated by *in vitro* analysis of cell-mediated and humoral immune reactions. This was early observed by Brawn (1970), who showed that lymph node cells from multiparous mice were cytotoxic *in vitro* for MCA-induced sarcoma cells as compared to the effect of lymph node cells from age-matched virgin female controls. Tumor-associated embryonic antigens on 7,12-dimethyl-benz[*a*]anthracene-induced murine sarcomas have similarly been detected by a $^{51}$Cr-release assay from plated tumor cells following exposure to spleen cells from syngeneic mice immunized against 10- to 14-day embryos (Ménard *et al.*, 1973*b*). Comparably, tumor-associated embryonic antigens have been detected in a range of chemically induced rat tumors by the *in vitro* cytotoxicity of lymph node cells or serum (in the presence of added complement) from multiparous female rats for tumor cells, and by membrane immunofluorescence staining of tumor cells by multiparous serum (Baldwin *et al.*, 1971*c*, 1972*a,b*). Initial studies were restricted to DAB-induced hepatomas and MCA-induced sarcomas, but the tumor types shown to express embryonic antigens have been extended to include FAA-induced mammary carcinomas and ear duct carcinomas (Baldwin and Vose, unpublished findings). Moreover, tumor-associated embryonic antigens have

368

ROBERT W.
BALDWIN
AND
MICHAEL R.
PRICE

been demonstrated on spontaneously arising mammary carcinomas, sarcomas and a squamous cell carcinoma, although not all of these tumor types express tumor rejection antigens at significant levels (Baldwin, 1966; Baldwin and Embleton, 1969a,b). Comparable with these studies, cross-reacting embryonic antigens have been detected on MCA-induced rat sarcomas by membrane immunofluorescence staining of suitably absorbed xenogeneic antisera and syngeneic tumor-immune sera (Thomson and Alexander, 1973). DENA-induced guinea pig hepatomas also express cross-reacting embryonic antigens which can be detected by complement fixation of rabbit antisera to hepatoma cells (Boros and Leonard, 1972). These findings suggest that embryonic expression may be a concomitant of neoplastic transformation, although a wider range of tumor types induced by different carcinomas need to be analyzed. It is pertinent, however, to note that embryonic antigens can be demonstrated on many virus-induced tumors including cells transformed by SV40 (Duff and Rapp, 1970; Coggin *et al.*, 1970, 1971; Baranska *et al.*, 1970; Girardi *et al.*, 1973; Ting *et al.*, 1972, 1973a,b), adenovirus (Coggin *et al.*, 1971; Hollinshead *et al.*, 1972), and Rauscher leukemia virus (Hanna *et al.*, 1971; Ishimoto and Ito, 1972). Moreover, the expression of embryonic antigens on human tumors is exemplified by the association of $\alpha$-fetoprotein with hepatocellular carcinoma and teratocarcinoma, and the presence of carcinoembryonic antigen in neoplastic disease, notably tumors of the gastrointestinal tract (reviewed by Laurence and Neville, 1972).

An important question raised by these investigations concerns whether the tumor rejection antigens demonstrable on many experimental tumors are, in fact, reexpressed embryonic antigens. This was postulated in SV40 tumors and adenovirus-induced tumors in hamsters, where significant resistance to tumor transplants could be induced following immunization with fetal tissues (Coggin *et al.*, 1971). There is, however, substantial evidence to indicate that this is not the case with chemically induced rat tumors, especially MCA-induced sarcomas and DAB-induced hepatomas (Baldwin *et al.*, 1971c, 1972a,b,c, 1974a,b; Thomson and Alexander, 1973). Thus the humoral antibody response elicited when these tumors are transplanted into syngeneic hosts is highly specific, being directed against cells of the immunizing tumor. This is evidenced by the specificity of membrane immunofluorescence (Baldwin and Barker, 1967b; Baldwin *et al.*, 1971a,c, 1972a,b) or cytotoxicity assay (Baldwin and Embleton, 1971a) of serum from tumor-immune rats, and in the immunofluorescence studies tumor-specific antibody could be absorbed only by cells of the immunizing tumor (Baldwin *et al.*, 1971a,c, 1972a). Similarly, lymph node cell cytotoxicity toward cultured tumor cells shows the individual specificity of the tumor-associated antigens (Baldwin and Embleton, 1971a). In contrast, serum or lymph node cells from multiparous rats react positively with a wide range of tumors (Baldwin *et al.*, 1971c, 1972a,b), suggesting that common, cross-reacting embryonic antigens are being detected. The possibility that each tumor may express an individual embryonic antigen which is being detected by multivalent antisera produced by sensitization of female rats during multiple pregnancies has further been discounted in absorption studies (Baldwin *et al.*, 1972a,b). These showed that absorption of multiparous sera with one tumor removed membrane immunofluorescence reactivity not only toward that tumor but also to cells of other previously cross-reacting tumors. This is markedly different from the result obtained with tumor-immune sera, where antibody demonstrable by membrane immunofluorescence can be absorbed only by cells of the immunizing tumor (Baldwin *et al.*, 1971*a*, 1972*a*).

369

NEOANTIGEN
EXPRESSION
IN CHEMICAL
CAR-
CINOGENESIS

Differentiation between tumor-specific and tumor-associated embryonic antigens expressed at the cell surface of carcinogen-induced rat hepatomas and sarcomas has also been possible by comparing the capacity of sera from tumor-immune and multiparous rats to block tumor cells from attack by sensitized lymph node cells (Baldwin *et al.*, 1974*a*). In this way, it was shown (Fig. 1) that the multiparous rat lymph node cells (sensitized against embryonic antigens) were no longer cytotoxic for plated tumor or embryo cells which had been pretreated with multiparous rat serum. This implies that the embryonic antigens expressed on both tumor and embryo cells are being "blocked" by preexposure to multiparous serum so that when lymph node cells sensitized to these antigens are added, there is no cytotoxic effect as measured by cell survival in the microcytotoxic assay. Lymph node cells from tumor-immune rats are also cytotoxic for both tumor and embryo cells, as assayed by reduced survival of plated target cells in the microcytotoxicity assay (Baldwin *et al.*, 1974*a*). In this case, the reaction of tumor-immune lymph node cells with embryo cells can be blocked by pretreating plated cells with multiparous serum. However, the reaction of tumor-immune lymph node cells with tumor cells is not blocked by pretreating target cells with multiparous rat serum. These results are interpreted as indicating that tumor immunization produces lymph node cell populations sensitized to the tumor-specific antigen and tumor-associated embryonic antigens, the latter reactivity being blocked when tumor cells are first exposed to multiparous rat serum (Baldwin *et al.*, 1974*a*).

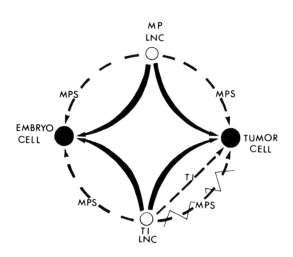

FIGURE 1. Schematic representation of serum blocking of lymph node cell cytotoxicity for rat tumor and embryo cells. Lymph node cells from multiparous rats or tumor-immune rats are cytotoxic for both cultured tumor and embryo cells (solid arrows). Serum from multiparous rats (MPS) has the capacity to block multiparous rat lymph node cell cytotoxicity (MP LNC) for embryo and tumor cells (broken-line arrows). Multiparous rat serum also blocks the cytotoxicity of lymph node cells from tumor-immune rats (TI LNC) for embryo cells (broken-line arrow) but not for tumor cells (crossed broken-line arrow). However, the cytotoxicity of tumor-immune lymph node cells (TI LNC) for tumor cells is blocked by serum from tumor-immune rats (TI) (broken-line arrow).

ROBERT W.
BALDWIN
AND
MICHAEL R.
PRICE

Comparable with these results, Thomson and Alexander (1973) were able to differentiate between individually distinct tumor antigens and tumor-associated embryonic antigens on an MCA-induced rat sarcoma by cross-absorption of tumor-specific antibody demonstrable by membrane immunofluorescence staining of tumor cells. In addition to these two tumor antigens, which were immunogenic in syngeneic hosts, they were also able to demonstrate two embryonic antigens using xenogeneic antisera prepared against tumor extracts. A complement fixation technique using xenogeneic antisera against two DENA-induced guinea pig hepatomas has similarly been used to demonstrate both tumor-specific and embryonic antigens in these tumors (Borsos and Leonard, 1972). It has also been reported that tumor-specific and embryonic antigens on polyoma or SV40-induced tumors can be differentiated using an isotope antiglobulin test (Ting et al., 1972, 1973a). These investigations established that the reactivity of antisera raised against tumors induced by SV40 or polyoma in syngeneic mice could be neutralized by absorption with cells of the appropriate tumor, but not with cells taken from embryos aged 1, 2, or 3 wk. However, antisera raised in syngeneic mice against irradiated (5000 R) fetal tissue of 1–2 wk gestation reacted with a range of tumor cells including SV40- and polyoma-transformed tumor cell lines. These studies were further extended to show that a multiplicity of embryonic antigens may be demonstrated on SV40-transformed cells. These antigens were also detected on SV40 "cryptic" transformants of BALB/c cell lines, which contain the SV40 genome but do not express SV40 coded antigens (T antigen, tumor-specific surface antigen, or tumor-specific rejection antigens).

The role of tumor-associated embryonic antigens in tumor rejection phenomena is still unresolved. As already described, immunization against embryonic antigens by implantation of irradiated (5000 R) fetal tissues or surgical excision of developing embryomas produces resistance to challenge with SV40- or adenovirus-induced tumors in hamsters (Coggin et al., 1971; Hollinshead et al., 1972; Girardi et al., 1973). At variance with these findings, immunization with mouse fetal tissues failed to produce protection against polyoma- or SV40-induced murine tumors (Ting, 1968; Kit et al., 1969), although as pointed out by Coggin et al. (1970) these negative findings may have been due to the use of nonirradiated fetal cells for immunization. In this case, it cannot be excluded that the fetal cells may rapidly mature, resulting in the loss of expression of embryonic antigens. The possibility was further analyzed by Ting et al. (1973b), who tried unsuccessfully to immunize BALB/c mice against SV40-transformed BALB/c cells with irradiated fetal tissue of 1–2 wk gestation. Nevertheless, tumor immunity could be induced following immunization with SV40-transformed cells or by SV40 virus.

It has similarly been established that embryonic antigens expressed on DAB-induced hepatomas and MCA-induced sarcomas do not function as tumor rejection antigens since immunization of syngeneic rats with irradiated (5000 R) midgestation fetal tissue did not result in the development of tumor immunity (Baldwin et al., 1972c, 1974b). Similarly, immunization by excision of embryomas produced by injection of fetal tissue failed to elicit significant tumor rejection. In these systems, it is known that the embryonic antigens are phase specific, showing only transient expression on fetal cells obtained approximately between 14 and 16 days of gestation, but this was taken into account so that the fetal tissues were used at a time when embryonic antigen was maximally expressed. Also, the challenge doses of tumor cells were only slightly larger than the threshold dose of cells necessary for progressive tumor growth. These observations reinforce the argument that the tumor-associated embryonic antigens on rat hepatomas and sarcomas differ from the individually distinct tumor rejection antigens since immunization by implantation of irradiated tumor cells or excision of tumor grafts readily elicits immunity. Although in these tumor systems the embryonic neoantigens do not appear to be contributing significantly to host resistance, it has clearly been established that syngeneic rats immunized with tumor cells do elicit a response against the embryonic antigens. Thus lymph node cells and serum (in the presence of added complement) from rats immunized against transplanted rat hepatomas and sarcomas are cytotoxic for embryo cells (Baldwin *et al.*, 1974*a*). Moreover, tumor-immune serum blocks plated embryo cells from attack by sensitized lymph node cells taken from multiparous rats (Baldwin *et al.*, 1974*a*). Host sensitization to tumor-associated embryonic antigens is further emphasized in studies on the immune responses to a range of rat tumors including FAA-induced mammary carcinomas and ear duct carcinomas as well as spontaneously arising mammary carcinomas and sarcomas (Baldwin and Embleton, 1974). These tumors are generally lacking in immunogenicity or at least are weakly immunogenic as assayed by the capacity to elicit tumor transplantation immunity in syngeneic rats (Baldwin and Embleton, 1969*a*,*b*, 1971*b*). Nevertheless, lymph node cells taken from tumor-bearing rats are cytotoxic for tumor cells *in vitro* when assayed by the microcytotoxicity test, although the specificities of the reactions differ from those observed with other carcinogen-induced and immunogenic tumors. In this case, lymph node cells from rats bearing a particular tumor reacted both with cells of the autochthonous tumor and with other tumors of similar histological type. These responses have been shown to reflect sensitization to tumor-associated embryonic antigens, since the cytotoxicity of tumor-bearer lymph node cells was blocked by preexposure of plated tumor cells to multiparous rat serum. Similarly, the cytotoxicity of lymph node cells from multiparous rats for plated embryo cells could be blocked by pretreating the embryo cells with tumor-bearer serum. These observations are consistent with the view that the tumor-associated embryonic antigens are immunogenic but do not function as rejection antigens. At variance with this conclusion, Le Mevel and Wells (1973) have reported that mice immunized with irradiated second-trimester embryo cells or exposed to these antigens during pregnancy develop transplantation resistance to an MCA-induced sarcoma. The conclusion that, in this case, tumor-associated rejection antigens are cross-reactive with embryonic antigens cannot be substantiated since no specificity tests were reported. These observations are contrary to the report of Basombrío and Prehn (1972*a*), who were unable to demonstrate tumor immunity to MCA-induced murine sarcomas following

371

NEOANTIGEN
EXPRESSION
IN CHEMICAL
CAR-
CINOGENESIS

372
ROBERT W.
BALDWIN
AND
MICHAEL R.
PRICE

immunization either with embryonic tissue from 12- to 20-day fetuses or with teratomas. Furthermore, multiparous pregnant mice were not protected against threshold challenge inocula of viable tumor cells. Also, Castro *et al.* (1973) noted that the most consistent response to immunization with 12-day fetal mouse tissue was an enhancement of MCA-induced tumor growth. These observations suggest, however, that in this case the immune response to fetal antigens has modified tumor growth. That an immune response to embryonic antigens expressed on fetal tissues or tumor cells occurs is further evidenced by the report of Parmiani and Della Porta (1973). In this case, immunization of syngeneic mice with either fetal tissues or an MCA-induced sarcoma was effective in reducing the pregnancy rate of BALB/c mice, indicating that a strong maternal immunity against an MCA-induced sarcoma or syngeneic embryo cells was harmful to the progeny.

As already discussed, with the DAB-induced rat hepatoma model, immunization of syngeneic rats either with attenuated fetal tissues or by excision of developing embryomas is apparently not effective in conferring tumor resistance, at least to strongly antigenic tumors. It has thus been proposed that antigen expression at the tumor cell surface may be transient and represent an inappropriate target for effective lymphocytotoxicity *in vivo* (Baldwin *et al.*, 1974a). Although it is evident by the very nature of the immunological methods used to identify embryonic antigens that these components are surface-expressed, the most abundant source of antigen for further purification is localized with the soluble cytoplasmic protein fraction (Cell sap) of tumor cell homogenates. This has been demonstrated by the capacity of cell sap fractions to neutralize the membrane immunofluorescence staining of viable tumor cells by antibody in multiparous rat serum (Baldwin *et al.*, 1974a). There are thus at least three possibilities regarding the nature of the expression and localization of embryonic antigens associated with these tumors:

1. The antigen is a soluble cytoplasmic component which is transiently expressed at the cell surface during secretion from the tumor cell.
2. The intracytoplasmic component is an antigenically active precursor of the macromolecule to be inserted within the plasma membrane.
3. The embryonic antigen is a plasma membrane–associated product which is not firmly integrated into the tumor cell surface and thus appears as a soluble component following tumor cell rupture.

Although it is clear that further investigations are required to elucidate which of these possibilities may be valid, some progress has been made on the isolation and characterization of the antigenic component present in the cell sap fraction of tumor cell homogenates (Baldwin, Price, and Vose, unpublished findings). A soluble, homogeneous component retaining the capacity to neutralize antibody in multiparous serum has been isolated following sequential fractionation hepatoma cell sap by fractional ammonium sulfate precipitation, ion exchange and gel filtration chromatography, and preparative polyacrylamide gel electrophoresis. The preparation exhibits several physical characteristics comparable to those of $\alpha$-fetoprotein such as a molecular weight of 65,000–70,000 and an isoelectric point of 4.8–5.0, although the fraction did not react in immunodiffusion tests with specific anti–rat α-fetoprotein antisera (kindly provided by Dr. Sell, University of California). It is worth noting that this preparation is biochemically distinguishable from the individual tumor-associated surface antigen isolated from the aminoazo dye–induced rat hepatoma (hepatoma D23) by papain solubilization of cell membrane fractions. For example, the individually specific surface antigen displays a lower molecular weight (50,000–60,000) and has a slower mobility on analytical polyacrylamide electrophoretic gels.

373
NEOANTIGEN
EXPRESSION
IN CHEMICAL
CAR-
CINOGENESIS

In a preliminary report by Bendich *et al.* (1973), embryonic antigens from an MCA-induced sarcoma or from murine embryos were isolated and purified chromatographically to give a fraction of molecular weight of 65,000–70,000, this being highly comparable to that of the embryonic antigen isolated from DAB-induced rat hepatomas. Similarly, Thomson and Alexander (1973) have detected an embryonic component of molecular weight 67,000–70,000 in an MCA-induced rat sarcoma using heterologous antisera raised against an aqueous extract of 9- to 11-day embryos and absorbed by extracts from normal adult tissues. In this study, two other embryonic components were also detected, these being identified by their reactvity with heterologous antisera.

It is considered that with the present availability of isolated embryonic antigen preparations from chemically induced tumors it will be possible to elucidate some of the more complex features of the expression of these components and their contribution to the immunological regulation of neoplastic disease.

## 2.3. Neoantigen Expression on Cells Transformed in Vitro By Chemical Carcinogens

One of the most promising aspects of contemporary studies in chemical carcinogenesis has been the induction and maintenance of cell lines transformed *in vitro* following exposure to carcinogens. An important advantage of these systems over tumors induced *in vivo* is that they permit the study of carcinogen-induced neoantigen expression under conditions where host immunosurveillance cannot modify these effects. Tumor-associated rejection and surface antigens have been detected on cultured C3H mouse prostate cells transformed *in vitro* by MCA or by nitrosoguanidine (Mondal *et al.*, 1970, 1971; Embleton and Heidelberger, 1972). Similarly, mouse 3T3 cells treated with MCA and maintained *in vivo* in the immunologically protective confines of Millipore chambers have been found to be immunogenic, eliciting tumor rejection responses in syngeneic mice (Basombrío and Prehn, 1972*b,c*). These MCA-transformed cells, like sarcomas induced *in vivo*, express individually distinct antigens even when derived from cloned cell lines. This was originally established by analysis of the specificity of the tumor rejection response induced following immunization of syngeneic mice (Mondal *et al.*, 1970, 1971; Basombrío and Prehn, 1972*b,c*). Furthermore individually distinct tumor-specific surface antigens have been demonstrated in MCA-transformed mouse prostrate cells by analysis of the cytotoxicity of serum and lymph node cells from immunized mice (Embleton and Heidelberger, 1972).

374

ROBERT W.
BALDWIN
AND
MICHAEL R.
PRICE

These findings provided strong evidence against the concept that the neoantigens detected on transformed cells are present on normal cells but become detectable only by clonal amplification of the neoplastic cell population (Burnet, 1970).

*In vitro* transformed cell lines have also been used to analyze variability of neoantigen expression and immunogenic potential. Although murine sarcomas induced *in vivo* show a gradual decline in immunogenicity with increasing latent induction time, no such correlation was obtained with tumors induced by MCA treatment of cells which were subsequently maintained *in vivo* in Millipore chambers (Bartlett, 1972). These findings support the concept that immunoselection by the host may be a contributory factor determining variability in neoantigen expression. Comparably, Parmiani *et al.* (1973) concluded that in MCA carcinogenesis immunological control was operative but was only one of the factors influencing tumor immunogenicity. This was based on the finding that the wide variability of immunogenicity of MCA-transformed cells did not correlate with latency period, length of exposure to carcinogen, or tumor growth rate. These findings were obtained with MCA-transformed newborn murine muscle cells in Millipore filter chambers maintained *in vivo* or *in vitro* so that host immunosuppression of neoantigens was prevented. It must be stressed, however, that in all these studies the carcinogen plays a central role in determining the immunogenicity of the transformed cell. Thus fibroblast cell lines spontaneously transformed *in vitro* in Millipore chambers (Parmiani *et al.*, 1971) are almost totally devoid of tumor-specific rejection antigens, and no tumor-specific surface antigens were detected on mouse prostate cells spontaneously transformed *in vitro* (Embleton and Heidelberger, 1972). This is comparable with the results obtained with tumors developing spontaneously *in vivo* since these are either nonimmunogenic or weakly so (Baldwin, 1966; Baldwin and Embleton, 1969*b*).

Although the immunology of cells transformed *in vitro* by chemical carcinogens has not yet been adequately studied, it is evident that individually distinct tumor rejection antigens and tumor-specific antigens are frequently present. Future studies will specify the conditions and types of carcinogen interaction which lead to this type of neoantigen expression. Furthermore, precise analysis of these antigens, using radioimmunoassay techniques, will provide specific quantitative methods for studying the extent of cellular derangement induced by particular carcinogens. It remains to be ascertained, however, whether cells transformed *in vitro* by chemical carcinogens express embryonic antigens comparable to those detected on tumors arising *in vivo*. Since these embryonic antigens are common to different tumor types, their assay may possibly be utilized to study early events in carcinogenesis. In this connection, neoantigens demonstrable by their capacity to elicit antibody responses in syngeneic hosts have been detected after treating cells of a line established from normal adult liver with N-methyl-N-nitrosourea (MNU) (Iype *et al.*, 1973). This antibody reacted in membrane immunofluorescence tests with cells of the immunizing line and also other MNU-treated liver cell lines, but not with untreated cells. This neoantigen was detected also on liver cells treated with MCA or 3-methyl-DAB but not on cells treated with N-acetoxy-2-fluorenylacetamide or aflatoxin so that its characteristics appear different from those of tumor-associated antigens hitherto studied on carcinogen-induced tumors.

375

NEOANTIGEN
EXPRESSION
IN CHEMICAL
CAR-
CINOGENESIS

## 3. Conclusions and Perspectives

The individually distinct neoantigens (TARA, TASA) which are frequently found within the plasma membrane of chemically induced tumors can be viewed as specific products arising as a consequence of carcinogen–DNA interactions or indirectly following carcinogen–cytoplasmic protein binding. It is apparent with some tumors, such as MCA-induced rat sarcomas and DAB-induced hepatomas, that these antigens differ from cross-reacting embryonic antigens which are also expressed at the plasma membrane. Even so, this does not exclude the possibility that the individually distinct neoantigens are reexpressed embryonic antigens which may be present on embryo cells at early stages of development and therefore not detectable by present methods of antigen assay. As well as the wide diversity in neoantigen specificities, there is comparable variability in the degree of immunogenicity even among tumors induced by the same carcinogen. This is influenced to some extent by host immunosurveillance mechanisms (Bartlett, 1972; Parmiani *et al.*, 1973), but it is likely that the degree of tumor immunogenicity is largely controlled by factors operative at the time of the carcinogen-induced transformation. These two features, variability of antigen expression and antigen specificity, represent important parameters for studying molecular mechanisms of carcinogenesis.

The characteristics of the individually specific neoantigens can be accommodated by the hypothesis that chemical carcinogens produce random changes within the neoplastic cell. On this basis, tumors deficient in neoantigens may arise through carcinogen interactions (directly or indirectly) at sites within the cell genome which do not code for cell surface specificities. It should be emphasized, however, that methods for detecting tumor-associated neoantigens are still relatively insensitive so that low levels of neoantigen expression may not be detected. The related question of whether carcinogen-treated but non-transformed cells express new cell surface antigens comparable to those detected on tumors has not yet been adequately studied. There is good evidence that MCA-induced skin papillomas (Lappé, 1968, 1969) and bladder papillomas (Taranger *et al.*, 1972*a,b*) express neoantigens comparable to those revealed on developing carcinomas. There is, however, little indication that these antigens can be detected on carcinogen-treated but nontransformed cells. Mouse skin treated with 7,12-dimethylbenz[*a*]anthracene has been reported to undergo rejection on transplantation to syngeneic recipients, suggesting the presence of neoantigens (Mathé, 1967). It is more likely that this reflects the cytotoxicity of the carcinogen, since Outzen *et al.* (1972) determined that accelerated rejection of mouse skin grafts treated with MCA or 7,12-dimethylbenz[*a*]anthracene occurred rapidly in both normal and immunosuppressed mice. Analysis of neoantigen expression on carcinogen-treated cells may be facilitated using *in vitro* systems, but, even so, it is

376

ROBERT W.
BALDWIN
AND
MICHAEL R.
PRICE

highly unlikely that individually distinct neoantigens will be demonstrable, because of technical problems in obtaining sufficient cells for immunological analysis. These systems should, however, be applicable for studying cross-reacting antigens such as the tumor-associated embryonic antigens.

Immune reactions in the autochthonous host to neoantigens associated with chemically induced tumors are well documented (Baldwin, 1973). These responses were originally detected in studies showing inhibition or suppression of growth of reimplanted biopsies of MCA-induced rat sarcomas following destruction of the primary tumor either by ligation of its blood supply (Takeda et al., 1966) or by complete surgical resection (Mikulska et al., 1966). Tumor-specific immunity in tumor-bearing animals has also been demonstrated by studies of "concomitant immunity," whereby a second challenge with the homologous tumor was rejected (Lausch and Rapp, 1969; Fisher et al., 1970; Vaage, 1971; Chandradasa, 1973). Furthermore in vitro studies of cell-mediated and humoral immunity have established that animals bearing chemically induced tumors are sensitized to tumor-associated neoantigens including both the individually specific surface antigens and the tumor-associated embryonic antigens (Hellström et al., 1970; Baldwin et al., 1973c, 1974a; Baldwin and Embleton, 1974).

These studies indicate that consideration must be given to the role of host immune reactivity in chemical carcinogenesis. This is further emphasized by a number of studies indicating that immunosuppression may inhibit or alter the response to chemical carcinogens (Baldwin, 1973; Ménard et al., 1973a; Denlinger et al., 1973; Rees and Symes, 1973). It should be stressed, however, that there is no simple correlation between immunosuppression and increased response to chemical carcinogenesis, and further studies are required. This may be because, as is now evident, the relationship between cellular and humoral responses to tumor-associated neoantigens is highly complex. This indicates that a variety of factors have to be taken into account in the tumor-bearing host, among which are the production and maintenance of various populations of sensitized lymphoid cells, including B and T cells and possibly a K cell activated by antigen–antibody binding as well as cells of the monocyte series. In addition, there is now definitive evidence that circulating humoral factors are present in tumor-bearing individuals which act antagonistically to inhibit cell-mediated immunity (reviewed by K. E. Hellström and Hellström, 1974). The nature of the humoral antagonistic factors has still not been fully elucidated, but a number of effects have now been demonstrated at least using in vitro assay systems. These include blocking of target cells by tumor-specific antibody or immune complexes so that the cells are not susceptible to attack by sensitized lymphoid cells. It has also been established that effector lymphoid cells can be specifically inhibited by contact with tumor antigen (I. Hellström and Hellström, 1969; K. E. Hellström and Hellström, 1974; Sjögren et al., 1971; Baldwin et al., 1972e, 1973c,e,f). In view of the complexity of the host response to tumor-associated antigens, it is not surprising that the effects of immunosuppression on chemical carcinogenesis are not clear-cut, and future studies must take into account all of the known immunological parameters.

Acknowledgments

This work was supported by grants from the Cancer Research Campaign and the Medical Research Council.

377

NEOANTIGEN
EXPRESSION
IN CHEMICAL
CAR-
CINOGENESIS

## 4. References

ABELEV, G. I., 1971, Alpha-fetoprotein in oncogenesis and its association with malignant tumors, *Advan. Cancer Res.* **14**:295.

ABELEV, G. I., PEROVA, S. D., KHRAMKOVA, N. I., POSTNIKOVA, Z. A., AND IRLIN, I. S., 1963, Production of embryonal α-globulin by transplantable mouse hepatomas, *Transplantation* **1**:174.

APFFEL, C. A., ARNASON, B. G., AND PETERS, J. H., 1966, Induction of tumor immunity with tumor cells treated with iodoacetate, *Nature (Lond.)* **209**:694.

BALDWIN, R. W., 1955, Immunity to methylcholanthrene-induced tumors in inbred rats following atrophy and regression of implanted tumors, *Brit. J. Cancer* **9**:652.

BALDWIN, R. W., 1966, Tumor-specific immunity against spontaneous rat tumours, *Int. J. Cancer* **1**:257.

BALDWIN, R. W., 1973, Immunological aspects of chemical carcinogenesis, *Advan. Cancer Res.*, **18**:1.

BALDWIN, R. W., AND BARKER, C. R., 1967a, Tumour-specific antigenicity of aminoazo-dye-induced rat hepatomas, *Int. J. Cancer* **2**:355.

BALDWIN, R. W., AND BARKER, C. R., 1967b, Demonstration of tumour-specific humoral antibody against aminoazo dye–induced rat hepatomata, *Brit. J. Cancer* **21**:793.

BALDWIN, R. W., AND EMBLETON, M. J., 1969a, Immunology of 2-acetylaminofluorene-induced rat mammary adenocarcinomas, *Int. J. Cancer* **4**:47.

BALDWIN, R. W., AND EMBLETON, M. J., 1969b, Immunology of spontaneously arising rat mammary adenocarcinomas, *Int. J. Cancer* **4**:430.

BALDWIN, R. W., AND EMBLETON, M. J., 1971a, Demonstration by colony inhibition methods of cellular and humoral immune reactions to tumour-specific antigens associated with aminoazo-dye-induced rat hepatomas, *Int. J. Cancer* **7**:17.,

BALDWIN, R. W., AND EMBLETON, M. J., 1971b, Tumor-specific antigens in 2-acetylaminofluorene-induced rat hepatomas and related tumors, *Israel J. Med. Sci.* **7**:144.

BALDWIN, R. W., AND EMBLETON, M. J., 1974, Neoantigens on spontaneous and carcinogen-induced rat tumours defined by *in vitro* lymphocytotoxicity assays, *Int. J. Cancer* **13**:433.

BALDWIN, R. W., AND GLAVES, D., 1972, Solubilization of tumour-specific antigen from plasma membrane of an aminoazo-dye-induced rat hepatoma, *Clin. Exp. Immunol.* **11**:51.

BALDWIN, R. W., AND MOORE, M., 1968, Isolation of membrane-associated tumour-specific antigens from rat hepatomas induced by aminoazo dye, *Nature (Lond.)* **220**:287.

BALDWIN, R. W., AND MOORE, M., 1969, Isolation of membrane-associated tumour-specific antigen from an aminoazo-dye-induced rat hepatoma, *Int. J. Cancer* **4**:753.

BALDWIN, R. W., AND MOORE, M., 1971, Tumour-specific antigens and tumour–host interactions, in: *Immunological Tolerance to Tissue Antigens* (N. W. Nisbet and M. W., Elves, eds.), pp. 299–313, Orthopaedic Hospital, Oswestry, England.

BALDWIN, R. W., BARKER, C. R., EMBLETON, M. J., GLAVES, D., MOORE, M., AND PIMM, M. V., 1971a, Demonstration of cell-surface antigens on chemically induced tumors, *Ann. N.Y. Acad. Sci.* **177**:268.

BALDWIN, R. W., GLAVES, D., HARRIS, J. R., AND PRICE, M. R., 1971b, Tumor-specific antigens associated with aminoazo dye-induced rat hepatomas, *Transpl. Proc.* **3**:1189.

BALDWIN, R. W., GLAVES, D., AND PIMM, M. V., 1971c, Tumor-associated antigens as expressions of chemically-induced neoplasia and their involvement in tumor–host interactions, in: *Progress in Immunology* (B. Amos, ed.), pp. 907–920, Academic Press, New York.

BALDWIN, R. W., GLAVES, D., PIMM, M. V., AND VOSE, B. M., 1972a, Tumour specific and embryonic antigen expression on chemically induced rat tumours, *Ann. Inst. Pasteur (Paris)* **122**:715.

BALDWIN, R. W., GLAVES, D., AND VOSE, B. M., 1972b, Embryonic antigen expression in chemically induced rat hepatomas and sarcomas, *Int. J. Cancer* **10**:233.

## 378

**ROBERT W. BALDWIN AND MICHAEL R. PRICE**

BALDWIN, R. W., GLAVES, D., AND VOSE, B. M., 1972c, Fetal antigen expression on chemically induced rat neoplasms, in: *Embryonic and Fetal Antigens in Cancer*, Vol. 2 (N. G. Anderson, J. S. Coggin, Jr., E. Cole, and J. W., Holleman, eds.), p. 193.

BALDWIN, R. W., HARRIS, J. R., AND PRICE, M. R., 1972d, Isolation of plasma-membrane-associated tumor-specific antigen from rat hepatoma cells, *Biochem. J.* **128**:130.

BALDWIN, R. W., PRICE, M. R., AND ROBINS, R. A., 1972e, Blocking of lymphocyte-mediated cytotoxicity for rat hepatoma cells by tumour-specific antigen–antibody complexes, *Nature New Biol.* **238**:185.

BALDWIN, R. W., BOWEN, J. G., AND PRICE, M. R., 1973a, Detection of circulating hepatoma D23 antigen and immune complexes in tumour bearer serum, *Brit. J. Cancer* **28**:16.

BALDWIN, R. W., EMBLETON, M. J., AND MOORE, M., 1973b, Immunogenicity of rat hepatoma membrane fractions, *Brit. J. Cancer,* **28**:389.

BALDWIN, R. W., EMBLETON, M. J., AND ROBINS, R. A., 1973c, Cellular and humoral immunity to rat hepatoma–specific antigens correlated with tumour status, *Int. J. Cancer* **11**:1.

BALDWIN, R. W., HARRIS, J. R., AND PRICE, M. R., 1973d, Fractionation of plasma membrane–associated tumour specific antigen from an aminoazo dye–induced rat hepatoma, *Int. J. Cancer* **11**:385.

BALDWIN, R. W., PRICE, M. R., AND ROBINS, R. A., 1973e, Significance of serum factors modifying cellular immune responses to growing tumours, *Brit. J. Cancer* **28**:37 (Suppl. 1).

BALDWIN, R. W., PRICE, M. R., AND ROBINS, R. A., 1973f, Inhibition of hepatoma immune lymph node cell cytotoxicity by tumour bearer serum and solubilized hepatoma antigen, *Int. J. Cancer* **11**:527.

BALDWIN, R. W., GLAVES, D., AND VOSE, B. M., 1974a, Differentiation between the embryonic and tumour specific antigens on chemically induced rat tumours, *Brit. J. Cancer,* **29**:1.

BALDWIN, R. W., GLAVES, D., AND VOSE, B. M., 1974b, Immunogenicity of embryonic antigens associated with chemically-induced rat tumours, *Int. J. Cancer,* **13**:135.

BARANSKA, W., KOLDOVSKY, P., AND KOPROWSKI, H., 1970, Antigenic study of unfertilized mouse eggs: Cross reactivity with SV-40-induced antigens, *Proc. Natl. Acad. Sci.* **67**:193.

BARTLETT, G. L., 1972, Effect of host immunity on the antigenic strength of primary tumors, *J. Natl. Cancer Inst.* **49**:493.

BARTLETT, G. L., AND ZBAR, B., 1972, Tumor-specific vaccine containing *Mycobacterium bovis* and tumor cells: Safety and efficiency, *J. Natl. Cancer Inst.* **48**:1709.

BASOMBRÍO, M. A., 1970, Search for common antigenicities among twenty-five sarcomas induced by methylcholanthrene, *Cancer Res.* **30**:2458.

BASOMBRÍO, M. A., AND PREHN, R. T., 1972a, Search for common antigenicities between embryonic and tumoral tissue, *Medicina (Arg.)* **32**:42.

BASOMBRÍO, M. A., AND PREHN, R. T., 1972b, Antigenic diversity of tumors chemically induced within the progeny of a single cell, *Int. J. Cancer* **10**:1.

BASOMBRÍO, M. A., AND PREHN, R. T., 1972c, Studies on the basis for diversity and time of appearance of antigens in chemically induced tumors, *Natl. Cancer Inst. Monogr.* **35**:117.

BENDICH, A., BORENFREUND, E., AND STONEHILL, E. H., 1973, Protection of adult mice against tumor challenge by immunization with irradiated adult skin or embryo cells, *J. Immunol.* **111**:284.

BLOOM, B. R., BENNETT, B., OETTGEN, H. F., MCLEAN, E. P., AND OLD, L. J., 1969, Demonstration of delayed hypersensitivity to soluble antigens of chemically induced tumors by inhibition of macrophage migration, *Proc. Natl. Acad. Sci.* **64**:1176.

BLOOM, E. T., 1970, Quantitative detection of cytotoxic antibodies against tumor-specific antigens of murine sarcomas induced by 3-methylcholanthrene, *J. Natl. Cancer Inst.* **45**:443.

BLOOM, E. T., AND HILDEMANN, W. H., 1970, Mechanisms of tumor-specific enhancement versus resistance toward a methylcholanthrene-induced murine sarcoma, *Transplantation* **10**:321.

BORBERG, H., OETTGEN, H. F., CHOUDRY, K., AND BEATTIE, E. J., 1972, Inhibition of established transplants of chemically induced sarcomas in syngeneic mice by lymphocytes from immunized donors, *Int. J. Cancer* **10**:539.

BORSOS, T., AND LEONARD, E. J., 1972, Simultaneous presence of tumor-specific and fetal antigens on guinea pig tumor cells, in: *Embryonic and Fetal Antigens in Cancer*, Vol. 2 (N. G. Anderson, J. H. Coggin, Jr., E. Cole, and J. W. Holleman, eds.), p. 206.

BRAWN, R. J., 1970, Possible association of embryonal antigen(s) with several primary 3-methylcholanthrene-induced murine sarcomas, *Int. J. Cancer* **6**:245.

BUBENÍK, J., PERLMANN, P., HELMSTEIN, K., AND MOBERGER, G., 1970a, Immune response to urinary bladder tumours in man, *Int. J. Cancer* **5**:39.

BUBENÍK, J., PERLMANN, P., HELMSTEIN, K., AND MOBERGER, G., 1970b, Cellular and humoral immune responses to human urinary bladder carcinomas, *Int. J. Cancer* **5**:310.

BURDICK, J. F., COHEN, A. M., AND WELLS, S. A., 1973, A simplified isotopic antiglobulin assay: Detection of tumor-cell antigens, *J. Natl. Cancer Inst.* **50:**285.

BURNET, F. M., 1970, A certain symmetry: Histocompatibility antigens compared with immunocyte receptors, *Nature (Lond.)* **226:**123.

CASTRO, J. E., LANCE, E. M., MEDAWAR, P. B., ZANELLI, J., AND HUNT, R., 1973, Foetal antigens and cancer, *Nature (Lond.)* **243:**225.

CHANDRADASA, K. D., 1973, The development of specific suppression of concomitant immunity in two syngeneic tumor–host systems, *Int. J. Cancer* **11:**648.

COGGIN, J. H., AMBROSE, K. R., AND ANDERSON, N. G., 1970, Fetal antigen capable of inducing transplantation immunity against SV40 hamster tumor cells, *J. Immunol.* **105:**524.

COGGIN, J. H., AMBROSE, K. R., BELLOMY, B. B., AND ANDERSON, N. G., 1971, Tumor immunity in hamsters immunized with fetal tissues, *J. Immunol.* **107:**526.

COHEN, A. M., MILLAR, R. C., AND KETCHAM, A. S., 1972, Host immunity to a growing transplanted methylcholanthrene-induced guinea pig sarcoma, *Cancer Res.* **32:**2421.

DELORME, E. J., AND ALEXANDER, P., 1964, Treatment of primary fibrosarcoma in the rat with immune lymphocytes, *Lancet* **1:**117.

DE NÉCHAUD, B., AND URIEL, J., 1973, Antigènes cellulaires transitoires du foie de rat. III. Mode de réapparition de l'α-foetoprotéine au cours de l'hepatocarcinogénèse chimique, *Int. J. Cancer* **11:**104.

DENLINGER, R. H., SWENBERG, J. A., KOESTNER, A., AND WECHSLER, W., 1973, Differential effect of immunosuppression on the induction of nervous system and bladder tumours by N-methyl N-nitrosourea, *J. Natl. Cancer Inst.* **50:**87.

DUFF, R., AND RAPP, F., 1970, Reactions of serum from pregnant hamsters with surface of cells transformed by SV40, *J. Immunol.* **105:**521.

EMBLETON, M. J., AND HEIDELBERGER, C., 1972, Antigenicity of clones of mouse prostate cells transformed *in vitro*, *Int. J. Cancer* **9:**8.

FISHER, B., SAFFER, E. A., AND FISHER, E. R., 1970, Comparison of concomitant and sinecomitant tumour immunity, *Proc. Soc. Exp. Biol. (N.Y.)* **135:**68.

FOLEY, E. J., 1953, Antigenic properties of methylcholanthrene-induced tumours in mice of the strain of origin, *Cancer Res.* **13:**835.

GIRARDI, A. J., REPUCCI, P., DIERLAM, P., RUTALA, W., AND COGGIN, J. H., 1973, Prevention of simian virus 40 tumors by hamster fetal tissue: Influence of parity status of donor females on immunogenicity of fetal tissue and on immune cell cytotoxicity, *Proc. Natl. Acad. Sci.* **70:**183.

GLOBERSON, A., AND FELDMAN, M., 1964, Antigenic specificity of benzo[a]pyrene-induced sarcomas, *J. Natl. Cancer Inst.* **32:**1229.

GORDON, J., 1965, Isoantigenicity of liver tumours induced by an azo dye, *Brit. J. Cancer* **19:**387.

HALLIDAY, W. J., 1971, Blocking effect of serum from tumor-bearing animals on macrophage migration inhibition with tumor antigens, *J. Immunol.* **106:**855.

HALLIDAY, W. J., AND WEBB, M., 1969, Delayed hypersensitivity to chemically-induced tumors in mice and correlation with an *in vitro* test, *J. Natl. Cancer Inst.* **43:**141.

HANNA, M. G., TENNANT, R. W., AND COGGIN, J. H., 1971, Suppressive effect of immunization with mouse fetal antigens on growth of cells infected with Rauscher leukemia virus on plasma cell tumours, *Proc. Natl. Acad. Sci.* **68:**1748.

HARDER, F. H., AND MCKHANN, C. F., 1968, Demonstration of cellular antigens on sarcoma cells by an indirect [125]I-labelled antibody technique, *J. Natl. Cancer Inst.* **40:**231.

HARRIS, J. R., PRICE, M. R., AND BALDWIN, R. W., 1973, The purification of membrane-associated tumour antigens by preparative polyacrylamide gel electrophoresis, *Biochim. Biophys. Acta* **311:**600.

HELLSTRÖM, I., AND HELLSTRÖM, K. E., 1969, Studies on cellular immunity and its serum mediated inhibition in Moloney-virus-induced mouse sarcomas, *Int. J. Cancer* **4:**587.

HELLSTRÖM, I., AND HELLSTRÖM, K. E., 1972, Murine bladder tumors as models for human tumor immunity, *Natl. Cancer Inst. Monogr.* **35:**125.

HELLSTRÖM, I., HELLSTRÖM, K. E., AND PIERCE, G. E., 1968, *In vitro* studies of immune reactions against autochthonous and syngeneic mouse tumors induced by methylcholanthrene and plastic discs, *Int. J. Cancer* **3:**467.

HELLSTRÖM, I., HELLSTRÖM, K. E., AND SJÖGREN, H. O., 1970, Serum mediated inhibition of cellular immunity to methylcholanthrene-induced murine sarcomas, *Cell. Immunol.* **1:**18.

HELLSTRÖM, K. E., AND HELLSTRÖM, I., 1969, Cellular immunity against tumor antigens, *Advan. Cancer Res.* **12:**167.

380

ROBERT W.
BALDWIN
AND
MICHAEL R.
PRICE

HELLSTRÖM, K. E., AND HELLSTRÖM, I., 1974, Lymphocyte mediated cytotoxicity and blocking serum activity to tumor antigens, *Advan. Immunol.* **18:**209.

HOLLINSHEAD, A., MCCAMMON, J. R., AND YOHN, D, S,, 1972, Immunogenicity of a soluble membrane antigen from adenovirus-12 induced tumor cells demonstrated in inbred hamsters (PD-4), *Canad. J. Microbiol.* **18:**1365.

HOLMES, E. C., KAHAN, B. D., AND MORTON, D. L., 1970, Soluble tumor-specific transplantation antigens from methylcholanthrene-induced guinea pig sarcomas, *Cancer* **25:**373.

HOLMES, E. C., MORTON, D. L., SCHIDLOWSKY, G., AND TRAHAN, E., 1971, Cross-reacting tumor-specific transplantation antigens in methylcholanthrene-induced guinea pig sarcomas, *J. Natl. Cancer Inst.* **46:**693.

HULL, E. W., CARBONE, P. P., GITLIN, D., O'GARA, R. W., AND KELLY, M. G., 1969, α-Fetoprotein in monkeys with hepatoma, *J. Natl. Cancer Inst.* **42:**1035.

ISHIMOTO, A., AND ITO, Y., 1972, Presence of antibody against mouse fetal antigen in the sera from C57Bl/6 mice immunized with Rauscher leukemia, *Cancer Res.* **32:**2333.

IYPE, P. T., BALDWIN, R. W., AND GLAVES, D., 1973, Cell surface antigenic changes induced in normal adult rat liver cells by carcinogen treatment *in vitro*, *Brit. J. Cancer* **27:**128.

JOHNSON, S., 1968, The effect of thymectomy and of the dose of 3-methylcholanthrene on the induction and antigenic properties of sarcomas in C57 Bl mice, *Brit. J. Cancer* **22:**93.

KIM, U., 1970, Metastasizing mammary carcinomas in rats: Induction and study of their immunogenicity, *Science* **167:**72.

KIT, S., KURIMURA, T., AND DUBBS, D. R., 1969, Transplantable mouse tumor line induced by injection of SV-40 transformed mouse kidney cells, *Int. J. Cancer* **4:**384.

KITAGAWA, T., YOKOCHI, T., AND SUGANO, H., 1972, α-Fetoprotein and hepatocarcinogenesis in rats fed 3-methyl-4-(dimethylamino) azo-benzene or *N*-2-fluorenylacetamide, *Int. J. Cancer* **10:**368.

KLEIN, G., 1973, Tumor immunology, *Transpl. Proc.* **5:**31.

KLEIN, G., SJÖGREN, H. O., KLEIN, E., AND HELLSTRÖM, K. E., 1960, Demonstration of resistance against methylcholanthrene-induced sarcomas in the primary autochthonous host, *Cancer Res.* **20:**1561.

KROES, R., WILLIAMS, G. M., AND WEISBURGER, J. H., 1972, Early appearance of serum α-fetoprotein during hepatocarcinogenesis as a function of age of rats and extent of treatment with 3-methyl-4-dimethylaminoazobenzene, *Cancer Res.* **32:**1526.

KROES, R., WILLIAMS, G. M., AND WEISBURGER, J. H., 1973, Early appearance of serum α-fetoprotein as a function of dosage of various hepatocarcinogens, *Cancer Res.* **33:**613.

KRONMAN, B. S., RAPP, H. J., AND BORSOS, T., 1969, Tumor-specific antigens: detection by local transfer of delayed skin hypersensitivity, *J. Natl. Cancer Inst.* **43:**869.

LAPPÉ, M. A., 1968, Evidence for the antigenicity of papillomas induced by 3-methylcholanthrene, *J. Natl. Cancer Inst.* **40:**823.

LAPPÉ, M. A., 1969, Tumour specific transplantation antigens: Possible origin in pre-malignant lesions, *Nature (Lond.)* **223:**82.

LAURENCE, D. J. R., AND NEVILLE, A. M., 1972, Foetal antigens and their role in the diagnosis and clinical management of human neoplasms: A review, *Brit. J. Cancer* **26:**335.

LAUSCH, R. N., AND RAPP, F., 1969, Concomitant immunity in hamsters bearing DMBA-induced tumor transplants, *Int. J. Cancer* **4:**226.

LEJNEVA, O. M., ZILBER, L. A., AND IEVLEVA, E. S., 1965, Humoral antibodies to methylcholanthrene sarcomata detected by a fluorescent technique, *Nature (Lond.)* **206:**1163.

LE MEVEL, B. P., AND WELLS, S. A., 1973, Foetal antigens cross-reactive with tumour-specific transplantation antigens, *Nature New Biol.* **244:**183.

LEONARD, E. J., 1973, Cell surface antigen movement: Induction in hepatoma cells by antitumor antibody, *J. Immunol.* **110:**1167.

LEONARD, E. J., MELTZER, M. S., BORSOS, T., AND RAPP, H. J., 1972, Properties of soluble tumor-specific antigen solubilized by hypertonic potassium chloride, *Natl. Cancer Inst. Monogr.* **35:**129.

MANN, D. L., 1972, The effect of enzyme inhibitors on the solubilization of HL-A antigens with 3M KCl, *Transplantation* **14:**398.

MATHÉ, G., 1967, Antigénicité nouvelle démontrée par isogreffe d'un fragment de peau prélevé 5 jours après injection intradermique de di-méthyl-benzenthracène, *Rev. Fr. Etudes Clin. Biol.* **12:**380.

MCCOLLESTER, D. L., 1970, Isolation of Meth A cell surface membranes possessing tumor-specific transplantation antigen activity, *Cancer Res.* **30:**2832.

MELTZER, M. S., LEONARD, E. J., RAPP, H. J., AND BORSOS, T., 1971, Tumor-specific antigen solubilized by hypertonic potassium chloride, *J. Natl. Cancer Inst.* **47**:703.

MELTZER, M. S., OPPEHEIM, J. J., LITTMAN, B. H., LEONARD, E. J., AND RAPP, H. J., 1972, Cell-mediated tumor immunity measured *in vitro* and *in vivo* with soluble tumor-specific antigens, *J. Natl. Cancer Inst.* **49**:727.

MÉNARD, S., COLNAGHI, M. I., AND CORNALBA, G., 1973a, Immunogenicity and immunoselectivity of urethane-induced murine lung adenomata, in relation to the immunological impairment of the primary tumour host, *Brit. J. Cancer* **27**:345.

MÉNARD, S., COLNAGHI, M. I., AND DELLA PORTA, G., 1973b, *In vitro* demonstration of tumor-specific common antigens and embryonal antigens in murine fibrosarcomas induced by 7,12-dimethylbenz[a]anthracene, *Cancer Res.* **33**:478.

MIKULSKA, Z. B., SMITH, C., AND ALEXANDER, P., 1966, Evidence for an immunological reaction of the host directed against its own actively growing primary tumor, *J. Natl. Cancer Inst.* **36**:29.

MONDAL, S., IYPE, P. T., GRIESBACH, L. M., AND HEIDELBERGER, C., 1970, Antigenicity of cells derived from mouse prostate after malignant transformation *in vitro* by carcinogenic hydrocarbons, *Cancer Res.* **30**:1593.

MONDAL, S., EMBLETON, M. J., MARQUARDT, H., AND HEIDELBERGER, C., 1971, Production of variants of decreased malignancy and antigenicity from clones transformed *in vitro* by methylcholanthrene, *Int. J. Cancer* **8**:410.

MORTON, D. L., GOLDMAN, L., AND WOOD, D., 1965, Tumor specific antigenicity of methylcholanthrene (MCA) and dibenzanthracene (DBA) induced sarcomas of inbred guinea pigs, *Fed. Proc. Fed. Am. Soc. Exp. Biol.* **24**:684.

MÜLLER, M., 1968, Versuche zur Erzeugung einer Transplantationsimmunität gegen o-Aminoazotoluol-Hepatome bei syngenen und F$_1$-Hybrid-Mäusen, *Arch. Geschwülstforsch.* **31**:235.

OETTGEN, H. F., OLD, L. J., MCLEAN, E. P., AND CARSWELL, E. A., 1968, Delayed hypersensitivity and transplantation immunity elicited by soluble antigens of chemically induced tumours in inbred guinea pigs, *Nature (Lond.)* **220**:295.

OLD, L. J., AND BOYSE, E. A., 1965, Antigens of tumors and leukemias induced by viruses, *Fed. Proc. Fed. Am. Soc. Exp. Biol.* **24**:1009.

OLD, L. J., BOYSE, E. A., CLARKE, D. A., AND CARSWELL, E. A., 1962, Antigenic properties of chemically induced tumors, *Ann. N.Y. Acad. Sci.* **101**:80.

O'TOOLE, C., PERLMANN, P., UNSGAARD, B., MOBERGER, G., AND EDSMYR, F., 1972a, Cellular immunity to human urinary bladder carcinoma. I. Correlation to clinical stage and radiotherapy, *Int. J. Cancer* **10**:77.

O'TOOLE, C., PERLMANN, P., UNSGAARD, B., ALMGARD, L. E., JOHANSSON, B., MOBERGER, G., AND EDSMYR, F., 1972b, Cellular immunity to urinary bladder carcinoma. II. Effect of surgery and preoperative irradiation, *Int. J. Cancer* **10**:92.

O'TOOLE, C., UNSGAARD, B., ALMGARD, L. E., AND JOHANSSON, B., 1973, The cellular immune response to carcinoma of the urinary bladder: Correlation to clinical stage and treatment, *Brit. J. Cancer* **28**:266 (Suppl. 1).

OUTZEN, H. C., ANDREWS, E. J., BASOMBRÍO, M. A., LITWIN, S., AND PREHN, R. T., 1972, Attempted induction of tumor antigens in carcinogen-treated cells, *J. Natl. Cancer Inst.* **49**:1295.

PARMIANI, G., AND DELLA PORTA, G., 1973, Effects of antitumour immunity on pregnancy in the mouse, *Nature New Biol.* **241**:26.

PARMIANI, G., CARBONE, G., AND PREHN, R. T., 1971, *In vitro* "spontaneous" neoplastic transformation of mouse fibroblasts in diffusion chambers, *J. Natl. Cancer Inst.* **46**:261.

PARMIANI, G., CARBONE, G., AND LEMBO, 1973, Immunogenic strength of sarcomas induced by methylcholanthrene in Millipore filter diffusion chambers, *Cancer Res.* **33**:750.

PASTERNAK, G., 1963, Die unterschiedliche Reaktionsfähigkeit zweier Mäuseinzuchtstämme gegen spezifische Antigene isolog transplantabler Carcinogentumoren, *Acta Biol. Med. Ger.* **10**:572.

PASTERNAK, G., GRAFFI, A., HOFFMANN, F., AND HORN, K. -H., 1964, Resistance against carcinomas of the skin induced by dimethylbenzanthracene (DMBA) in mice of the strain XVII/*Bln*, *Nature (Lond.)* **203**:307.

PASTERNAK, G., HOFFMANN, F., AND GRAFFI, A., 1966, Growth of diethylnitrosamine-induced lung tumours in syngeneic mice specifically, pre-treated with X-ray killed tumour tissue, *Folia Biol. (Prague)* **12**:299.

PILCH, Y. H., 1968, The antigenicity and immunogenicity of cell-free extracts of chemically induced murine sarcomas, *Cancer Res.* **28**:2502.

381

NEOANTIGEN
EXPRESSION
IN CHEMICAL
CAR-
CINOGENESIS

382

ROBERT W.
BALDWIN
AND
MICHAEL R.
PRICE

PREHN, R. T., 1960, Tumor-specific immunity to transplanted dibenz[a,h]anthracene-induced sarcomas, Cancer Res. 20:1614.

PREHN, R. T., 1962, Specific isoantigenicities among chemically induced tumors, Ann. N. Y. Acad. Sci. 101:107.

PREHN, R. T., AND MAIN, J. M., 1957, Immunity to methylcholanthrene-induced sarcomas, J. Natl. Cancer Inst. 18:769.

REES, J. A., AND SYMES, M. O., 1973, Immunodepression as a factor during 3-methylcholanthrene carcinogenesis and subsequent tumour growth in mice, Int. J. Cancer 11:202.

REINER, J., AND SOUTHAM, C. M., 1967, Evidence of common antigenic properties in chemically induced sarcomas of mice, Cancer Res. 27:1243.

REINER, J., AND SOUTHAM, C. M., 1969, Further evidence of common antigenic properties in chemically induced sarcomas of mice, Cancer Res. 29:1814.

REISFELD, R. A., AND KAHAN, B. D., 1970, Biological and chemical characterization of human histocompatibility antigens, Fed. Proc. Fed. Am. Soc. Exp. Biol. 29:2034.

REISFELD, R. A., AND KAHAN, B. D., 1972, Markers of biological individuality, Sci. Am. 226: No. 6:28.

RÉVÉSZ, L., 1960, Detection of antigenic differences in isologous host–tumor systems by pretreatment with heavily irradiated tumor cells, Cancer Res. 20:443.

SJÖGREN, H. O., HELLSTRÖM, I., BANSAL, S. C., AND HELLSTROM, K. E., 1971, Suggestive evidence that the "blocking antibodies" of tumor-bearing individuals may be antigen–antibody complexes, Proc. Natl. Acad. Sci. 68:1372.

STANISLAWSKI-BIRENCWAJG, M., URIEL, J., AND GRABAR, P., 1967, Association of embryonic antigens with experimentally-induced hepatic lesions in the rat, Cancer Res. 27:1990.

SUTER, L., BLOOM, B. R., WADSWORTH, E. M., AND OETTGEN, H. F., 1972, Use of the macrophage migration inhibition test to monitor fractionation of soluble antigens of chemically induced sarcomas of inbred guinea pigs, J. Immunol. 109:766.

TAKASUGI, M., AND KLEIN, E., 1970, A microassay for cell-mediated immunity, Transplantation 9:219.

TAKEDA, K., 1969, Immunology of Cancer, Hokkaido University, Sapporo, Japan.

TAKEDA, K., AIZAWA, M., KITUCHI, Y., YAMAWAKI, S., AND NAKAMURA, K., 1966, Tumour autoimmunity against methylcholanthrene-induced sarcomas of the rat, Gann 57:221.

TARANGER, L. A., CHAPMAN, W. H., HELLSTRÖM, I., AND HELLSTRÖM, K. E., 1972a, Immunological studies on urinary bladder tumors of rats and mice, Science 176:1337.

TARANGER, L. A., HELLSTRÖM, I., CHAPMAN, W. H., AND HELLSTRÖM, K. E., 1972b, In vitro demonstration of common tumor antigens in mouse and rat bladder carcinomas, Proc. Am. Assoc. Cancer Res. 13:56.

THOMSON, D. M. P., AND ALEXANDER, P., 1973, A cross-reacting embryonic antigen in the membrane of rat sarcoma cells which is immunogenic in the syngeneic host, Brit. J. Cancer 27:35.

THOMSON, D. M. P., STEELE, K., AND ALEXANDER, P., 1973, The presence of tumor-specific membrane antigen in the serum of rats with chemically induced sarcomata, Brit. J. Cancer 27:27.

TING, R. C., 1968, Failure to induce transplantation resistance against polyoma tumor cells with syngeneic embryonic tissue, Nature (Lond.) 217:858.

TING, C. C., LAVRIN, D. H., SHIU, G., AND HERBERMAN, R. B., 1972, Expression of fetal antigens in tumor cells, Proc. Natl. Acad. Sci. 69:1664.

TING, C. C., ORTALDO, J. R., AND HERBERMAN, R. B., 1973a, Expression of fetal antigens and tumor-specific antigens in SV40-transformed cells. I. Serological analysis of antigenic specificities, Int. J. Cancer 12:511.

TING, C. C., RODRIGUES, D., AND HERBERMAN, R. B., 1973b, Expression of fetal antigens and tumor-specific antigens in SV40-transformed cells. II. Tumor transplantation studies, Int. J. Cancer 12:519.

TUFFREY, M. A., AND BATCHELOR, J. R., 1964, Tumour specific immunity against murine epitheliomas induced with 9,10-dimethyl-1,2-benzanthracene, Nature (Lond.) 204:349.

URIEL, J., AUSSEL, C., BOUILLON, D., DE NÉCHAUD, B., AND LOISILLIER, F., 1973, Localization of rat liver α-foetoprotein by cell affinity labelling with tritiated oestrogens, Nature New Biol. 244:190.

VAAGE, J., 1971, Concomitant immunity and specific depression of immunity by residual or re-injected tumour tissue, Cancer Res. 31:1655.

WATABE, H., HIRAI, H., AND SATOH, H., 1972, α-Fetoprotein in rats transplanted with ascites hepatoma, Gann 63:189.

WEPSIC, H. T., ZBAR, B., RAPP, H. J., AND BORSOS, T., 1970, Systemic transfer of tumor immunity: delayed hypersensitivity and suppression of tumor growth, J. Natl. Cancer Inst. 44:955.

WOLF, A., AND AVIS, P. J. G., 1970, Preparation and purification of plasma membranes from murine lymphoma cells carrying tumour-specific antigenicity, *Transplantation* **9**:18.

ZBAR, B., WEPSIC, H. T., RAPP, H. J., BORSOS, T., KRONMAN, B. S., AND CHURCHILL, W. H., 1969, Antigenic specificity of hepatomas induced in strain-2 guinea pigs by diethylnitrosamine, *J. Natl. Cancer Inst.* **43**:833.

ZBAR, B., WEPSIC, H. T., RAPP, H. J., STEWART, L. C., AND BORSOS, T., 1970, Two-step mechanism of tumor graft rejection in syngeneic guinea pigs. II. Initiation of reaction by a cell fraction containing lymphocytes and neutrophils, *J. Natl. Cancer Inst.* **44**:701.

ZBAR, B., BERNSTEIN, I. D., AND RAPP, H. J., 1971, Suppression of tumor growth at the site of infection with living bacillus Calmette Guérin, *J. Natl. Cancer Inst.* **46**:831.

ZBAR, B., BERNSTEIN, I. D., BARTLETT, G. L., HANNA, G., AND RAPP, H. J., 1972a, Immunotherapy of cancer: Regression of intradermal tumors and prevention of growth of lymph node metastases after intralesional injection of living *Mycobacterium bovis*, *J. Natl. Cancer Inst.* **49**:119.

ZBAR, B., RAPP, H. J., AND RIBI, E. E., 1972b, Tumor suppression by cell walls of *Mycobacterium bovis* attached to oil droplets, *J. Natl. Cancer Inst.* **48**:831.

383

NEOANTIGEN
EXPRESSION
IN CHEMICAL
CAR-
CINOGENESIS

# Physical
# Carcinogenesis

# Physical Carcinogenesis: Radiation—History and Sources

ARTHUR C. UPTON

## 1. Introduction

More than half a century has elapsed since the carcinogenic effects of radiation were first recorded. Study of such effects has since received continuing impetus from the early and expanding uses of radiation in diagnosis and therapy, and from the far-reaching applications of nuclear technology in science, medicine, and industry. In historical perspective, the effects of radiation have received greater study than those of any other physical agent of comparable environmental significance. As such, our experience with radiation is applicable to the study and control of other environmental carcinogens.

It is beyond the scope of this report to review in detail the vast literature on biological and carcinogenic effects of radiation. An attempt will be made herein merely to survey those historical aspects which are of major relevance to the accompanying chapters on carcinogenesis.

## 2. Types of Radiations

Carcinogenic activity has been documented for radiations of the electromagnetic spectrum (Fig. 1) and for corpuscular, or particulate, radiations. Of the electromagnetic radiations, only ultraviolet radiations and the ionizing radiations

ARTHUR C. UPTON ● Health Sciences Center, State University of New York at Stony Brook, Stony Brook, New York.

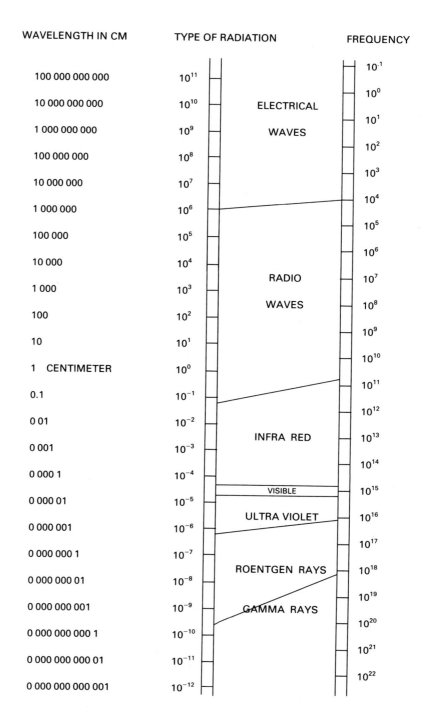

FIGURE 1. The electromagnetic spectrum, showing wavelength and frequency of the different bands. From Glasser (1944).

($\gamma$-rays, X-rays) are known to possess carcinogenic properties, whereas corpuscular radiations ($\alpha$-particles, $\beta$-particles, protons, neutrons), which are also ionizing, have been found to be carcinogenic in every case investigated.

As is discussed elsewhere, the carcinogenic effects of ultraviolet radiation (Urbach, this volume) and of the ionizing radiations (Kellerer and Rossi, this volume; Storer, this volume) are attributed to their production of physicochemical changes in critical macromolecular constituents (e.g., DNA) of cells in which they are absorbed. Only small amounts of energy need be involved, the lethal dose of ionizing radiation for mammals being of the order of $10^{-3}$ cal/g, deposited randomly in discrete events averaging about 60 eV each (Hutchinson and Rauth, 1962). Although the biological effects of radiation cannot be defined fully as yet at the molecular level, knowledge of the effects of radiation on DNA has advanced rapidly, and it is now known that effects on DNA may be influenced profoundly by biological repair processes. Among the changes in DNA attributable to ultraviolet irradiation, formation of pyrimidine dimers is considered to be foremost in importance, while the changes in DNA attributable to ionizing radiation include base alteration, base destruction, sugar–phosphate bond cleavage, chain breakage (single-strand and double-strand), crosslinking of strands (intrastrand and interstrand), and degradation (Kanazir, 1969). Double-strand breaks, which are thought to constitute roughly 7–10% of all the breaks induced by X-irradiation in mammalian cells, are estimated to require approximately 600 eV per break (Corry and Cole, 1968), compared to 44 eV per break for single-strand breaks (Lehman and Ormerod, 1970). Either type of strand break may, if repaired incorrectly, lead to more complicated changes in the affected DNA, including base-pair alterations and deletions such as have been implicated in radiation mutagenesis (Malling and De Serres, 1969).

It is now amply clear that the induction of a mutagenic or carcinogenic effect in DNA must be viewed as the end result of a sequence of reactions, the outcome of which may depend as much on the influence of repair mechanisms as on the nature of the primary lesion itself (Fox and Lajtha, 1973). At least three types of DNA repair have been noted in bacteria: (1) photoenzymatic repair, (2) excision repair, and (3) postreplication (recombinational) repair (United Nations, 1972; Fox and Lajtha, 1973). Excision repair, through which pyrimidine dimers are removed from affected DNA, is deficient in many patients suffering from xeroderma pigmentosum, the deficiency itself presumably accounting for their photosensitivity (see Urbach, this volume). This type of repair also varies in effectiveness among different mammalian cell lines. Photoenzymatic repair has not been found in mammals other than marsupials. Because both types of repair involve enzyme systems that are affected by genetic, physiological, metabolic, and environmental factors (Fox and Lajtha, 1973), their role in mutagenesis and carcinogenesis can be characterized only in a general way. Further complicating assessment of their role is our uncertainty concerning the relationship between the DNA in mammalian cells and its associated nucleoprotein, which also appears to undergo alteration and repair following irradiation (United Nations, 1972; Fox and Lajtha, 1973).

*3. Sources and Levels of Radiation in the Environment*

ARTHUR C.
UPTON

Man has evolved in the continuous presence of radiations, which vary with altitude, latitude, and other environmental factors (Bener, 1969; Stair, 1969; National Academy of Sciences, 1972; United Nations, 1972; Urbach, this volume). The levels of ionizing radiation received by the general population from various sources are summarized in Table 1. From inspection of the table, it is evident that

TABLE 1

*Estimated Average Annual Whole-Body Dose Rates in the United States (1970)*

| Source | Average dose rate[a] (mrem/yr) |
|---|---|
| Environmental | |
| Natural | |
| Cosmic rays | 44 |
| Terrestrial radiation | |
| External | 40 |
| Internal (mostly from $^{40}$K) | 18 |
| Subtotal | 102 |
| Global fallout | 4 |
| Nuclear power | 0.003 |
| SUBTOTAL | 106 |
| Medical | |
| Diagnostic | 72[b] |
| Radiopharmaceuticals | 1 |
| SUBTOTAL | 73 |
| Occupational | 0.8 |
| Miscellaneous | 2 |
| TOTAL | 182 |

From NAS–NRC (1972).

[a] The numbers shown are average values only. For given segments of the population, dose rates considerably greater than those may be experienced.
[b] Based on the abdominal dose.

the major source of exposure to manmade radiation is the use of X-rays in medical diagnosis. Other manmade sources contribute as yet only such a minute percentage to the overall exposure that even though they may be expected to increase in magnitude within the foreseeable future, their total importance is likely to remain relatively small (National Academy of Sciences, 1972; United Nations, 1972).

4. *Historical Developments in Carcinogenesis by Ionizing Radiation*     391

PHYSICAL
CAR-
CINOGENESIS:
RADIATION—
HISTORY AND
SOURCES

## 4.1. Observations in Humans

Study of radiation carcinogenesis in human populations is complicated by several difficulties: (1) Cancer is sufficiently rare that large populations must be studied to define the incidence of neoplasms at any one site, few populations being large enough or exposed to high enough doses to yield quantitative dose-incidence data for specific malignancies. (2) Even in such populations, the latent period intervening between irradiation and the appearance of neoplasms is so long that it hampers the follow-up of exposed individuals and the evaluation of their absorbed dose. (3) Because of the length of the latent period, none of the irradiated populations investigated to date has been followed long enough to disclose the cumulative lifetime effects of radiation on the incidence of cancer. (4) Many of the existing dose–incidence data have been derived from patients exposed to radiation for medical purposes, in whom the effects of radiation are complicated by effects of other forms of treatment or by effects of the underlying disease itself. (5) Some of the existing data are based on effects of internally deposited radionuclides, interpretation of which is complicated by variations of the radiation dose in space and time. (6) The natural incidence of cancer varies so widely from one organ to another and under the influence of so many variables (e.g., genetic background, age, sex, geographic location, diet, socioeconomic factors) that dose–incidence data derived from one population may not be strictly applicable to another.

### 4.1.1. Early Radiologists and Radiation Workers

The first neoplasm attributed to radiation was an epidermoid carcinoma on the hand of a radiologist (Frieben, 1902), followed by dozens of similar cases in ensuing decades, owing in part to the practice among pioneer radiographers of exposing their hands repeatedly in focusing their primitive fluoroscopic equipment. The manifestations of injury in such victims commonly began with reddening and blistering of the skin, often within weeks after exposure. Whether or not exposure was then discontinued, the lesions frequently remained painful and were accompanied by paresthesia, anesthesia, throbbing, and tenderness. Within a few years, they were characteristically followed by atrophy of the epidermis and development of keratoses from which malignant cells frequently extended into the dermis. Many of the carcinomas arising in this way were multiple and occurred on both hands. Within 15 yr after Roentgen's discovery of the X-ray, 94 cases of skin cancer had been attributed to radiation among physicians, X-ray technicians, and radium handlers in America, England, and Germany (Hesse, 1911). The neoplasms were predominantly squamous cell and basal cell carcinomas but also included fibrosarcomas (Furth and Lorenz, 1954). Because the development of such tumors characteristically required a long induction period (averaging 10–39 yr), with radiation dermatitis preceding the appearance of the tumors themselves, it was generally thought that tumor induction would not occur unless preceded by gross radiation damage to the skin (see Furth and Lorenz, 1954). Although tumors have since been reported to follow irradiation in normal-appearing skin (see International Commission on Radiological Protection, 1969), they have ceased to be an occupational disease of radiologists. Radiodermatitis and skin cancer may continue to occur, however among those using radiation equipment without adequate safeguards (Mohs, 1952).

The induction of leukemia by ionizing radiation was also first tentatively reported because of clustering of 5 cases of leukemia in pioneer radiation workers (von Jagie *et al.*, 1911). Since then, the leukemogenic action of ionizing radiation has been amply confirmed by epidemiological studies in radiation workers and in other irradiated populations, over 200 cases of "radiation-induced" leukemia appearing in the world literature between 1911 and 1959 (Cronkite *et al.*, 1960).

### 4.1.2. Dial Painters

The induction of bone tumors by radiation was first observed in dial painters (see Martland, 1931; Looney, 1958) who had ingested radium in applying luminous paint to clock and watch dials, through the practice of pointing their brushes between their lips. In addition to osteosarcomas, such victims showed an excess of fibrosarcomas and carcinomas of paranasal and mastoid sinuses (Aub *et al.*, 1952; Marinelli, 1958; Looney, 1958). The development of the tumors was usually preceded by radiation osteitis, characterized by coarsening of trabeculae and necrosis of bone, with rarefaction, formation of atypical osseous tissue, and localized calcification (Aub *et al.*, 1952; Looney, 1958). The latent period for induction of the tumors varied inversely with the radium content of the skeleton, being as short as 10 yr in patients with 6–50 $\mu$g of radium and more than 25 yr in those with smaller radium burdens (Evans, 1966). The incidence of bone tumors has been interpreted to vary roughly as the square of the terminal concentration of radium in the skeleton, exceeding 20% at levels of 5 $\mu$Ci or more, but with no evidence of tumor induction at levels of less than 0.5 $\mu$Ci (National Academy of Sciences, 1972; United Nations, 1972). Interpretation of the dose–incidence relation is complicated by the inhomogeneity of the radiation dose in space and time, the radium being localized in hot spots, and the amount present in the skeleton at the time the tumors have been detected being only a small percentage of that present earlier.

### 4.1.3. Miners of Radioactive Ore

Carcinoma of the lung, long known to be an occupational disability of pitchblend miners in Saxony and Bohemia, has only recently been attributed to irradiation by radon in this population (Weller, 1956). U.S. uranium miners have likewise shown an excess of pulmonary carcinomas, varying with the duration and intensity of their exposure, even after correction for such variables as age, cigarette smoking,

393
PHYSICAL
CAR-
CINOGENESIS:
RADIATION—
HISTORY AND
SOURCES

heredity, urbanization, self-selection, diagnostic accuracy, prior hard-rock mining, nonradioactive-ore constituents, including silica dust" (Lundin *et al.*, 1971). A comparable excess of bronchial carcinoma has been noted in other hard-rock miners who are similarly exposed to radon and its radioactive disintegration products (National Academy of Sciences, 1972; United Nations, 1972).

The duration of exposure among affected U.S. uranium miners averages 15–20 yr; however, the cumulative dose responsible for tumorigenesis in any given individual cannot be estimated precisely, owing to the following sources of uncertainty: (1) The miners received their irradiation primarily from inhaling radon and its radioactive disintegration products present in the atmosphere of the mines in concentrations which were measured only infrequently within the 2500 mines in question. (2) The concentration of radioactivity in the air of a given mine varied from time to time and from one part of the mine to another, depending on operating conditions, ventilation, meteorological factors, the quality of the ore being extracted, and other variables. (3) The dose of radiation delivered by the radon and its radioactive decay products varied from one region of the respiratory tract to another, depending on the extent to which the radionuclides were adsorbed to aerosols, dust, or other particulates, and on the physiochemical properties of the inhaled atmosphere and any aerosols or particulates it may have contained. (4) The radiation dose received from a given level of total radioactivity—expressed in "working level" (WL) units or "working level months" (WLM)—varied, depending on the relative proportions of radon and its several radioactive decay products which were inhaled and subsequently cleared from the lung. (5) The dose of radiation delivered to the cancer-forming cells may be expected to have varied, depending on (a) the identity of the cells in question (which is uncertain, although such cells are generally presumed to be the basal cells of the bronchial epithelium), (b) the thickness of the bronchial epithelium and overlying mucous layers in different segments of the respiratory tract (which may vary in the presence of bronchitis or other inflammation), and (c) the rate of clearance of adsorbed radioactive particulates. (6) The fraction of the total dose that was responsible for tumor induction in a given miner cannot be distinguished from that part of his dose which he received after his tumor had been elicited and which was to that extent superfluous. (7) Most miners worked in more than one mine during their careers, often intermittently and irregularly, receiving a considerable fraction of their total cumulative radiation exposure in hard-rock mines other than uranium mines. (8) The radiation received by the miners consisted of a complex mixture of $\gamma$-rays, $\beta$-radiations, and $\alpha$-particles, the relative contributions of which cannot be assessed precisely, owing in part to uncertainty about the relative biological effectiveness of the $\alpha$-particles. (9) Most of the miners were cigarette smokers, necessitating correction for the known carcinogenic effects of smoking (Lundin *et al.*, 1969; National Academy of Sciences, 1972; United Nations, 1972), and the data have suggested that the combined effects of smoking and irradiation exceeded those to be expected from simple additivity of the effects of each factor alone (Lundin *et al.*, 1969).

### 4.1.4. Patients Exposed to Radiation for Medical Purposes

A number of patients exposed to large doses of radiation delivered therapeutically to various regions of the body have been evaluated for subsequent changes in cancer incidence. These populations include (1) patients given X-ray therapy to the mediastinum in infancy for enlargment of the thymus or other conditions, in whom an excess of thyroid tumors, leukemias, osteochondromas, salivary gland tumors, and other neoplams in irradiated sites has been observed (Hempelmann, 1969; National Academy of Sciences, 1972); (2) patients given X-ray therapy to the spine for ankylosing spondylitis, in whom an excess of leukemias and tumors in certain irradiated sites (e.g., lung, bone, pharnx, pancreas, stomach) has been observed (Court Brown and Doll, 1957, 1965); (3) patients sterilized by pelvic X-irradiation for treatment of menorrhagia, in whom an excess of leukemias and gastrointestinal tumors has been observed (see Pochin, 1972; National Academy of Sciences, 1972); (4) patients treated with X-rays for various nonneoplastic disorders, in whom solid tumors (chiefly sarcomas) have been observed to arise subsequently at the site of irradiation Cade, 1957); (5) patients treated with phosphorus-32 for polycythemia vera, in whom an excess of leukemias has been observed (see Wald et al., 1962: National Academy of Sciences, 1972); (6) patients treated with radium-226 for ankylosing spondylitis or tuberculosis of the skeleton, in whom an excess of osteosarcomas and osteochondromas has been observed (Spiess and Mays, 1970); (7) patients given X-ray therapy to the mammary gland for postpartum mastitis, in whom an excess of carcinomas of the breast has been observed (National Academy of Sciences, 1972); (8) patients treated with iodine-131 for adenocarcinoma of the thyroid gland, in whom an excess of leukemias has been observed (Pochin, 1969); and (9) patients treated for various other conditions in whom an excess of malignancies has been observed (National Academy of Sciences, 1972; United Nations, 1972).

Certain groups of patients exposed to radiation for diagnostic examination have also revealed an excess of some types of cancer, e.g. (1) women subjected to repeated fluoroscopic examination of the lung in the treatment of pulmonary tuberculosis, who have been observed to show an excess of carcinoma of the breast (Mackenzie, 1965; Myrden and Hiltz, 1969); (2) children exposed prenatally in the diagnosic examination of their mothers, who have been found to show an excess incidence of leukemia and other childhood malignancies (Stewart et al., 1958; MacMahon and Hutchison, 1964; National Academy of Sciences, 1972); (3) patients injected intravascularly with thorium oxide (thorotrast) for angiographic examination, who have shown an increased incidence of leukemia, hemangioendotheliomas of the liver, and certain other tumors (de Silva Horta et al., 1965); and (4) patients examined radiographically for various other conditions (National Academy of Sciences, 1972).

### 4.1.5. Japanese Atomic Bomb Survivors

The incidence of leukemia in Japanese atomic bomb survivors appeared to become elevated within 5 yr after irradiation and to remain elevated to a lesser degree 25 yr later (Ishimaru *et al.*, 1971; National Academy of Sciences, 1972; 395

PHYSICAL
CAR-
CINOGENESIS:
RADIATION—
HISTORY AND
SOURCES United Nations, 1972). As in other irradiated human populations, the leukemias included all types except the chronic lymphocytic type (National Academy of Sciences, 1972). The data for Hiroshima implied a linear dose–incidence relationship, whereas the data for Nagasaki implied a sigmoid dose–incidence relationship, differences which are consistent with experiments on leukemia induction in mice, in view of the differences in the relative proportions of fast neutrons and $\gamma$-rays received in the two cities, fast neutrons predominating at Hiroshima but making a negligible contribution to the dose in Nagasaki (National Academy of Sciences, 1972).

The incidence of malignancies other than leukemia became elevated in the survivors after a latency substantially longer than the latency for leukemias (National Academy of Sciences, 1972). The neoplasms appearing in excess include thyroid carcinomas, carcinomas of the breast, bronchial carcinomas, and tumors of gastrointestinal organs (National Academy of Sciences, 1972).

Dose–induction data, although preliminary, imply that susceptibility to the induction of cancer was higher in children than in those who were irradiated as adults (Jablon and Kato, 1970; National Academy of Sciences, 1972).

### 4.1.6. Marshallese Exposed to Fallout

Among natives of the Marshall Islands who were accidentally exposed to nuclear fallout from a weapon test in 1954, the incidence of thyroid nodules increased from zero to more than 80% between 8 and 16 yr after exposure in those who were heavily irradiated at less than 10 yr of age (Conard *et al.*, 1970). In some victims, the development of tumors was associated with hypothyroidism. The dose to the thyroid in such cases was estimated to approximate 700–1400 rads from internally deposited radioiodine and 175 rads from external $\gamma$-rays. Less than 10% of persons exposed at ages older than 10 yr developed tumors, and no tumors were observed in unexposed controls.

### 4.2. Observations in Experimental Animals

Within less than a decade after the first observations of radiation-induced cancer in humans, studies on the experimental induction of tumors in laboratory animals were reported (Table 2). Since then, neoplasms of virtually every type have been induced experimentally. The early literature on the subject has been reviewed by Lacassagne (1945a,b), Brues (1951), and Furth and Lorenz (1954). More recent reviews have been published by Casarett (1965), Upton (1967), and the United Nations (1972).

From experimental studies on radiation carcinogenesis, the following conclusions can be made: (1) Neoplasms of virtually any type can be induced, given appropriate conditions of irradiation and animals of suitable susceptibility. (2) Irradiation may influence the pathogenesis of neoplasia through a variety of

TABLE 2

Early Experiments on Radiation Carcinogenesis

| Author | Date | Radiation or isotope | Species | Type of tumor |
|---|---|---|---|---|
| Marie et al. | 1910 | X-ray | Rat | Sarcoma, spindle-celled |
| Marie et al. | 1912 | X-ray | Rat | Sarcoma, spindle-celled |
| Lazarus-Barlow | 1918 | Ra | Mouse, rat | Carcinoma of skin |
| Bloch | 1923 | X-ray | Rabbit | Carcinoma |
| Bloch | 1924 | X-ray | Rabbit | Carcinoma |
| Goebel and Gérard | 1925 | X-ray | Guinea pig | Sarcoma, polymorphous |
| Daels | 1925 | Ra | Mouse, rat | Sarcoma, spindle-celled |
| Jonkhoff | 1927 | X-ray | Mouse | Carcinoma-sarcoma |
| Lacassagne and Vinzent | 1929 | Ra | Rabbit | Fibrosarcoma, osteosarcoma, rhabdomyosarcoma |
| Schürch | 1930 | X-ray | Rabbit | Carcinoma |
| Daels and Biltris | 1931 | Ra | Rat | Sarcoma of cranium, kidney, spleen |
| Daels and Biltris | 1931 | Ra | Guinea pig | Sarcoma of cranium, kidney, spleen |
| Daels and Biltris | 1937 | Ra | Chicken | Carcinoma of biliary tract, osteosarcoma |
| Schürch and Uehlinger | 1931 | Ra | Rabbit | Sarcoma of bone, liver, spleen |
| Uehlinger and Schürch | 1935–1947 | Ra, Ms-Th | Rabbit | Sarcoma of bone, liver, spleen |
| Sabin et al. | 1932 | Ra, Ms-Th | Rabbit | Osteosarcoma |
| Lacassagne | 1933 | X-ray | Rabbit | Sarcoma, spindle-celled, myxosarcoma |
| Petrov and Krotkina | 1933 | Ra | Guinea pig | Carcinoma of biliary tract |
| Sedginidse | 1933 | X-ray | Mouse | Carcinoma, spindle-celled |
| Ludin | 1934 | X-ray | Rabbit | Chondrosarcoma |

From Lacassagne (1945a,b), Furth and Lorenz (1954), and Upton (1968).

changes, some of which involve direct effects on the tumor-forming cells themselves, and others indirect effects on distant cells or organs (Cole and Nowell,
1965; Upton, 1967). (3) In certain experimentally induced neoplasms, oncogenic
viruses may be implicated, but the nature of their role and their general
significance for radiation carcinogenesis remain to be disclosed (Upton, 1967;
United Nations, 1972). (4) The dose–effect relation for carcinogenesis is not
precisely known for any neoplasm over a wide range of dose, dose rate, and linear
energy transfer (LET); however, radiations of higher LET, such as $\alpha$-particles and
fast neutrons, are generally more effective than radiations of low LET, such as
X-rays and $\gamma$-rays, and their effectiveness is less dependent on dose and dose rate
(Upton, 1967; United Nations, 1972). (5) The process of neoplasia involves a
series of alterations, some of which may precede conception and any of which may
conceivably be caused by radiation; hence the dose required for inducing cancer
in a given individual may be postulated to depend on the extent to which
mechanisms other than radiation contribute to the process. (6) The
dose–incidence relation in experimental animals is generally curvilinear, with the
following features: (a) in the high dose region, the incidence tends to reach a
plateau or to decline with increasing dose, presumably because of excessive injury
(Upton, 1967; United Nations, 1972); (b) in the intermediate dose region, the
incidence tends to rise more steeply with increasing dose than at lower or higher
dose levels; (c) with decreasing dose and dose rate, the curve tends to become
shallower, at least in the case of low-LET radiation.

From the foregoing, the cancer biologist is tempted to infer that at low dose
levels (1) "initiating" effects of radiation predominate, which are to some extent
reversible in incipient stages; (2) these effects may be magnified by other types of
effects ("enhancing," "promoting," etc.) at intermediate dose levels; and (3) both
types of carcinogenic effects fail to be expressed fully at high dose levels, because
of side-effects or excessive injury.

## 5. Evolution of Radiation Protection Standards

Although it was recognized within months after Roentgen's discovery of the X-ray
in 1895 that this form of radiation could cause serious injury to the skin and
deeper tissues (Table 3), the first organized efforts to promote radiation safety
standards were those of the Roentgen Society in 1916 (Morgan, 1967).

In 1921, the newly formed British X-Ray and Radium Protection Committee
considered establishing a maximum tolerance dose, to be defined in terms of a
reproducible biological standard and to be expressed insofar as possible in
physical units (Stone, 1959). In 1928, the International Committee on Radiological Protection (ICRP) was established, and 1 yr later the Advisory Committee on
X-Ray and Radium Protection was formed in the United States, under the
sponsorship of leading radiological organizations. In 1931, this committee
recommended a tolerance dose of 0.2 R/day (measured in air), which was
endorsed in 1934 by IRCP. Two years later, the United States committee reduced

397

PHYSICAL
CAR-
CINOGENESIS:
RADIATION—
HISTORY AND
SOURCES

TABLE 3

*Early Reports of Radiation Injury Following Discovery of X-Rays by Roentgen in 1895*

| Date | Type of injury | Reported by |
|------|----------------|-------------|
| 1896 | Dermatitis of hands | Grubbé |
| 1896 | Smarting of eyes | Edison |
| 1896 | Epilation | Daniel |
| 1897 | Constitutional symptoms | Walsh |
| 1899 | Degeneration of blood vessels | Gassman |
| 1902 | Cancer in X-ray ulcer | Frieben |
| 1903 | Bone growth inhibited | Perthes |
| 1903 | Sterilization produced | Albers-Schonberg |
| 1904 | Blood changes produced | Milchner and Mosse |
| 1906 | Bone marrow changes demonstrated | Warthin |
| 1911 | Leukemia in five radiation workers | Jagie |
| 1912 | Anemia in two X-ray workers | Bélére |

From Stone (1959).

its recommended tolerance level to 0.1 R/day, in order to conform more closely with the tolerance level in Europe, where the dose was customarily measured on the skin, thus including backscatter, rather than in air as was customary in the United States, and to compensate for the growing prevalence of 200-kv X-ray machines and the resulting increase in the percentage of the surface dose penetrating to deeper parts of the body (Stone, 1959).

Selection of the tolerance level of 0.1 R/day, as opposed to higher or lower levels, was based on study of the occupational exposures of people who had worked with radiation for many years without detectable injury. The number of such people was relatively small, however, and the estimation of their exposure levels highly uncertain. With the advent of nuclear fission, and expansion in the number of radiation workers, it became increasingly important to establish a more reliable tolerance dose, without unnecessarily restricting the development of atomic energy and allied fields. The ensuing stepwise reduction of the maximum permissible dose (Tables 4 and 5) occurred not because of newly documented evidence of injury at previous tolerance levels, but because new knowledge about the effects of low-level radiation implied a need for greater margins of safety.

The large-scale atmospheric testing of nuclear weapons in the 1950s caused growing concern about the hazards of radioactive fallout to the general public. As a result of this concern, a number of national and international groups were formed to consider the risks of low-level irradiation to the general population. In 1955, the United States National Academy of Sciences–National Research Council (NAS–NRC) established a Committee on the Biological Effects of Atomic Radiation, which made a thorough study of the hazards of radiation (see NAS–NRC, 1956, 1960). Similar studies were carried out by the Medical Research Council in England (1956, 1960), and by the United Nations Scientific Committee on the Effects of Atomic Radiation (see United Nations, 1958, 1962, 1964, 1966, 1969). In 1959, the U.S. Congress established the Federal Radiation Council (FRC) (see Palmiter and Tompkins, 1965); this council, in contrast to the aforementioned

399
PHYSICAL
CAR-
CINOGENESIS:
RADIATION—
HISTORY AND
SOURCES

TABLE 4
*Some Historical Highlights in the Evolution of Radiation Protection Standards*

| | |
|---|---|
| 1902 | Rollins established photographic indication of "safe" intensity |
| 1921 | British X-Ray and Radium Protection Committee considered "establishing a maximum tolerance dose" |
| 1925 | First attempt was made by Mutscheller to define a "tolerance dose" |
| 1931 | U.S. Advisory Committee on X-Ray and Radium Protection recommended a dose limit of 0.2 R/day |
| 1936 | U.S. Advisory Committee on X-Ray and Radium Protection reduced dose limit to 0.1 R/day |
| 1950 | International Commission on Radiological Protection recommended a dose limit of 0.3 R/wk |
| | 1956    International Commission on Radiological Protection recommended an occupational dose limit of 5 R/yr |
| 1956 | National Academy of Sciences recommended 10 R/30 yr for gonadal dose limit of general population |
| 1960 | Federal Radiation Council Recommended 5 R/yr dose limit for radiation workers and 0.17 R/yr dose limit for general population, exclusive of natural background and medical radiation |

From Stone (1959) and Upton (1969).

TABLE 5
*Historical Sequence of Reductions in Maximum Permissible Doses for Radiation Workers*

| Exposure period | Maximum permissible doses (R) | | | |
|---|---|---|---|---|
| | 1931–1936 | 1936–1948 | 1948–1956 | 1956 |
| Per day | 0.2 | 0.1 | 0.05 | |
| Per 6-day week | 1.2 | 0.6 | 0.3 | 0.3 |
| Per 50-wk year | 60 | 15 | 15 | 5 |
| Per decade | 600 | 300 | 150 | 50 |
| Up to age 60 | 2400 | 1200 | 600 | 200 |

From Stone (1957).

groups which had no statutory authority, was mandated to advise the President on radiation matters affecting health. Although legislative responsibility for the regulation of radiation health remained with the states, the Federal Radiation Council was designated as the policy-forming body to advise in the recommendation of radiation standards for all federal agencies.

In its first report (1960), the Federal Radiation Council stated its philosophy about radiation protection policy as follows:

> There is a particular uncertainty with respect to the biological effects at very low doses and dose rates. It is not prudent, therefore, to assume that there is a level of radiation exposure below which there is absolute certainty that no effect may occur.
>
> This consideration, in addition to the adoption of the conservative hypothesis of a linear relation between biological effect and the amount of dose, determines our basic approach to the formulation of radiation protection guides.

Fundamentally, setting basic radiation protection standards involves passing judgment on the extent of the possible health hazards society is willing to accept in order to realize the known benefits of radiation.

There should not be any man-made radiation without the expectation of benefit resulting from such exposure.

The safety standards established by the Federal Radiation Council conformed with the recommendations of the ICRP and the NCRP in stipulating that occupational exposure of the whole body and the most radiosensitive organs of the body (the bone marrow, lens of the eye, and gonads) should not deliver a cumulative dose (in rems) exceeding 5 times the age of the worker (in years) beyond 18 (Table 6). A worker aged 28, for example, would be allowed a

TABLE 6
*Radiation Protection Guides*

| Type of exposure | Duration or condition of exposure | Maximum permissible dose (rems) |
|---|---|---|
| Exposure of radiation worker | | |
| Whole body, head and trunk, active blood-forming organs, gonads, or lens of eye | Accumulated dose | 5 times number of years beyond age 18 |
| | 13 wk | 3 |
| Skin of whole body and thyroid | Year | 30 |
| | 13 wk | 10 |
| Hands and forearms, feet and ankles | Year | 75 |
| | 13 wk | 25 |
| Bone | Body Burden | 0.1 μg of radium–226 or its biological equivalent |
| Other organs | Year | 15 |
| | 13 wk | 5 |
| Exposure of general population | | |
| Individual | Year | 0.5 (whole body) |
| Average | 30 yr | 5 (gonads) |

From FRC Report No. 1 (1960).

cumulative total dose of up to 50 rems. A larger dose was considered permissible to a part of the body, such as the thyroid or the skin, since it was presumed to entail less risk than exposure of the whole body or its more radiosensitive organs. The radiation guide for bone was based largely on accumulated knowledge of the effects of internally deposited radium. For the public as opposed to the radiation worker, the protection standards were more conservative, and exposure of the gonads was regarded as the most important consideration. An average gonad dose of only 5 rems per generation (or 30 yr) was specified as the maximum permissible limit because it was thought that this level, which amounted to roughly a doubling of the natural background radiation level, would affect the mutation

401

PHYSICAL CAR-
CINOGENESIS:
RADIATION—
HISTORY AND
SOURCES

rate only slightly and would not therefore involve serious genetic risk (see NAS–NRC, 1960; ICRP, 1966, United Nations, 1966).

Since publication of the first report of the Federal Radiation Council, epidemiological studies of irradiated populations have disclosed greater evidence of carcinogenic effects of irradiation at low dose levels than had been suspected. As a result of this new evidence, risk estimates imply the possibility that the risk of cancer associated with low-level radiation may be comparable in magnitude to the risk of genetic effects (NAS–NRC, 1972), i.e., that up to 1–2% of the natural cancer incidence may be attributable to background radiation (NAS–NRC, 1972). It is considered increasingly important, therefore, that the dose to the individual, as well as the average dose to the population, be kept as low as is practicable (NAS–NRC, 1972).

Since the average gonadal dose to the population from medical exposure nearly equals that from natural background (Table 1), growing attention is being given to limitation of the doses involved in medical and dental practice (NAS–NRC, 1972). Methods for reducing the dose to the patient from medical exposure include (1) reduction of the number of radiographs per patient with avoidance of all unnecessary exposure, (2) reduction of the duration and intensity of exposure per radiograph, (3) use of radiography in preference to fluoroscopy whenever possible, (4) reduction of field size to a minimum, (5) shielding of tissues outside the field to be examined, especially the gonads, (6) proper training of staff engaged in radiological examinations, and (7) proper calibration and optimal operation of radiological apparatus (IRCP, 1960).

# 6. References

AUB, J. C., EVANS, R. D., HEMPELMANN, L. H., AND MARTLAND, H. S., 1952, The late effects of internally-deposited radioactive materials in man, *Medicine* **31**(3):221–329.

BENER, P., 1969, Spectral intensity of natural ultraviolet radiation and its dependence on various parameters, in: *The Biologic Effects of Ultraviolet Radiation* (F. Urbach, ed.), pp. 351–358, Pergamon Press, New York.

BRUES, A. M., 1951, Carcinogenic effects of radiation, *Advan. Biol. Med. Phys.* **2**:171–191.

CADE, S., 1957, Radiation induced cancer in man, *Brit. J. Radiol.* **30**:393–402.

CASARETT, G. W., 1965, Experimental radiation carcinogenesis, *Prog. Exp. Tumor Res.* **7**:82.

COLE L. J., AND NOWELL, P. C., 1965, Radiation carcinogenesis: The Sequence of events, *Science* **150**:1782.

CONARD, R. A., DOBYNS, B. M., AND SUTOW, W. W., 1970, Thyroid neoplasia as a late effect of acute exposure to radioactive iodines in fallout, *JAMA* **214**:316–324.

CORRY, P. M., AND COLE, A., 1968, Radiation-induced double strand scission of the DNA mammalian metaphase chromosomes, *Radiation Res.* **36**:528–543.

COURT BROWN, W. M., AND DOLL, R., 1957, *Leukemia and Aplastic Anemia in Patients Irradiated for Ankylosing Spondylitis*, Medical Research Special Report Series, No. 295, H.M.S.O., London.

COURT BROWN, W. M., AND DOLL, R., 1965, Mortality from cancer and other causes after radiotherapy for ankylosing spondylitis, *Brit. Med. J.* **2**:1327–1332.

CRONKITE, E. P., MOLONEY, W., AND BOND, V. P., 1960, Radiation leukemogenesis, an analysis of the problem, *Am. J. Med.* **5**:673–682.

DE SILVA HORTA, J., ABBAT, J. D., CAYOLLA DA MOTTA, L. A. R. C., AND RORIZ, M. L., 1965, Malignancy and other late effects following administration of thorotrast, *Lancet* **2**:201.

EVANS, R. D., 1966, The effects of skeletally deposited alpha-ray emitters in man, *Brit. J. Radiol.* **39**:881–895.

FEDERAL RADIATION COUNCIL, 1960, *Report No. 1: Background Material for the Development of Radiation Protection Standards*, Government Printing Office, Washington, D.C.

FOX, B. W., AND LAJTHA, L. G., 1973, Radiation damage and repair, *Brit. Med. Bull.* **29**:16–22.

FRIEBEN, A., 1902, Demonstration lines cancroids des rechten Handrückens, das sich nach lang-dauernder Einwirkung von Röntgenstrahlen entwickelt hatte, *Fortschr. Geb. Röntgenstr.* **6**:106.

FRUTH, J., AND LORENZ, E., 1954, Carcinogenesis by ionizing radiations, in: *Radiation Biology*, Vol. 1 (A. Hollaender, ed.), pp. 1145–1201, McGraw-Hill, New York.

GLASSER, O., 1944, Radiation spectrum, in: *Medical Physics* (O. Glasser, ed.), p. 1969, Year Book Publishers, Chicago.

HEMPELMANN, L. H., 1969, Risk of thyroid neoplasms after irradiation in childhood, *Science* **160**:159–163.

HESSE, O., 1911, *Symptomalologie, Pathogenese und Therapie des Röntgenkarzinoms*, J. A. Barth, Leipzig.

HUTCHINSON, F., AND RAUTH, A. M., 1962, The characteristics of the energy loss of spectrum for fast electrons which are important in radiation biology, *Radiation Res.* **16**:598.

INTERNATIONAL COMMISSION ON RADIOLOGICAL PROTECTION, 1960, *Report of Committee III: Protection Against X-Rays up to Energies of 3 Mev and Beta- and Gamma-Rays from Sealed Sources*, Pergamon Press, New York.

INTERNATIONAL COMMISSION ON RADIOLOGICAL PROTECTION, 1966, The evaluation of risks from radiation, *Health Phys.* **12**:239–302.

INTERNATIONAL COMMISSION ON RADIOLOGICAL PROTECTION, 1969, *Publication 14: Radiosensitivity and Spatial Distribution of Dose*, Reports prepared by Two Task Groups of Committee 1 of the International Commission on Radiological Protection, Pergamon Press, New York.

ISHIMARU, T., HOSHIMO, T., ICHIMARU, M., OKADA, A., TOMIYASU, T., TSUCHIMOTO, T., AND YAMAMOTO, T., 1971, Leukemia in atomic bomb survivors, Hiroshima and Nagasaki, 1 October 1950–30 September, 1966, *Radiation Res.* **45**:216–233.

JABLON, S., AND KATO, H., 1970, Childhood cancer in relation to prenatal exposure to A-bomb radiation, *Lancet* **2**:1000–1003.

KANAZIR, D. T., 1969, Radiation-induced alterations in the structure of deoxyribonucleic acid and their biological consequences, in: *Progress in Nucleic Acid Research and Molecular Biology*, Vol. 9, pp. 117–122, Academic Press, New York.

LACASSAGNE, A., 1945a, Les cancers produits par les rayonnements corpusculaires; mécanisme présumable de la cancerisation par les rayons, in *Actualities Scientifiques et Industrielles*, No. 981, Hermann et Cie, Paris.

LACASSAGNE, A., 1945b, Les cancers produits par les rayonnements électromagnétiques, in *Actualités Scientifiques et Industrielles*, No. 975, Hermann et Cie, Paris.

LEHMAN, A. R., AND ORMEROD, M. G., 1970, The replication of DNA in murine lymphoma cells (L5178Y). 1. Rate of replication, *Biochim. Biophys. Acta* **204**:128–143.

LOONEY, W. B., 1958, Effects of radium in man, *Science* **127**:630–633.

LUNDIN, F. E., LLOYD, J. W., SMITH, E. M., ARCHER, V. E., AND HOLADAY, D. A., 1969, Mortality of uranium miners in relation to radiation exposure, hard rock mining, and cigarette smoking—1950 through September, 1967, *Health Phys.* **16**:571–578.

LUNDIN, F. E., JR., WAGONER, J. K., AND ARCHER, V. E., 1971, *Radon Daughter Exposure and Respiratory Cancer: Quantitative and Temporal Aspects*, NIOSH–HIEHS Joint Monograph No. 1, U.S. Public Health Service, Bethesda, Md.

MACKENZIE, I., 1965, Breast cancer following multiple fluoroscopies. *Brit. J. Cancer* **19**:1–8.

MACMAHON, B., AND HUTCHISON, G. B., 1964, Prenatal X-ray and childhood cancer: A review, *Acta Unio Int. Contra Cancrum* **20**:1172–1174.

MALLING, H. V., AND DE SERRES, E. J., 1969, Identification of the spectrums of X-ray-induced intragenic alterations at the molecular level in *Neurospora crassa*, *Jap. J. Genet.* **44**:61 (Suppl. 2).

MARINELLI, L. D., 1958, Radioactivity and the human skeleton, *Am. J. Roentgenol.* **80**:729–739.

MARTLAND, H. S., 1931, The occurrence of malignancy in radioactive persons: A general review of data gathered in the study of the radium dial painters, with special reference to the occurrence of osteogenic sarcoma and the interrelationship of certain blood diseases, *Am. J. Cancer* **15**:2435–2516.

MEDICAL RESEARCH COUNCIL, 1956, *The Hazards to Man of Nuclear and Allied Radiations*, H.M.S.O., London.

403

PHYSICAL
CAR-
CINOGENESIS:
RADIATION—
HISTORY AND
SOURCES

MEDICAL RESEARCH COUNCIL, 1960, *The Hazards to Man of Nuclear and Allied Radiations: A Second Report to the Medical Research Council*, H.M.S.O., London.

MOHS, T. B., 1952, Roentgen-ray cancer of the hands of dentists, *J. Am. Dent. Assoc.* **45:**160–164.

MORGAN, K. Z., 1967, History of damage and protection from ionizing radiation, in *Principles of Radiation Protection: A Textbook of Health Physics* (K. Z. Morgan and J. E. Turner, eds.), pp. 1–75, Wiley, New York.

MYRDEN, J. A., AND HILTZ, J. E., 1969, Breast cancer following multiple fluoroscopies during artificial pneumothorax treatment of pulmonary tuberculosis, *Canad. Med. Assoc. J.* **100:**1032–1034.

NATIONAL ACADEMY OF SCIENCES–NATIONAL RESEARCH COUNCIL, 1956, *The Biological Effects of Atomic Radiation: Summary Reports*, Washington, D.C.

NATIONAL ACADEMY OF SCIENCES–NATIONAL RESEARCH COUNCIL, 1960, *The Biological Effects of Atomic Radiation: Summary Reports*, Washington, D.C.

NATIONAL ACADEMY OF SCIENCES–NATIONAL RESEARCH COUNCIL, 1972, *The Effects on Populations of Exposure to Low Levels of Ionizing Radiation*, Report of the Advisory Committee on the Biological Effects of Ionizing Radiations, Washington, D.C.

PALMITER, C. C., AND TOMPKINS, P. C., 1965, Guides, standards, and regulations from the Federation Radiation Council point of view, *Health Phys.* **2:**865–868.

POCHIN, E. E., 1969, Long-term hazards of radioiodine treatment of thyroid cancer in: *Thyroid Cancer*, UICC Monograph Series, Vol. 12, pp. 293–304, Springer, Berlin.

POCHIN, E. E., 1972, Frequency of induction of malignancies in man by ionizing radiation, in: *Encyclopedia of Medical Radiology* (A. Zuppinger and O. Hug, eds.), pp. 341–355, Springer, Berlin.

SPIESS, H., AND MAYS, C. W., 1970, Bone cancers induced by 224 ra (Th X) in children and adults, *Health Phys.* **19:**713–720.

STAIR, R., 1969, Measurement of natural ultraviolet radiation: Historical and general introduction, in: *The Biologic Effects of Ultraviolet Radiation* (F. Urbach, ed.), pp. 377–390, Pergamon Press, New York.

STEWART, A., WEBB, J., AND HEWITT, D. A., 1958, A survey of childhood malignancies, *Brit. Med. J.* **1:**1495–1508.

STONE, R. S., 1957, Common sense in radiation protection applied to clinical practice, *Am. J. Roentgenol. Radium Ther. Nuclear Med.* **78:**993–999.

STONE, R. S., 1959, Maximum permissible exposure standards, in: *Protection in Diagnostic Radiology*, Rutgers University Press, New Brunswick, N.J.

UNITED NATIONS, 1958, *Report of the United Nations Scientific Committee on the Effects of Atomic Radiation*, General Assembly, Official Records: 13th Session, Suppl. No. 17 (A/3838), New York.

UNITED NATIONS, 1962, *Report of the United Nations Scientific Committee on the Effects of Atomic Radiation*, General Assembly, Official Records: 17th Session, Suppl. No. 16 (A/5216), New York.

UNITED NATIONS, 1964, *Report of the United Nations Scientific Committee on the Effects of Atomic Radiation*, General Assembly, Official Records: 19th Session Suppl. No. 14 (A/5814), New York.

UNITED NATIONS, 1966, *Report of the United Nations Scientific Committee on the Effects of Atomic Radiation*, General Assembly, Official Records: 21st Session, Suppl. No. 14 (A/6314), New York.

UNITED NATIONS, 1969, *Report of the United Nations Scientific Committee on the Effects of Atomic Radiation*, Official Records of the General Assembly, 24th Session, Suppl. No. 13 (A/7613), New York.

UNITED NATIONS, 1972, *Ionizing Radiation: Levels and Effects, A Report of the United Nations Scientific Committee on the Effects of Atomic Radiation*, General Assembly, Official Records: 27th Session, Suppl. No. 25 (A/8725), New York.

UPTON, A. C., 1967, Comparative observations on radiation carcinogenesis in man and animals, in: *Carcinogenesis: A Broad Critique* pp. 631–675, University of Texas, M. D. Anderson Hospital and Tumor Institute, Williams and Wilkins, Baltimore.

UPTON, A. C., 1968, Radiation carcinogenesis, in: *Methods in Cancer Research*, Vol. IV (H. Busch, ed.), pp. 53–82, Academic Press, New York.

VON JAGIE, N., SCWARZ, G., AND VON SIENBENROCK, L., 1911, Blutbefunde bei Rontgenologon, *Berl. Klin. Wschr.* **48:**1220–1222.

WALD, N., THOMA, G. E., JR., AND BROWN, G., 1962, Hematologic manifestations of radiation exposure in man, in: *Progress in Hematology*, Vol. 3, pp. 1–52, Grune and Stratton, New York.

WELLER, C. V., 1956, *Causal Factors in Cancer of the Lung*, pp. 43–47, Thomas, Springfield, Ill.

# Biophysical Aspects of Radiation Carcinogenesis

ALBRECHT M. KELLERER AND HARALD H. ROSSI

## 1. Introduction

Although radiation carcinogenesis was recognized some 75 years ago, we still know virtually nothing of the mechanisms involved. Because of its profoundly important theoretical and practical aspects, the phenomenon has been very extensively studied, but most of the information obtained has been of a phenomenological nature.

Between the two extremes of a purely descriptive treatment of a process and the detailed knowledge of the causal chain of events responsible for it can be intermediate levels of understanding. Sometimes these can be based on generally observed or otherwise deduced basic features of the process which permit the formulation of its kinetics. This in turn can furnish clues concerning its mechanism.

The application of radiation biophysics to the phenomenon of carcinogenesis has yielded some insights of this kind. Most of the arguments employed are stochastic, and in the following sections dealing with physics and theoretical radiobiology the influence of random factors is stressed. In a final section, the concepts developed in the previous sections are applied to two types of radiation carcinogenesis.

ALBRECHT M. KELLERER AND HARALD H. ROSSI ● Department of Radiology, Columbia University College of Physicians and Surgeons, New York, New York. This investigation was supported by Contract AT(11-1)-3243 from the United States Atomic Energy Commission and by Public Health Service Research Grant No. CA12536-03 from the National Cancer Institute.

406

ALBRECHT M.
KELLERER
AND
HARALD H.
ROSSI

Because of practical limitations, much of the information contained in the second section is condensed and simplified. General literature references have been provided for more exhaustive study.

## 2. Interaction of Radiation and Matter

### 2.1. Mechanisms

Radiation is termed "ionizing" when its interactions are so energetic that they remove electrons from the atoms that constitute the irradiated matter. In the case of many materials—including tissues—this leads to permanent changes which are produced with far greater efficiency than is obtained with radiations that merely induce electronic or molecular excitations.

In nearly all cases of practical interest, ionization occurs through the agency of electrically charged particles that may be high-speed electrons or nuclear constituents such as protons and α-particles. These are *directly ionizing radiations* that may originate in external or internal sources, or be generated inside the irradiated matter by *indirectly ionizing radiations*. The latter include high-frequency electromagnetic quanta (or photons) such as X- and γ-rays and electrically neutral particles such as neutrons.

Although the energies of ionizing particles can vary by an enormous factor which is at least $10^{20}$, the energies of principal practical importance range roughly from 0.1 to 10 MeV. In this energy interval, the range of directly ionizing particles is generally much less than the dimensions of the human body or even the dimensions of organs of small animals. Consequently, irradiation by directly ionizing particles arising from external sources is of limited significance, but it is important in the case of radioactive substances that are deposited within the irradiated tissues by physiological processes. Examples include location of ingested or injected radium in bone and concentrations of radioactive iodine isotopes in the thyroid. With a few exceptions (such as the presence of water containing tritium, the radioactive isotope of hydrogen), internal irradiations tend to be quite nonuniform. More or less uniform irradiation of organs of whole animals usually occurs when the more penetrating indirectly ionizing radiations are applied.

It may be useful to provide numerical indications of the degree of penetration of some of these radiations. Figure 1 depicts the mean free path, $\lambda$, and its inverse, the linear absorption coefficient, $\mu$, in water for protons and neutrons of energies between 10 keV and 10 MeV; $\mu$ is defined by the equation

$$N = N_0\, e^{-\mu d} \tag{1}$$

where $N_0$ is the number of incident particles and $N$ the number of particles that arrive at a depth $d$. The mean free path $\lambda$ is equal to $1/\mu$. When $d$ is equal to $1/\mu$, the fraction of particles that have not interacted is $e^{-1}$, which is approximately 0.37. For example, $\mu$ for 1 MeV photons is approximately 0.07/cm, which means that a

407
BIOPHYSICAL
ASPECTS OF
RADIATION
CAR-
CINOGENESIS

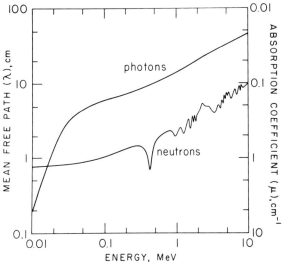

FIGURE 1. Mean free path, $\lambda(E)$, and absorption coefficient, $\mu(E)$, as a function of energy for photons and neutrons in water.

thickness of about 1/0.07 or approximately 14 cm of water will transmit 37% of incident 1 MeV photons without interactions.

It must be noted that these curves cannot be used to derive immediately energy deposition as a function of depth in irradiated material because in many instances the interactions lead to the production of secondary radiations which have appreciable penetration of their own, with the result that more energy arrives at any given depth than that merely carried by the primary radiation. In the case of photons, the three principal types of interaction reflected in Fig. 1 are the *photoelectric effect*, the *Compton effect*, and *pair* (and to some extent *triplet*) *production*. The first of these processes is of importance only at the low end of the energy scale and results in the ejection of a photoelectron and of fluorescent radiation, both of which are locally absorbed. Pair production, which occurs only at the upper end of the energy scale, results in the production of an electron–positron pair. Following the annihilation of the positron, about 1 MeV of the original photon energy appears as the shared energy of two new photons which have appreciable penetration. The main section of the photon curve in Fig. 1 is due to the Compton effect, in which varying fractions of the incident photon energy appear in the form of scattered photons, particularly near the low end of the energy scale.

In the case of neutrons, by far the most important reaction responsible for the shape of the curve in Fig. 1 is *elastic scattering* (principally by hydrogen), in which the neutron can retain a substantial fraction of its energy. Thus also in this case appreciable radiation energy can penetrate beyond the site where primary radiation has been absorbed.

In order to illustrate the far more restricted penetration of directly ionizing radiations, Fig. 2 shows the range of what are perhaps the two most important charged particles in radiobiology, the electron and the proton. In contrast to the indirectly ionizing radiations, which tend to be absorbed exponentially and cannot

408

ALBRECHT M.
KELLERER
AND
HARALD H.
ROSSI

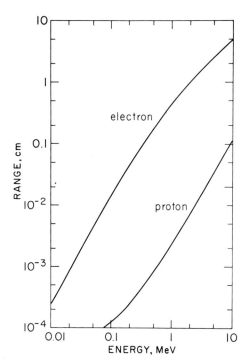

FIGURE 2. Range of electrons and protons in water as a function of energy (ICRU, 1970).

be characterized by a well-defined range of penetration, charged particles have as a rule a reasonably well-defined distance of penetration.

The principal process determining the range of charged particles is electronic collision. The electrons of atoms located in the vicinity of the particle trajectory are subject to electrical impulses that excite them, or eject them from their parent atom with varying energy. To a good first approximation, the interaction is proportional to the square of the charge of the incident particle and inversely proportional to the square of its velocity. Both the electron and the proton carry unit charge, but because of its far greater mass a proton moves much more slowly than an electron of equal energy. This results in a much higher rate of energy loss and consequently a much shorter range for the proton.

The rate of energy loss of charged particles is known as the *linear energy transfer* (LET), and it is usually specified in terms of kiloelectron-volts per micrometer in the medium of interest (usually water of tissue). Figure 3 shows the LET in water of electrons and protons as a function of the energy.

### 2.2. Dosimetry

The physical quantity which is of central importance in radiobiology is the *absorbed dose, D*, which is defined as

$$D = E/m \qquad (2)$$

where $E$ is the energy deposited in a volume element and $m$ is the mass contained

409
BIOPHYSICAL
ASPECTS OF
RADIATION
CAR-
CINOGENESIS

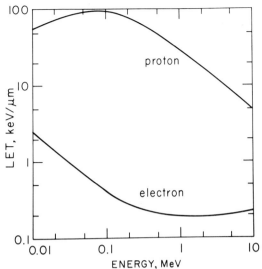

FIGURE 3. Linear energy transfer, LET, for electrons and protons in water as a function of energy (ICRU, 1970).

in the volume element. $E$ is proportional to the product of the number of charged particles traversing the element and to their LET.

In the case of indirectly ionizing radiation, the absorbed dose evidently depends on the fraction of the incident energy that is transformed into kinetic energy of charged particles. A useful quantity in this connection is the *kerma*, which is the kinetic energy of directly ionizing radiations released per unit mass in a specified material (here usually tissue). Figure 4 shows this quantity per unit fluence (number of indirectly ionizing particles per unit cross-sectional area) for electromagnetic radiation and neutrons. In irradiated matter, kerma and the absorbed dose frequently have nearly the same numerical value. Because of the short range of charged particles, the energy absorbed per unit mass at some point in the medium is nearly the same as the kinetic energy of the charged particles

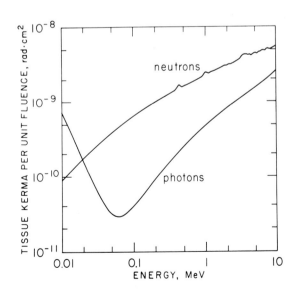

FIGURE 4. Tissue kerma per unit fluence for photons and neutrons as a function of energy. Based on Bach and Caswell (1968).

410

ALBRECHT M.
KELLERER
AND
HARALD H.
ROSSI

released. This is the condition known as *radiation equilibrium*. It does not exist when the absorption of indirectly ionizing radiations is comparable to that of the directly ionizing radiations or when one is near interfaces of different materials. For example, in the case of X-irradiation soft tissues in proximity to bone receive a higher dose than those more distant because of the more copious electron emission from the irradiated bone.

The unit generally employed for both absorbed dose and kerma is the *rad*, which represents an energy absorption of 100 ergs per gram of irradiated material. The reason for the magnitude of this unit is largely historical and relates to another quantity, the *exposure*, and its special unit, the *roentgen*. The exposure is a measure of X- and γ-radiations based on their ability to ionize air. Its exact definition is not necessary here, but it may be noted that in almost all cases of interest exposure of tissues to 1 roentgen results in an absorbed dose that is equal to 1 rad within less than 10%. It appears very likely that within a few years these units will be replaced by those of the International System of Units (SI), which has been adopted by virtually all nations. In this system, the appropriate unit for absorbed dose and kerma is the *joule per kilogram* (J/kg), which is equal to 100 rads.

Under well-defined conditions, doses can be measured and often also calculated within an accuracy of a few percent. However, in some instances, and in particular those relating to human carcinogenesis, doses must often be determined retrospectively on the basis of incomplete information. Under these conditions, major uncertainties arise.

## 2.3. Microdosimetry

Many radiobiological phenomena and probably at least one type of radiation carcinogenesis (see Section 5.1) are due to multicellular response to radiation injury. However, in all instances individual cells are injured randomly, and it is consequently the energy absorbed by individual cells that governs all radiobiological phenomena. It appears to be established that virtually all of the radiation sensitivity of the eukaryotic cell resides in its nucleus, and it is quite probable that the ultimate target is DNA. The biological effect of ionizing radiations is therefore determined by energy concentrations in domains of cellular dimensions.

As explained above, radiation energy is deposited by discrete, directly ionizing particles. Its concentration is therefore subject to statistical fluctuations. These fluctuations can be appreciable in small volumes for doses that are sufficiently large to produce marked biological effects. Consider, for example, a region with a diameter of 1 μm in tissue that receives an absorbed dose of 100 rads (1 J/kg). In the case of γ-rays, the mean number of electrons traversing this volume is near 10; in the case of fast neutrons, the frequency of particle traversals is only of the order of $\frac{1}{10}$. Any radiation effects are, of course, determined by the energy actually deposited, and it is plain that this can differ greatly from the *mean* or *expectation value* which is represented by the absorbed dose. In the example just quoted, there is no neutron secondary and therefore no energy deposition in nine out of ten cases, but in the remaining one the energy density is typically 10 times larger than might be expected on the basis of the absorbed dose. Such fluctuations are the principal subject of microdosimetry.

The central variable in microdosimetry is the *specific energy, z*, which is defined as

$$z = \Delta E / \Delta m \tag{3}$$

where $\Delta E$ is the energy actually deposited in the region of mass $\Delta m$.

Unlike the absorbed dose, the specific energy is a *stochastic* quantity which has a range of values in uniformly irradiated matter. The variability of $z$ is expressed by the distribution function $f(z)$, which represents the probability that the specific energy is equal to $z$. The width of this distribution depends on three factors:

1.  The volume containing $\Delta m$. Strictly speaking, this involves both the size and the shape of this volume, but as a rule shape is of secondary importance and it is usually assumed that the volume is at least approximately spherical and that it can therefore be characterized by its *diameter, d*.
2.  The absorbed dose.
3.  The LET of the charged particles traversing $\Delta m$.

The influence of these factors is illustrated in Figs. 5 and 6, which are logarithmic representations of $f(z)$ vs. $z$ for various absorbed doses of 5.7 MeV neutrons and $^{60}$Co-$\gamma$-rays for spheres having diameters of 0.5 or 12 $\mu$m. Neutrons of energy 5.7 MeV are somewhat more energetic and therefore slightly less densely ionizing than fission neutrons. The average LET is somewhat higher for natural $\alpha$-emitters and somewhat lower for more energetic neutrons. Electrons produced by $^{60}$Co-$\gamma$-rays exhibit minimal variance of energy deposition. In the case of X-rays, the statistical fluctuations are somewhat larger.

The curves in Figs. 5 and 6 have common characteristics. At high doses the number of particles is large, particularly for $\gamma$-radiation and the larger diameter. Consequently, statistical fluctuations are small and $z$ is unlikely to differ greatly from $D$. As the dose is reduced, fluctuations become greater because the number of particle traversals is correspondingly lessened. At low doses, a distribution is observed that has a shape largely independent of dose but has an amplitude proportional to dose. This occurs when the average number of events is less than 1. In this case, one is dealing with the energy-deposition spectrum generated by single particles (indicated by the broken lines in Figs. 5 and 6). A reduction of dose merely results in a decrease of the amplitude of the spectrum with the remainder of the distribution appearing at $z = 0$.

For any distribution, $f(z)$, the mean value of $z$ is defined by

$$\bar{z} = \int_0^\infty z f(z) \, dz \tag{4}$$

In Figs. 5 and 6, and at high doses, it is evident that $z$ is equal to $D$. Although the shape of the distribution for finite energy losses does not change with decreasing dose when only single events are of importance, the decreasing frequency of events and the corresponding increase of instances in which there is no event result in equality between $\bar{z}$ and $D$ at all doses.

ALBRECHT M.
KELLERER
AND
HARALD H.
ROSSI

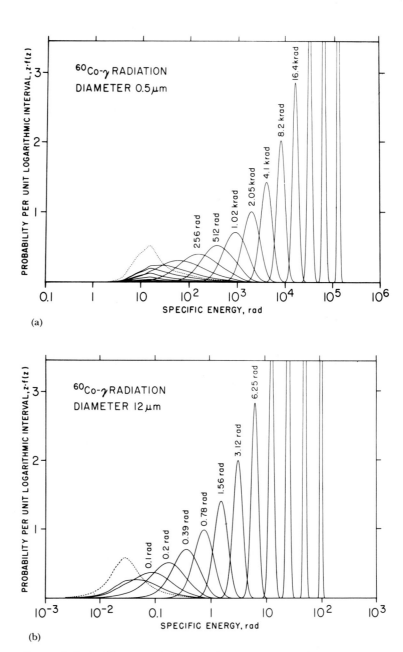

FIGURE 5. Probability per unit logarithmic interval of specific energy, z, at various doses of $^{60}$Co-γ-rays in a spherical tissue region of diameter (a) 0.5 μm and (b) 12 μm. The distributions of the increments of z produced in single events are given as broken lines.

413
BIOPHYSICAL
ASPECTS OF
RADIATION
CAR-
CINOGENESIS

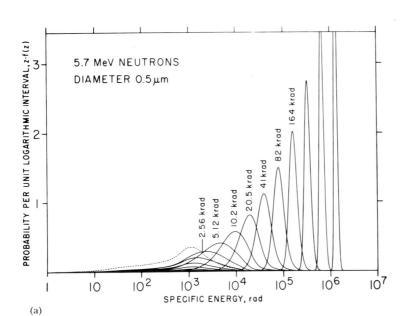

(a)

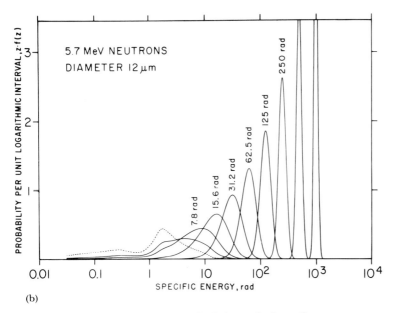

(b)

FIGURE 6. Probability per unit logarithmic interval of specific energy, z, at various doses of 5.7 MeV neutrons in a spherical tissue region of diameter (a) 0.5 μm and (b) 12 μm. The distributions of the increments z produced in single events are given as broken lines.

414

ALBRECHT M.
KELLERER
AND
HARALD H.
ROSSI

The biological effect of radiation on the cell must be due to deposition of energy in one or several sensitive sites. Consider one of these sites and assume that the probability of it being affected is $E(z)$. Any dose $D$ produces a corresponding distribution $f(z)$ and $E(D)$. The effect produced by this dose is given by

$$E(D) = \int_0^\infty E(z)f(z)\,dz \tag{5}$$

Comparison of equations (3) and (4) indicates that if

$$E(z) = kz \tag{6}$$

i.e., if the effect probability is proportional to $z$, then

$$E(D) = k\bar{z} = kD \tag{7}$$

Thus $\bar{z}$ and therefore also the absorbed dose are meaningful averages of specific energy provided that the effect probabilities are proportional to $z$. As will be seen in the next section, most if not all somatic radiation effects on higher organisms are characterized by a dependence which is not proportional to $z$ but rather to $z^2$. This statement applies in particular to the two instances where the induction of malignancies by ionizing radiation could be studied in adequate detail. This nonlinear dependence is the ultimate reason for the need to employ micro-dosimetry in the analysis of the primary steps in radiation carcinogenesis.

## 3. General Stochastic Considerations

### 3.1. The Linear Dose–Effect Relation at Small Doses

As has been pointed out in the preceding section, the absorbed dose determines only the mean value of the energy absorbed in a cell or in its sensitive nuclear region. The energy actually absorbed in microscopic volumes may widely deviate from this mean value. It has also been concluded in the preceding section that the statistical fluctuations in energy deposition play no role if the cellular damage is proportional to the specific energy, $z$; in this case, the average effect observed at a given absorbed dose is proportional to this absorbed dose.

In all effects on higher organisms, one finds, however, that densely ionizing radiations are more effective than sparsely ionizing radiations, such as X-rays or $\gamma$-rays. All commonly employed ionizing radiations work by the same primary physical processes, namely by electronic excitations and by ionizations. The unequal biological effectiveness of different types of ionizing radiations can therefore only be explained by the different spatial distribution of absorbed energy on a microscopic scale. Specifically, the increased biological effectiveness of densely ionizing radiations must be due to the high local concentration of absorbed energy in the tracks of heavy charged particles. Accordingly, one concludes that the dependence of cellular damage on specific energy, z, is steeper than linear. The actual form of the nonlinear dependence, $E(z)$, will be considered later. One can, however, draw certain important conclusions which follow from microdosimetry and are valid regardless of the actual form of $E(z)$. Such conclusions will be dealt with in the remainder of this section.

415

BIOPHYSICAL
ASPECTS OF
RADIATION
CAR-
CINOGENESIS

One general conclusion which follows from microdosimetry is that in the limit of small absorbed doses the average cellular effect is always proportional to dose. Such a linear relation between observed cellular effect and absorbed dose must be expected regardless of the dependence of cellular effect on specific energy; it is due to the fact that even at smallest doses finite amounts of energy are deposited in a cell when this cell is traversed by a charged particle. The energy deposited in such single events does not depend on the dose; accordingly, the effect in those cells which are traversed by a charged particle does not change with decreasing dose. The only change which occurs with decreasing absorbed dose is the decrease in the fraction of cells which are subject to an event of energy deposition. This can be treated quantitatively, and microdosimetry can furnish conclusions as to the range of absorbed doses in which the statement applies for different radiation qualities.

The effect probability, $E(D)$, at a given dose $D$ is equal to the sum of all products of the probabilities for various numbers, $v$, of events (charged particle traversals) in the sensitive sites and the effect probabilities, $E_v$, under the condition that $v$ events occur:

$$E(D) = \sum_{v=1}^{\infty} p_v E_v \qquad (8)$$

The equation is written in the form which does not include the spontaneous incidence, $E_0$; i.e., it is assumed that $E(D)$ is corrected for the spontaneous incidence and that the latter need therefore not be considered.

Because energy deposition events are by definition statistically independent, their number follows Poisson statistics; i.e., the probability, $p_v$, that exactly $v$ events occur is

$$p_v = e^{-\phi D} (\phi D)^v / v! \qquad (9)$$

The term $\phi D$ is the mean number of events per site. Event frequencies, $\phi$, for various radiation qualities and site sizes will be given below.

It will in the present context not be necessary to evaluate equation (8) in its complete form. Instead, it will be sufficient to consider the case of small event frequencies, $\phi D$, which occurs at small doses especially of densely ionizing radiations.

In order to evaluate the case where the number, $\phi D$, of events is small compared to 1, equation (9) can be expanded into a power series. Because it is assumed that $\phi D \ll 1$, the term $e^{-\phi D}$ can be set equal to 1, and with this simplification one obtains

$$E(D) = E_1 \phi D + E_2 (\phi D)^2 / 2 + \cdots \qquad (10)$$

416

ALBRECHT M.
KELLERER
AND
HARALD H.
ROSSI

$E_1$ is the probability for the effect if exactly one event has taken place; $E_2$ is the effect probability if two events have taken place. The probability $E_2$ will normally exceed $E_1$, but if $\phi D$ is sufficiently small the quadratic term and higher terms can be neglected in comparison with the linear term.

A possible objection to this conclusion is that $E_1$ may be zero, while $E_2$ is not zero; i.e., one could assume that the effect cannot be produced by a single charged particle, while it can be produced by two particles. However, this assumption is inconsistent with microdosimetric evidence. It has been found that for both sparsely ionizing and densely ionizing radiation there is a broad distribution of the increments of specific energy produced in single events. There is always a probability, although it may be small, that the same amount of energy deposited in two events can also be deposited in one event. One can therefore quite generally state that in the limiting case of small absorbed doses the cellular effect is proportional to dose. If, as pointed out above, the spontaneous incidence is eliminated by subtraction from the observed effect, one has the simple linear relation

$$E(D) = E_1\phi D \qquad \text{for } \phi D \ll 1 \qquad (11)$$

This relation implies that in the action of ionizing radiation on individual cells there is no threshold as far as absorbed dose is concerned. The probability $E_1$ may be small if one deals with sparsely ionizing radiation, but ultimately in the limiting case of very small absorbed doses the effect must be proportional to dose. It is important to realize that this is the case whether there is a threshold or no threshold in the dependence of the cellular effect on specific energy z. The absence of a threshold with regard to absorbed dose is merely due to the fact that even at the smallest doses some of the cells receive relatively large amounts of energy when they are traversed by a single charged particle.

The preceding considerations apply only to objects which are small enough that at the lowest doses of practical interest the number of absorption events is small. That this is the case for cells or subcellular units but not for multicellular organisms can be seen from the following example. The exposure to environmental radioactivity and to cosmic radiation leads to absorbed doses of the order of 100 mrad/yr. This background exposure corresponds to a large number of events for a multicellular organism. For man, several charged particle traversals occur per second. For a smaller animal, such as a mouse, a few events may occur per minute. For a single mammalian cell, however, only a few events per year will occur, and if one considers only the nucleus of the cell less than one event per year will take place. These are the frequencies which result mainly from sparsely ionizing radiations, such as the $\gamma$ component of the environmental radiation or the relativistic mesons from the cosmic radiation. If one were to consider the densely ionizing radiation, event frequencies would be considerably lower.

Table 1 gives event frequencies per rad for microscopic regions of various diameters and for different qualities. The largest region included in this table corresponds approximately to the size of a mammalian cell. Various radiobiological studies have shown that for most cellular effects only energy deposition within

TABLE 1
*Event Frequencies per rad in Spherical Tissue Regions Exposed to Different Radiations*

417

BIOPHYSICAL
ASPECTS OF
RADIATION
CAR-
CINOGENESIS

| Diameter of critical region $d\ (\mu m)$ | $^{60}$Co-$\gamma$-rays $\phi(\text{rad}^{-1})$ | Type of radiation | | |
|---|---|---|---|---|
| | | Neutrons, $\phi(\text{rad}^{-1})$ | | |
| | | 0.43 MeV | 5.7 MeV | 15 MeV |
| 12 | 20 | 0.55 | 0.51 | 0.61 |
| 5 | 3.6 | 0.042 | 0.086 | 0.11 |
| 2 | 0.58 | $3.9 \times 10^{-3}$ | $1.2 \times 10^{-2}$ | $1.6 \times 10^{-2}$ |
| 1 | 0.12 | $8 \times 10^{-4}$ | $3.2 \times 10^{-3}$ | $3.8 \times 10^{-3}$ |
| 0.5 | 0.017 | $2 \times 10^{-4}$ | $7.3 \times 10^{-4}$ | $9 \times 10^{-4}$ |

the cell nucleus is relevant; therefore, a region of 5 $\mu$m diameter, which corresponds approximately to the cell nucleus, is included in Table 1. In Section 4, evidence will be given that for most effects in eukaryotic cells the effective site diameter is somewhat less than the size of the nucleus; diameters of 1 $\mu$m and 2 $\mu$m are therefore also of interest.

One can generally state that the linear component in the dose–effect relation must be dominant whenever the event frequencies are substantially below 1 or, in other words, if the absorbed dose is considerably smaller than $1/\phi$. This defines the dose region in which proportionality between effect and absorbed dose can be assumed. For the whole cell, the value of $1/\phi$ is approximately 0.05 and 2 rads for $\gamma$-rays and 5.7 MeV neutrons, respectively. If one considers only the nucleus of the cell as the sensitive region, the values of $1/\phi$ are approximately 0.3 and 24 rads for these two radiation qualities. As mentioned earlier, a recent analysis (see Section 4) has shown that the actual sensitive sites in the cell are somewhat smaller than the cellular nucleus, and one deals therefore with even larger values of $1/\phi$. It is a very important result for all considerations regarding radiation protection that below fractions of a rad, and for densely ionizing radiations at considerably higher doses, a linear relation must hold if one deals with effects on individual cells. As pointed out, this is because even at the smallest doses appreciable amounts of energy are deposited in those cells which are subject to an event of energy deposition. The mean specific energy produced in a single event in the cell or in its sensitive site is equal to the reciprocal, $1/\phi$, of the event frequency; i.e., one deals with fractions of a rad in the nucleus of the cell for sparsely ionizing radiations and with tens of rads for densely ionizing radiations, such as neutrons. In Section 4, it will be shown that the effective event size produced in single events is even higher because the relevant average of the specific energy produced in single events is larger than the frequency average, which corresponds to the values of $\phi$.

## 3.2. Dose–Effect Relation and the Number of Absorption Events

The considerations in this section are of a more abstract nature and require a certain amount of mathematical formalism. The essential result which links the

418

ALBRECHT M.
KELLERER
AND
HARALD H.
ROSSI

logarithmic slope of the dose–effect relation with the number of absorption events in the cell can, however, be understood and applied without detailed knowledge of the mathematical derivation. This derivation is therefore given in the Appendix, and only the main conclusions are discussed in this section. A practical application of the result will be dealt with in Section 5. For the purpose of the present discussion, rigorous definitions of some of the quantities involved are necessary.

The considerations in the preceding subsection are valid regardless whether the effect, $E$, is considered as the probability for a quantal effect, i.e., an effect which either takes place or does not take place in the cell, or whether it is considered as the average value within the irradiated cellular population of a gradual effect. The following considerations will be restricted to the former case; i.e., only the occurrence or nonoccurrence of certain cellular effects will be considered. The coefficients $E(D)$, $E(z)$, and $E_v$ stand therefore for probabilities and can only take values between 0 and 1. Examples of such quantal effects, which include the survival of irradiated cells or the occurrence of certain cytogenic alterations, are of great practical importance in quantitative radiobiology. Another example is transformation of irradiated cells, which underlies carcinogenesis. This latter case will be further discussed in Section 5.

A clarification is also necessary concerning the concepts *sensitive site* and *gross sensitive region*. The concept of a sensitive site has frequently been invoked in biophysical models of radiation-induced cytogenetic alteration such as chromosome aberrations (e.g., see Lea, 1946; Wolf, 1954; Savage, 1970; however, it is not confined to radiation effects on chromosomal structure. In the next section, it will be shown that various effects on eukaryotic cells can be understood if one postulates sites which are somewhat smaller than the cell nucleus and which are affected with a probability dependent on the square of the energy actually deposited in these sites. In such considerations, it is not necessarily implied that the cell contains only one of these sites, and it is therefore useful to apply a concept which is somewhat more general. This is the concept of the so-called gross sensitive region (Rossi, 1964). The term is used to designate that part of the cell which contains all the sensitive structures or all the structures whose sensitivity has to be considered with regard to the experimental end point studied. The concept of a gross sensitive region is not necessarily equivalent to that of a sensitive site since a cell may contain several sites subject to damage produced by ionizing radiations; the gross sensitive region would then include all the different sensitive structures. In many practical cases, it will be a reasonable approximation to assume that the gross sensitive region of the cell is the cellular nucleus.

In the following, a slightly different term will be used: *critical region*. The reason for introducing yet another term is that it will be convenient in the following considerations to deal with a reference volume which contains all the sensitive structures of the cell but may be even larger than the gross sensitive region itself. The concept is useful, first, because it can be applied to a population of irradiated cells which are not all equal or are not all in the same stage of the generation cycle. In such an inhomogeneous population, the gross sensitive region and its size may vary from cell to cell; however, their critical region can be chosen in such a way that it is equal for all irradiated cells. Furthermore, it is convenient to obtain certain conservative estimates in the absence of precise knowledge concerning the gross sensitive region; this can be done by equating the critical region either with the cell nucleus or with the whole cell.

419

BIOPHYSICAL
ASPECTS OF
RADIATION
CAR-
CINOGENESIS

Another concept which has to be further explained is that of an *energy deposition event*, for brevity *event*. This is defined (ICRU, 1971) as energy deposition by a charged particle or by a charged particle together with its associated secondary particles in the region of interest. Two ionizing particles which pass the region are counted as separate events only if they are statistically independent. Usually, for example in the case of neutron irradiation, one can identify an absorption event with the appearance of a charged particle in the reference region.

These definitions are of interest in connection with an important theorem concerning the number of absorption events in the cell and the slope of the dose–effect curves in a logarithmic representation of effect probability as function of absorbed dose.

Assume that $c$ is the slope of the dose–effect relation in a logarithmic representation; then

$$c = \frac{d \ln E(D)}{d \ln D} \tag{12}$$

$E(D)$ stands for the effect probability at dose $D$; it is assumed that this probability is corrected for spontaneous incidence, which need therefore not be considered.

It can be shown, and the detailed derivation is given in the Appendix, that the slope $c$ is equal to the difference of the mean event number, $\bar{n}_E$, in the critical region of those cells which show the effect and the mean event number, $\bar{n}$, in the critical region of the cells throughout the exposed population regardless of whether they show the effect or not:

$$c = \bar{n}_E - \bar{n} \tag{13}$$

This equation holds at any value of absorbed dose. The relation remains valid if a critical region larger than the actual gross sensitive volume is considered. The sole condition is that energy deposition outside the critical region does not affect the cell. As pointed out above, it is often sufficient to identify the critical region with the nucleus of the cell. It is also important to note that biological variability, e.g., the variation of sensitivity throughout the cellular population, does not invalidate the result.

The theorem is fundamental for the application of microdosimetry to the analysis of dose–effect relations. If for certain values of the absorbed dose the effect probability $E(D)$ and the slope $c$ of the dose–effect curve in logarithmic representation are known, one can derive the minimum size of the critical structure. Although $\bar{n}_E$, the frequency of traversals in the affected cells may not be known, it is evident from equation (13) that it cannot be less than $c$. One can therefore ask how large the sensitive structure must be so that at the dose $D$ the cell is traversed by at least $c$ charged particles with a probability $E(D)$. The answer to

420

ALBRECHT M.
KELLERER
AND
HARALD H.
ROSSI

this question is given by microdosimetric data for various radiation qualities and for different sizes of the critical region. In this way, one can derive lower limits for the dimensions of the sensitive structures in the cell and for the interaction distances of elementary lesions in the cell.

Equation (13) contains as a limiting case a statement which is of significance to the analysis of dose–effect curves at smallest doses. The relation implies that in the region of small doses the slope $c$ of the effect curve in the logarithmic representation is equal to the order of the reaction kinetics which determines the effect. In the limit where the absorbed dose $D$ (and consequently $\bar{n}$) approaches 0, this fact may appear obvious. According to the considerations in the previous section, it is to be expected that at least in the case of radiation action on individual cells first-order kinetics apply at low doses; this corresponds to a value of $c = 1$ when $\bar{n} \ll 1$.

In connection with basic aspects of radiation carcinogenesis, it is of interest to determine whether $c$ can in fact be less than 1. The degree to which this can occur is limited by the fact that $\bar{n}_E$ cannot be less than 1 since the number of absorption events in affected cells must be at least 1. Consequently,

$$c \geq 1 - \phi D \qquad (14)$$

This inequality follows directly from the more general relation expressed in equation (13).

Studies performed by Vogel (1969) and by Shellabarger et al. (1973) on the induction of mammary tumors in Sprague-Dawley rats show a logarithmic slope $c$ of the dose–effect curve for neutrons in the range of very small doses which is considerably less than 1. This fact will be further discussed in Section 5 and it will be concluded that in these experiments the observed tumor frequencies in the irradiated animals cannot reflect the action of radiation on individual cells which give rise to the observed tumors without mutual interaction or interference.

## 4. The Quadratic Dependence of the Cellular Effect on Specific Energy

### 4.1. Dose–Effect Relations

It has been pointed out in the preceding sections that the dependence, $E(z)$, of the cellular effect on specific energy is not identical to the observed dependence, $E(D)$, of the cellular effect on absorbed dose. This would be the case only if the cellular damage was a linear function of specific energy. In the preceding section, general statements have been derived which are valid regardless of the actual form of the dependence of effect on specific energy. Particularly it has been pointed out that at very low doses the cellular effect must always be linearly related to absorbed dose. It has also been possible to derive a relation which connects the mean number of charged particles traversing the affected and unaffected cells with the slope of the dose–effect curve in the logarithmic representation. In the present section, the actual dependence of cellular effect on specific energy will be analyzed. It will be seen that dose–effect relations, as well as RBE–effect relations, for higher organisms point to a quadratic dependence of the primary cellular damage on specific energy.

As far as the production of two-break chromosome aberrations is concerned, a quadratic dependence of the yield of the observed effect on energy deposited in sensitive sites of the cell has been postulated as early as in the works of Sax (1938, 1941) and in numerous other studies, particularly those by Lea (1946). In this case, the quadratic dependence is merely due to the fact that two-break chromosome aberrations are assumed to result from the interaction of two "single breaks." The yield of single breaks is assumed to be proportional to energy absorbed in the cell, and the average number of single breaks per cell is therefore simply proportional to dose. Statistical fluctuations in energy deposition in the cell are, however, highly relevant if the probability for the production of a two-break aberration depends on the square of the concentration of single breaks in the cell. A two-break aberration can result from two single breaks which are produced in the same charged particle track, or it can result from the interaction of two single breaks produced by independent particle tracks. In the former case one expects a linear relation to absorbed dose, in the latter case one expects a quadratic dependence on absorbed dose. For densely ionizing radiations, such as neutrons or α-particles, the increments of specific energy produced in the critical sites of the cell are so large that the linear component is dominant. For sparsely ionizing radiations, such as X-rays or γ-rays, on the other hand, the ionization density in the charged particle tracks is so low that neighboring single breaks are usually produced by independent particle tracks. One must therefore expect the quadratic component to be dominant in the latter case. This characteristic difference between densely ionizing radiation and sparsely ionizing radiation has been borne out by experimental results.

While the quadratic dependence of the yield of the chromosome aberrations on absorbed dose is approximately valid for sparsely ionizing radiation, it must be concluded from microdosimetric data that at very small doses the dose-effect relation must be linear even for such radiations. Until recently, it has not been possible to assess the magnitude of this linear component because of limitations in the statistical accuracy of the experimental data. However, recent work performed in different laboratories (see Brewen et al., 1973; Schmid et al., 1973; Brenot et al., 1973 with X-rays and with fast electrons has indeed shown a linear relation at small doses of X-rays which turns into a quadratic dependence only at somewhat higher doses. These studies thus confirm the predictions made on general microdosimetric principles. As will be shown, the relative contributions of the linear and quadratic components can be accounted for on the basis of microdosimetric data. In the following, it will be seen that such considerations apply also to other radiation effects on eukaryotes. Furthermore, the quantitative relation of the site diameter, the radiation quality, and the ratio between linear and quadratic components of the cellular damage will be discussed.

Figure 7 represents as an example dose–effect relations for the yield of pink mutations in *Tradescantia* (Sparrow et al., 1972. Curves are given for 430 keV

422

ALBRECHT M.
KELLERER
AND
HARALD H.
ROSSI

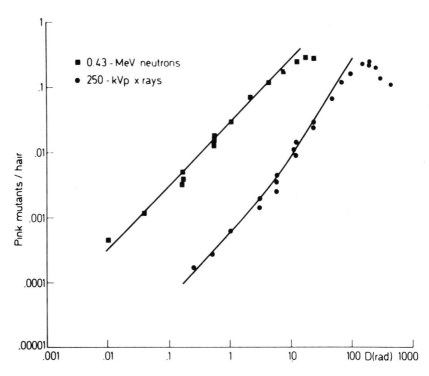

FIGURE 7. Induction of pink mutant cells in the stamen hairs of *Tradescantia* by X-rays and 430 keV neutrons (Sparrow *et al.*, 1972). The spontaneous incidence is subtracted from the observed values.

neutrons and for X-rays. For the purpose of the present discussion, the saturation and the ultimate decline of the yield in the range of higher doses will not be considered. This latter effect may be connected to cell killing, but as a recent study on the transformation of cells *in vitro* (Borek and Hall, 1973) has indicated it may involve a complex interrelation between the observed cellular alterations and cell killing.

It should be pointed out that a logarithmic representation has been used for these curves in order to represent the experimental data in the range of low doses and small observed yields of mutations with sufficient accuracy. The logarithmic representation has the further advantage that proportionality of the effect to a power, $n$, of the absorbed dose expresses itself in the slope, $n$, of the effect curve. In their initial parts, both the curve for neutrons and the curve for X-rays have the slope 1; i.e., effect and absorbed dose are proportional in both cases. The slope of the X-ray curve approaches the value 2 at somewhat higher doses, and the observations are therefore consistent with the statement that in an intermediate dose range the yield of mutations produced by X-rays is proportional to the square of absorbed dose. The accuracy with which the linear component in the dose–effect curve for X-rays has been established in this experiment is due to the fact that this particular experimental system permits the scoring of extremely large numbers of irradiated cells in the stamen hairs of *Tradescantia*.

While the example given in Fig. 7 supports the general conclusions drawn from microdosimetric considerations, it remains to be seen whether these results are also quantitatively in agreement with predictions based on microdosimetry. For this reason, the quadratic dependency of cellular damage on specific energy and the resulting dose–effect relation will be analyzed in detail.

If one assumes that the degree of cellular damage or the probability for a certain effect in the cell is proportional to the square of specific energy:

$$E(z) = kz^2 \tag{15}$$

then the average effect observed at a certain absorbed dose is obtained by averaging the square of the specific energy in the sensitive sites of the cells over its distribution throughout the irradiated population:

$$E(D) = k \int_0^\infty z^2 f(z) \, dz \tag{16}$$

It can be shown, and the mathematical details have been given elsewhere (Kellerer and Rossi, 1972) that the integral in equation (16) has a simple solution. One finds that this integral, which is the expectation value of $z^2$, is equal to the square of the absorbed dose plus the product of absorbed dose and the energy average, $\zeta$, of the increments of specific energy produced in single events in the site:

$$\overline{z^2} = \int_0^\infty z^2 f(z) \, dz = \zeta D + D^2 \tag{17}$$

Accordingly, one has

$$E(D) = k(\zeta D + D^2) \tag{18}$$

The ratio of the linear component to the quadratic component is therefore equal to the ratio $\zeta/D$ of the characteristic increment $\zeta$ of specific energy to the absorbed dose. If the absorbed dose $D$ is smaller than $\zeta$, the linear component dominates; if the absorbed dose is larger than $\zeta$, the quadratic component dominates; if the absorbed dose is equal to $\zeta$, both components are equal. The value of $\zeta$ is determined by the size of the site and by the type of the ionizing radiation. It is largest for smallest site diameters, and it is considerably larger for densely ionizing radiation than for sparsely ionizing radiation, such as $\gamma$-rays or X-rays.

Figure 8 represents the value of $\zeta$ for different radiation qualities as a function of the diameter of the reference volume. These values are obtained from experimental microdosimetric determinations as well as from theoretical calculations. In the example represented in Fig. 7, one finds that for X-rays the linear component is equal to the quadratic component at a dose of approximately 10 rads. According to Fig. 8, the value of 10 rads for $\zeta$ corresponds to a site diameter of approximately 2 $\mu$m. According to the microdosimetric determinations, the quantity $\zeta$ for neutrons should be approximately 35 times larger than for X-rays, and this is indeed borne out in Fig. 7, where the initial part of the neutron curve is

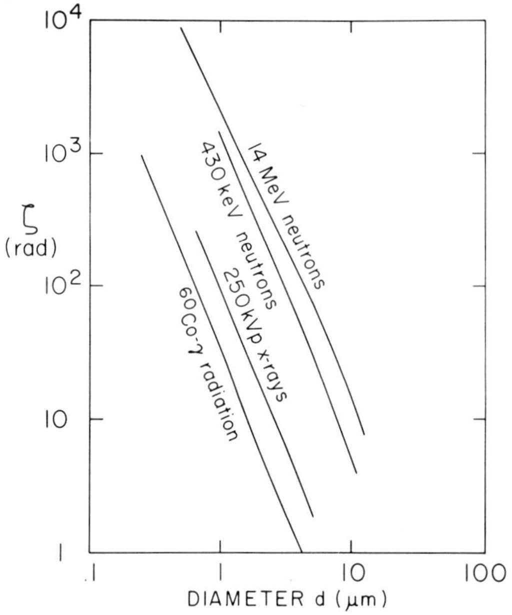

ALBRECHT M.
KELLERER
AND
HARALD H.
ROSSI

FIGURE 8. Energy mean, $\zeta$, of the specific energy produced in single events by different radiation qualities in spherical tissue regions of diameter $d$.

shifted vertically by about this factor with regard to the initial part of the X-ray curve.

The analysis of dose–effect relations for two-break chromosome aberrations (Kellerer and Rossi, 1972; Schmid et al., 1973; Brenot et al., 1973) has led to somewhat larger values of $\zeta$, namely to values which correspond to site diameters of approximately 1 $\mu$m.

Survival curves for mammalian cells in vitro can to a good approximation be represented by an exponential which contains a linear and a quadratic term in dose:

$$S(D) = S_0 \, e^{-k\,(\zeta D + D^2)} \tag{19}$$

where $S(D)$ is the survival at dose $D$ and $S_0$ is the survival at zero dose. If one uses this equation, which has earlier been invoked by Sinclair (1968), one obtains values which also correspond to site diameters of 1 to several micrometers for cells in $S$ phase. For cells in $G_1$ and $G_2$ and in mitosis, the initial linear component is more pronounced and the values of $\zeta$ correspond therefore to smaller site diameters of only a fraction of a micrometer. Whether this latter observation corresponds to a more condensed state of the DNA in these stages of the generation cycle of the cell (see observations of Dewey et al., 1972, and earlier results by Cole, 1967) or whether the initial linear component in the survival curve is partly due to a type of cellular damage which is linearly related to specific energy in the sensitive sites of the cell remains an open question.

One concludes that in certain cases, and in particular in such cases as cytogenetic effects where the observed experimental end point is closely related to the primary damage in the cell, the quadratic dependence of cellular damage on specific energy can be directly inferred from the dose–effect relations. In other cases, the situation is more complicated. Particularly this is the case for effects on the tissue level, where the interaction of damaged cells may play a role. Such cases are complicated also because the scale used to measure the effect may often be arbitrary. There are, for example, many ways in which the degree of lens opacification after exposure of the eye to ionizing radiation can be measured. Similar complications arise if in a system, such as the Sprague-Dawley rat, mammary tumors occur with high spontaneous rate so that their incidence is merely accelerated after exposure of the animals to ionizing radiations. In all such cases, the numerical form of dose–effect curves has little absolute meaning. One can, however, assume that complicating factors such as the interaction of damaged cells or the arbitrary construction of the effect scale cancel if one considers equal effects of different radiation qualities.

The relative biological effectiveness (RBE) of radiation B relative to radiation A is defined as the ratio $D_A/D_B$ of the respective absorbed doses for equal effect. It may be expected that this ratio of physical quantities is a measure of the effectiveness of energy distribution on the cellular or subcellular level only.

## 4.2. Dose–RBE Relations

The preceding considerations have indicated that the dose–effect relation is an expression of the combined influences of primary cellular (or subcellular) lesions and their interactions. If, however, according to the considerations put forward at the end of the last section, only the primary cellular damage depends on radiation quality, the value of the RBE is not determined by interaction processes between damaged cells. Equality of the observed effect for two different radiation qualities then implies equal levels of primary damage.

In the following, the example of neutrons and X-rays will be used, but the considerations are equally valid for any two types of radiation. If one assumes the quadratic dependence of cellular damage on specific energy, the condition for equal effectiveness of X-rays and neutrons is

$$k(\zeta_x D_x + D_x^2) = k(\zeta_n D_n + D_n^2) \tag{20}$$

Where $\zeta_x$ and $\zeta_n$ are the values of $\zeta$ for X-rays and neutrons, and $D_x$ and $D_n$ the absorbed doses for X-rays and neutrons. Since the relative biological effectiveness of neutrons relative to X-rays is defined as the ratio of the X-ray dose to the equivalent neutron dose:

$$RBE = D_x/D_n \tag{21}$$

one can express the RBE as function of either the X-ray dose or the neutron dose. In the following, the relative biological effectiveness of neutrons will be expressed as a function of the neutron dose. Inserting equation (21) into equation (20), one obtains

$$\zeta_x \cdot RBE \cdot D_n + RBE^2 \cdot D_n^2 = \zeta_n D_n + D_n^2 \tag{22}$$

426

ALBRECHT M.
KELLERER
AND
HARALD H.
ROSSI

or

$$RBE = \frac{2(\zeta_n + D_n)}{\zeta_x + [\zeta_x^2 + 4(\zeta_n + D_n)D_n]^{1/2}} \qquad (23)$$

It is easy to identify certain general characteristics of this dependence of RBE on dose. At very low doses, the linear components are dominant both for neutrons and for X-rays, and RBE must then have a constant value equal to the ratio $\zeta_n/\zeta_x$ of the values $\zeta$ for neutrons and for X-rays. This plateau of RBE corresponds to the region in the example of Fig. 7 where the initial part of the X-ray curve runs parallel to the neutron curve. In the range of intermediate doses, one can neglect the linear component for X-rays, while the linear component for neutrons is still dominant. In this case, the RBE of neutrons is inversely proportional to the square root of the neutron dose; in a logarithmic plot of RBE vs. neutron dose, one obtains curves of slope $-1/2$. At the high doses, finally, one should expect that RBE tends toward the value 1. It is, however, not easy to obtain meaningful biological data with neutrons at doses which are large enough that the linear component can be neglected.

The dose–RBE relation expected on the basis of a quadratic dependence of primary cellular damage on specific energy has been compared with the experimental observations for a wide spectrum of radiation effects on mammalian cells. Figure 9, together with Table 2, is a compilation of such results. One must draw the general conclusion that in the intermediate dose range in which the available data are most complete the observed dose–RBE relations are in agreement with the dependence theoretically predicted. In the example of the mutations in *Tradescantia*, it has been possible to find the plateau of the values of RBE at low doses, and this value agrees well with microdosimetric data. It is not surprising that relatively few data are available in the range of extremely small doses, because

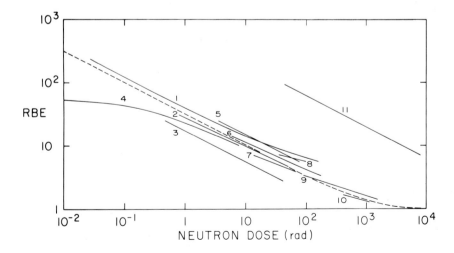

FIGURE 9. Relative biological effectiveness of neutrons as a function of absorbed dose of neutrons for various biological end points. The experimental curves belong to the cases listed in Table 2. The dotted line corresponds to equation (23) with $\zeta_x = 0$ and $\zeta_n = 1000$ rad.

**427**

BIOPHYSICAL
ASPECTS OF
RADIATION
CAR-
CINOGENESIS

TABLE 2

| Author and number of curve in Fig. 9 | | End point | Neutron energy | Estimate of $\zeta_n$(rad) | Diameter $d$ ($\mu$m) |
|---|---|---|---|---|---|
| Bateman *et al.* (1972) | 1 | Opacification of the murine lens | 430 keV | 150 | 3 |
| | 2 | Opacification of the murine lens | 1.8 MeV | 840 | 2 |
| | 3 | Opacification of the murine lens | 14 MeV | 260 | 3 |
| Sparrow *et al.* (1972) | 4 | Mutations of *Tradescantia* stamen hairs (blue to pink) | 430 keV | 800 | 1.8 |
| Vogel (1969) | 5 | Mammary neoplasm in the Sprague-Dawley rat | Fission | 2200 | 1 |
| Biola *et al.* (1971) | 6 | Chromosome aberrations in human lymphocytes | Fission | 1300 | 1.4 |
| Hall *et al.* (1973) | 7 | Growth reduction of *Vicia faba* root, aerated | 3.7 MeV | 600 | 2 |
| | 8 | Growth reduction of *Vicia faba* root, anoxic | 3.7 MeV | 2000 | 1.3 |
| Field (1969) | 9 | Skin damage (human, rat, mouse, pig) | 6 MeV | 1200 | 1.5 |
| Withers *et al.* (1970) | 10 | Inactivation of intestinal cryptic cells in the mouse | 14 MeV | 800 | 2 |
| Smith *et al.* (1968) | 11 | Various effects on seeds of *Zea mays* | Fission | 400,000 | 0.15 |

428

ALBRECHT M.
KELLERER
AND
HARALD H.
ROSSI

only few experimental systems permit the necessary statistical accuracy at small doses. It is however, remarkable that in two experimental systems, namely in the lens opacification studies and in the system for induction of mammary tumors in the rat, extremely high values of the RBE of neutrons have been found at low doses. These values exceed the predictions made on the basis of microdosimetric data, and they may be taken as evidence that, in addition to the quadratic dependence of the effect on energy concentration over regions of the order of magnitude of 1 to several micrometers diameter, one deals with a dependence of the effectiveness of ionizing radiation on the distribution of energy in regions of the order of only a few nanometers. Formally, this would correspond to a dependence of the coefficients $k$ in equation (18) on radiation quality.

The examples of the induction of mammary tumors by neutrons and X-rays and the study of leukemia incidence after neutron irradiation and exposure to $\gamma$-rays will be discussed in the next section. As an example of a dose–RBE relation which extends over an extremely wide range of doses, the studies on the opacification of the murine lens may be presented in detail. Figure 10 contains this relation together with its 95% confidence limits. One should note that the inverse relationship between the RBE of neutrons and the square root of the neutron dose extends over more than 4 orders of magnitude of the neutron dose in this example. These results obtained in a multicellular system are therefore in good agreement with the various other observations which support the assumption that the primary cellular damage is proportional to the square of the specific energy in sites whose diameter is of the order of 1 to several micrometers.

These observations formed the basis of what has been termed the theory of dual radiation action, which is an interpretation in terms of the site concept or in terms of the interaction of pairs of cellular lesions with a characteristic interaction distance of the order of magnitude of micrometers. This is covered in an earlier

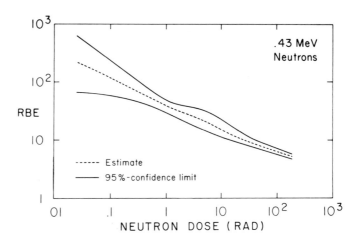

FIGURE 10. RBE of 430 keV neutrons relative to X-rays for the induction of lens opacification in the mouse (Bateman *et al.*, 1972; Kellerer and Brenot, 1973).

publication (Kellerer and Rossi, 1972). In the next section, the main conclusions of the preceding section will be applied to experimental findings relevant to the etiology of tumors.

## 5. Applications to Radiation Carcinogenesis

The subjects covered in the preceding sections of this chapter are of relatively recent origin. In particular, the theory of dual radiation action was developed only a few years ago. Practical applications are few in number, and the results tend to be notable more because of the proof they adduce for the theory than because of their disclosure of new facts. In each of the two instances where data relating to radiation carcinogenesis were analyzed, other useful results have nevertheless been obtained. In the case of an experimental animal tumor it could be deduced that the observed incidence depends not only on lesions in individual cells but also on radiation-induced changes in several cells or in tissues, and in an analysis of data on the induction of human leukemia conclusions were reached which are of importance to risk estimates.

### 5.1. Mammary Neoplasms in the Sprague-Dawley Rat

Bond *et al.* (1960) and Shellabarger *et al.* (1969, 1974) discovered that moderate doses of γ-radiation or X-rays produce a high incidence of mammary neoplasms in the Sprague-Dawley rat. The majority of the tumors are not malignant (fibroadenomas), but an appreciable proportion are adenocarcinomas. It was found that the incidence of these tumors is approximately proportional to γ- or X-ray dose up to a few hundred rad, where the incidence curve flattens and finally declines when doses in excess of 500 rad are applied. This is a phenomenon that is common in radiation carcinogenesis. It was also concluded that the effect is not abscopal—i.e., it requires irradiation of the tissue in which the neoplasms are to arise—and it was moreover demonstrated that the effect can be produced by *in vitro* irradiation of excised mammary tissue when it is subsequently grafted onto unirradiated animals. A related finding is that the incidence of multiple tumors follows Poisson statistics, supporting the view that the neoplasms arise independently from individual foci.

Vogel (1969), as well as Shellabarger *et al.* (1974), investigated the effectiveness of neutrons for this phenomenon and found it to be high in relation to that of γ-rays or X-rays, particularly at low levels of incidence. A number of comparatively large-scale experiments in which Shellabarger employed 0.43 MeV neutrons down to doses as low as about 0.1 rad yielded results of sufficient accuracy to permit the analysis shown in Fig. 11. This shows the dependence of RBE on neutron dose and the confidence limits of this dependence. The broken line indicates the best estimate of the dose–RBE relation. The vertical bars cover those ranges of RBE which can be excluded with statistical certainty exceeding 95%.

430

ALBRECHT M.
KELLERER
AND
HARALD H.
ROSSI

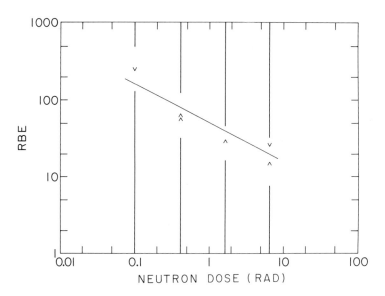

FIGURE 11. RBE of 430 keV neutrons relative to sparsely ionizing radiation for the induction of mammary tumors in the Sprague-Dawley rat (Shellabarger *et al.*, 1974). The vertical bars indicate the ranges of RBE values which are excluded with statistical significance exceeding 95%.

The statistical analysis is based on the direct comparison of the effect of each neutron dose applied in the experiment with that of each X-ray dose. Details of this procedure are described by Kellerer and Brenot (1973). Earlier results obtained by Bond *et al.* (1960) with $\gamma$-rays are also utilized in the analysis. As seen from Fig. 11, the slope of $-1/2$ postulated by the theory of dual radiation action applies for RBE values as high as 100, where the incidence approaches levels that are at the border of experimental detection.

It is one of the major assumptions of the theory that beginning with the production of elementary lesions the series of steps leading to the effect under observation is the same regardless of the radiation type involved. The validity of this assumption is difficult to assess. However, one necessary (although certainly not sufficient) condition is that the time course of incidence be the same. The curves in Figs. 12 and 13 represent the mean number of mammary tumors per animal as a function of time after exposure to neutrons and to X-rays. No systematic differences in the time course of incidence are suggested by these results. Except near the levels of spontaneous incidence, where the dependence appears to be somewhat steeper, the curves seem to be consistent with straight lines of slope 1. Since in these logarithmic plots the abscissa scale has been chosen twice as wide as the ordinate scale, straight lines of slope 1 would correspond to proportionality between the mean number of tumors and the square of the time after irradiation. Such a relation would be obtained if the tumor rate were constant during the interval of observation. Although further experimental studies and a detailed statistical analysis might lead to some modifications, one must conclude that at present there is no evidence of characteristic differences

431
BIOPHYSICAL
ASPECTS OF
RADIATION
CAR-
CINOGENESIS

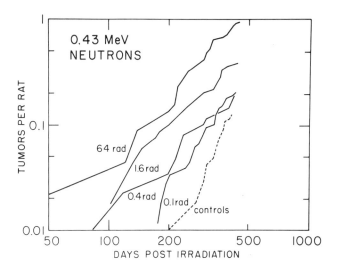

FIGURE 12. Mean number of mammary tumors in the Sprague-Dawley rat as function of time after exposure to different doses of 430 keV neutrons (Shellabarger *et al.*, 1974). The representation is logarithmic; the unit chosen for the abscissa scale is twice as wide as that for the ordinate.

between the neutron- and the X-ray-induced effects. This is further supported by the analysis of the relative frequency of different tumor types produced by the different radiations (Shellabarger *et al.*, 1973).

The information presented thus far corroborates the postulates of the theory. However, there is another aspect of the results that is of significance with regard to

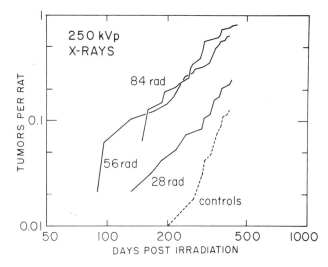

FIGURE 13. Mean number of mammary tumors in the Sprague-Dawley rat as function of time after exposure to different doses of 250 kVp X-rays (Shellabarger *et al.*, 1974). The representation is logarithmic; the unit chosen for the abscissa scale is twice as wide as that for the ordinate.

432

ALBRECHT M.
KELLERER
AND
HARALD H.
ROSSI

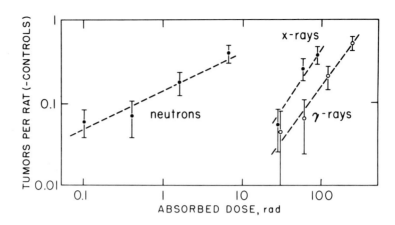

FIGURE 14. Mean number of tumors per rat minus spontaneous incidence 400 days after exposure to neutrons (Shellabarger *et al.*, 1973), to X-rays (Shellabarger *et al.*, 1974), and to γ-rays (Bond *et al.*, 1960). The broken lines have no mathematical significance and are merely inserted to indicate the trend of the data. The vertical bars represent the standard deviations.

the mechanism of tumor inductions. The RBE–dose relation shown in Fig. 11 puts certain constrictions on the dose–effect relations for both X-rays and neutrons, although it does not determine their shape. If dose–effect relations are plotted explicitly as in Fig. 14, it is at once apparent that in this logarithmic representation the slope of the line for neutrons is less than 1, indicating that tumor production is not proportional to dose. This has become especially indicative with the recent availability of the data at very low doses, although even when an earlier analysis (Rossi and Kellerer, 1972) was carried out it was already necessary to conclude that the nonproportionality extends to doses that are so low that multiple traversal of cells is improbable. As mentioned above, the average number of particles traversing a cell nucleus is of the order of 1 for a neutron dose of about 25 rad. The lowest dose used in these experiments was about 0.1 rad, where only one in about 240 cell nuclei experiences the traversal by a neutron secondary; i.e., where the mean number, $\bar{n}$, of events per nucleus is roughly 0.004. If one considers the whole cell, the mean number, $n$, of events at 0.1 rad of 430 keV neutrons is about 0.05. In Section 3.2, it has been concluded that in a logarithmic plot of the effect probability vs. dose the slope of the resulting curve can never be smaller than $1 - \bar{n}$, provided that the effect depends only on the lesions in individual cells. Because in the present experiments the slope is considerably less, one must conclude that the observed incidence depends not only on the transformation of individual cells but also on radiation-induced changes in adjacent cells or on dose-dependent changes at the tissue level. At this time, no further statement can be made, but one may consider factors such as virus release by lysed cells with some local saturation or with attendant increase in immune reactions even at low dose levels of the order of fractions of a rad.

*5.2. Radiation Leukemogenesis*

433

BIOPHYSICAL
ASPECTS OF
RADIATION
CAR-
CINOGENESIS

For man, the principal somatic hazard of ionizing radiation is carcinogenesis. Although it is now established that radiation can induce a variety of neoplasms in humans, the most frequently observed and the most extensively documented is leukemia. However, even in this disease the available information is insufficient to permit firm conclusions regarding the magnitude of the hazard, especially for doses near the maximum permitted by various recommendations, codes, or laws.

The most important source of information on radiation-induced leukemia is data obtained from studies on survivors of the Japanese cities bombed with nuclear weapons at the end of World War II. Not only are the populations involved far larger than those in other studies, but also special efforts have been made by the Atomic Bomb Casualty Commission to achieve maximum follow-up in order to select optimum control populations and to determine as accurately as possible the doses received by individuals.

Another important aspect of these observations is that they were obtained for two types of radiations. In Hiroshima, a substantial neutron dose was delivered which was primarily responsible for the biological effects observed. In Nagasaki, the relative neutron dose was very low and virtually negligible at greater distances from the epicenter of the explosion (Ishimaru *et al.*, 1971). Dosimetric information for both radiations has been derived for both cities. What is said to be the "dose" or "air dose" is actually the tissue kerma in free air (see Section 2). At any distance from the epicenter of the explosion, the free-air ratio of neutron kerma to $\gamma$-ray kerma must have been higher than the ratio of the respective absorbed doses in the blood-forming organs since the overlying body tissues attenuate neutrons more strongly than the prompt $\gamma$-radiation emitted by a burst. This necessitates a correction of perhaps a factor of 2 for the absolute value of the RBE but should have a minor effect on relative values.

The availability of data for both neutron and $\zeta$-radiations provides an opportunity to address the question of whether the dose dependence of RBE regularly found in other systems can be shown to apply also to human leukaemia. This is a question of importance to risk estimates, because a dose-dependent RBE makes it impossible that such estimates can be meaningfully carried out by linear extrapolation from high doses for *both* radiations since the shapes of their dose–effect curves must be different.

The establishment of the RBE–dose relation is difficult not only because of considerable statistical uncertainties but also because the neutrons at Hiroshima were accompanied by $\gamma$-radiation which in terms of kerma was from about 1.5 to 2.5 times as intense between the inner and the outer perimeters of the zone of interest in this analysis. Consequently, if it is assumed that all of the radiation at Hiroshima was neutrons and all the radiation at Nagasaki was $\gamma$-rays, one obtains an underestimate of the neutron RBE which becomes progressively larger at lower values of kerma. Accordingly, one observes less of an increase of RBE at low levels of effect than if one dealt either with a pure neutron radiation or with a constant mixture of neutrons and $\gamma$-rays.

434

ALBRECHT M.
KELLERER
AND
HARALD H.
ROSSI

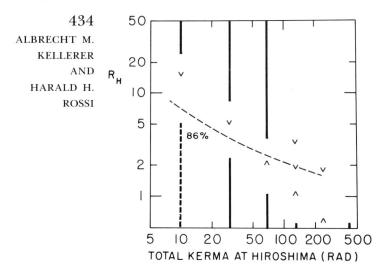

FIGURE 15. Relative biological effectiveness of the radiation in Hiroshima for the induction of leukemia compared to that in Nagasaki as a function of kerma in Hiroshima (Rossi and Kellerer, 1974). The bars indicate those values which can be excluded with 95% confidence; the broken bar stands for a level of confidence of 86%. The broken curve is the result of a least-squares fit.

If one nevertheless analyzes the data with this assumption utilizing the same technique discussed in the previous section, one obtains the relation depicted in Fig. 15.* Although the most crucial of the limits (the lower bound as 10 rad) is established with 86% rather than 95% significance, this value seems sufficiently large, particularly in view of the conservative assumption made. It may thus be concluded that the neutron RBE for human leukemia, like that for all other somatic effects investigated, increases with decreasing level of effect.

While this finding is of interest, it is of course even more desirable to determine the shapes of the dose–effect relations. In particular, the very important question arises of whether, as in the case of mammary neoplasms, the neutron dose–effect relation rises with a power of the dose that is less than 1 or whether the power is 1 or exceeds 1. Linear extrapolations would in the former case underestimate the neutron hazard but in the latter case overestimate the γ-ray hazard.

In order to gain information on this point, it was assumed that for both cities the dose–effect can be approximated by

$$I(K) = I_0 + aK + bK^2 \tag{24}$$

where $I$ is the incidence and $I_0$ its control level, $K$ is the total kerma, and $a$ and $b$ are constants. Utilizing a statistical treatment described elsewhere (Kellerer and Brenot, 1974), it was established that for Hiroshima the quadratic component has to be rejected and only a linear component need be assumed. For Nagasaki, the most probable value for $a$ turned out to be negative, and only the quadratic component was therefore considered in the further analysis. It thus appears that

---

* In this as well as in the other analysis, the information for the highest kerma level at Nagasaki and the two highest kerma levels at Hiroshima has been ignored. This has two reasons. One is that survivors in these categories must represent a highly selected and uncertain group because $LD_{50}$ levels are approached or even exceeded. The other reason is that, in accord with all other experience with radiation carcinogenesis, it must be expected that the dose–effect curve should at such high doses saturate or even decrease.

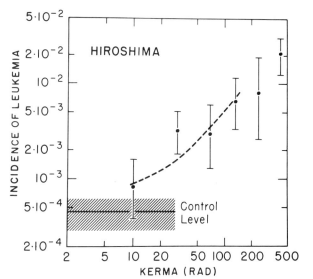

435

BIOPHYSICAL
ASPECTS OF
RADIATION
CAR-
CINOGENESIS

FIGURE 16. Incidence of leukemia for the period from October 1950 to September 1966 vs. kerma at Hiroshima (Rossi and Kellerer, 1974). The bars represent 95% confidence ranges; the shaded area is the 95% confidence region for the unirradiated population of the city. The broken curve is the result of a least-squares fit.

at Hiroshima, where the biological effect of the neutrons was dominant (because of their higher RBE), radiation induced leukemia at a rate proportional to kerma, while at Nagasaki, where neutrons could be all but neglected, the incidents increased with the square of kerma.

In a final step, a more accurate treatment was utilized by assuming that in both cities the incidence could be expressed by

$$I = I_0 + aK_N + bK_x^2 \qquad (25)$$

where $K_N$ and $K_x$ are the kermas of neutrons and X-rays and the parameters $I_0$, $a$, and $b$ are the same for both cities. The least-squares fit obtained on this basis is shown in Figs. 16 and 17 together with the observed incidences and their standard

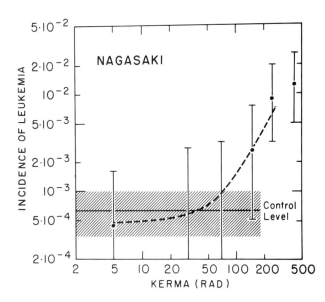

FIGURE 17. Incidence of leukemia for the period from October 1950 to September 1966 vs. kerma at Nagasaki (Rossi and Kellerer, 1974). The bars represent 95% confidence ranges; the shaded area is the 95% confidence region for the unirradiated population of the city. The broken curve is the result of a least-squares fit.

436

ALBRECHT M.
KELLERER
AND
HARALD H.
ROSSI

deviations. The resulting values of the estimated parameters are $I_0 = 4.8 \times 10^{-4}$, $a = 2.2 \times 10^{-4}$ (rad$^{-1}$), and $b = 8.7 \times 10^{-8}$ (rad$^{-2}$). The data are for leukemias of all types and relate to incidence within the observational period from October 1950 to September 1966. Because of the small numbers involved, a meaningful study of individual types seems impractical.

It is noteworthy that in the two types of carcinogenesis considered in this section the dose–effect relations turn out to be quite different. The question of whether this is because the experimental animal tumors have a high spontaneous incidence while the normal incidence of human leukemia is much lower is intriguing, but it cannot at this time be answered with any certainty.

## 6. Appendix

In the following, a formal derivation will be given of the theorem which is expressed in equation (13) of Section 3.2. As exemplified in Section 5.1, this theorem can be utilized to decide whether an observed dose–effect relation is compatible or incompatible with the assumption that the effect is due to independent alterations in individual cells.

Let $E_v$ be the probability of observing the effect in a cell after exactly $v$ energy deposition events have occurred. As pointed out earlier, an event is energy transfer to the critical region of the cell by a charged particle and/or its secondaries. The cells are assumed to belong to an irradiated population in which no interaction of cellular damage occurs; i.e., energy deposition in one cell does not influence the effect probability for another cell.

Energy deposition events are by definition statistically independent; their number is therefore distributed according to Poisson statistics. According to equation (8), the effect probability at dose $D$ is

$$E(D) = \sum_{v=1}^{\infty} p_v E_v = \sum_{v=1}^{\infty} e^{-\phi D}(\phi D)^v/v! E_v \tag{A1}$$

It is important to note that this equation holds even for an inhomogeneous population. The sole condition is that the critical regions for the individual cells are chosen to be of equal size. Without this condition, Poisson statistics would not apply. Since the critical regions can be larger than the sensitive sites of the cells or even than the cells themselves, the condition of equality of critical regions can always be met even for a population of unequal cells. It is furthermore essential to note that the coefficients $E_v$ do not depend on absorbed dose. This is the case because, by definition, energy deposition outside the critical region does not influence the fate of the cell; the effect is determined solely by the number of events taking place within the critical region and by the amount of energy imparted by these events.

The slope of the dose–effect relation in the logarithmic representation is

$$c = \frac{d \ln E}{d \ln D} = \frac{D}{E} \frac{dE}{dD} \tag{A2}$$

If one inserts equation (A1) into this expression, one obtains

437
BIOPHYSICAL
ASPECTS OF
RADIATION
CAR-
CINOGENESIS

$$c = \frac{D}{E(D)} \sum_{v=1}^{\infty} E_v \, e^{-\phi D} \left( \frac{(\phi D)^{v-1}}{(v-1)!} \phi - \phi \frac{(\phi D)^v}{v!} \right)$$

$$= \frac{\sum\limits_{v=1}^{\infty} E_v \, e^{-\phi D}[(\phi D)^v/v!](v - \phi D)}{\sum\limits_{v=1}^{\infty} E_v \, e^{-\phi D}[(\phi D)^v/v!]} \qquad (A3)$$

$$= \frac{\sum\limits_{v=1}^{\infty} v p_v E_v}{\sum\limits_{v=1}^{\infty} p_v E_v} - \phi D$$

The term

$$\pi_v = \frac{p_v E_v}{\sum\limits_{v=1}^{\infty} p_v E_v} \qquad (A4)$$

can be understood as a conditional probability, namely as the fraction of cells with exactly $v$ events among those cells which are affected. From equations (A3) and (A4),

$$c = \sum_{v=1}^{\infty} v \pi_v - \phi D \qquad (A5)$$

This form of the equation for the logarithmic slope of the dose–effect curves has a highly interesting interpretation. The sum $\sum_{v=1}^{\infty} v \pi_v$ is the mean number of events in those cells which show the effect; one can symbolize this mean value by $\bar{n}_E$. On the other hand, the mean number of absorption events throughout the cell population, regardless of whether the cells will show the effect or not, is equal to $\phi D$; this latter quantity can therefore be symbolized as $\bar{n}$. Thus the difference of the mean event numbers in those cells which show the effect and in the cells throughout the population is equal to the slope of the dose–effect curve in the logarithmic representation at the particular value of the absorbed dose which is considered. This is the theorem discussed in Sections 3 and 5:

$$c = \bar{n}_E - \bar{n} \qquad (A6)$$

A somewhat more general formulation of the relation can be found elsewhere (Kellerer and Hug, 1972).

## 7. References

BACH, R. L., AND CASWELL, R. S., 1968, Energy transfer to matter by neutron, *Radiation Res.* **35**:1–25.
BATEMAN, J. L., ROSSI, H. H., KELLERER, A. M., ROBINSON, C. V., AND BOND, V. P., 1972, Dose dependence of fast neutron RBE for lens opacification in mice, *Radiation Res.* **51**:381–390.
BIOLA, M. T., LeGO, R., DUCATEZ, G., AND BOURGUIGNON, M., 1971, *Formation de Chromosomes Dicentriques dans les Lymphocytes Humains Soumis in Vitro a un Flux de Rayonnement Mixte (Gamma, Neutrons)*, pp. 633–645, IAEA, Vienna.

438

ALBRECHT M.
KELLERER
AND
HARALD H.
ROSSI

BOND, V. P., CRONKITE, E. P., LIPPINCOTT, S. W., AND SHELLABARGER, C. J., 1960, Studies on radiation induced mammary gland neoplasia in the rat, *Radiation Res.* **12**:276–285.

BOREK, C., AND HALL, E. J., 1973, Transformation of mammalian cells *in vitro* by low doses of X-rays, *Nature (Lond.)* **244**:450–453.

BRENOT, J., CHEMTOB, M., CHMELEVSKY, D., FACHE, P., PARMENTIER, N., SOULIE, R., BIOLA, M. T., HAAG, J., LEGO, R., BOURGUIGNON, M., COURANT, D., DACHER, J., AND DUCATEZ, G., 1973, Aberrations chromosomiques et microdosimetrie, in: *Proceedings of the IV Symposium of Microdosimetry, Verbania, 1973*, Euratom, Brussels.

BREWEN, J. G., PRESTON, R. J., JONES, K. P., AND GOSSLEE, D. C., 1973, Genetic hazards of ionizing radiations: Cytogenetic extrapolations from mouse to man, *Mutation Res.* **17**:245–254.

COLE, A., 1967, Chromosome structure, in: *Theoretical and Experimental Biophysics*, Vol. I (A. Cole, ed.), Dekker, New York.

DEWEY, W. C., NOEL, J. S., AND DETTOR, C. M., 1972, Changes in radiosensitivity and dispension of chromatin during the cell cycle of synchronous Chinese hamster cells, *Radiation Res.* **52**:373–394.

FIELD, ST. B., 1969, The relative biological effectiveness of fast neutrons for mammalian tissues, *Radiology* **93**:915–920.

HALL, E. J., ROSSI, H. H., KELLERER, A. M., GOODMAN, L. J., AND MARINO, S., 1973, Radiobiological studies with monoenergetic neutrons, *Radiation Res.* **54**:431–443.

HUGHES, D. J., AND SCHWARTZ, R. B., 1958, *Neutron Cross Sections*, Brookhaven National Laboratory, Document 325, Government Printing Office, Washington, D.C.

ICRU, 1970, *Report 16: Linear Energy Transfer*, International Commission on Radiation Units and Measurements, Washington, D.C.

ICRU, 1971, *Report 19: Radiation Quantities and Units*, International Commission on Radiation Units and Measurements, Washington, D.C.

ISHIMARU, T., HOSHINO, T., ICHIMARU, M., OKADA, H., TOMIYASU, T., AND TSUCHIMOTO, T., 1971, Leukemia in atomic bomb survivors, Hiroshima and Nagasaki, 1 October 1950–30 September 1966, *Radiation Res.* **45**:216–233.

KELLERER, A. M., AND BRENOT, J., 1973, Nonparametric determination of modifying factors in radiation action, *Radiation Res.* **55**:28–39.

KELLERER, A. M., AND BRENOT, J., 1974, On the statistical evaluation of dose-response functions, *Rad. Environm. Biophys.* **11**:1–13.

KELLERER, A. M., AND HUG, O., 1972, Theory of dose–effect relations, in: *Encyclopedia of Medical Radiology*, Vol. II/3, 1–42, Springer, New York.

KELLERER, A. M., AND ROSSI, H. H., 1972, The theory of dual radiation action, in: *Current Topics in Radiation Research*, Vol. 8, pp. 85–158, North-Holland, Amsterdam.

LEA, D. E., 1946, *Actions of Radiations on Living Cells*, Cambridge University Press, Cambridge.

ROSSI, H. H., 1964, Correlation of radiation quality and biological effect, *Ann. N.Y. Acad. Sci.* **114**:4–15 (Art. 1).

ROSSI, H. H., AND KELLERER, A. M., 1972, Radiation carcinogenesis at low doses, *Science* **175**:200–202.

ROSSI, H. H., AND KELLERER, A. M., 1974, The validity of risk estimates of leukemia incidence based on Japanese data, *Radiation Res.* **58**:131–140.

SAVAGE, J. R. K., 1970, Sites of radiation induced chromosome exchanges, in: *Current Topics in Radiation Research*, pp. 131–194, North-Holland, Amsterdam.

SAX, K., 1938, Chromosome aberrations induced by X-rays, *Genetics* **23**:494–516.

SAX, K., 1941, Types and frequencies of chromosomal aberrations induced by X-rays, *Cold Spring Harbor Symp. Quant. Biol.* **9**:93.

SCHMID, E., RIMPL, G., AND BAUCHINGER, M., 1973, Dose–response relation of chromosome aberrations in human lymphocytes after *in vitro* irradiation with 3 MeV electrons, *Radiation Res.* **57**:228–238.

SHELLABARGER, C. J., BOND, V. P., CRONKITE, E. P., AND APONTE, G. E., 1969, Relationship of dose of total-body $^{60}$Co radiation to incidence of mammary neoplasia in female rats. *Radiation-Induced Cancer*, IAEA-SM–118/9.

SHELLABARGER, C. J., KELLERER, A. M., ROSSI, H. H., GOODMAN, L. J., BROWN, R. D., MILLS, R. E., RAO, A. R., SHANLEY, J. P., AND BOND, V. P., 1974, Rat mammary carcinogenesis following neutron or X-irradiation, in: *Biological Effects of Neutron Irradiation*, IAEA, Vienna.

SINCLAIR, W. K., 1968, The shape of radiation survival curves of mammalian cells cultured *in vitro*, in: *Biophysical Aspects of Radiation Quality*, IAEA, Vienna.

439

BIOPHYSICAL
ASPECTS OF
RADIATION
CAR-
CINOGENESIS

SMITH, H. H., COMBATTI, N. C., AND ROSSI, H. H., 1968, Response of seeds to irradiation with X-rays and neutrons over a wide range of doses, in: *Neutron Irradiation of Seeds*, Vol. II, Technical Report Series No. 92, pp. 3–8, IAEA, Vienna.

SPARROW, A. H., UNDERBRINK, A. G., AND ROSSI, H. H., 1972, Mutations induced in *Tradescantia* by small doses of X-rays and neutrons. Analysis of dose-response curves, *Science* **176**:916–918.

VOGEL, H. H., 1969, Mammary gland neoplasms after fission neutron irradiation, *Nature (Lond.)* **222**:1279–1281.

WITHERS, H. H., BRENNAN, J. T., AND ELKIND, M. M., 1970, The response of stem cells of intestinal mucosa to irradiation with 14 MeV neutrons, *Brit. J. Radiol.* **43**:796–801.

WOLF, S., 1954, Delay of chromosome rejoining in *Vicia faba* induced by irradiation, *Nature (Lond.)* **173**:501–502.

## 8. Selected General References

*Section 2*

ATTIX, F. H., AND ROESCH, W. C., 1968, *Radiation Dosimetry*, Vol. I: *Fundamentals*, Academic Press, New York.

HINE, G. J., AND BROWNELL, G. L., 1956, *Radiation Dosimetry*, Academic Press, New York.

ICRU, 1970, *Report 16: Linear Energy Transfer*, International Commission on Radiation Units and Measurements, Washington, D.C.

ICRU, 1971, *Report 19: Radiation Quantities and Units*, International Commission on Radiation Units and Measurements, Washington, D.C.

ROSSI, H. H., 1967, Energy distribution in the absorption of radiation, *Advan. Biol. Med. Phys.* **11**:27–85.

WHYTE, G. N., 1959, *Principles of Radiation Dosimetry*, Wiley, New York.


*Section 3*

ELKIND, M., AND WHITMORE, G., 1967, *The Radiobiology of Cultured Mammalian Cells*, Gordon and Breach, London.

FISZ, M., 1965, *Probability Theory and Mathematical Statistics*, Wiley, New York.

HUG, O., AND KELLERER, A. M., 1966, *Stochastik der Strahlenwirkung*, Springer, New York.

KELLERER, A. M., AND HUG, O., 1972, Theory of dose–effect relations, in: *Encyclopedia of Medical Radiology*, Vol. II/3, pp. 1–42, Springer, New York.

ZIMMER, K. G., 1961, *Studies on Quantitative Radiation Biology*, Oliver and Boyd, London.


*Section 4*

KELLERER, A. M., AND ROSSI, H. H., 1972, The theory of dual radiation action, in: *Current Topics in Radiation Research*, Vol. 8, pp. 85–158, North-Holland.

LEA, D. E., 1946, *Actions of Radiations on Living Cells*, Cambridge University Press, Cambridge.

ROSSI, H. H., 1970, The effects of small doses of ionizing radiation, *Phys. Med. Biol.* **15**:255–262.

SAVAGE, J. R. K., 1970, Sites of radiation induced chromosome exchanges, in: *Current Topics of Radiation Research*, pp. 131–194, North-Holland, Amsterdam.


*Section 5*

NATIONAL ACADEMY OF SCIENCES–NATIONAL RESEARCH COUNCIL, 1972, *The Effects on Populations of Exposure to Low Levels of Ionizing Radiation*, Washington, D.C.

U.S. ATOMIC ENERGY COMMISSION, 1973, *Radionuclide Carcinogenesis*, CONF-720505, AEC Symposium Series 29, Washington, D.C.

UNITED NATIONS, 1972, *Ionizing Radiation: Levels and Effects*, Vol. I, New York.

UNITED NATIONS, 1972, *Ionizing Radiation: Levels and Effects*, Vol. II, New York.

# 15

# Ultraviolet Radiation: Interaction with Biological Molecules

FREDERICK URBACH

## 1. Introduction

Solar radiation is a very important element in our environment and yet, because of its ubiquity, the wide scope of its chemical and biological effects is often not fully appreciated. That solar energy fixation makes life possible is a generally known fact. It is not so generally appreciated that many of the effects of solar radiation are detrimental. Most people are aware that a painful sunburn can be caused by excessive exposure to the sun, and that colors fade and materials age in the sun. There also are more subtle effects of sunlight on living cells, including the production of mutations and the development of skin cancer following sufficient chronic exposure to sunlight.

Recent work has shown that plant and animal cells are able to repair radiation-induced genetic damage. Evidently, plants and animals have evolved in such a way as to be able to protect themselves from the detrimental radiations of the sun, while at the same time allowing themselves to receive the benefit of other portions of the solar spectrum. The situation is one of balance: sunlight is necessary for life, yet in excess it is harmful.

The short-wave portion of the solar spectrum is potentially very detrimental to plant and animal cells. A small amount of ozone in the atmosphere filters out these harmful wavelengths of ultraviolet light and thus prevents most such radiation

FREDERICK URBACH ● Temple University Health Sciences Center, Skin and Cancer Hospital, Philadelphia, Pennsylvania.

from reaching the surface of the earth. The formation of this ozone shield in geological time was most likely a prerequisite for the evolution of terrestrial life. However, even in the presence of this ozone layer, a biologically significant amount of ultraviolet radiation does reach the surface of the earth.

Ample evidence indicates that the sun's illumination possesses carcinogenic activity. Many geographic and population studies correlate fair skin plus degree and intensity of sun exposure with skin cancer (Segi, 1963; Urbach *et al.*,1972). Controlled experiments in animals have proven that ultraviolet radiation can be carcinogenic (multiple exposures lead to cancer; Blum, 1959) as well as a tumor initiator (a high dose of ultraviolet radiation followed by promotion with chemical cocarcinogens; Epstein, 1966; Pound, 1970). The observation that reduced ability to repair ultraviolet (UV) induced damage of cells occurs in patients genetically predisposed to extremely high incidence of skin cancer has stimulated great interest among investigators dealing with the etiology of cancer (Cleaver, 1968, 1970).

## 2. Effects of Ultraviolet Radiation on Biological Systems

The first observation of UV effects on living systems dates back to 1877, when Downes and Blunt reported that bacteria were inactivated by light. A large variety of UV effects on many cell types and organisms were reported in the next 50 years, but the early work suffered from a lack of appreciation of the necessity for controlling the wavelengths of the light as well as from a lack of understanding of the importance of the physiological state of the biological system before, during, and after the radiation. Gates discovered that the relative effectiveness of different wavelengths in killing bacteria paralleled the absorption spectrum of nucleic acid. The chemical basis for some of the deleterious effects of UV on nucleic acids did not become evident until the late 1940's. The most recent discovery of Beukers and Berents (1960) of UV-induced thymine dimers in DNA stimulated a resurgence of interest in UV photobiology.

It has now become apparent that in addition to thymine dimers there are many other types of photoproducts produced in the nucleic acid of cells, and some of these have been isolated and characterized (Smith and Hanawalt, 1969). In a number of cases, their relative biological importance has also been determined.

One area in which photobiology has been particularly useful has been in the study of cellular repair mechanisms *per se*: not merely to learn more about mechanisms of recovery from light-induced damage, but also to understand the broader aspects of the mechanisms that may operate to protect cells from many of the hazards of their natural environment.

Among the major effects of UV radiation on biological systems are inhibition of cell division, inactivation of enzymes, induction of mutation, and killing of cells and tissues.

3. *Photochemistry of Nucleic Acids*

443

ULTRAVIOLET
RADIATION:
INTERACTION
WITH
BIOLOGICAL
MOLECULES

Some of the biological effects of UV radiation can now be explained in terms of specific chemical and physical changes produced in DNA. Structural defects are produced in DNA by chemical mutagens and by radiations. This defective DNA may be repaired by cellular enzyme systems and thus serves as the substrate for repair enzymes (see below). Although our knowledge of the possible types of induced structural changes is far from complete, it may be useful to discuss briefly the most frequently formed products whose actions are best understood. Some structural defects can disrupt the continuity of the molecule, while others interfere with replication or transcription by changing hydrogen bonding. single-strand breaks, and DNA–DNA crosslinks are induced by UV, but these usually occur only at high doses, so that their practical importance is questionable (Smith, 1966). Pyrimidine hydrates do not seem to be formed efficiently in double-stranded DNA, but are formed in single-stranded DNA and may be of possible importance in the induction of mutations (Smith, 1966). The cyclobutane-type dimers formed by pyrimidines (separately and as mixed dimers) are chemically the most stable and well-defined lesions readily produced by UV in DNA (Beukers and Berends, 1960; Smith and Hanawalt, 1969). Dimers can also be formed between thymine and cytosine, or between cytosine pairs alone (Setlow *et al.*, 1965). Their formation involves linking the 5,6-unsaturated bonds to form a cyclobutane ring and must distort the phosphodiester backbone of the twin helix in the vicinity of each dimer. In bacteria, a UV dose of 1 erg/mm$^2$ will produce about six pyrimidine dimers in a DNA molecule containing 10$^7$ nucleotides. This is the approximate number of nucleotides in the genome of *Escherichia coli* (Cairns, 1963). The biological importance of this type of dimer has been demonstrated in certain situations (Cleaver, 1968), but this type of photoproduct is not formed in DNA under all conditions and thus other types of photoproducts must also be of significance. Under certain conditions, DNA can crosslink with protein (Smith, 1966). One chemical mechanism for this crosslinking may involve the attachment of amino acid residues through their SH or OH groups to the 5- or 6-carbon of cytosine and thymine.

The sensitivity of DNA to alteration by UV can be changed by a variety of factors, notably changes in the environment of physical state, or change in base composition.

Finally, the biological importance of any given photochemical alteration of nucleic acid depends on whether or not it is formed under a particular set of experimental conditions, and, if formed, whether the biological system can repair the lesion (Smith and Hanawalt, 1969).

## 4. *Photochemistry of Proteins*

UV irradiation of proteins results in the formation of both lower and higher molecular weight products. In the presence of oxygen, higher molecular weight aggregates begin to decompose and thus the protein solubility increases. Irradiated proteins are much more susceptible to enzymatic digestion.

Two different theories of the mechanism of UV inactivation of enzymes have evolved over a period of years. One holds that the alteration of any amino acid residue causes inactivation of an enzyme (McLaren and Sugar, 1964). The other theory states that enzyme inactivation is the consequence of disruption of specific cystine residues and of hydrogen bonds responsible for the spatial integrity of the active center of the enzyme (Augenstein and Riley, 1967).

## 5. Photoinactivation of Cells and Tissues

As might be expected, application of the knowledge of the photochemistry of DNA and proteins to interpretation of effects on metabolizing, living cells is fraught with great difficulty. Living cells have a variety of mechanisms specifically designed for dealing with potentially injurious events and exhibit different sensitivities to the same stimulus at different stages in the growth cycle. DNA is the principal target for most injurious effects of photons on growing cells. Damage to a single nucleotide may kill a cell, or result in a nonlethal mutation, or be not detectable by any biological assay. Most of the insight into photobiological events has been obtained from studies of bacteria, particularly *E. coli* and a variety of more or less sensitive mutants of this organism (for review, see Howard-Flanders, 1968; Smith and Hanawalt, 1969). In recent years, the virus has become a most useful biological tool for photobiological investigations. Extensive studies have been made on bacteriophages and plant and animal viruses (Luria, 1955; McLaren and Sugar, 1964).

Effects of light become even much more complex in large eukaryotic cells or in multicellular organisms. Such systems have much more redundancy of genetic information, so that inactivation of a particular gene may not be consequential. The nuclei are shielded by surrounding cytoplasm or even light-absorbing materials (pigments, chitin, etc.) and there are fewer critical functions necessary for survival of a particular cell.

The UV sensitivity of eukaryotic cells varies during the mitotic cycle, they being more resistant in metaphase and telophase. In such cells, selective irradiation of parts of the cell has provided much useful information, e.g., that, as expected, irradiation of the nucleus is more deleterious to survival of the cell than irradiation of the cytoplasm (Giese, 1964).

## 6. DNA Repair

Since biologically important amounts of UV radiation reach earth, and must have done so since the beginning of evolution, mechanisms must have arisen very early in biological time to protect cells and to aid in the recovery from the damaging effects of photons.

445

ULTRAVIOLET
RADIATION:
INTERACTION
WITH
BIOLOGICAL
MOLECULES

In recent years, three major kinds of recovery have been described:

1. The damaged molecule or part of a molecule can be restored to its functional state *in situ*. This is accomplished either by an enzymatic mechanism or by "decay" of the damage to some innocuous form.
2. The damaged part can be removed and replaced with undamaged material to restore normal function.
3. The damage may remain unrepaired, but the cell may either bypass or ignore the damage.

Because of the importance of the sequence of events necessary for appropriate biological replication and normal function of DNA molecules, conditions favorable to survival of a cell usually require that any molecular repair process be completed within some narrowly defined period of time to be effective. Furthermore, the type of recovery as well as the extent of recovery will depend on the nature of the molecule that has been damaged.

A large number of different repair mechanisms have been described to date, and other kinds are being discovered with increasing frequency as new methods for photoinjury and analysis of repair are studied. An excellent review of presently known repair mechanisms can be found in Smith and Hanawalt (1969) and in the proceedings of a symposium on molecular and cellular repair processes (Beers et al., 1972).

Here, only the most important and best-studied repair processes will be described.

## 7. Enzyme-Catalyzed Photoreactivation

Enzyme-catalyzed photoreactivation is the best-known form of *in situ* repair. In this system, illumination with visible light facilitaties the direct repair *in situ* of photoproducts produced by absorption of UV photons in DNA. It has been clearly shown that most nonmammalian cells contain an enzyme system which splits pyrimidine dimers, thus restoring a normal DNA strand *in situ*. The enzyme binds specifically to UV-irradiated DNA to form a complex that is stable in the dark. If the complex is illuminated with long UV (330 nm or longer) or visible light, it separates into the active enzyme and a repaired DNA which can no longer bind to the enzyme. Illuminating the enzyme or the damaged DNA prior to complex formation has no effect on UV damage repair (Kelner, 1953, 1969).

The photoreactivation mechanism is of greatest importance for the survival of plants and small animals (such as insects) in the field, accounting for the capability of such cells to survive in tropical and mountainous areas.

FREDERICK
URBACH

The studies of Setlow (1968) provided the first experimental evidence leading to a model for repair of UV-damaged in the dark. A repair mechanism was postulated in which defective regions in one of the two DNA strands could be excised and then subsequently replaced with normal nucleotides, Utilizing the complementary base-pairing information in the intact strand. This mechanism (Fig. 1), which

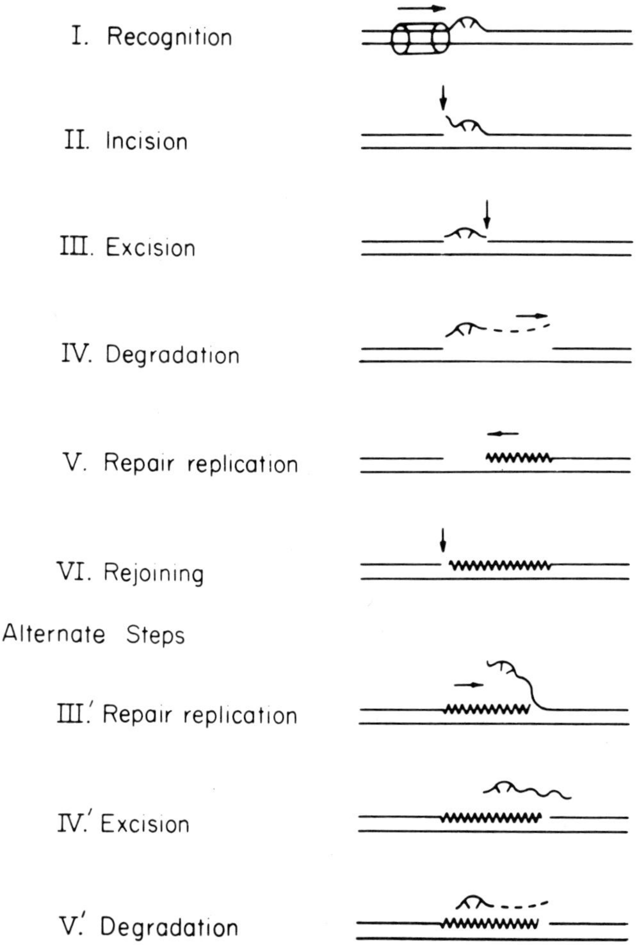

FIGURE1. Schematic representation of the postulated steps in the excision repair of damaged DNA. Steps I through VI illustrate the "cut and patch" sequence. An initial incision in the damaged strand is followed by local degradation before the resynthesis of the region has begun. In the alternative "patch and cut" model, the resynthesis step III begins immediately after the incision step II and the excision of the damaged region occurs when repair replication is complete. In either model, the final step (VI) involves a rejoining of the repaired section to the contiguous DNA of the original parental strand. From Smith and Hanawalt (1969), by permission.

has come to be known as "cut and patch," has turned out to be of widespread significance for the repair of a variety of structural defects of DNA.

447
ULTRAVIOLET
RADIATION:
INTERACTION
WITH
BIOLOGICAL
MOLECULES

Excision repair involves (Smith and Hannawalt, 1969) the following:

1. Recognition—This system is capable of recognizing a variety of structural defects in DNA, including those which do not involve pyrimidines and those not due to UV effects (usually caused by alkylating agents, etc.). The exact nature of the recognition mechanism is not known.
2. Incision—Following recognition of DNA damage, a single-strand break near the damage point must be produced. This is most likely done by an enzymatic process.
3. Excision and repair replication—These processes may occur as separate steps or concurrently. It is thought that the known enzymes exonuclease III and DNA polymerase may be responsible for these steps.
4. Rejoining—Completion of the repair process requires rejoining of the repaired segment to the continuous DNA strand. Polynucleotide ligase may well be the enzyme responsible for this step.

Evidence for excision repair mechanisms has been found in microorganisms, viruses, and mammalian cells (Lieberman and Forbes, 1973).

## 9. Recombination Repair

The observation of Howard-Flanders (1968) that double mutant strains of E. coli, deficient in both excision and recombination, were more sensitive to UV than either of the single mutant strains alone suggested the existence of a dark repair mechanism other than "cut and patch." The nature of DNA synthesis on unrepaired templates is not yet clear, but studies in various mutant strains of bacteria support the presence of at least one and perhaps more than one dark repair system in addition to the excision repair mode.

It is important to note that the known DNA repair systems in bacteria are under genetic control and that genetic loci control the extent of DNA degradation and may control gene products needed for the correct functioning of the repair enzymes. The finding by Cleaver and Carter (1973) of a genetic defect of excision repair in a heritable disease in man (xeroderma pigmentosum) and the fact that variants of this disorder involve different abilities to repair UV damage to the cells are of considerable importance for the hypothesis that heritable characteristics may be involved in the liability for cancer production in man.

## 10. Ultraviolet Light, DNA Repair, and Carcinogenesis

Since the end of the nineteenth century, when the earliest suggestions were made that frequent and prolonged exposure to sunlight is the cause of skin cancer

(Unna, 1894; Dubreuilh, 1896; Shield, 1899), substantial experimental, epidemiological and clinical observations have changed these earlier suspicions to virtual certainty (Blum, 1959; Urbach, 1966; Gordon *et al.*, 1972).

The evidence for the assumption that exposure to sunlight, particularly the midultraviolet component, is an essential and major factor in the development of most human skin cancers can be briefly summarized as follows:

1. Skin cancer appears on parts of the body most exposed to sunlight, particularly the head, neck, arms, and hands (Silverstone and Gordon, 1966).
2. Squamous cell carcinoma in particular (and basal cell carcinoma to a lesser degree) occurs primarily on skin sites most heavily exposed to solar radiation (Urbach, 1966).
3. There is greater prevalence of skin cancer in outdoor workers (Blum, 1959), and in a particular community greater frequency of skin cancer (and occasionally the only incidence of skin cancer) is found in those who have spent the longest periods outdoors (Urbach *et al.*, 1972; O'Beirn *et al.*, 1970).
4. For similar types of skin, skin cancer increases fairly rapidly with decrease in latitude, particularly in the middle latitudes (mid 50s to low 20s). This tendency is not shown for any other cancer except malignant melanoma (Dorn, 1944; Blum, 1959; Gordon *et al.*, 1972).
5. Susceptible racial types, particularly those of Celtic origin, are more prone to skin cancer than other whites, and especially to multiple lesions. The characteristic skin has little pigment, or scattered freckles, and susceptible individuals seem more often to have fair hair and blue or gray eyes and to sunburn easily, severely, and often (O'Beirn *et al.*, 1970; Gellin *et al.*, 1966; Silverstone and Searle, 1970; Urbach *et al.*, 1972).
6. In extensive, carefully controlled experiments with UV on animal (primarily mouse) skin, it has been shown without any doubt that skin cancer is produced by repeated exposure to wavelengths between 320 and 250 nm, with the 320–280 nm range being most effective (Findlay, 1928; Blum, 1959; Epstein, 1966). Tumors have also been induced by massive single doses of UV (Hsu *et al.*, 1975), and tumor cells have been initiated by a single, modest UV exposure and promoted into cancers by chemical substances (Epstein, 1966; Pound, 1970).

Despite these and numerous other biological and biochemical studies, the pathogenetic mechanism of UV carcinogenesis on the cellular level remains obscure. Basic data about the molecular effect of UV on DNA had not helped either, until recently when pyrimidine dimer formation, excision, and repair by unscheduled DNA replication were demonstrated in mammalian cells *in vitro* (Evens and Norman, 1968) and *in vivo* (Epstein *et al.*, 1968) and in cultured cells from skin cancer–prone patients (Cleaver, 1968). This last observation resulted in a flurry of research activity because the possible implication of unrepaired DNA damage in cancer production hit a responsive chord—a "Zeitgeist" phenomenon. However, xeroderma pigmentosum variants were soon discovered in which

449

ULTRAVIOLET
RADIATION:
INTERACTION
WITH
BIOLOGICAL
MOLECULES

excision repair systems were apparently normal, although the patients were as exquisitely cancer prone as those showing little or no DNA repair (Cleaver and Carter, 1973).

Excision repair is now known to occur after damage with both carcinogenic and noncarcinogenic agents (Roberts, 1972) as well as in the skin of man and mice (Epstein *et al.*, 1971), rat liver and kidney, rabbit brain, UV-induced squamous cell carcinoma of hairless mouse skin (Lieberman and Forbes, 1973), and human tumor cell suspensions (Norman *et al.*, 1972). It is thus clear that a great variety of mammalian cells and at least some malignant cells have excision repair capacity.

In addition to the well-documented capability of UV radiation to induce cancer of the skin in man and mice, Setlow (1973) has been able to show that *in vitro* UV-irradiated fish liver cells, reinjected into isogeneic recipients, give rise to tumors. The tumor induction is UV dose dependent, and illumination of the irradiated cells with visible light before injection markedly reduces tumor production. Since fish cells possess the photoreactivating enzyme, these data imply that pyrimidine dimers induced in cellular DNA by UV are related to the development of the tumors.

The available evidence suggests that injury to DNA is somehow related to carcinogenesis. In view of the evidence that DNA damage encourages mutagenesis in cells, this is a tenable assumption. However, in mouse skin and in most cancer patients, the DNA repair systems seem to be capable of repairing UV damage; thus lack of DNA repair cannot be the basis of most skin cancers. An elegant experiment of Zajdela and Latarjet (1973) suggests a possible reason for this dilemma. They painted a solution of caffeine, a potent inhibitor of DNA repair, on the skin of mice during irradiation with UV. The caffeine-treated skin developed fewer skin cancers than an unpainted control area on the same animal.

Epstein *et al.* (1971) and Zajdela and Latarjet (1973) suggest that the production of skin cancer by UV is initiated by repair of DNA, allowing the cell to survive, yet leaving in place or even favoring subsequent errors in DNA replication, resulting in a greater likelihood of malignant change. Further experiments are needed to sort out the mechanisms involved and the relative contribution of DNA damage and DNA repair to carcinogenesis.

## 11. References

AUGENSTEIN, L., AND RILEY, P., 1967, The inactivation of enzymes by UV light: The effect of environment on cystine disruption by UV light, *Photochem. Photobiol.* **6**:423.

BEERS, R. F., JR., HERRIOTT, R. M., AND TILGHMAN, R. C., eds., 1972, *Molecular and Cellular Repair Processes,* Johns Hopkins University Press, Baltimore.

BEUKERS, R., AND BERENDS, W., 1960, Isolation and identification of the irradiation product of thymine, *Biochim. Biophys. Acta* **41**:550–551.

BLUM, H. F., 1959, *Carcinogenesis by Ultraviolet Light,* Princeton University Press, Princeton, N.J.

CAIRNS, J., 1963, The chromosome of *Escherichia coli, Cold Spring Harbor Symp. Quant. Biol.* **28**:43–46.

CLEAVER, J. E., 1968, Defective repair replication of DNA in xeroderma pigmentosum, *Nature (Lond.)* **218**:652.

CLEAVER, J. E., 1970, DNA damage and repair in light sensitive human skin disease, *J. Invest. Dermatol.* **54:**181.

CLEAVER, J. E., AND CARTER, P. M., 1973, Xeroderma pigmentosum: Influence of temperature on DNA repair, *J. Invest. Dermatol.* **60:**29–32.

DORN, H. F., 1944, Illness from cancer in the United States, *U.S. Public Health Rep.* **59:**33–48, 65–77, 97–115.

DUBREUILH, W., 1896, Des Hyperkeratoses Circonscriptes, *Ann. Dermatol. Syph. (Ser. 3)* **7:**1158–1204.

EPSTEIN, J. H., 1966, Ultraviolet light carcinogenesis, in: *Advances in Biology of Skin,* Vo. VII: *Carcinogenesis* (W. Montagna and R. L. Dobson, eds.), Appleton-Century-Crofts, New York.

EPSTEIN, J. H., 1970, Ultraviolet carcinogenesis, in: *Photophysiology: Current Topics,* Vol. 5 (A. C. Giese, ed.), p. 235*ff,* Academic Press, New York.

EPSTEIN, J. H., FUKUYAMA, K., AND EPSTEIN, W. L., 1968, UVL induced stimulation of DNA synthesis in hairless mouse epidermis, *J. Invest. Dermatol.* **51:**445.

EPSTEIN, W. L., FUKUYAMA, K., AND EPSTEIN, J. H., 1971, UV light, DNA repair and skin carcinogenesis in man. *Fed. Proc.* **30:**1766–1771.

EVANS, R. G., AND NORMAN, A., 1968, Unscheduled incorporation of thymidine in ultraviolet irradiated human lymphocytes, *Radiation Res.* **36:**287.

FINDLAY, G. M., 1928, Ultraviolet light and skin cancer, *Lancet* **215:**1070–1073.

FITZPATRICK, T. B., PATHAK, M. A., AND LANE-BROWN, M. M., 1972, Prevention of solar degeneration and sun induced carcinoma of the skin, in: *Melanoma and Skin Cancer* (W. H. McCarthy, ed.), NSW Government Printer, Sydney.

GELLIN, G. A., KOPF, A. W., AND GARFINKEL, L., 1966, Basal cell epithelioma: A controlled study of associated factors, in: *Advances in Biology of Skin,* Vol. VII: *Carcinogenesis* (W. Montagna and R. L. Dobson, eds.), Pergamon Press, Oxford.

GIESE, A. C., 1964, Studies on UV radiation action upon animal cells, in: *Photophysiology* Vol. 2 (A. C. Giese, ed.), pp. 203*ff,* Academic Press, New York.

GORDON, D., SILVERSTONE, H., AND SMITHHURST, B. A., 1972, The epidemiology of skin cancer in Australia, in: *Melanoma and Skin Cancer* (W. H. McCarthy, ed.), NSW Government Printer, Sydney.

HOWARD-FLANDERS, P., 1968, DNA repair. *Am. Rev. Biochem.* **37:**175–199.

HSU, T., FORBES, P. D., HARBER, L. C., AND LAKOW, E., 1975, Induction of skin tumors in hairless mice following single exposure to ultraviolet radiation, Photochemistry and Photobiology (in press).

KELNER, A., 1953, Growth, respiration and nucleic acid synthesis in UV-irradiated and in photoreactivated *E. coli, J. Bacteriol.* **65:**252–262.

KELNER, A., 1969, Biological aspects of UV damage, photoreactivation and other repair systems in micro-organisms, in: *The Biologic Effects of UV Radiation* (F. Urbach, ed.), Pergamon Press, Oxford.

LIEBERMAN, M. W., AND FORBES, P. D., 1973, Demonstration of DNA repair in normal and neoplastic tissues after treatment with proximate chemical carcinogens and UV radiation, *Nature New Biol.* **241:**199–201.

LURIA, S. E., 1955, Radiation and viruses, in: *Radiation Biology,* Vol. 2 (A. Hollander, ed.), p. 333*ff,* McGraw-Hill, New York.

McLAREN, A. D., AND SUGAR, D., 1964, *Photochemistry of Proteins and Nucleic Acids,* Pergamon Press, Oxford.

NORMAN, H., OTTOMAN, R. E., CHAN, P., AND KILSAK, I., 1972, Unscheduled DNA synthesis, *Mutation Res.* **15:**358.

O'BEIRN, S. F., JUDGE, P., URBACH, F., MacCON, C. F., AND MARTIN, F., 1970, The prevalence of skin cancer in County Galway Ireland, in: *Proceedings of the 6th National Cancer Conference,* pp. 489–500, Lippincott, Philadelphia.

POUND, A. W., 1970, Induced cell proliferation and the initiation of skin tumor for motion in mice by ultraviolet light, *Pathology* **2:**269–275.

ROBERTS, J. J., 1972, in: *Molecular and Cellular Repair Processes* (R. F. Beers, R. M. Herriott, and R. Tilghman, eds.), p. 238*ff,* Johns Hopkins University Press, Baltimore.

SEGI, M., 1963, World incidence and distribution of skin cancer, in: *Monograph No. 10, National Cancer Institute* (F. Urbach and H. L. Stewart, eds.), Government Printing Office, Washington, D.C.

SETLOW, R. B., 1968, The photochemistry, photobiology and repair of polynucleotides, *Prog. Nucleic Acid Res. Mol. Biol.* **8:**257*ff.*

SETLOW, R. B., 1973, Personal communication.

SETLOW, R. B., CARRIER, W. L., AND BOLLUM, F. J., 1965, Pyrimidine dimers in UV-irradiated poly dI:dC, *Proc. Natl. Acad. Sci.* **53:**1111–1118.

SHIELD, A. M., 1899, A remarkable case of multiple growths of the skin caused by exposure to the sun, *Lancet* **1**:22–23.

SILVERSTONE, H., AND GORDON, D., 1966, Regional studies in skin cancer, 2nd report: Wet tropical and sub-tropical coast of Queensland, *Med. J. Austral.* **2**:733–740.

SILVERSTONE, H., AND SEARLE, J. H. A., 1970, The epidemiology of skin cancer in Queensland: The influence of phenotype and environment, *Brit. J. Cancer* **24**:235–252.

SMITH, K. C., 1966, Physical and chemical changes induced in nucleic acids by UV light, *Radiation Res. Suppl.* **6**:54–79.

SMITH, K. C., AND HANAWALT, P. C., 1969, *Molecular Photobiology*, Academic Press, New York.

UNNA, P. G., 1894, *Die Histopathologie der Hautkrankheiten*, A. Hirschwald, Berlin.

URBACH, F., 1966, Ultraviolet radiation and skin cancer in man in: *Advances in Biology of Skin*, Vol. VII: *Carcinogenesis* (W. Montagna and R. L. Dobson, eds.), Pergamon Press, Oxford.

URBACH, F., ROSE, D. B., AND BONNEM, M., 1972, Genetic and environmental interactions in skin carcinogenesis, in: *Environment and Cancer*, pp. 355–371, Williams and Wilkins, Baltimore.

ZAJDELA, F., AND LATARJET, R., 1973, The inhibiting effect of caffeine on the induction of skin cancer by UV in the mouse, *Compt. Rend. Acad. Sci. Paris*, 29 Aug.

451

ULTRAVIOLET
RADIATION:
INTERACTION
WITH
BIOLOGICAL
MOLECULES

# 16

# Radiation Carcinogenesis

John B. Storer

## 1. Introduction

Ionizing radiation in sufficiently high dosage acts as a complete carcinogen in that it serves as both initiator and promoter. Further, cancers can be induced in nearly any tissue or organ of man or experimental animals by the proper choice of radiation dose and exposure schedule. Principal interest in radiation as an environmental carcinogen is not at very high dosage levels, however, since relatively few individuals receive such high dosages and in most cases where they do the radiation is received as localized treatment for a malignant tumor. Additionally, radiation delivered to the entire body, as is usually the case for environmental exposure, is acutely fatal (within weeks) at doses higher than a few hundred rads. For these reasons, the major goal of studies on radiation as a carcinogen is the determination of its cancerogenic effectiveness in the extremely low to moderate dosage range. Because radiation can be easily delivered in precisely measured quantities and because it is a fairly potent carcinogen, it has also been widely used as an experimental tool in cancer research.

Information on the effects of radiation on man has been obtained from a variety of sources. These include persons or populations receiving (1) occupational exposure (radiologists and uranium miners), (2) accidental exposure, (3) therapeutic exposure, (4) diagnostic exposure (X-rays or radioisotopes), and (5) wartime exposure (Hiroshima and Nagasaki). Summary information and an evaluation of the data so far obtained from these sources have been recently summarized in the 1972 reports of the United Nations Scientific Committee on the Effects of Atomic Radiation (UNSCEAR Report) and the NAS-NRC Advisory Committee on the Biological Effects of Ionizing Radiations (BEIR Report).

John B. Storer ● Biology Division, Oak Ridge National Laboratory, Oak Ridge, Tennessee. Research sponsored by the U.S. Atomic Energy Commission under contract with the Union Carbide Corporation.

Information from experimental animals has been accumulating for over 70 yr
although at a greatly accelerated rate over the past 25 yr. Because of this rapid
proliferation of information, any review of the subject that deals with specific
conclusions is likely to become obsolete rapidly. General principles emerging
from animal experimentation are likely to stand the test of further research,
however, and for this reason emphasis in this chapter is on principles rather than
specific details.

## 2. Tissue Sensitivity

### 2.1. Man

As indicated earlier, cancer of nearly any tissue can be induced by the proper
choice of radiation dose and treatment schedule. The question, then, is not
whether some tissues are absolutely refractory to carcinogenic effects but whether
there are differences in sensitivity to the induction of cancer. There is ample
evidence at the present time to conclude that human tissues do indeed show a very
wide range in susceptibility to radiation-induced cancers. This conclusion is based
on published studies of all the exposed populations enumerated earlier but leans
most heavily on data from the two largest populations, namely the survivors of the
atomic bombings in Japan as reported by the Atomic Bomb Casualty Commission
(ABCC) and the patients with ankylosing spondylitis treated with therapeutic
radiation in Great Britain as reported by Court Brown and Doll (1965).

A number of scientific committees have studied this question and have
attempted to classify various tissues according to relative sensitivity. These
committees include the United Nations Scientific Committee on the Effects of
Atomic Radiation (1972), the NAS-NRC Advisory Committee on the Biological
Effects of Ionizing Radiations (1972), and a task group for the International
Commission on Radiological Protection (ICRP) (1969). These groups, although
basing their conclusions on essentially the same data reached slightly different
conclusions. In turn, the conclusions I have reached are also somewhat different.
The reason for these differences is that each individual or committee attempting
to classify relative sensitivity must make judgments on the following points. First,
is there consistency between and among the various studies with respect to the
induction of a particular type of tumor? For example, if a slight excess incidence
of cancer of a particular type is found in one irradiated population but not in any
of the others, then the suspicion of a chance sampling variation arises, particularly
if the positive population has a small sample size. Second, are the control data
adequate to reach the conclusion of a radiation-induced excess of cases? This
consideration is particularly important in studies on cancer incidence following
therapeutic radiation, where the patient population is already ill with a disease
which might itself be associated with an increased cancer risk. Third, is the
number of cases sufficient to conclude that there is a significant excess of a
particular cancer? An observed incidence of one case when the expected number

s 0.21 yields a relative risk of 4.8* but does not inspire much confidence in the validity of the risk estimate. Finally, is the observed increased incidence of cancer likely due to factors other than ionizing radiation? It is virtually impossible to match perfectly between control and irradiated populations such factors as economic status, medical history, personal habits, occupation, and dietary preferences, all of which could contribute to predilection to the development of cancer.

While there is an impressive amount of data on radiation carcinogenesis in human populations, the data are inadequate for most types of cancer to permit a clear-cut classification of tissue sensitivities. For this reason, any such classification (with the exception of a few tissues) must be tentative and reflect the best judgment of the reviewer or the reviewing committee. Fortunately, it seems unlikely that the data will be improved in view of the widespread awareness of the hazards of unnecessary radiation exposure.

### 2.1.1. Leukemia

Myeloid leukemia and the acute leukemias are probably the most easily induced of all radiation-induced neoplasms. All studies in which the sample sizes were sufficiently large, the radiation doses were higher than about 50 rads, and an appreciable fraction of the body was irradiated have shown an excess of leukemia over the control group (Seltser and Sartwell, 1965; Court Brown and Doll, 1965; Doll and Smith, 1968; Ishimaru et al., 1971).

There have also been a number of reports of an association between in utero exposure to diagnostic X-rays and an increased risk of leukemia. In these cases, the radiation doses were very small, amounting only to a few rads. Because the evidence is somewhat conflicting, these studies will be considered in more detail in Section 6 under the heading of "host factors."

Unlike solid tumors of other tissues, where the latent period between exposure and development of the tumor may be very long (and the period of increased risk perhaps also correspondingly long), the leukemias occur early, show a high incidence, and then fall to close to the control incidence. Perhaps the best source of information on the human leukemias is the population of Japanese exposed to radiation from the atomic bomb (Ishimaru et al., 1971; Jablon and Kato, 1972). By 5 yr after their exposure, they showed a significantly increased leukemia incidence in the higher-dose groups. This increase was sustained for several years, but by 25 yr after exposure the incidence had fallen to close to control values. Barring an unanticipated second wave of leukemias, then, the data are essentially complete for this disease in the ABCC studies. For this reason, it is not premature to try to evaluate the shape of the dose–response curve, and this will be done in a later section. Briefly, the Hiroshima survivors who were exposed to a mixture of neutrons and $\gamma$-rays showed an increased leukemia incidence at doses of 50 rads

---

* This example is taken from Table 2-1, p. 164, of the Report of the NAS-NRC Advisory Committee on the Biological Effects of Ionizing Radiations (NAS-NRC, 1972).

and above. In Nagasaki, where the exposure was to γ-rays, no increase was detectable at doses below about 100 rads, although the sample size was about one-half that of Hiroshima.

In contrast to the acute and myeloid leukemias, other neoplasms of reticular tissues, such as chronic lymphatic leukemia and Hodgkin's disease, are resistant to radiation induction.

### 2.1.2. Cancer of the Thyroid

The other relatively easily induced tumor in human populations is cancer of the thyroid, particularly when the radiation is delivered to juveniles. It should be noted that, in contrast to leukemia, thyroid cancer is relatively infrequently fatal. Roughly 10–20% of the cases are fatal depending on age at onset. In general, those cancers occurring late in life tend to be more malignant. For these reasons, it is necessary to establish incidence rates (preferably confirmed by biopsy) for thyroid cancers rather than to depend on death rates. This requirement makes it more difficult to determine precisely the relationship between radiation dose and response.

The principal populations studied to date have been persons receiving therapeutic radiation (usually as infants) for thymic enlargement (Hempelmann et al., 1967), the Marshallese people inadvertently exposed to fallout radiation (Conard et al., 1970), and the survivors of the Japanese bombings (Wood et al., 1969). These studies indicate that at doses in excess of about 50 rads there is a significantly elevated risk of thyroid neoplasms. In one of the studies of children irradiated for thymic enlargement, the dose to the thyroid was estimated at less than 30 rads (Pifer et al., 1968). Over an observation period of about 30 yr, there was a slight but not statistically significant increase in thyroid cancer. Benign tumors appeared to be significantly increased, but the validity of this conclusion is questionable because of the great uncertainty in estimating the frequency of benign lesions in the control population. The duration of the period of elevated risk is not known, and studies such as those at ABCC cannot be considered complete at the present time.

Interestingly, patients receiving very large doses of radiation from [131]I (5000–10,000 rads) do not show an increased incidence of thyroid cancer. Presumably these high doses kill the thyroid cells, and neoplasms cannot develop (Conard et al., 1970).

### 2.1.3. Cancer of the Breast

Breast cancer can also be induced by radiation exposure, but in contrast to leukemias and thyroid cancer, where an excess incidence has been reported following relatively small radiation doses, higher doses (in excess of about 100 rads) are required for its induction. Wanebo et al. (1968a) reported the incidence in women periodically examined in the Adult Health Study at the ABCC. This group consists of a subsample of the much larger Life Span Study, but because of the repeated medical examinations it is possible to ascertain incidence of a disease, whereas the Life Span Study detects mortality from various

diseases. At radiation doses in excess of 90 rads, the incidence was significantly
increased, although the total number of cases was small. This observation was
subsequently verified by mortality data from the Life Span Study (Jablon and
Kato, 1972). A significant increase in mortality was seen only in the period of more
than 20 yr after exposure, reflecting the slow time course of the fatal progression
of the disease.

Independent verification of susceptibility of the breast to radiation-induced
cancer is provided by earlier studies of women exposed to repeated fluoroscopic
examinations in the course of treatment of tuberculosis by pneumothorax
(Mackenzie, 1965; Myrden and Hiltz, 1969) and by studies of women treated with
X-rays for acute postpartum mastitis (Mettler et al., 1969). In both studies, there
was a significant excess incidence of breast cancer. The radiation doses are not
very well known in the fluoroscopy cases, but at least some of the women must
have received very large doses since they showed evidence of severe radiodermatitis. The majority of the women must have received at least several hundred
roentgens based on the output of the machine, number of fluoroscopies, and
exposure time for each procedure. In the series treated for mastitis, the tumor
incidence was about twice that found in the general population. The radiation
doses ranged from about 100 to 600 rads, with a mean dose to the irradiated
breast (most patients received unilateral radiation) of about 350 rads.

On the basis of these studies, it is concluded that the breast is moderately
sensitive to the induction of cancer by radiation.

### 2.1.4. Cancer of the Lung

Evidence that the lung is moderately sensitive to cancer induction is provided
principally from studies of uranium miners occupationally exposed to radon and
radon daughters, the patients treated for ankylosing spondylitis by X-rays, and
the studies at the ABCC. However, there are difficulties in the interpretation of all
these studies, that make quantitative conclusions difficult. First of all, cancer of the
lung is common and its incidence is known to be affected by such variables as
smoking habits and urban as opposed to rural living. Additionally, the incidence
rate in various populations has been changing rapidly, making it difficult to
interpret the effect of an additional variable such as radiation exposure.

There is no question that uranium miners whose lungs were occupationally
exposed to α-particle radiation from radon and radon daughters showed an
increased incidence of lung cancer (Lundin et al., 1971). Further, those believed to
be more heavily exposed showed a higher incidence. The difficulty is that the
radiation dosages are not at all well known. Estimates of dose are based on work
histories and on infrequent determinations of the radon content in air samples
obtained in the mines. Continuous monitoring of work areas was not practiced. It
is known that radon concentrations vary greatly by location within the same mine
and that there are large temporal variations in concentrations at the same location
within a mine. Attempts have been made to estimate the extent of exposure of the

miners, but these are at best only rough approximations. α-Particles are densely ionizing (they have a high value for linear energy transfer or LET) and, in general densely ionizing radiations are biologically more effective on a dose-for-dose basis than lightly ionizing radiations such as X- or γ-rays. This point is of importance when we consider the data for the Japanese since the people in Hiroshima were exposed to radiation with a large component of neutrons, which also have a high LET.

In the patients treated for ankylosing spondylitis, the relative risk of developing lung cancer was approximately twice that in the general population (Court Brown and Doll, 1965). The average dose to the lung of these patients has recently been reestimated as about 400 rads (BEIR Report, NAS-NRC, 1972). There is some uneasiness about accepting this incidence figure at face value, however, for the following reasons. The patient population was ill with a seriously debilitating disease. Medications and treatments other than radiation were undoubtedly administered. The smoking habits of the patients may very well have differed from those of the general population, and, finally, the disease interferes with free motion of the rib cage. This interference could conceivably affect the clearance rate of inhaled materials from the lung and thus contribute to susceptibility to cancer.

Perhaps the best population in which to evaluate carcinogenic effect is the Japanese survivors (Beebe *et al.*, 1971; Wanebo *et al.*, 1968b; Jablon and Kato, 1972), but even here there are serious problems. The segment of the population in Hiroshima which received significant radiation exposure (part of which was at high LET) showed about twice the risk of cancer than did those receiving negligible exposures (median dose of 0 rads). This control group itself and the group "not-in-city" at the time of the bombing both showed consistently higher rates than the general population of Japan. Further, the significantly irradiated population in Nagasaki (low LET radiation) did not show an excess risk over those negligibly exposed.

Tuberculous patients in Israel who presumably were exposed to more diagnostic radiation from fluoroscopy than the general population have been reported to show an increased risk of lung cancer (Steinitz, 1965). Radiation doses are not known, however, nor have other variables been evaluated, such as the primary disease itself, which might lead to an increased cancer risk. It is interesting that excessive lung cancer risk in the patients repeatedly fluoroscoped in connection with pnemothorax treatment of tuberculosis was not reported.

In view of the above uncertainties, it seems fair to conclude that the lung is probably moderately sensitive to radiation-induced cancer, but precise quantitative relationships remain to be established.

### 2.1.5. Salivary Gland Tumors

Salivary gland tumors are relatively rare, and few have been reported as being radiation induced. On the basis of the available evidence, however, it is concluded that the salivary gland is moderately sensitive to cancer induction. Belsky *et al.*

1972) have reported from the ABCC on 30 cases in their study population. Of these, three occurred in patients exposed to more than 300 rads, whereas the expected number in this group was 0.4. This difference is statistically significant.

Supporting evidence of radiation-induced salivary gland tumors is found in the studies on children irradiated for thymic enlargement (Hempelmann et al., 1967) and in other patients receiving radiation to areas which included the salivary glands (Saenger et al., 1960; Hazen et al., 1966).

### 2.1.6. Skin

Cancer of the skin was a frequent sequela to exposure to very large doses of radiation received by earlier X-ray workers who were unaware of the hazards of radiation exposure. These cancers usually arise in areas of chronic radiation dermatitis, and X-ray doses must have been well in excess of 1000 rads. In the two largest populations studied to date, namely the spondylitics (Court Brown and Doll, 1965) and the Japanese survivors (Johnson et al., 1969), no excess of skin cancer has been found even at doses of several hundred rads. Initially it appeared that skin cancer in children treated with 450–805 rads for ringworm of the scalp might be increased (Albert and Omran, 1968; Schulz and Albert, 1968). According to the BEIR Report (NAS-NRC, 1972), a recent reevaluation of the data by Albert indicates no significant effect.

In view of the fact that skin cancer is induced only by very high doses, we conclude that this tissue is relatively resistant to radiation-induced cancer.

### 2.1.7. Bone

Like skin, bone is resistant to cancer induction, even though a large number of radiation-induced sarcomas have been reported. These tumors have occurred principally in persons with internally deposited radium and mesothorium as a result of occupational exposure (radium dial painters) or therapeutic administration for various diseases including bone tuberculosis and ankylosing spondylitis (Evans et al., 1969, 1972; Spiess and Mays, 1970, 1971). The radium isotopes selectively localize near the cells of interest. In general, bone cancers have not been seen at doses below about 500 rads, and the great majority have occurred at doses well in excess of a 1000 rads. Since, as pointed out earlier, the $\alpha$-particle radiation from these isotopes has a high LET and therefore would be expected to be appreciably more effective than X- or $\gamma$-radiation, it is apparent that bone must be relatively resistant to cancer induction.

Studies of the two principal populations exposed to an external source of penetrating radiation where the dosimetry problem is much less complex support this conclusion. No excess bone cancers have been found in the Japanese survivors (Yamamoto and Wakabayaski, 1968). Five bone cancers were found in the spondylitic patients treated with X-rays, whereas only 1.1 were expected at control rates (Court Brown and Doll, 1965). However, many of these patients received well over 1000 rads to the spine, and this small number of excess cases is therefore not unexpected.

Bone tumors have been reported in other patients receiving radiotherapy, but again the radiation doses to bone were very high (Bloch, 1962).

### 2.1.8. Stomach

Court Brown and Doll (1965) reported an excess number of cases of gastric cancer in the spondylitics treated with X-rays. In the Japanese survivors, however, no evidence of an increased incidence has been found (Yamamoto *et al.*, 1970). Because of the lack of independent confirming evidence from the various other study populations, it is concluded that the stomach is relatively resistant to radiation-induced cancer and that the excess in the spondylitics may be related either to their primary disease or to its treatment by other medications.

### 2.1.9. Other Tissues

There have been reports of excess cancers of other specific tissues in some of the irradiated populations. These sites include the pancreas, larynx, pharynx, and esophagus. Other studies have been unable to confirm these reports, and it is concluded therefore that the tissues other than those specifically discussed in earlier paragraphs are probably relatively resistant.

Cancers of these other types occur sufficiently infrequently that it is a common practice to pool them in a category of "all other cancers." When such pooling is done, it is often possible to demonstrate an excess over the control population. Because the excess risk is usually small, however, amounting to considerably less than the risk for leukemia, it follows that each individual site or tissue must be relatively resistant.

The classification of tissues into rough categories of relative sensitivity is shown in Table 1. These classifications must be considered as approximate and subject to

TABLE 1
*Relative Sensitivity of Various Human Tissues to the Induction of Radiogenic Cancer*

| High sensitivity | Moderate sensitivity | Low sensitivity |
|---|---|---|
| Myelopoietic tissue (Acute leukemia and myeloid leukemia) | Breast | Skin |
| Thyroid | Lung | Bone |
| | Salivary gland | Stomach |
| | | Other tissues (including other lymphomas) |

change as the period of follow-up of the various irradiation populations is increased. It is conceivable that some cancers have a very long latent period (in excess of 25 yr) and that they will show a dramatic increase as follow-up continues. This possibility seems unlikely, and if latency is very much greater than 25 yr it may exceed the normal remaining life expectancy of many members of the irradiated populations and therefore never become manifest.

There is a pronounced lack of uniformity of tissue sensitivities to cancer induction among the various species of experimental animals or even within strains of the same species. In general, most animals, like man, are sensitive to the induction of leukemia. There seem to be special sensitivities to many other tumor types. Some lines of rats are exquisitely sensitive to mammary tumor induction (Shellabarger *et al.*, 1969). Mice are very sensitive to ovarian tumors (Furth *et al.*, 1959), and burros seem resistant to any type of tumor (Brown *et al.*, 1965). For these reasons, it is not possible to classify precisely the relative tissue sensitivities for experimental animals as a whole. The important point to determine is whether animals behave like man in the sense of showing marked variations in susceptibility without regard to whether there is precise correspondence in terms of specific tumor types. This appears to be the case for all species so far studied.

No attempt will be made to tabulate and summarize the very extensive literature on experimental animals. Instead, we will consider a single large experiment in one mouse strain which clearly establishes that there are differences in sensitivity. The data shown in Table 2 are from an experiment initiated in the Oak Ridge National Laboratory by Upton and his colleagues and completed by me and my colleagues. The experiment is now complete, but the data are not yet completely analyzed. Certain conclusions can be drawn, however, and these form the basis of the following discussion. A total of 12,000 female mice of the RFM/Un strain were irradiated at the age of 10 wk with γ-rays. Doses ranged from 10 to 400 rads. A total of 4000 mice served as unirradiated controls, giving a total sample size of 16,000. The mice were then set aside to live out their lives. Over 97% were autopsied, and of these about 40% were subjected to histological examination. There was excellent correspondence between tumor diagnoses based on gross autopsy and those verified histologically.

In Table 2, the tissues classified as highly sensitive were those where a significant increase in tumor incidence over control values was seen at 25 rads. (No significant increase in any tumor type occurred at 10 rads in a group of about 3000 mice.) The column headed "moderate sensitivity" refers to tumors showing a significant increase at 50–150 rads, and the "resistant" category includes tumors showing either no increase at any dose or an increase only at doses greater than 150 rads.

TABLE 2
*Relative Tissue Sensitivities in RFM Female Mice to the Induction of Radiogenic Cancer*

| High sensitivity | Moderate sensitivity | Low sensitivity |
|---|---|---|
| Thymus | Pituitary | Bone |
| Ovary | Uterus | Skin |
| | Breast | Stomach |
| | Myelopoietic tissue (myeloid leukemia) | Liver |
| | Lung | Gastrointestinal tract |
| | Harderian gland | Other tissues |

Unlike man, female mice of this strain are susceptible to the induction of endocrine-associated tumors (ovary, pituitary, uterus), but like man the various tissues show a wide range of sensitivity. It would be unreasonable to expect that the mouse (or dog, monkey, rat, or burro) would show a precise one-to-one correspondence of tissue sensitivity to cancer induction. There is excellent agreement, however, in terms of the general principle that all tissues are not equally radiosensitive.

## 3. Dose–Response Relationships

There are two rather divergent philosophies of approach to the problem of the relationship of radiation dose to the probability of tumor induction. These approaches might be characterized as administrative and scientific. The administrative approach has been used by those concerned with health protection. In order to insure that hazards are not underestimated, this approach assumes that any amount of radiation exposure, no matter how small, is potentially deleterious. Further, it is assumed that the risk is directly proportional to dose; i.e., twice the dose yields twice the risk. These two assumptions lead to the so-called linear no-threshold hypothesis. In support of this hypothesis, the argument is often made that since data from human populations are not sufficiently precise to exclude a linear relationship with a great deal of confidence (the level usually unspecified), the hypothesis should be accepted. Since many other relationships such as quadratic, sigmoid, and higher polynomials also cannot be excluded, this does not constitute an adequate evaluation of the most likely true dose–response curve.

Two other assumptions are usually made in the administrative approach, even though they conflict with a considerable body of scientific evidence. These assumptions are that there is no effect of dose rate and that the relative biological effectiveness (RBE) of densely ionizing radiations is constant regardless of dosage level. Taken altogether, these various assumptions result in a system having both the virtue of conservatism (it is unlikely that risks are underestimated) and a simplified method of bookkeeping (weighting factors for total dose, dose rate, and variable RBE need not be applied).

The scientific approach, unencumbered with the thorny problems of health protection or the serious consequences of underestimating risk, seeks to establish the true functional relationship of dose and response. It is important to establish this relationship since, by knowing the true functional form, it is possible to draw inferences about the nature of the carcinogenic mechanisms and factors involved in the expression of neoplasms.

### 3.1. Theoretical Considerations

The initiating cellular change in radiation carcinogenesis must result directly or indirectly from ionizations produced in the cell. The change itself almost surely is in the informational content of the cell, whether somatic mutation, viral activation, or whatever. If a single ionizing event is adequate to produce the change and if, further, the change itself is sufficient to produce cancer uninfluenced by host factors or promoting effects, then the dose–response relationship should be linear, with no dose rate effect at least in a restricted dosage range. Further, if the initiating change is a somatic mutation, one would expect all tissues to be roughly equally sensitive to cancer induction since it is unlikely that there are major differences in resistance to mutation in the various tissues.

If, on the other hand, host factors such as immune competence, endocrine function, cellular proliferation rate, and level of repair enzymes play a predominant role in whether the transformed cells ultimately produce neoplasms, it is difficult to visualize a linear relationship. Most quantitative biological characteristics in populations show an approximately normal or log normal distribution. Presumably a characteristic such as the immune competence of individuals within a population would show a similar distribution, as would other host characteristics which might influence the induction of cancer. In this case, a sigmoid rather than a linear dose–response curve would be anticipated. To obtain a linear relationship under these circumstances would require a rectangular distribution of the relevant host factor in the population. Such distributions must be extremely rare in biological materials. For radiation-induced skin tumors in rats (Burns *et al.*, 1968), kidney tumors in rats (Maldague, 1969), and osteogenic sarcomas in patients exposed to internally deposited radium (Evans *et al.*, 1969), a sigmoid relationship adequately fits the data over a restricted dosage range. The relationship breaks down at very high doses, where either cell killing or intercurrent mortality from other cancers reduces the cancer incidence.

There are other cases where variability in host factors appears to play a relatively minor role in determining the outcome of radiation exposure. These cases would include the induction of mammary cancers in rats (Shellabarger *et al.*, 1969) and thymic lymphomas in mice (Storer, 1973). If the dose–response relationship is truly sigmoid, the "tail" at the low dose end is very short and the incidence rises rapidly at low to moderate doses. For intermediate cases, the dose–response curve may represent a complex interaction between the curve for induction of the initiating event and the population distribution of relevant host factors. In those cases where host factors or promoting factors play a significant role, it is likely that the dose–response curve deviates from simple linearity, with less effectiveness per rad at the low dose end.

Even if induction of the initiating event is of overriding importance, as it may be in very sensitive tissues, it can be argued on physical grounds that the dose–response curve for low LET radiation cannot be linear. If a single ionizing event in the cell initiates the neoplastic change, then low LET radiation delivered at very low dose rates should be at least as effective as low LET radiation at high dose rates. The reason for this is that at very low rates the vast majority of ionizations are of the single-hit variety. The fact is that in nearly all (perhaps all) cases adequately studied, low dose rate radiation is less effective than high dose rate radiation (e.g., see Upton *et al.*, 1970). At moderate to high doses of low LET radiation, a large fraction of the cells are subjected to multiple ionizing events (two or more hits) within a brief time span. Since exposure under these circumstances is more effective than under conditions of low dose rates, multiple ionizing events in the cell must be more efficient in inducing the neoplastic change. This argument is supported by studies of high LET radiations, such as neutrons, where fewer cells are "hit" per unit dose but those that are hit receive multiple ionizing events. This is true whether the radiation is delivered at low rates or at high rates because of the nature of the ionizing tracks. Neutrons tend to show effects that are very much less dependent on dose rate than low LET radiations. Further, on a dose-for-dose basis they are more effective than X- or $\gamma$-rays (Upton *et al.*, 1970). These observations argue strongly that multiple event injury is usually required to produce the neoplastic change. If this were not the case, then high LET radiations would be less effective than low LET radiations because most of their ionizations would be wasted.

If we accept the hypothesis of multiple ionizations being required for neoplastic change, then the dose–response curve for low LET radiations at high dose rates cannot be linear. The reason is that at low total doses most of the events will be of the single-hit variety, and as the dose increases an increasing number of multiple hits will occur. With high LET radiation, on the other hand, the relationship will be linear since the proportion of multiple hits does not vary with dose. These physical considerations lead to the prediction that the RBE for neutrons should vary with dose, being higher at low doses than at high doses. This prediction has not been adequately tested for cancer induction, although the data from the Japanese survivors (see UNSCEAR Report, United Nations, 1972) are compatible with this prediction. In a wide variety of other experimental test systems, it has been demonstrated that RBE does indeed vary with dose and in the way predicted (see Kellerer and Rossi, 1972).

A final complication in the theoretical prediction of dose–response curves is the role of cell killing by radiation. In one respect, cell transformation and cell killing are working at cross purposes since transformed cells that are killed cannot produce cancers. It is unlikely that the curves for these two responses are identical or even similar, leading to problems in prediction. It is known that cell-killing curves for mammalian cells and low LET radiation are not linear. What effect this would have on the composite curve for cancer yield is not clear. Cell killing may also act in the opposite direction by serving as a promoting agent if the stimulus to proliferation of transformed cells originates from the killing of other cells in the tissue. In this case, the dose–cancer relationship should be concave because of the low efficiency of cell killing at low doses.

In view of all the factors discussed above, it would seem little short of miraculous if the true dose–response curve for cancer induction by X- or $\gamma$-rays turns out to be the administratively convenient simple linearity. It is more likely that different relationships will be found for different tumors and different radiation qualities, with the majority of cases being sigmoid or concave (which could represent one end of a sigmoid) particularly for low LET radiation.

There are only two populations and two tumor types where the information is adequate to make it worthwhile considering the dose–response curves, namely, leukemia in the Japanese survivors (Ishimaru *et al.*, 1971) and bone tumors in the persons exposed to internally deposited radium (Evans *et al.*, 1969; Spiess and Mays, 1970, 1971).

As indicated earlier, barring an unexpected second wave of leukemia, the data are essentially complete for this disease in the Japanese. For Hiroshima, the increase in incidence appears to increase linearly with dose. For Nagasaki, the relationship appears sigmoid or curvilinear upward at the lower dose end, with no excess at doses less than 100 rads. A simple linear relationship cannot be excluded on statistical grounds for either population. The difference may very well be real, however, and possible explanations for it should be considered.

The chief radiobiological difference between the two populations is that those in Hiroshima received a mixture of neutrons and γ-rays while those in Nagasaki received essentially γ-rays. If an RBE of 5 is assigned to the neutron component of the Hiroshima radiation, the two dose–response relationships come into much closer alignment (Ishimaru *et al.*, 1971). If a variable RBE, ranging from 10 at the lowest doses to 1 at the high doses is applied, the correspondence of the curves is improved further (UNSCEAR Report, United Nations, 1972). If it is assumed the neutrons show a linear dose–response relationship, which is reasonable from the data, then it follows that the γ-ray line is curvilinear upward. A similar conclusion has been reached by Rossi and Kellerer (this volume) using a different method of analysis.

The other population, where the period of follow-up has been sufficiently long and the incidence of tumors sufficiently high to justify an analysis of the shape of the dose–response curve, consists of persons carrying appreciable skeletal burdens of radium isotopes. The group which has been studied the longest is comprised of persons in the United States who ingested radium in the course of painting luminous instrument dials ("radium dial painters") and patients who ingested nostrums containing radium for a variety of diseases. These exposures occurred in the early part of the century. The period of intake of radium was quite variable, but since the radium isotopes avidly deposit in bone the radiation exposure has been continuous. The complex problem of dosimetry has been and continues to be actively studied and for our purposes can be considered reasonably accurate. There are, of course, inhomogeneities in dose from one part of the skeleton to another and very pronounced variations within a bone. The usual method of expressing dose is to average the energy absorption over the entire skeleton and sum the dose received over the relevant period of exposure.

A plot of the incidence of bone tumors as a function of dose yields two very distinct regions (Evans *et al.*, 1969, 1972). At doses below about 1000 rads, no bone tumors have been observed. At doses above 1000 rads, there is a high incidence of tumors (roughly 30%), but the incidence does not increase with further increases in dose. The function best describing the relationship is a sigmoid curve with a precipitously rising segment in the region between about 900 and 1200 rads. The radiation from radium and its decay products is principally α-particles. If, as is generally agreed, this high LET radiation has a high RBE, it is obvious that bone is relatively refractory to tumor induction and massive doses of low LET radiation such as X- or γ-rays would be required for a major increase in tumor incidence.

A more recent study from Germany on patients treated for tuberculosis (principally of the bone) or ankylosing spondylitis in the period 1946–1951 indicates tumor induction at considerably lower total doses (Spiess and Mays, 1970, 1971). A sigmoid dose–response curve appears to describe the relationship adequately, however. There are two major differences between this and the U.S. study. In the German series, many of the patients were treated as juveniles and the authors have been able to demonstrate a greater sensitivity of juveniles to bone tumor indication. The second difference is that the German patients were treated with nearly pure $^{224}$Ra, while in the U.S. series the exposure was principally to $^{226}$Ra or $^{228}$Ra (mesothorium). Because of the short half-life of $^{224}$Ra, most of the radiation dose is absorbed near the surface of bone and in actively growing sites. This inhomogeneity results in far higher doses to the relevant cells at risk than would be suggested by averaging over the entire skeletal mass. For this reason, it is likely that $^{224}$Ra and $^{226}$Ra are about equally cancerogenic at the microdosimetry level and the apparent greater effectiveness of the $^{224}$Ra at the macrodosimetry level is spurious.

It was indicated earlier that the high LET neutron component of the radiation in Hiroshima may very well have yielded a linear dose–response curve for leukemia induction. On the other hand, an even higher LET from α-particles appeared to yield a sigmoid curve for bone tumor induction in the dial painters. How can this apparent paradox be resolved? In the first place, there is no *a priori* reason to believe that the dose–response curves for the induction of all tumors should necessarily have the same shape. Different curves would be expected if host factors were involved unequally in the induction of different tumors. For example, if the initiating cellular change is of overriding importance in the induction of leukemia and host defense or promoting factors are of little importance, then a high LET radiation might very well yield a linear relationship since the probability of producing the initiating event should be proportional to dose. On the other hand, host factors may be of great importance in the induction of bone sarcomas and a sigmoid curve result. This would be particularly true if cell killing and tissue regeneration serve as promoting agents for these two tumor types. Lymphopoietic and myelopoietic cells are very sensitive to cell killing, and significant numbers are killed at low doses. Bone cells are considerably more resistant. It it were necessary to kill a sufficient number of bone cells so that extensive regeneration and remodeling of bone had to occur before the promoting effect was manifest, then the observed sigmoid curve could result.

Despite the very large number of studies conducted on the effects of ionizing radiation on experimental animals, there are only a limited number suitable for examination of the shape of the dose–response curve for cancer induction. There are a number of reasons for this relative paucity of data. In many cases, end points other than cancer incidence were looked for and careful necropsies were not performed. When external sources of radiation have been employed, it has been a common practice to perform total-body exposures. This limits the size of the dose that can be used, and further, in the case of mice in particular, there tends to be a "swamping" effect of a high incidence of early-occurring lymphomas and leukemias which preclude the development of later-occurring solid tumors. Unless sample sizes are very large, too few solid tumors of specific sites are seen to evaluate dose and response. Another common problem has been the failure of the investigator to provide data corrected for competing causes of death (see UNSCEAR Report, United Nations, 1972). At high radiation doses, there may actually be an apparent decrease in the incidence of late-occurring tumors, which is an artifact arising from the depletion of the population by incidence of earlier-occurring diseases such as thymic lymphoma so that few of the initial population remain at risk for developing the late tumor. Correction procedures to circumvent this problem are available (for example, Hoel and Walburg, 1972), but only recently has the need for their use been widely recognized.

Some of the most useful studies have been those which employ partial-body or single-organ irradiation. High doses can be achieved and the complication of competing risks is greatly reduced. Partial-body exposure has been achieved by either feeding or injecting radioisotopes that selectively localize in specific tissues or by shielding much of the body from radiation from external sources. When low LET radiations have been used, the majority of studies have shown dose–response curves that are curvilinear upward or a sigmoid relationship. Mays and Lloyd (1972a) have reviewed the incidence of bone sarcomas in a wide variety of species exposed to $^{90}Sr$ (a low LET bone-seeking isotope). In all cases, a curvilinear relationship gave the best fit. In the larger studies, a linear, no-threshold fit could be convincingly rejected.

External irradiation to limited areas of the skin of rats (Burns *et al.*, 1968) resulted in sigmoid dose–response curves over a portion of the dose range. When the optimally carcinogenic dose was exceeded, the incidence decreased significantly. A similar effect has been reported for renal cancers in rats (Maldague, 1969). The reason for the decline is undoubtedly cell killing. If an organ is completely ablated by radiation, it obviously cannot undergo neoplastic change.

In test systems showing a high sensitivity to tumor induction, the dose–response relationship may appear linear in the low dose range. For example, female Sprague-Dawley rats are exquisitely sensitive to the induction of mammary tumors, and a linear relationship at the low dose end followed by a plateau at higher doses describes the data (Shellabarger *et al.*, 1969). Similarly, in the as yet unreported studies in Oak Ridge that were referred to earlier, the incidence of thymic lymphoma appears linear in a restricted dose range beginning at 25 rads. Extrapolation of the line back to 0 dose predicts reasonably well the control incidence. If a large sample had not been irradiated at 10 rads, a conclusion that the dose–response curve is linear would have been justified. However, the 10-rad group showed no increase in thymic lymphomas, and it appears that the relationship is probably sigmoid with a very short tail in the low dose region. This points up the difficulty in choosing among various alternative curves for tumors that are easily induced. Very large samples are required and even then the choice of one function over another may be tenuous.

On a dose-for-dose basis, high LET radiations are more effective carcinogens than low LET radiations. Most animal studies at high LET values have been conducted using internally deposited α-emitters such as radium or plutonium (both bone seekers). Except for the case of neutrons, it is extremely difficult to use external sources of high LET radiation. The mass and charge of the particles (protons, α-particles, and heavier ions) that yield densely ionizing tracks makes them very poorly penetrating except at very high energies. Once they are accelerated to high enough energies to become penetrating, they give up most of their energy in tissue at low LET. There are exceptions, but the necessary hardware for external sources of high LET radiation is not commonly available. Neutrons, because of their lack of charge, penetrate reasonably well, and their interactions in tissue yield a high proportion of high LET radiation. The difficulty is that partial-body or single-organ exposure is extremely difficult because the beam cannot be focused (neutrons are uncharged) and body shielding is extraordinarily difficult. Most, if not all, neutron studies therefore have utilized total-body radiation with the attendant problem of restricted dose range and a "swamping" effect of easily induced tumors.

The studies with internally deposited α-emitters have yielded two types of dose–response curves for the induction of bone tumors, namely linear and curvilinear upward (see review by Mays and Lloyd, 1972b). The principal species studied have been mice and beagle dogs. Within each species both types of curves have been found, so the effect is not species specific. Curiously, the same investigators (Finkel and Biskis, 1962; Finkel et al., 1969), using the same mouse strain, found both types of curve depending on the choice of isotope (Mays and Lloyd, 1972b). In the studies with dogs, the sample sizes are too small and the follow-up is insufficiently long to choose either type of function with confidence. It is concluded that high LET radiation yields dose–response curves that are more nearly linear than those for low LET radiation, but the data are inadequate to determine which, if any, functional form is characteristic.

One unusual characteristic of the dose–response curve for any tumor type so far studied over a sufficiently wide dose range is that the incidence plateaus in the higher dose range. This indicates that even in genetically homogeneous populations such as mice there are individuals apparently refractory to induction of the cancer, suggesting that host factors that are not genetically determined may play a role in determining whether the malignancy becomes manifest.

In the summary, the true form of most dose–response curves for cancer induction is probably sigmoid (the curvilinear form representing one tail of the distribution). For easily induced tumors, where host factors may play a minor role in the outcome, it is extremely difficult to distinguish between linearity and a rapidly rising sigmoid with a very short "tail" at the low dose end. Very large sample sizes are required and the benefits to be derived by such a distinction may not be worth the bother.

## 4. Threshold or Minimum Effective Doses

Most experienced investigators agree that it is a futile exercise to attempt to establish the dose of radiation or any other known carcinogen below which there is absolutely no increased probability of developing cancer. There are a number of reasons why this is so. The first of these has to do with proving a negative effect, something much more difficult than proving a positive effect. If, for example, one conducted a meticulously controlled study in 10,000 or 100,000 animals exposed to, say, 5 rads and found precisely the same number (or even fewer) cancers in the treated group as in an equal-sized control group, one could still not conclude that at 5 rads there is absolutely no possibility of increased risk. Suppose one found no cancers of a particular type in either group (an unlikely possibility, as will be shown below). The value of 0 in 10,000 still has a statistically calculable upper confidence limit which is greater than zero. One might then feel confident that with a certain probability the risk does not exceed this upper limit, but zero risk could not be assumed. To complicate matters further, radiation does not produce unique cancers that are identifiable as being radiation induced. It simply changes the overall incidence of naturally occurring cancers (or perhaps cancers induced by other agents). For this reason, there is always a variable background "noise" level in the population which reduces the statistical certainty that the radiation risk does not exceed some specified value. The unanswerable argument can also be raised that in a heterogeneous population such as man there may be a uniquely sensitive population subset that will respond at doses which are ineffective in the majority of the population.

While it is virtually impossible to demonstrate empirically that there is an absolute threshold, there is an alternative approach which suggests that for certain tumors there may be a "practical" threshold (Evans *et al.*, 1969). This approach is based on the fact that for many tumors the latent period, i.e., the time between radiation exposure and appearance of the tumor, increases as the dose decreases. This appears to be the case for radiogenic bone sarcomas in the dial painters (Evans *et al.*, 1969) and for a number of different types of tumors in experimental animals (Furth *et al.*, 1959; Upton, 1964; Hulse, 1967; Burns *et al.*, 1968; Dougherty and Mays, 1969; Hug *et al.*, 1969; Shellabarger *et al.*, 1969; Nilsson, 1970). If one extrapolates to low doses, the latent period may exceed the remaining life expectancy and a practical threshold is therefore predicted. The difficulty with this approach is that it requires extrapolation beyond the range of dosages where reasonably good data exist into the low dosage region of statistical uncertainty, and the same objections can be raised as with predictions of absolute thresholds. Nevertheless, if risk estimates in the low dose range can be made by extrapolations from data at high doses (BEIR Report, NAS-NRC, 1972), it would seem equally valid (or invalid) to predict practical thresholds by the same procedure.

In summary, the preferred approach to more realistic risk estimates at low doses is not to attempt to demonstrate thresholds but to elucidate the most likely shape of the dose–response curves by as many independent lines of evidence as possible. Examples of such independent lines of approach include empirical studies, studies of RBE as a function of dose, evaluation of latency with dose, and research on mechanisms of cancer induction including the role of host factors.

## 5. Physical Factors

### 5.1. Dose Rate

There are no data on the effectiveness of low LET radiation delivered at low rates over long periods of time to human populations. All the studied populations, including those receiving multiple fractionated exposures, received the radiation at high rates. On physical grounds, it would not be expected that fractionated exposure would be the equivalent of continuous low rate exposure unless the dose per fraction was very small. The reason for this has to do with the likelihood of two or more ionizing events occurring in the target of interest in a brief time interval. At low dose rates, most of the injury will be of the single-hit variety. Multiple very small doses would also yield the same type of injury. The only human population in which doses per fraction and multiplicity of fractions would be expected to simulate continuous exposure is the occupationally exposed radiologists. Radiologists practising in the United States in the earlier part of this century indeed showed an excess of leukemia and other tumors (Seltser and Sartwell, 1965). The problem is that their radiation doses are not at all well known and there must have been major inhomogeneities of dose. Braestrup (1957) attempted to estimate their dosages based on the type of equipment employed and work practices. He has estimated an average dose of 2000 rads accumulated over many years. It can be calculated that the excess risk of leukemia in this group (relative risk of 2.5) amounts to considerably less than what would be expected from 200 rads of high dose rate exposure. Because of the great uncertainties in dose estimates and factors associated with the radiation quality, this line of evidence can be considered only as suggestive of a much lessened effectiveness of protracted exposure.

The dial painters and the patients treated with radium received their exposure continuously over a long period of time. There is no comparable group, however, that received a single brief exposure for comparison. Further, in experimental studies, high LET radiations have been shown to exert their effects relatively independently of dose rate, presumably because the majority of injury is of the multiple ionizing event type and dose rate does not affect the proportion of this type of injury with high LET radiations. It must be concluded that there are no suitable studies to evaluate the dose rate effect on carcinogenesis in man.

With very few exceptions, studies on experimental animals have shown that low LET radiation delivered at low dose rate is far less effective in producing cancer than the same total dose given at high dose rates. This general rule also applies to mutation induction.

Grahn and Sacher have systematically investigated the effects of dose rate on survival time and have shown that the lower rates are less effective by a factor of at least 5 (see review by Grahn et al., 1972) in shortening longevity. Since in the low total dose domain life shortening was entirely explainable on the basis of tumor induction, it follows that the cancerogenic effect is reduced at low rates. Leukemias and ovarian tumors, both of which are easily induced in mice, show a lower incidence at low dose rates than at high dose rates (Upton et al., 1970).

One problem in interpreting some of the experimental studies is that no correction procedures have been applied to the incidence figures. If the animals exposed at low rates survive longer than those at high rates, the observed final incidence of tumors might be the same or even higher at low rates. This could result from the animals being at risk longer or more animals being at risk in the critical period, and uncorrected values can therefore be misleading. This problem is discussed in detail by UNSCEAR (United Nations, 1972).

One notable exception to the rule of lessened effectiveness at low rates is the report by Shellabarger and Brown (1972) that the incidence of benign mammary tumors in Sprague-Dawley rats was the same whether $\gamma$-radiation was delivered at 0.03 R/min or at 10 R/min. The incidence of carcinomas was lower at the lower rate. This test system is an unusual one in many respects and apparently does not represent the general case.

Many of the reported studies have compared the effectiveness of only two dose rates, and the difference between them is often not great. Further, the lower rate is often not very low. Yuhas (1973) is currently studying the relative effectiveness in mice of $\gamma$-rays at eight different dose rates ranging from 1 rad/day to 100 rads/min. Terminated exposures are used so as to reduce the amount of wasted radiation. Four total doses are being used. A preliminary analysis shows that for some tumors the highest dose rate is not always the most effective but the lowest dose rate is always the least effective. Thus there appears to be an optimum rate for the induction of certain tumors which lies in the moderately high dose range. Some of the confusion in the literature may result from investigators not choosing low enough dose rates for making comparisons.

It is not possible to assign a single value to the effectiveness factor for low dose rate exposures with much confidence. Most studies suggest that such exposures are perhaps one-fifth to one-tenth as effective as high dose rate exposures, depending on the end point. On physical grounds, one would expect low dose rates to yield more nearly linear dose–response curves because the injury is primarily single hit and the probability of such injury should be proportional to dose. If host factors do not intervene, the effectiveness factor might then vary with dose in much the manner the RBE of neutrons varies with dose. At very low doses, the effectiveness might approximate that for high dose rates, with a progressive divergence as dose increases until some limiting value is reached. This speculation presupposes nonlinearity of response at high rates and a closer approximation to linearity at low rates. For purposes of risk estimation, linearity is assumed at high rates (BEIR Report, NAS-NRC, 1972), which would lead to a constant factor for relative effectiveness at low rates if linearity is also assumed at low rates. While committees concerned with health protection assume an effectiveness factor of unity (no effect of dose rate), the experimental studies indicate that radiation is far less effective when delivered at low rates.

## 5.2. Radiation Quality

In general, high LET radiations such as neutrons and $\alpha$-particles are more effective than low LET radiations such as X- and $\gamma$-rays. The precise value of the RBE appears to vary with total dose, dose rate, and biological end point. The data from human populations are not adequate to sort out the contribution of each of these variables, but the data are at least consistent with the general conclusion. Better concordance of the dose–response curves for leukemia induction in Nagasaki and Hiroshima is obtained if the neutron component of the radiation at Hiroshima is assigned an RBE of 5 (Ishimaru et al., 1971). The concordance is further improved if a sliding scale of RBEs ranging from 10 to 1, depending on the total dose, is applied (UNSCEAR Report, United Nations, 1972). For other tumors as well, the agreement between the data from the Japanese populations and those from other populations is improved by using an RBE of 5 for neutrons (BEIR Report, NAS-NRC, 1972). The data are not adequate, however, to reach a firm conclusion that the RBE is precisely 5. It could range from 1 to 10.

In the case of lung cancer in uranium miners exposed to $\alpha$-particles from radon and radon daughters, the risk estimates agree better with those from populations exposed to low LET radiations if an RBE of 10 is applied to the estimated $\alpha$-particle dose BEIR Report, NAS,-NRC, 1972).

It is difficult to assign an RBE to the radiation received by the radium dial painters and patients receiving radium internally because of the lack of a suitable comparison group. An RBE of 10, however, is not inconsistent with the fragmentary data from other groups.

Evidence from animals and plants strongly supports the concept that the RBE of neutrons increases with decreasing dose (see Kellerer and Rossi, 1972, for a summary). Unfortunately, data are as yet limited with respect to the RBE in carcinogenesis, although fragmentary data are consistent with this conclusion (UNSCEAR Report, United Nations, 1972).

It was pointed out earlier that high LET radiations tend to exert their effect relatively independently of dose rate (Upton, 1964; Upton et al., 1970). Since this is the case and since low LET radiation is less effective at low dose rates, it follows

that the apparent RBE for high LET radiation will increase at low dose rates, not
because these radiations are more effective, but because the baseline low LET radiation is less effective.

### 5.3. Internal Emitters vs. External Exposure

There is no evidence to suggest and no reason to believe that a cell or tissue can distinguish whether the ionizing energy it absorbs originated from radionuclides within the body or from an external radiation source. If the tissue dosages and dose rates are similar, then one would expect similar results. With few exceptions, however, it is difficult to simulate the dose distribution from an internal emitter with external sources. The reason is that the various isotopes are differentially taken up by various tissues, resulting in marked macroscopic differences in dose as well as microdosimetric differences. Despite the problems in dosimetry, studies with internal emitters have provided some of the most useful experimental data in radiation carcinogenesis since very large doses can be delivered to the organs showing a high affinity for the isotope. This gets the tumor incidence up out of the background range and dose–response relationships can be examined. Similar studies could be conducted using external beams by selective organ irradiation, but it would be most difficult to accomplish other than a brief high dose rate exposure.

### 5.4. Total-Body Exposure vs. Partial-Body Exposure

With the exception of the Japanese survivors and children receiving radiation exposure while *in utero*, the human populations studied to date received essentially partial-body irradiation. From these studies, certain general principles have emerged. The risk of induction of solid tumor at any specified site is increased only if the site is included in the radiation field. In the case of leukemia, it is necessary only to irradiate a certain fraction (as yet unspecified) of the bone marrow to increase the risk. Further, if the dose to this fraction of the marrow is averaged over the entire marrow, the leukemia risk is about the same as if the entire marrow had received this average dose. The exception to this conclusion occurs when a very limited part of the marrow receives a very high dose. Presumably in this case there is sufficient cell killing to preclude leukemic transformation. An apparent example of this effect is provided by the study on women treated intensively with radiation for cancer of the uterine cervix. Despite a high average marrow dose, there was no evidence of an increase in leukemia (Hutchison, 1968). Data are not adequate to determine whether the risk of a tumor at a particular site is greater if a specified dose is delivered to the entire body or only to the particular site of interest. If generalized host factors such as immune competence are involved in determining the outcome, it might be expected that whole-body radiation would be more effective.

As indicated in the preceding section, studies of carcinogenesis with internally deposited radionuclides are usually studies on partial-body irradiation. Not unexpectedly, tumors occur in the tissues and organs where the isotopes concentrate. Similarly, in studies with external beams, cancers occur only in the areas included in the radiation field. The situation is not as clear-cut in the case of leukemia. In contrast to the case in man, shielding of a portion of the marrow of mice greatly reduces the incidence of leukemia (see review by Upton and Cosgrove, 1968). This may result from a greater mobility of stem cells in the mouse and a consequent greater ability to repopulate irradiated areas with normal cells. It could also mean that the immune state is of more importance in mouse than in man. This could be particularly true if viral action plays a greater role in the mouse. As in man, the data are not adequate to determine whether a total-body dose is more effective in producing solid tumors of specific sites than radiation restricted to that site. Despite the experimental problems associated with this approach, particularly in mice where total-body doses can be delivered that are insufficient to produce more than a small increase in a limited number of cancer types, it should be possible to resolve this point.

## 6. Host Factors

Persons exposed to radiation as juveniles have a higher risk of leukemia and most other cancers than do persons exposed as adults. This conclusion seems amply supported by the data of Jablon and Kato (1972) for the Japanese survivors and of Spiess and Mays (1970, 1971) for patients treated with radium. The precise factor by which the risk is increased probably varies with tumor type and is difficult to estimate. It is probably highest for thyroid cancer since adults seem relatively refractory to induction of this cancer while children are quite sensitive. For osteogenic sarcomas, leukemia, and some other tumors the risk may be higher by about a factor of 2.

There have also been reports suggesting an extreme sensitivity of the human fetus to the induction of leukemia and perhaps other types of tumors (Stewart *et al.*, 1958; MacMahon and Hutchison, 1964; MacMahon, 1962; Gibson *et al.*, 1968; Stewart and Kneale, 1970; Bross and Natarajan, 1972). If the reported association between diagnostic radiation exposure and the likelihood of developing leukemia represents a causal relationship, prenatal radiation sensitivity must be astonishing since a dose of a few rads at most would increase leukemia incidence by about 50%. These reports are based on retrospective studies in which children dying from leukemia are usually identified from a tumor registry. The cases are then matched with suitable normal controls and an attempt is made to determine whether there is a difference in the previous histories of the two groups with respect to some specified variable or variables. This type of approach has been very useful in epidemiology since the study can be done reasonably quickly and the enormous sample sizes needed for prospective studies (discussed later) are not required. Studies on radiation as a possible etiological agent vary, of course, in the method of selecting the control group and in the ascertainment of whether radiation has been delivered. In a typical study, the investigator might find that 15% of the mothers of leukemic children had received diagnostic radiation (usually pelvimetry) during the relevant pregnancy, while only 10% of the mothers of control children had been so exposed, this leads to a relative risk estimate of 15/10 or 1.5.

Stewart *et al.* (1958), who appear to have been the first to report the association between *in utero* exposure and childhood cancer, initially examined the history of other factors as well and identified some (history of reproductive wastage, childhood infections) that other workers (Gibson *et al.*, 1968) subsequently confirmed as being positively associated with leukemia risk. In later reports by Stewart and her colleagues (Stewart, 1961; Stewart and Kneale, 1968, 1970), the other factors were ignored and emphasis was placed on radiation as the most likely etiological agent. It is interesting that in a study predating Stewart's, Manning and Carroll (1957) did not consider radiation history but did determine that a history of allergies leads to an increased estimate of risk. This has also been confirmed subsequently (Bross and Natarajan, 1972).

Following these early reports, a large number of studies were conducted ro attempt to confirm or refute the reported association of radiation and leukemia. Relative risk estimates, ranging from 0.42 (Lewis, 1960) to 1.72 (Kaplan, 1958), were reported, but most of these studies were conducted on a relatively modest scale. MacMahon (1962) undertook a reasonably large-scale study of the problem that differed from the earlier studies in that he used hospital records rather than interviews to determine whether radiation exposures had been given. He found a relative risk of about 1.4. MacMahon and Hutchison (1964) reviewed the earlier studies and concluded that the pooled data from all studies to that time gave a weighted best estimate of relative risk of 1.4. In 1968, Gibson *et al.* reported on a very large-scale study of this problem. They identified four factors as being associated with an increased risk of leukemia. These were a history of (1) *in utero* radiation, (2) preconception radiation to either parent, (3) reproductive wastage (earlier stillbirths or abortions), and (4) childhood viral disease. When each was considered singly and in the absence of any of the others, the risk estimates were greatly reduced. for example, if there was only a history of *in utero* radiation and none of the other factors, the relative risk was only 1.06. It was only when the variables were combined that the risk estimates increased, with a maximum risk in the group having a history of all four factors. Bross and Natarajan (1972) have recently reanalyzed the same data and reported somewhat higher risk estimates.

For establishing cause and effect rather than identifying an association, prospective studies are preferred. In prospective studies, a population exposed to the factor and a control population are first identified and then the determination is made of what subsequently happened with respect to the incidence of the disease in question. Such studies are enormously difficult in the case of a rare disease like leukemia because of the very large sample sizes required. Three such studies have been made in the case of children receiving *in utero* radiation. Court Brown *et al.* (1960) studied a population of about 40,000 such children. Based on the incidence of leukemia in the general population, they expected an incidence of 10.5 cases in their treated population but observed only 9. Griem *et al.* (1967) studied about 1000 cases in which women were subjected to routine X-ray pelvimetry (and thus there was no selection which might bias the results) and found no leukemia, but, of course, the population size was quite small. Diamond (1968) evaluated leukemia incidence in a population of 20,000 irradiated children and 40,000 controls. He found an increase of the disease in the irradiated white segment of the population but a decrease in blacks. Thus the three prospective studies were negative, but the sample sizes were probably not large enough to detect less than a 40 or 50% increase in risk.

More recently, Stewart and Kneale (1970) reported a linear increase in relative risk of cancer with the number of X-ray films taken (radiation dose). From this, they estimated the excess cancer risk at 572 cases per million per rad of exposure. Jablon and Kato (1970) examined the validity of this estimate in light of the Japanese experience. About 1300 Japanese children received significant *in utero* exposure at the time of the bombing. Although the number is small, the product of number of people times the average dose is large, about 35,000 man-rads. (If a linear, no-threshold relationship is assumed, the expected number of cases can be calculated from the product of people times dose or man-rads. Thus the expected number of cases is the same if 1 million people are exposed to 1 rad or if 10,000 people are exposed to 100 rads. This can lead to some unusual conclusions if the dose–response curve is clearly non-linear as in the case of epilation; e.g., see Evans *et al.*, 1972.) From Stewart and Kneale's estimate, about 20 cases of cancer in the Japanese children would have been expected. No cases of leukemia were observed. Only one case of cancer of any type (liver) was seen in this population, while the expectation at national rates was about 0.75.

In view of the above uncertainties and particularly in view of the fact that leukemia induction may result from the complex interplay of a number of factors, it is concluded that the question of extreme sensitivity of parental children to leukemia induction by radiation remains unresolved. Certainly risk estimates based on the available evidence are very tenuous at best.

Juvenile experimental animals, particularly mice, are, like man, more susceptible to a number of radiogenic neoplasms (Kaplan, 1948; Upton *et al.*, 1960; Lindop and Rotblat, 1962). In contrast to the suggested very high susceptibility of prenatal children, the fetal stages in animals do not show increased sensitivity and in some cases have appeared to be refractory (Upton *et al.*, 1960; Upton, 1964; Upton *et al.*, 1966; Rugh *et al.*, 1966; Warren and Gates, 1969). When very old animals (mice) are irradiated, they do not show an increased tumor incidence (Storer, 1973), probably because the latent period exceeds the remaining life expectancy. This lack of effect is probably also true for man but is ignored if the period of follow-up is short (due to death from other causes).

## 7. Relationship to Spontaneous Incidence Rate

Radiation either could induce an absolute number of new tumors independent of the spontaneous incidence rate or could act multiplicatively with the spontaneous rate. In the former case, the appropriate method of expressing risk would be the "absolute" risk; i.e., a specified dose of radiation would be expected to yield some number of tumors independently of whether the spontaneous incidence is high or low. If, on the other hand, radiation acts multiplicatively and the increase in number of cases depends on natural incidence, then the "relative" risk is the proper expression. The difference in these two concepts is of more than trivial significance. For administrative convenience, one would hope that the absolute risk concept is correct because then risk estimates would be independent of race, geography, epoch, and presence or absence of cocarcinogenic factors. Nature rarely takes cognizance of administrative convenience, however, and it seems likely that for some tumors, at least, the relative risk may be proper. This could depend on what factors are involved in the so-called natural incidence.

Data from human populations are inadequate to choose between these two alternatives and both methods are used in risk estimates, although perhaps the majority of epidemiologists use the relative risk because of convenience. The issue could perhaps be resolved by animal experimentation, although at the present time experimental data are also inadequate for the evaluation.

## 8. Effect on Longevity

It has long been believed by many investigators that radiation causes a nonspecific life shortening that might be the equivalent of premature or accelerated aging. This is formally equivalent to an increased mortality rate, particularly at later ages. Dublin and Spiegelman (1948) reported a mortality ratio of 1.3 for U.S. radiologists compared to other physicians. In 1956, Warren estimated a loss of longevity in radiologists practicing before 1942 of about 5 yr. Seltser and Sartwell (1965) reexamined this question and found excess mortality from all causes in the radiologists as compared to ophthalmologists-otolaryngologists. Court Brown and Doll (1958), however, did not find such an effect in British radiologists, but possibly their radiation exposures were lower because of differences in safety practices. Court Brown and Doll (1965) found excess mortality from a variety of causes in the irradiated spondylitics. Since the excess incidence of cancer and leukemia in the U.S. radiologists and in the spondylitics did not account for the loss of longevity, this seemed good evidence of nonspecific life shortening, a conclusion in apparently good agreement with studies in many species of experimental animals.

More recently, Jablon and Kato (1972) in a report on the mortality experience at ABCC through 1970 in persons exposed to more than 200 rads did not find excess mortality for several categories of disease including cerebrovascular disease and circulatory disease, two very common causes of death. Mortality from leukemia and from other cancers was significantly increased, as was death from all causes (which includes neoplasms). Deaths from all diseases except neoplasms were increased slightly (mortality ratio of 1.12) but nothing like the extent of the increase for neoplasms. Thus the concept of nonspecific life shortening in man is called into serious question.

Based on studies in mice where careful autopsies were performed, Walburg and Cosgrove (1970), Grahn et al. (1972), and Storer (1973) have concluded that in the low to moderate dose range, the loss of longevity in mice can be accounted for solely on the basis of increased tumor incidence. At higher doses, particularly in female mice, there is a component of life shortening that has not yet been accounted for (Storer, 1973), but it seems likely that it results from specific radiogenic diseases as yet unrecognized rather than an across-the-board premature aging.

## 9. Interactions with Other Agents

When studies on the interaction of radiation with chemical, physical, or biological agents are undertaken, there are myriad (almost infinite) possible combinations and permutations of agents, dosages, and treatment schedules. This is perhaps the reason that interest in studying such interactions has been limited. A classic example of a synergistic effect in human populations is provided by studies on lung cancer in uranium miners. Nearly every case of lung cancer occurred in cigarette smokers (see review by Bair, 1970). Examples of experimental studies of interactions are provided by the reports of Shubik et al. (1953), Upton et al. (1961), Lindsay and Chaikoff (1964), Lindop and Rotblat (1966), Berenblum et al. (1968), Cole and Foley (1969), Telles et al. (1969), Segaloff and Maxfield (1971), Epstein (1972), and Shellabarger and Straub (1972). In general, the two-stage concept of cancer induction, namely initiation and promotion, as advanced by Berenblum (1941) seems to apply reasonably well to these interaction studies (see Berenblum, this volume). Radiation at sufficiently high doses is a complete carcinogen in that it serves as both initiator and promotor. There are a number of strong chemical carcinogens that act the same way. When large doses of radiation are combined with high doses of a strong carcinogen, it would be expected that no particular synergism would be obtained and the resulting tumor yield would be that predicted by independent action. This was found to be the case in a study by Shellabarger and Straub (1972) in which breast tumors in rats were induced by neutrons combined with methylcholanthrene. If initiating doses of radiation are combined with a promoting agent such as croton oil or urethan, one would predict synergism, and such effects have been reported (Shubik et al., 1953; Cole and Foley, 1969). There are problems in interpreting much of the existing experimental data because it is not always clear that the sequence of administration of the agents was optimal, full dose–response curves are rarely run, and in cases of fatal tumors the data are usually not corrected for competing risks. It is probably possible to predict the outcome of combining radiation and other agents based on the characteristics of each agent (if these are adequately known) and the dose level used. However, such predictions have not been adequately tested.

The mechanism by which ionizing radiation induces tumors remains obscure, although increasing evidence is accumulating which implicates a number of variables. In certain murine tumors, the activation or release of oncogenic viruses must play a major role. For man, however, there is no good evidence that an effect mediated through viruses occurs. In recent years, there has been intensive investigation of the role of the immune system in carcinogenesis. Since radiation is a potent immunosuppressor, it is apparent that this could be a factor in radiation carcinogenesis. Radiation effects on the immune system have been extensively reviewed in the recent UNSCEAR Report (United Nations, 1972). The concept that somatic cell mutations are the initiating change in cancer induction is widely supported, but direct experimental proof remains elusive. Many carcinogens are also potent mutagens, which supports but does not prove the somatic mutation hypothesis. Endocrine imbalances are almost certainly involved in the induction of some tumors of experimental animals, particularly female mice.

One thing that confounds the interpretation of experiments in the general areas mentioned above is the role of cell killing and subsequent increased rate of cellular proliferation. For example, immunosuppression is attained only by killing immunocompetent cells, and it may be significant that the principal induced tumors in immunosuppressed patients are reticulum cell sarcomas. Radiation may activate latent endogenous viruses, but cellular proliferation is apparently necessary for amplification of the effect. Carcinogens are capable of cell killing or at least inhibition of mitosis, both of which lead to a later increase in cellular proliferation. Potent mutagens are also capable of cell killing, and mutational change is very likely a major mechanism of cell death. A cancer-producing endocrine imbalance in irradiated female mice apparently results from killing of the very sensitive oocytes. In view of these considerations, it seems likely that cell killing plays a primary role in radiation carcinogenesis even though the intermediate steps (immune suppression, viral amplification, endocrine effects, etc.) may be varied.

## 11. References

ALBERT, R. E., AND OMRAN, A. R., 1968, Follow-up study of patients treated by X-ray epilation for tinea capitis. 1. Population characteristics, post-treatment illnesses, and mortality experience, *Arch. Environ. Health* **17**:899.

BAIR, W. J., 1970, Inhalation of radionuclides and carcinogenesis, in: *Inhalation Carcinogenesis* (P. Nettesheim, M. G. Hanna, Jr., and J. R. Gilbert, eds.), pp. 77–97, USAEC Division of Technical Information, Symposium Series 18, National Technical Information Service, Springfield, Va., CONF–691001.

BEEBE, G. W., KATO, H., AND LAND, C. E., 1971, Studies on the mortality of A-bomb survivors. 4. Mortality and radiation dose, 1950–1966, *Radiation Res.* **48**:613.

BELSKY, J. L., TACHIKAWA, K., CIHAK, R. W., AND YAMOMOTO, T., 1972, Salivary gland tumors in atomic bomb survivors, Hiroshima–Nagasaki, 1957 to 1970, *JAMA* **219**:864.

BERENBLUM, I., 1941, The mechanism of carcinogenesis: A study of the significance of carcinogenic action and related phenomena, *Cancer Res.* **1**:807.

BERENBLUM, I., CHEN, L., AND TRAININ, N., 1968, A quantitative study of the leukemogenic action of whole-body x-irradiation and urethane, *Israel J. Med. Sci.* **4:**1159.

BLOCH, C., 1962, Osteogenic sarcoma: Report of a case and review of literature, *Am. J. Roentgenol.* **87:**1157.

BRAESTRUP, C. B., 1957, Past and present radiation exposure to radiologists from the point of view of life expectancy, *Am. J. Roentgenol.* **78:**988.

BROSS, I. D. J., AND NATARAJAN, N., 1972, Leukemia from low level radiation, *New Engl. J. Med.* **287:**107.

BROWN, D. G., JOHNSON, D. F., AND CROSS, F. H., 1965, Late Effects observed in burros surviving external whole-body gamma irradiation, *Radiation Res.* **25:**574.

BURNS, F. J., ALBERT, R. E., AND HEIMBACH, R. D., 1968, RBE for skin tumors and hair follicle damage in the rat following irradiation with alpha particles and electrons, *Radiation Res.* **36:**225.

COLE, L. J., AND FOLEY, W. A., 1969, Modification of urethan–lung tumor incidence by low x-radiation doses, cortisone and transfusion of isogenic lymphocytes, *Radiation Res.* **39:**391.

CONRAD, R. A., DOBYNS, B. M., AND SUTOW, W. W., 1970, Thyroid neoplasia as late effect of exposure to radioactive iodine in fallout, *JAMA* **214:**316.

COURT BROWN, W. M., AND DOLL, R., 1958, Expectation of life and mortality from cancer among British radiologists, *Brit. Med. J.* **2:**181.

COURT BROWN, W. M., AND DOLL, R., 1965, Mortality from cancer and other causes after radiotherapy for ankylosing spondylitis, *Brit. Med. J.* **2:**1327.

COURT BROWN, W. M., DOLL, R., AND HILL, A. B., 1960, Incidence of leukemia after exposure to diagnostic radiation *in utero, Brit. Med. J.* **2:**1539.

DIAMOND, E. L., 1968, Unpublished studies. Cited by Kessler, I. I., and Lilienfeld, A. M., 1969, Perspectives in the epidemiology of leukemia, in: *Advances in Cancer Research*, Vol. 12 (G. Klein and S. Weinhouse, eds.), pp. 225–302, Academic Press, New York.

DOLL, R., AND SMITH, P. G., 1968, The long-term effects of x irradiation in patients treated for metropathia haemorrhagica, *Brit. J. Radiol.* **41:**362.

DOUGHERTY, T. F., AND MAYS, C. W., 1969, Bone cancer induced by internally-deposited emitters in beagles, in: *Radiation-Induced Cancer*, pp. 361–367, IAEA, Vienna.

DUBLIN, L. I., AND SPIEGELMAN, M., 1948, Mortality of medical specialists 1938–1942, *JAMA* **137:**1519.

EPSTEIN, J. H., 1972, Examination of the carcinogenic and cocarcinogenic effects of Grenz radiation, *Cancer Res.* **32:**2625.

EVANS, R. D., KEANE, A. T., KOLENKOW, R. J., NEAL, W. R., AND SHANAHAN, M. M., 1969, Radiogenic tumors in the radium and mesothorium cases studied at M.I.T., in: *Delayed Effects of Bone-Seeking Radionuclides* (C. W. Mays, W. S. S. Jee, R. D. Lloyd, B. J. Stover, J. H. Dougherty, and G. N. Taylor, eds.), pp. 157–194, University of Utah Press, Salt Lake City.

EVANS, R. D., KEANE, A. T., AND SHANAHAN, M. M., 1972, Radiogenic effects in man of long-term skeletal alpha-irradiation, in: *Radiobiology of Plutonium* (B. J. Stover and W. S. S. Jee, eds.), pp. 431–468, The J. W. Press, Salt Lake City.

FINKEL, M. P., AND BISKIS, B. O., 1962, Toxicity of plutonium in mice, *Health Phys.* **8:**565.

FINKEL, M. P., BISKIS, B. O., AND JINKINS, P. B., 1969, Toxicity of radium-226 in mice, in: *Radiation-Induced Cancer*, pp. 369–391, IAEA, Vienna.

FURTH, J., UPTON, A. C., AND KIMBALL, A. W., 1959, Late pathologic effects of atomic detonation and their pathogenesis, *Radiation Res. Suppl.* **1:**243.

GIBSON, R. W., BROSS, I. D. J., GRAHAM, S., LILIENFELD, A. M., SCHUMAN, L. M., LEVIN, M. L., AND DOWD, J. E., 1968, Leukemia in children exposed to multiple risk factors, *New Engl. J. Med.* **279:**906.

GRAHN, D., FRY, R. J. M., AND LEA, R. A., 1972, Analysis of survival and cause of death statistics for mice under single and duration-of-life gamma irradiation, in: *Life Sciences and Space Research*, Vol. X (A. C. Strickland, ed.), Akademie-Verlag, Berlin.

GRIEM, M. D., MEIER, P., AND DOBBEN, G. D., 1967, Analysis of the morbidity and mortality of children irradiated in fetal life, *Radiology* **88:**347.

HAZEN, R. W., PIFER, J. W., TAYOOKA, T., LIVENGOOD, J., AND HEMPELMANN, L. H., 1966, Neoplasms following irradiation of the head, *Cancer Res.* **26:**305.

HEMPELMANN, L. H., PIFER, J. W., BURKE, G. W., TERRY, R., AND AMES, W. R., 1967, Neoplasms in persons treated with X-rays in infancy for thymic enlargement: A report of third follow-up survey, *J. Natl. Cancer Inst.* **38:**317.

HOEL, D. G., AND WALBURG, H. E., JR., 1972, Statistical analysis of survival experiments, *J. Natl. Cancer Inst.* **49:**361.

HUG, O., GÖSSNER, W., MÜLLER, W. A., LUZ, A., AND HINDRINGER, B., 1969, Production of osteosarcomas in mice and rats by incorporation of radium-224, in: *Radiation-Induced Cancer*, pp. 393–409, IAEA, Vienna.

HULSE, E. V., 1967, Incidence and pathogenesis of skin tumors in mice irradiated with single external doses of low energy beta particles, *Brit. J. Cancer* **21**:531.

HUTCHISON, G. B., 1968, Leukemia in patients with cancer of the cervix uteri treated with radiation: A report covering the first 5 years of an international study, *J. Natl. Cancer Inst.* **40**:951.

International Commission on Radiological Protection, 1969, *Publication 14: Radiosensitivity and Spatial Distribution of Dose*, Pergamon Press, Oxford.

ISHIMARU, T., HOSHINO, T., ICHIMARU, M., OKADA, H., TOMIYASU, T., TSUCHIMOTO, T., AND YAMAMOTO, T., 1971, Leukemia in atomic bomb survivors, Hiroshima and Nagasaki, 1 October 1950–30 September 1966, *Radiation Res.* **45**:216.

JABLON, S., AND KATO, H., 1970, Childhood cancer in relation to prenatal exposure to atomic-bomb radiation, *Lancet* **2**:1000.

JABLON, S., AND KATO, H., 1972, Studies of the mortality of a-bomb survivors. 5. Radiation dose and mortality, 1950–1970, *Radiation Res.* **50**:649.

JOHNSON, M. L. T., LAND, C. E., GREGORY, P. B., TAURA, T., AND MILTON, R. C., 1969, *Effects of Ionizing Radiation on the Skin, Hiroshima–Nagasaki*, ABCC TR 20–69.

KAPLAN, H. S., 1948, Influence of age on susceptibility of mice to the development of lymphoid after irradiation, *J. Natl. Cancer Inst.* **9**:55.

KAPLAN, H. S., 1958, An evaluation of the somatic and genetic hazards of the medical uses of radiation, *Am. J. Roentgenol.* **80**:696.

KELLERER, A. M., AND ROSSI, H. H., 1972, The theory of dual radiation action, *Curr. Topics Radiation Res. Quart.* **8**:85.

LEWIS, T. L. T., 1960, Leukemia in childhood after antenatal exposure to X-rays, *Brit. Med. J.* **2**:1551.

LINDOP, P. J., AND ROTBLAT, J., 1962, The age factor in the susceptibility of man and animals to radiation, I. The age factor in radiation sensitivity in mice, *Brit. J. Radiol.* **35**:23.

LINDOP, P. J., AND ROTBLAT, J., 1966, Induction of lung tumors by the action of radiation and urethane, *Nature (Lond.)* **210**:1392.

LINDSAY, S., AND CHAIKOFF, 1964, The effects of irradiation on the thyroid gland with particular reference to the induction of thyroid neoplasms: A review, *Cancer Res.* **24**:1099.

LUNDIN, F. E., JR., WAGONER, J. K., AND ARCHER, V. E., 1971, *Radon Daughter Exposure and respiratory Cancer: Quantitative and Temporal Aspects*, Report from the epidemiological study of United States uranium miners, NIOSH-NIEHS Joint Monograph No. 1., U.S. Public Health Service, National Technical Information Service, Springfield, Va., P.B. 204–871.

MACKENZIE, I., 1965, Breast cancer following multiple fluoroscopies, *Brit. J. Cancer* **19**:1.

MACMAHON, B., 1962, Prenatal x ray exposure and childhood cancer, *J. Natl. Cancer Inst.* **28**:1173.

MACMAHON, B., AND HUTCHISON, G. B., 1964, Prenatal x-ray and childhood cancer: A review, *Acta Unio. Int. Contra Cancrum* **20**:1172.

MALDAGUE, P., 1969, Comparative study of experimentally induced cancer of the kidney in mice and rats with x-rays, in: *Radiation-Induced Cancer*, pp. 439–458, IAEA, Vienna.

MANNING, M. D., AND CARROLL, B. E., 1957, Some epidemiological aspects of leukemia in children, *J. Natl. Cancer Inst.* **19**:1087.

MAYS, C. W., AND LLOYD, R. D., 1972a, Bone sarcoma risk from $^{90}$Sr, in: *Biomedical Implications of Radiostrontium Exposure* (M. Goldman and L. K. Bustad, eds.), pp. 352–370, USAEC Division of Technical Information, Symposium Series 25, National Technical Information Service, Springfield, Va., CONF-710201.

MAYS, C. W., AND LLOYD, R. D., 1972b, Bone sarcoma incidence vs. alpha particle dose, in: *Radiobiology of Plutonium* (B. J. Stover and W. S. S. Jee, eds.), pp. 409–430, The J. W. Press, Salt Lake City.

METTLER, F. A., HEMPELMANN, L. H., DUTTON, A. M., PIFER, J. W., TOYOOKA, E. T., AND AMES, W. R., 1969, Breast neoplasms in women treated with X-rays for acute post-partum mastitis: A pilot study, *J. Natl. Cancer Inst.* **43**:803.

MYRDEN, J. A., AND HILTZ, J. E., 1969, Breast cancer following multiple fluoroscopies during artificial pneumothorax treatment of pulmonary tuberculosis, *Canad. Med. Assoc. J.* **100**:1032.

NATIONAL ACADEMY OF SCIENCES–NATIONAL RESEARCH COUNCIL, 1972, *The Effects on Populations of Exposure to Low Levels of Ionizing Radiation*, Report of the Advisory Committee on the Biological Effects of Ionizing Radiations, Washington, D.C.

NILSSON, A., 1970, Pathologic effects of different doses of radiostrontium in mice: Dose effect relationship in $^{90}$Sr-induced bone tumors, *Acta Radiol. Ther. Phys. Biol.* **9**:155.

PIFER, J. W., HEMPELMANN, L. H., DODGE, H. J., AND HODGES, F. J., II, 1968, Neoplasms in the Ann Arbor series of thymus irradiated children; a second survey, *Am. J. Roentgenol. Radium Ther. Nuclear Med.* **103**:13.

RUGH, R., DUHAMEL, L., AND SKAREDOFF, L., 1966, Relation of embryonic and fetal x irradiation to life time average weights and tumor incidence in mice, *Proc. Soc. Exp. Biol. Med.* **121**:714.

SAENGER, E. L., SILVERMAN, F. N., STERLING, T. D., AND TURNER, M. E., 1960, Neoplasia following therapeutic irradiation for benign conditions in childhood, *Radiology* **74**:889.

SAENGER, E. I., SILVERMAN, F. N., STERLING, T. D., AND TURNER, M. E., 1960, Neoplasia following therapeutic irradiation for benign conditions in childhood, *Radiology* **74**:889.

SCHULZ, R. J., AND ALBERT, R. E., 1968, III. Dose to organs of the head from the X-ray treatment of tinea capitis, *Arch. Environ. Health* **17**:935.

SEGALOFF, A., AND MAXFIELD, W. S., 1971, The synergism between radiation and estrogen in the production of mammary cancer in the rat, *Cancer Res.* **31**:168.

SELTSER, R., AND SARTWELL, P. E., 1965, The influence of occupational exposure to radiation on the mortality of American radiologists and other medical specialists, *Am. J. Epidemiol.* **81**:2.

SHELLABARGER, C. J., AND BROWN, R. D., 1972, Rat mammary neoplasia following $^{60}$Co irradiation at 0.03 R or 10 R per minute, *Radiation Res.* **51**:493.

SHELLABARGER, C. J., AND STRAUB, R., 1972, Effect of 3-methylcholanthrene and fission neutron irradiation, given singly or combined, on rat mammary carcinogenesis, *J. Natl. Cancer Inst.* **48**:185.

SHELLABARGER, C. J., BOND, V. P., CRONKITE, E. P., AND APONTE, G. E., 1969, Relationship of dose of total-body $^{60}$Co radiation to incidence of mammary neoplasia in female rats, in: *Radiation-Induced Cancer*, pp. 161–172, IAEA, Vienna.

SHUBIK, P., GOLDFARB, A. R., RITCHIE, A. C., AND LISCO, H., 1953, Latent carcinogenic action of beta-irradiation on mouse epidermis, *Nature (Lond.)* **171**:934.

SPIESS, H., AND MAYS, C. W., 1970, Bone cancers induced by $^{224}$Ra(ThX) in children and adults, *Health Phys.* **19**:713.

SPIESS, H., AND MAYS, C. W., 1971, Erratum, *Health Phys.* **20**:543.

STEINITZ, R., 1965, Pulmonary tuberculosis and carcinoma of the lung, *Am. Rev. Resp. Dis.* **92**:758.

STEWART, A., 1961, Aetiology of childhood malignancies, *Brit. Med. J.* **1**:452.

STEWART, A., AND KNEALE, G. W., 1968, Changes in the cancer risk associated with obstetric radiography, *Lancet* **1**:104.

STEWART, A., AND KNEALE, G. W., 1970, Radiation dose effects in relation to obstetric X-rays and childhood cancers, *Lancet* **1**:1185.

STEWART, A., WEBB, J., AND HEWITT, D., 1958, A survey of childhood malignancies, *Brit. Med. J.* **1**:1495.

STORER, J. B., 1973, Unpublished data.

TELLES, N. C., WARD, B. C., WILLENSKY, E. A., AND JESSUP, G. L., 1969, Radiation–ethionine carcinogenesis, in: *Radiation-Induced Cancer*, pp. 233–245, IAEA, Vienna.

UNITED NATIONS, 1972, *Ionizing Radiation: Levels and Effects*, Vol. II: *Effects*, Report of the United Nations Scientific Committee on the Effects of Atomic Radiation, United Nations, New York.

UPTON, A. C., 1964, Comparative aspects of carcinogenesis by ionizing radiation, *Natl. Cancer Inst. Monogr.* **14**:221.

UPTON, A. C., AND COSGROVE, G. E., 1968, Radiation induced leukemia, in: *Experimental Leukemia* (M. Rich, ed.), pp. 131–158, Appleton-Century-Crofts, New York.

UPTON, A. C., ODELL, T. T., JR., AND SNIFFEN, E. P., 1960, Influence of age at time of irradiation on induction of leukemia and ovarian tumors in RF mice, *Proc. Soc. Exp. Biol. Med.* **104**:769.

UPTON, A. C., WOLFF, F. F., AND SNIFFEN, E. P., 1961, Leukemogenic effect of myleran on the mouse thymus, *Proc. Soc. Exp. Biol. Med.* **108**:464.

UPTON, A. C., JENKINS, V. K., AND CONKLIN, J. W., 1964, Myeloid leukemia in the mouse, *Ann. N.Y. Acad. Sci.* **114(1)**:189.

UPTON, A. C., CONKLIN, J. W., AND POPP, R. A., 1966, Influence of age at irradiation on susceptibility to radiation-induced life-shortening in RF mice, in: *Radiation and Ageing* (P. J. Lindop and G. A. Sacher, eds.), pp. 337–344, Taylor & Francis, London.

UPTON, A. C., RANDOLPH, M. L., AND CONKLIN, J. W., 1970, Late effects of fast neutrons and gamma-rays in mice as influenced by the dose rate of irradiation: Induction of neoplasia, *Radiation Res.* **41**:467.

WALBURG, H. E., JR., AND COSGROVE, G. E., 1970, Life shortening and cause of death in irradiated germ free mice, in: *Proceedings of the First European Symposium on Late Effects of Radiation* (P. Metalli, ed.), pp. 51–67, Comitato Nazionale Energia Nucleare, Roma.

WANEBO, C. K., JOHNSON, K. G., SATO, K., AND THORSLUND, T. W., 1968a, Breast cancer after exposure to the atomic bombings of Hiroshima and Nagasaki, *New Engl. J. Med.* **279**:667.

WANEBO, C. K., JOHNSON, K. G., SATO, K., AND THORSLUND, T. W., 1968b, Lung cancer following atomic radiation, *Am. Rev. Resp. Dis.* **98**:778.

WARREN, S., 1956, Longevity and causes of death from irradiation in physicians, *JAMA* **162**:464.

WARREN, S., AND GATES, O., 1969, Effects of continuous irradiation of mice from conception to weaning, in: *Radiation Biology of the Fetal and Juvenile Mammal* (M. R. Sikov and D. D. Mahlum, eds.), pp. 419–437, USAEC Technical Information Division, Symposium Series 17, National Technical Information Service, Springfield, Va., CONF–690501.

WOOD, J. W., TAMAGAKI, H., NERIISKI, S., SATO, T., SHELDON, W. F., ARCHER, P. G., HAMILTON, H. B., AND JOHNSON, K. G., 1969, Thyroid carcinoma in atomic bomb survivors Hiroshima and Nagasaki, *Am. J. Epidemiol.* **89**:4.

YAMAMOTO, T., AND WAKABAYASKI, T., 1968, *Bone Tumors Among the Atomic Bomb Survivors of Hiroshima and Nagasaki*, ABCC TR 26–68.

YAMAMOTO, T., KATO, H., ISHIDA, K., TAHARA, E., AND MCGREGOR, D. H., 1970, Gastric carcinoma in fixed population, Hiroshima and Nagasaki, *Gann* **61**:473.

YUHAS, J. M., 1973, Personal communication.

# 17

# Foreign Body Induced Sarcomas

K. Gerhard Brand

## 1. Introduction

Several reviews on foreign body (FB) induced tumors have been published in recent years, notably those of Bischoff and Bryson (1964), who proposed the term "solid state carcinogenesis," Bryson and Bischoff (1969), Ott (1970), and Bischoff (1972). The reader is referred to these monographs, which, taken together, provide a complete bibliography on this subject up to early 1972. There are some differences in the selection of references since the reviewers concentrated on diverse aspects of FB tumorigenesis such as histopathology, chemical and physical properties of implant materials, biocompatibility, methodology of safety testing, or historical accounts. Most of the references listed there have been omitted from the reference section of this chapter because it was not intended to create an updated all-encompassing version of earlier reviews. Instead, the emphasis is on etiological aspects, in accordance with the general orientation of this volume. By elaboration of this perspective, the scope of preceding reviews is extended and a new spectrum of relevant literature is drawn into the discussion.

## 2. Historical Background

Tumors in man associated with FBs, chronic sclerosing FB reactions, chronic inflammation, or scars have been reported occasionally since 1888 (Ott, 1970). These were singular observations, however, and the question of an etiological

K. Gerhard Brand ● Department of Microbiology, University of Minnesota Medical School, Minneapolis, Minnesota.

relationship was always left open, although it was raised. Around the 1940s, several investigators found (Bischoff and Bryson, 1964) that rats may develop sarcomas in connection with plastic materials implanted for various experimental purposes at various body sites. This observation was explored during the 1950s by a number of research groups, especially Oppenheimer *et al.*, Nothdurft, Zollinger, Druckrey and Schmähl, Alexander, and Kogan *et al.* The etiological role of FBs was established beyond any doubt. By excluding chemical factors, the conclusion was reached that the physical presence and nature of the FB were singularly responsible for tumorigenesis. In view of the fact that artificial implants of various kinds were increasingly employed by surgeons for anatomical, functional, or cosmetic reasons, most of the research work during the 1960s was concerned with problems of biocompatibility (Bischoff, 1972). Only in recent years has FB tumorigenesis been used as a method for etiological studies of cancer in general.

### 3. Foreign Body-Associated Tumors in Man

Considering the increasing frequency of FB implantations in humans during the preceding two decades, the actual number of FB-associated tumors is surprisingly small compared to experimental FB tumorigenicity in mice and rats. This is documented by several follow-up reports on patients who had received artificial implants. No tumors were detected by Rubin *et al.* (1971) among 281 patients with facial prostheses, nor by de Cholnoky (1970) among 11,000 women who underwent mamma augmentation by various techniques with various materials. Negative reports were also submitted by Spence (1954), Dutton (1959), Dukes and Mitchley (1962), Johnson (1965), Hoopes *et al.* (1967), Howe and Rastelli (1969), and Calnan (1970).

Apparently true differences exist between the human and murine species regarding general susceptibility to FB tumorigenesis, as will be discussed later in more detail. The statistical difference in tumor incidence may relate at least in part to differences in average tumor latency. Whereas in mice FB tumor latency ranges from 6 to 24 months (depending on various determining factors), in man it is a matter of years. Since artificial implantations are more often performed in older patients, tumor latency may actually exceed life expectancy in many cases. A tumor latency of 10 yr was reported by Burns *et al.* (1969) for a sarcoma following arterial repair by means of a Teflon–Dacron graft. A chondrosarcoma developed 18 yr after implantation of Lucite spheres for the purpose of lung plombage (Thompson and Entin, 1969). Ott (1970) has tabulated all cases published until 1966, several of them with latencies of over 40 yr. In these cases, the responsible FBs were mainly metal implants, bullets, shrapnel pieces, bone transplants, etc. Recently, sarcomas were observed in connection with implanted plastic materials (Bischoff, 1972). Ott (1970) includes in this etiological category sarcomas which reportedly developed from extensive chronic scars, especially as a result of deep burns. He also mentions a few carcinomas connected with chronic purulent inflammation around FBs.

Despite the rarity of FB tumors in man, it would be irresponsible to look at the situation with complacency. Several measures are at our disposal which would minimize the probability of FB tumors in man (Bauer, 1963 ; Brand, 1970; Brand and Brand, 1973). These include (1) a more restrictive approach to artificial implantations, especially the exclusion of medically unnecessary cosmetic procedures, unless they are indicated for psychiatric reasons; (2) smallest possible size of implants; (3) reexaminations of implant carriers at frequent intervals; (4) a centralized registry for gathering information on general complications as well as instances of neoplasia; (5) continued research (a) on implant materials regarding their suitability for specific surgical purposes and (b) on etiological questions concerning this type of neoplasia.

Two human tumor entities which are of great concern, asbestosis of the lung and bladder cancer resulting from chronic *Schistosoma haematobium* infection, have several features in common with FB-induced tumorigenesis, as will be discussed later in more detail (Bryson and Bischoff, 1967; Milne, 1969; Wagner and Berry, 1969; McDonald *et al.*, 1970; Roberts, 1970; Pott and Friedrichs, 1972; Stanton and Wrench, 1972; Maroudas *et al.*, 1973; Domingo and Warren, 1968; von Lichtenberg *et al.*, 1971; Kuntz *et al.*, 1972). It is to be expected, therefore, that research on FB sarcomas may contribute to the elucidation of those types of cancer as well.

## 4 Characteristics of Foreign Body-Sarcomas

### 4.1. Histopathology

A conspicuous characteristic of FB sarcomas is that they appear in a great variety of histological types. In man, these include fibrosarcomas (Burns *et al.*, 1969), chondrosarcomas (Thompson and Entin, 1969), meningiomas (Bischoff, 1972), as well as asbestos-induced mesotheliomas (Milne, 1969; McDonald *et al.*, 1970; Roberts, 1970; Stanton and Wrench, 1972). The findings in rats are similar (Oppenheimer *et al.*, 1955, 1964; Alexander and Horning, 1959; Carter and Roe, 1969; Wagner and Berry, 1969), including rhabdomyosarcomas, mesenchymomas, liposarcomas, reticulosarcomas, plasmocytomas, and histiocytomas (Ott, 1970). In mice, Langvad (1968) and Johnson *et al.* (1973b) found anaplastic sarcomas with myxoid areas, hemangiosarcomas, bone-forming sarcomas, and reticulosarcomas.

FB sarcomas can be grouped according to degree of anaplasticity (Johnson *et al.*, 1970). Four classes have been proposed and defined as follows: (I) well-differentiated sarcomas with low mitotic rate and minimal pleomorphism, usually containing some collagen; (II) spindle cell sarcomas with slightly higher mitotic rate and greater pleomorphism, containing little or no collagen; (III) anaplastic invasive round cell sarcomas with areas of necrosis and hemorrhage, and with high mitotic rate and hyperchromatic nuclei; (IV) anaplastic sarcomas as in (III), but with numerous multinucleated cells. The majority of tumors examined by Johnson *et al.* (1970, 1973*b*) fell into classes (III) and (IV).

### 4.2. Ultrastructure

Electron microscopic studies were carried out on a large selection of FB-sarcomas induced in mice (Johnson *et al.*, 1973*b*). Cells of all tumors contained nonbranching microfilaments, about 60 Å in width, which were scattered diffusely throughout the cytoplasmic matrix or were arranged in perinuclear or cytoplasmic bundles. Extracellularly they formed irregular deposits resembling basal laminae. Ample numbers of lysosomes were also regularly evident. Smooth-surfaced endoplasmic reticulum was found restricted to the Golgi region. In many but not all tumors, and most abundantly in hemangiosarcomas, intercellular junctions of the adherens type were found manifested as electron densities along the cytoplasmic surfaces of adjacent cell membranes.

Specifically in sarcomas with higher degrees of anaplasticity, rough endoplasmic reticulum presented itself in the form of short irregular profiles, often with dilated cisternae. Large numbers of polyribosome-like structures were always present. Nuclear pockets or blebs were occasionally identified. Mitochondria were numerous and often appeared swollen or filled with dense myelin-like configurations. Cells of some highly anaplastic sarcomas contained large cytoplasmic masses of microfilaments.

Tumors of low anaplasticity were comprised primarily of stellate or elongated cells that had fewer mitochondria, fewer polyribosome-like structures, and longer profiles of rough endoplasmic reticulum.

### 4.3. Growth Characteristics, Metastasibility, Transplantability

Some pathologists have questioned the true malignant nature of FB tumors (Ott, 1970) because metastases are rarely observed, even in the regional lymph tissue. Especially the tumors of classes (I) and (II) (Johnson *et al.*, 1970) remain encapsulated and noninvasive for some time. However, most FB sarcomas grow rapidly and cause death of animals within a few weeks by spreading invasively and destructively (Ott, 1970; Brand *et al.*, 1967*b*). The latter found that all FB sarcomas which they had induced in mice were transplantable to isogeneic recipients. When kept in serial transplantation passages, the tumors may gain in malignancy as expressed by degree of histological anaplasticity, growth rate, invasiveness, and metastasibility. They may even become transplantable to allogeneic recipients (Ott, 1970).

### 4.4. Antigenicity

In mice or rats which develop FB sarcomas, no immune reaction against the tumor has been detected. To some extent, this may be the result of a direct immunosuppressive effect of the FB, as demonstrated in Balb/c mice by Kripke and Weiss (1970) and Saal *et al.* (1972). However, the main reason seems to lie in the fact that only extremely weak tumor-specific antigens, if any, emerge in conjunction with FB tumorigenesis. This was confirmed by several investigators *in vitro* and *in vivo* (Klein *et al.*, 1963; Prehn, 1963; Old and Boyse, 1964; Sjögren, 1965; Horn *et al.*, 1966; Hellström and Hellström, 1967; Hellström *et al.*, 1968). Only in very sensitive experiments was it possible to find traces of specific immune resistance. In such experiments, animals were hyperimmunized against isogeneic FB sarcoma cells and then challenged with few viable cells of the same tumor.

Recently it was shown that FB sarcomas have a pronounced tendency to lose antigens (Brand *et al.*, 1972). Tumors induced in $F_1$ hybrids of congeneic CBA/Br and CBA/H mice threw off tumor variants which lacked the antigen responsible for the histocompatibility barrier between the parents. This occurred at a rate of 80%, which is higher than that observed with chemically induced tumors.

## 4.5. Karyological Aberrations

Karyological analyses have been carried out on FB sarcomas of mice (Banerjee and Bates, 1966; Brand *et al.*, 1967a,b; Buoen and Brand, 1968; Johnson *et al.*, 1970). It was found that chromosome numbers deviated from normal virtually without exception. Also frequently recognized were certain morphological aberrations of chromosomes, e.g., metacentrics and double minutes (Buoen and Brand, 1968), which are conspicuous because the normal chromosomal complement of mice consists exclusively of telocentrics. Most karyotypes of FB sarcomas were found in the hyperdiploid or in the hypo- to hypertetraploid range, but no singular chromosomal characteristic was identified as being specific for murine FB sarcomas in general.

It became apparent in these studies that tumors with greater anaplasticity tended to tetraploidy. The same observation was made on sarcomas induced in various mouse strains by means of methylcholanthrene (Biedler, 1962) or Rous sarcomas virus (Mark, 1968), as well as on plasma cell tumors induced by intraperitoneal injection of Freund's adjuvant (Yosida *et al.*, 1967). The shift in ploidy level was interpreted as a consequence of anaplastic growth behavior, possibly related to the presence of multinucleated cells or of cells with excessively enlarged nuclei (Johnson *et al.*, 1970).

## 5. Factors Determining Tumor Incidence and Latency

### 5.1. Genetic Background of Host Species

The strikingly low incidence of FB sarcomas in humans as compared to that in rats and mice has already been emphasized. Whether tumor latency generally parallels life expectancy of a species is a matter of controversy, although similar observations in other fields of experimental carcinogenesis add a certain measure of support to this presumption. Like man, some other species have been shown to be relatively resistant to FB tumorigenesis. Chickens, which have a life expectancy of 10 yr, did not develop FB sarcomas during an observation time of 2 yr (Oberling, 1960). Attempts to induce FB sarcomas in guinea pigs, which are known to be less susceptible to chemical carcinogenesis than mice, have also been unsuccessful (Stinson, 1964). However, FB sarcomas occurred, in dogs (Ott, 1970) and in Syrian hamsters (Bering *et al.*, 1955; Bering and Handler, 1957), although the incidence in the latter species proved to be low, as was also found for Chinese and Armenian hamsters in the author's laboratory.

## 5.2. Genetic Background of Inbred Animal Strains

No data from systematic comparative experiments on FB tumorigenesis in different inbred animal strains are available as yet. Such investigations are presently underway in the author's laboratory, and it appears that inbred mouse strains do differ with regard to latency of FB sarcomas. It is hypothesized that these differences relate to hormonal, metabolic, or other constitutional factors which may be accessible to experimental analysis.

Of interest in this context is the observation that FB sarcomas of CBA/H mice were often more anaplastic than those of CBA/H-T6 animals. Yet both substrains are genetically identical, at least with regard to histocompatibility. The only known difference is the T6 chromosome pair, which presumably resulted from a break of the No. 15 chromosome without deletion or gain of genetic material. Nevertheless, CBA/H-T6 animals were found to be more temperamental and motoric than CBA/H mice (Johnson *et al.*, 1970). This behavioral difference may have an influence on, or may be linked to, the factor that determines anaplasticity.

## 5.3. Influence of Sex

It has been shown for different species and various kinds of tumors that sex can influence incidence and latency of tumors (Ashley, 1969*a,b*). Such differences exist also in both CBA/H and CBA/H-T6 mice in that females were found to reach the $TI_{50}$ (tumors in 50% of the animals) about 2 months earlier than males (Brand *et al.*, 1967*b*). On the other hand, males of either strain produced more tumors of high anaplasticity than females did (Johnson *et al.*, 1970). These studies are being extended to other inbred mouse strains. So far, it appears that sex influence on FB tumor latency is not uniformly seen in all strains.

## 5.4. Histopathology of Foreign Body Reaction

It was realized by many early workers in the field that species differences regarding FB tumor incidence may provide clues as to the etiological factors involved in FB tumorigenesis (Dobberstein, 1960). Although comparative investigations were carried out with diverse FB materials including plastics, metals, glass, membrane filters, and asbestos fibers, species differences regarding FB reactivity were found to be consistent.

Tumor-resistant chickens form a very thin membrane around the FB (Oberling, 1960). The reaction complex is not well anchored in the tissue, which points to a lack of vascular connections.

The findings on FB reactions of guinea pigs are similar in some respects (Virenque *et al.*, 1947; Coronel and Kerneis, 1948; Stinson, 1964; Davis, 1970). During the first few weeks following implantation, the reaction is cellular and proliferative, resulting in a capsule up to ten cell layers thick. But then the development of the capsule is regressive. By the third month, it comprises no more than three to five cell layers.

Foreign body reactions in rats and mice, which have the highest tumor incidence, are significantly at variance with those described for chickens and guinea pigs. Cellular activity around the implant, predominantly of macrophages, subsides after 1–2 months and is followed by pronounced fibrosis and collagen formation (Davis, 1970; Murphy, 1971; Rigdon, 1973). Sequential studies by light microscopy (Vasiliev *et al.*, 1962; Contzen, 1963; Brand *et al.*, 1967b; Murphy, 1971; Johnson *et al.*, 1972; Karp *et al.*, 1973b) and electron microscopy (Johnson *et al.*, 1972; Karp *et al.*, 1973b) on tumorigenic FB reactions of mice or rats established the following chain of events. Investigators who used solid plastic film implants found that during the first 2 wk monocytic macrophage-type cells infiltrated the implant site and actually settled down onto the implant surface, forming a monolayer with numerous binucleated or mitotic cells, interdispersed with a few polymorphonuclear leukocytes, fibroblast-like cells, and thin elongated spindle cells resembling smooth muscle cells. At this stage, a very thin coherent fibroblastic collagenous membrane with few capillary vessels was in existence and formed a fine intermediate space between the cell layers on the implant surface and the inner aspect of the developing capsule. During the following weeks, the capsule thickened because of collagenization and hence became relatively less cellular. After 3 months, the fibrotic capsule appeared stagnant and quiescent, a finding which most investigators considered significant. Electron microscopic studies during this stage showed dormant-appearing macrophage-like cells of variable morphology attached to the implant as a continuous monolayer. The organelles in these cells were sparse and poorly differentiated. Lysosome-like structures were, however, a characteristic feature. The space between implant-attached cells and the inner aspect of the surrounding capsule was mostly inconspicuous, but contained free macrophage-type cells in some areas, and occasionally neutrophils and eosinophils when debris of degenerated or necrotic cells had accumulated. The capsule was sharply separated from this intermediate zone by a continuous layer of greatly extended fibroblast-like cells. The capsule itself was composed predominantly of parallel planes of fibroblasts or fibrocytes separated by bands of collagen fibrils. Blood vessels and mast cells were always restricted to the outermost perimeter of the capsule.

In man (Ott, 1970), subcutaneous FB reactions remain active for a long time with pronounced cellularity and vascularization. Collagenization is slow and leads to a scarlike fibrous capsule only gradually after 1–2 yr. Whereas tumor formation in response to FB implantation is a rare occurrence in man, chronic asbestosis and schistosomiasis lead to cancer in a high and predictable proportion of patients. It appears that specifically the intrapleural site and the bladder wall and generally the serous membranes of man may respond to minute corpuscles such as asbestos fibers and schistosoma eggs with tumorigenic FB reaction. In animal experiments, it was shown (Stanton and Wrench, 1972) that asbestos fibers and glass fibers of comparable size and shape were equally tumorigenic. They caused vigorous granulomatous reactions investing the particles with dense fibrous capsules. The capsule tissue was poorly vascularized and was composed of immature spindle cells with abundant collagen and frequent hyalin or necrotic foci. The extent of fibrosis correlated with tumor incidence. In tumor-negative controls with larger glass fibers, the FB reaction was characterized by an abundance of mononuclear macrophages, giant cells, and capillary vessels, while the extent of fibrosis was negligible. In schistosomiasis, as in certain parasitic infections of rodents which cause FB sarcomas (Dobberstein, 1960; Salyamon, 1961), granuloma formation is greatly enhanced by antigens which evoke delayed hypersensitivity reactions (Domingo and Warren, 1968; von Lichtenberg *et al.*, 1971; Kuntz *et al.*, 1972). The result is a firm fibrotic encapsulation of worm eggs stuck in the bladder wall.

These comparative morphological investigations led to the conclusion that extent and chronicity of fibrosis may be correlated with FB tumor incidence (Vasiliev *et al.*, 1962; Bischoff and Bryson, 1964; Grasso and Goldberg, 1966; Bryson and Bischoff, 1969; Carter *et al.*, 1970; Davis, 1970; Ott, 1970; Schmitt and Beneke, 1971; Bischoff, 1972; Stanton and Wrench, 1972; Pott and Friedrichs, 1972).

The conclusion received support from various other avenues of research. As mentioned above, sex of animals affects tumor incidence, which may also be related to FB activity. It is known (Bashey *et al.*, 1964) that in female mice and rats the number of cells per volume of connective tissue is double that in males. To offset this imbalance, collagen synthesis in female fibroblasts is half as rapid as that in male fibroblasts.

Another relevant observation was made by Nothdurft (1962). He found that FBs implanted near the head of Wistar rats gave a higher tumor yield than FBs implanted near the tail. Dizon and Southam (1968) and Carter (1970) related this phenomenon to the presence of larger amounts of metabolically active brown fat in the shoulder region of rats and mice. However, Ott (1970) was unable to reproduce these results in E3 rats. He found histologically that Wistar rats developed a thicker and more fibrous FB capsule in the neck region than near the tail. This peculiar difference in local FB reactivity was not apparent in E3 rats.

Several investigators have reported (Nothdurft, 1960; Salyamon, 1961; Brand *et al.*, 1967b; Johnson *et al.*, 1972) that in mice and rats tumor latency was prolonged and tumor incidence on the whole diminished if FB reactions were complicated by persistent irritation or by recurrent inflammations. In these cases, the tissue reactions remained in an acute phase, showing prominent granulocytic cellularity and a high degree of vascularization. Fibrosis was suppressed and

delayed, which is consistent with the assumption that chronic fibrosis is indeed a
significant factor in FB tumorigenesis. This also explains why tumors usually arise
at the center of implant surfaces and rarely along the rim where irritation and
granulocytic infiltration are often histologically evident (Nothdurft, 1960; Bischoff and Bryson, 1964; Ott, 1970; Johnson et al., 1972).

### 5.5. Chemical and Physicochemical Properties of Foreign Bodies

Zollinger (1952) was probably the first investigator to suggest that the chemical
nature of an FB is not responsible for its tumorigenicity. Although most FB
materials are not completely inert chemically, e.g., plastics may contain plasticizers, remnant monomers, or free radicals (Oppenheimer et al., 1955; Leininger,
1965; Tomatis, 1966; Bischoff, 1972), they do not cause tumors when implanted
in powdered, finely shredded, or perforated form (Bischoff and Bryson, 1964).
On the other hand, absolutely inert materials such as glass, metals, or certain
polymers proved to be fully tumorigenic (Nothdurft, 1955a, 1960; Klärner, 1962;
Tomatis, 1963; Bischoff and Bryson, 1964; Hueper, 1964; Stinson, 1964; Bryson
and Bischoff, 1965; Grasso and Goldberg, 1966; Furst and Haro, 1969; Bischoff,
1972). But even chemically inert materials show considerable variations with
regard to surface properties such as wettability, electrostatic load, hardness, and
smoothness. These factors greatly affect tissue reactions in that they determine
degrees of irritation, inflammation, cellularity, blood clotting, etc. They are
therefore of main concern in reconstructive surgery (Hoopes et al., 1967;
Straumann and Paschke, 1967; Bischoff, 1972). By the same token, they influence
the degree of FB tumorigenicity. Andrews (1972) observed that tumor incidence
in mice is increased when the surfaces of implanted Millipore filters are hydrophobic. Carter et al. (1971) likewise found physicochemical surface properties of
importance, although his results did not entirely conform with those of Andrews.
When implant surfaces were roughened, the tumor incidence in mice or rats
decreased markedly. This was demonstrated by using sandpapered plastic films
(Bates and Klein, 1966), corroding iron platelets (O'Gara and Brown, 1967), or
wax pellets with low melting point (Shubik et al., 1962). The explanation for these
phenomena probably again goes back to FB reactivity in that FB reactions around
soft, rough, or hydrophilic surfaces were found less fibrotic and more cellular
than implants with the opposite surface properties.

### 5.6. Size and Shape of Foreign Bodies

Tumor incidence is greatly influenced by the size of FBs, as was first suspected by
Alexander (1954) and Alexander and Horning (1959) and subsequently proven
by many investigators (Bischoff and Bryson, 1964; Ott, 1970). Statistical evaluations indicated a direct correlation between tumor incidence and surface area of
implants (Brand et al., 1973). Since size of FBs determines magnitude of FB
reactions, it follows that a basic quantitative relationship exists between tumor
incidence and some tumorigenic component participating in FB reaction.

Also, the shape of an FB may have an influence on tumor incidence, although this relationship has not yet been explored systematically. Nothdurft (1960) obtained higher tumor yields in rats by employing concave button-like implants, which seemed to cause more extensive fibrosis to fill the indentations (Straumann and Paschke, 1967; Ott, 1970).

### 5.7. Porosity of Foreign Bodies

As already mentioned, tumor incidence decreases and eventually reaches zero when implants are perforated with holes in increasing number or having increasing diameter (Nothdurft, 1955b; Oppenheimer et al., 1955; Bischoff and Bryson, 1964; Ott, 1970). The same phenomenon was observed in experiments with sponges (Oppenheimer et al., 1955; Alexander et al., 1960; Dukes and Mitchley, 1962; Roe et al., 1967; Straumann and Paschke, 1967; Ott, 1970; Schmitt and Beneke, 1971) or Millipore filters of graded pore sizes (Merwin and Algire, 1959; Goldhaber, 1961, 1962; Bischoff and Bryson, 1964; Ott, 1970; Karp et al., 1973b). Sequential histological and ultrastructural studies have been performed (Karp et al., 1973b) to compare the FB reactions caused by tumorigenic and nontumorigenic Millipore filters, about 150 $\mu$m in width. With pore sizes of 0.22 $\mu$m and larger, filter implants did not induce any tumors. The FB-reactive capsules were poorly developed. Filter pores were invaded by highly active macrophages or their cytoplasmic processes, phagolysosomes being present inside the macrophages as evidence of phagocytic activity. These features were always missing in tumorigenic FB reactions around filter implants with pore sizes below 0.22 $\mu$m. Filter pores were never invaded and macrophages appeared dormant, similar to those described in tumorigenic FB reactions around solid plastic films. Fibrosis, however, was pronounced and resulted in thicker collagenous capsules.

### 5.8. Concluding Remark

Various factors have been identified which determine or influence FB tumorigenicity. They uniformly and specifically affect the primary FB reaction, which therefore must be suspected to hold the key or one of the keys to the etiology of FB tumorigenesis.

## 6. Exploration of Preneoplastic Events in Foreign Body Tumorigenesis

### 6.1. Histologically Suspected Preneoplastic Foci

Attempts were made by numerous investigators to identify preneoplastic and early neoplastic foci in FB-reactive capsule tissue (Mohr and Nothdurft, 1958; Oppenheimer et al., 1958; Hueper, 1959; Raykhlin and Kogan, 1961; Vasiliev et al., 1962; Bischoff and Bryson, 1964; Murphy, 1971; Johnson *et al.*, 1972). Such studies were done on rats or mice using a wide variety of implant materials. Particular attention was focused on "nodules" or "patches" of atypical fibroblastic proliferation which regularly appeared after the FB reaction had gone through the period of quiescence and relative inactivity (Oppenheimer *et al.*, 1959; Danishefsky *et al.*, 1959) for several months, i.e., about 6–12 months after implantation. These atypical proliferations were believed by most investigators to represent actual preneoplastic foci. However, the interpretations by Carter and Roe (1969) and Carter (1970) were more cautious. They observed that many such foci regressed or remained unchanged, a situation which they considered entirely normal in chronic FB reactions. Yet they granted that some foci may fail to resolve and eventually become the grounds for neoplastic transformation.

### 6.2. *Monoclonal Origin of Preneoplastic Cells (Fig. 1)*

A new dimension in the study of preneoplastic events was opened by the demonstration (Brand *et al.*, 1967*a,b*) that preneoplastic cells reside not just in the capsule tissue but predominantly in firm attachment on the implant surface. This finding made it possible to approach the problem more analytically in the following way. Plastic films subcutaneously implanted in CBA/H or CBA/H-T6 mice were excised after various times and cut into smaller segments. Each of these was transferred subcutaneously to a recipient mouse which, although fully histocompatible, was easily distinguished from the donor mouse on the basis of the T6 chromosomes. Sarcomas of donor origin developed in the recipients up to 2 yr later. Tumors that arose from segments of the same original implant were often identical or closely related ("homologous") with regard to (1) tumor latency in that neoplastic growth commenced in recipients at closely spaced points in time, (2) specific chromosome aberrations in terms of number and morphology, (3) histopathology in terms of sarcoma type and degree of anaplasticity (Johnson *et al.*, 1970), (4) growth characteristics and cell generation times *in vivo* and *in vitro*. Segments of tissue capsules were likewise transferred in the same manner. However, tumors were only rarely obtained from these transfers unless a new piece of plastic film was inserted in the capsule pocket (Brand and Buoen, 1968). In the latter situation, tumors were again mostly of donor origin, but they were usually not homologous with the tumors obtained from the corresponding original film implant.

These results led to the following conclusions. In the case of "homology," the tumors must have arisen from cells with the same neoplastic specificity, which points to their clonal nature. Specific tumor properties must have been predetermined in these clonal cells long before they actually started neoplastic proliferation. In fact, specific clones must have been in existence before implants were cut and the segments transferred. Demonstration of such clones implies prior existence of "parent cells" in which the initial event must have taken place, the event which not only created the neoplastic potential but moreover predetermined specific tumor properties as well as duration of latency.

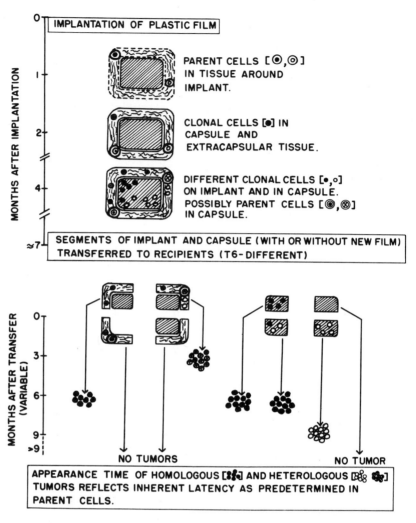

FIGURE 1. Exploration of preneoplastic events. A summary of typical experimental results. After Brand *et al.* (1967b, 1971), and Brand and Buoen (1968).

## 6.3. *Appearance Time and Location of Preneoplastic Parent Cells and Clones in Relation to Foreign Body Reaction (Fig. 1)*

Extended experiments (Brand *et al.*, 1971) similar to those described in the foregoing showed that in 30% of animals preneoplastic parent cells had arrived at the FB reaction site within 4 wk following implantation, in 80% within 8 wk. Immediately after their arrival, they seemed to expand into clones. This was shown to occur especially in the tissue of the developing capsule, but also in the extracapsular areas. During the third month after implantation and later, clonal progeny were found mainly adhering to the implant surface, and less frequently in the capsule proper, which at that time had become consolidated and well demarcated.

Although many millions of cells engage in experimental tumorigenic FB reactions, only very few seem to actually possess the properties of preneoplastic parent cells. By applying the maximum likelihood estimate, it was calculated (Brand *et al.*, 1973) that in CBA mice the Most Probable Number of preneoplastic parent cells is 1.0 in response to a single 7- by 15- by 0.2-mm plastic film. It is 3.0 in response to a single 15- by 22- by 0.2-mm implant. These values are in good agreement with results obtained by more direct experimental methods (Brand *et al.*, 1967*a,b*; Brand and Buoen, 1968; Brand *et al.*, 1971; Thomassen *et al.*, 1975).

### 6.5 Evidence for the Existence of Several Classes of Preneoplastic Cells According to Inherent Neoplastic Latency

Noncumulative tumor incidence curves in relation to time from experiments performed on large groups of animals consistently showed several distinct peaks (Brand *et al.*, 1971). The type of curve obtained did not conform with a single normal distribution curve but was interpreted as a composite of several subpopulations, each with a normal distribution curve of its own. This same phenomenon was described and mathematically confirmed with the help of computer analyses by Iversen *et al.* (1968) and Turusov *et al.* (1971) for chemically induced tumors. It was concluded (Brand *et al.*, 1971) that FB tumors fall into several distinct categories according to inherently different ranges of latency. As a consequence, it must be assumed that fixed class differences exist already among the population of preneoplastic parent cells since tumor latency is one of their predetermined properties.

### 6.6. Cell Type of Origin and Identification of Preneoplastic Parent Cells (Fig. 2)

Macrophage-type cells represent the predominant cell type found in FB-reactive tissue and especially in firm attachment on the surfaces of FB implants (Brand *et al.*, 1967*c*; Carter, 1969*a,b*; Kanazawa *et al.*, 1970; Ryan and Spector, 1970). The normal life span and turnover of these cells in the body as well as in active granulation tissue are of short duration (Spector and Lykke, 1966), but the cells may become long-lived in chronic granulomas and FB reactions (Spector and Ryan, 1969; Ryan and Spector, 1969), characteristically without dividing, which makes them resemble the dormant macrophages seen in tumorigenic FB reactions (Johnson *et al.*, 1972). Macrophage-type cells have been suspected to be the progenitor cells of FB sarcomas (Richmond, 1959; Haddow and Horning, 1960), particularly in view of claims that they can transform into fibroblast-like cells (Maximow, 1927; Stout, 1960; Davis, 1963, 1967; van Winkle, 1967; Noack, 1970; McDougal and Azar, 1972) besides being able to synthesize collagen (McDougal and Azar, 1972). However, macrophages had to be excluded from consideration not only on morphological grounds (Carter, 1970) but especially on the basis of

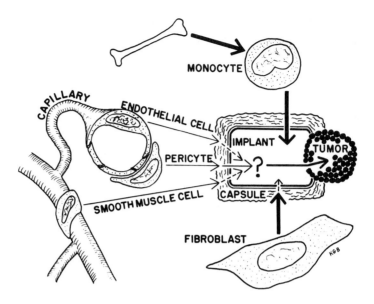

FIGURE 2. Cell types involved in foreign body reaction and in foreign body tumorigenesis. From Johnson *et al.* (1973*b*), with permission of *Cancer Research.*

recent experimental findings. First of all, it was established beyond doubt that macrophage-type cells, including giant cells and fixed histiocytes, are derived from blood monocytes (Cronkite *et al.*, 1960; Goldman and Walker, 1962; Kosunen *et al.*, 1963; Spector *et al.*, 1965; Volkman and Gowans, 1965*a,b*; Sutton and Weiss, 1966; Volkman, 1966; Leder, 1967; Spector *et al.*, 1967; Spector and Willoughby, 1968; Spector, 1969; Ryan and Spector, 1970; Bell and Shand, 1972; Shand and Bell, 1972), which, in turn, are descendants of radiosensitive stem cells in the bone marrow. These findings led to the following kind of experiment (Barnes *et al.*, 1971; Johnson *et al.*, 1972, 1973*b*). Radiation chimeras of CBA/H and CBA/H-T6 mice were produced by lethally irradiating animals of one substrain and then reconstituting their bone marrow with that of the other substrain, being distinguishable by T6 chromosome markers. Subsequently, FB sarcomas were induced in such chimeras and it was found that the tumor cells never showed the chromosome marker of the bone marrow donor. This led to the conclusion that in FB tumorigenesis the cell of origin is radioresistant and most likely not derived from bone marrow.

As a consequence, attention was shifted to another candidate, the fibroblast, which represents the predominant cell type engaged in the formation of the fibrous capsule. Most investigators agree that the true fibroblast originates from fibroblastic precursors, probably radioresistant resting fibrocytes (van Winkle, 1967) present throughout the body tissues (Gillman and Wright, 1966; van Winkle, 1967; Barnes and Khruschchov, 1968; Spector, 1969; Ross *et al.*, 1970). Support for the progenitor role of fibroblasts in FB tumorigenesis comes from the fact, discussed earlier, that FB tumor susceptibility of animals and incidence are directly related to the extent of chronic fibrosis in FB reactions. It was further suggested that random chromosomal aberrations, such as those regularly observed in FB sarcomas, occur with relative frequency in proliferating fibroblasts (Higurashi and Conen, 1971).

However, results and interpretations of more recent investigations (Johnson *et al.*, 1973*b*) pointed in still another direction. It was noted that FB sarcomas vary greatly not only in the degree of anaplasticity, spanning the whole range from a fibrosarcoma to a highly undifferentiated sarcoma, but also regarding the basic sarcoma type, as in myxosarcomas, hemangiosarcomas, osteogenic sarcomas, and leiomyosarcomas. Moreover, as was pointed out, many sarcomas are mixed in that they most often contain undifferentiated, fibrosarcomatous, myxoid, or osteogenic elements side by side despite their monoclonal origin. Histological and ultrastructural studies (Johnson *et al.*, 1973*b*) on such varied FB-induced sarcomas showed that certain features were always present: (1) Pericellular, PAS-positive, argyrophilic, and filamentous substance characteristic of basal laminae; (2) cytoplasmic accumulations of 60 Å microfilaments; (3) relative sparsity of collagen production, if there was any. These findings brought into focus particularly those mesenchymal cell types which produce basal laminae: endothelial cells, pericytes, and smooth muscle cells, all being a fixed structural part of the microvasculature. Especially the pericyte is considered a possible common progenitor in FB tumorigenesis because it fulfills the following key criteria: (1) The pericyte is a local mesenchymal cell with pluripotentiality (van Winkle, 1967; Crocker *et al.*, 1970; Rossi *et al.*, 1973) and capacity to serve as precursor of various mesenchymal cell types, probably including smooth muscle cells (Rhodin, 1968). These properties would fully account for the histological and subcellular variety within and between sarcomas. (2) The pericyte is functionally involved in the FB reaction by way of angiogenesis. (3) The pericyte possesses subcellular morphological features which are compatible with those seen in the sarcoma cells.

These conclusions link up with related findings and interpretations in some other areas. Mesenchymal stem cells in the microvasculature were also incriminated as the progenitor cells of sarcomas which developed *in vitro* from a variety of normal tissues (Franks and Wilson, 1970; Franks *et al.*, 1971; Franks and Cooper, 1972; Wilson and Franks, 1972). Smooth muscle cells (Wissler, 1967; Fritz *et al.*, 1970; McDougal and Azar, 1972; Rossi *et al.*, 1973) and their clonal progeny (Benditt and Benditt, 1973) are etiologically involved in the formation of atherosclerotic plaques.

## 7. The Tumorigenic Process: Experimental Findings in Mice and Attempts at Interpretation

### 7.1. Acquisition of a Specific Neoplastic Potential by "Parent Cells" During Early Foreign Body Reaction

*Finding:* Preneoplastic parent cells and their clonal progeny are present at the site of the FB reaction within 4–8 wk after implantation. The clonal cells uniformly carry the information for the specific characteristics which are subsequently exhibited by homologous tumors, including tumor latency, karyological aberrations, histopathological classification, degree of anaplasticity, and *in vitro* and *in vivo* growth characteristics.

*Interpretation:* The parent cell is already endowed with the information for specific tumor characteristics. The determining key event must occur before the parent cell expands into a clone, i.e., during the first 4–8 wk of FB reaction, and many months, if not years, before the start of actual neoplastic proliferation. The initial tumorigenic key event not only occurs early in the FB reaction, but it is also definite and final. It creates determinants of tumor characteristics that are stable throughout the entire preneoplastic period, even despite transfer of preneoplastic clonal cells to different recipient animals. Hereditary transmission and stability of tumor-specific determinants through several cell generations during clonal expansion implicate the genetic–regulatory apparatus of the cell as the primary tumorigenic site.

*Finding:* At the time when the tumorigenic key event takes place, the parent cells affected are present in the developing capsule and in the extracapsular tissue, but are not demonstrable directly on the FB surface. The preneoplastic cells that are found on the FB surface at a later time are clonal progeny of the parent cells.

*Interpretation:* Direct contact of parent cells with the FB is not required for the tumorigenic key event to be initiated.

*Finding:* The Most Probable Number of parent cells with neoplastic potential is directly related to the size of the FB surface area. This number is very low, i.e., in the neighbourhood of 1, although millions of cells are generally mobilized in response to the FB.

*Interpretation:* The tumorigenic key event is an extremely rare event. There is no indication of a "field effect," which would be expected to involve a larger proportion of cells on exposure to the same inducing factor or mechanism. The total number of cells mobilized in an FB reaction as well as the Most Probable Number of cells with neoplastic potential is determined by the size of the FB, i.e., by the extent of the FB reaction. This means that, regardless of FB size, the ratio of preneoplastic parent cells to nonpreneoplastic cells remains constant. It appears, therefore, that the tumorigenic key event is a statistical chance event, or else that a small constant proportion of the cell population has a primary neoplastic susceptibility or disposition which manifests itself under the condition of a chronic FB reaction.

*Finding:* The determination of tumor latency is a fixed property of preneoplastic parent and clonal cells. However, the population of preneoplastic parent cells is heterogeneous in that several subpopulations can be distinguished on account of differences in tumor latency.

*Interpretation:* If one assumes that preneoplastic determination of tumor latency is linked to the tumorigenic key event, as many different etiological factors or events may be singularly responsible for initiating the tumorigenic process as there are distinct latency classes of preneoplastic parent cells.

*Finding:* When implanted FBs are removed during the preneoplastic period, the probability is low that sarcomas will develop from the empty capsules. Only if the removed cell-laden FBs are replaced by fresh cell-free ones is the appearance of sarcomas assured. However, these tumors are usually not homologous to the tumors that arise from the original FBs on transfer to recipient animals.

*Interpretation:* Continued presence of the FB is generally a prerequisite for neoplastic maturation, which apparently takes place in cells of a specific clone that is attached to the FB surface and usually present only there. Other clones (or parent cells) residing in the capsule tissue can, as a rule, not fully mature to the point of neoplasia unless a free FB surface becomes available for attachment. Hence cellular contact with an FB surface seems to be a prerequisite for neoplastic maturation. Note that this is in contrast to the initial tumorigenic key event, which seems to have occurred in parent cells before contact with the FB surface is established.

*Finding:* In rare instances, sarcomas develop from empty capsules after FBs have been removed during the preneoplastic period. However, in mouse experiments (Thomassen *et al.*, 1975) this was observed only when the FB reaction had advanced at least into the ninth month after implantation.

*Interpretation:* Preneoplastic cells may come off the FB surface when the FB is pulled out of the capsule. If this happens at an advanced stage of FB reaction, neoplastic maturation may have reached a point of no return, and may have become independent of cell attachment to a FB surface. Also, the fibrosis of the capsule may have developed at this time to a permanent scar, preventing a speedy resolution of the process, possibly even assuming the place of a FB.

*Finding:* Preneoplastic parent cells originate from mesenchymal precursor cells of the microvasculature, probably pericytes.

*Interpretation:* Pericytes and their descendants participate in the formation of the FB capsule as building elements of the capillary net. The initial tumorigenic event may have occurred in one or few pericytes, but neoplastic maturation progresses only after the descendants have attached to the FB surface. Here, the functional situation must be fundamentally abnormal for these cells. By being flattened out as part of a monolayer on a smooth surface, they are obviously incapacitated to fulfill their programmed task, the construction of a three-dimensional vascular system. Could this relate to the process of neoplastic maturation?

*Finding:* The main cell populations seen on FB surfaces as well as in capsule tissue take on an appearance of inactivity and quiescence approximately by the third month following FB implantation. This phenomenon is positively related to the tumorigenicity of FB reactions.

*Interpretation:* The cells showing this phenomenon in tumorigenic FB reactions are the macrophages which are most likely not the preneoplastic ones. Whether pericytes and their clonal descendants, suspected to be the preneoplastic cells, are likewise dormant during this time is not known. Therefore, it could be a fallacy to conclude that dormancy of preneoplastic cells is a requirement for their neoplastic maturation. However, dormancy of the macrophage population as well as chronicity of fibrosis definitely creates or expresses the conditions which are essential for neoplastic maturation to proceed in cells destined to become sarcomatous.

### 7.3. Switch to Autonomous Tumor Growth

*Finding:* All member cells of the same preneoplastic clone, whether still residing in the original FB carrier animal or having been transferred with FB segments to a recipient animal, often start neoplastic proliferation simultaneously or at closely spaced points in time.

   *Interpretation:* This phenomenon seems to reflect a precisely timed molecular process which eliminates the last barrier of growth control and turns the preneoplastic cells into autonomous tumor cells. It is to be remembered that this specific occurrence and its exact timing were predetermined months or years earlier in the parent cell by an initial tumorigenic key event at the molecular level.

## 8. Etiological Hypotheses of Foreign Body Tumorigenesis: A Critical Appraisal

Various hypotheses have been proposed through the years to explain FB tumorigenesis. Research progress in the field, described and discussed in the foregoing, has clarified a number of issues and eliminated several hypotheses altogether. Crucial is the finding that the initial tumorigenic key event occurs during the first 4–8 wk of FB reaction in parent cells before they have made contact with the FB surface. Some hypotheses require cellular contact with the FB or an advanced state of FB reaction for the proposed etiological factors to become operative. Such factors appear to be out of consideration as inducers of the etiological key event, although they may effectively influence the process of neoplastic maturation and in this way determine tumor incidence secondarily to some extent.

### 8.1. Chemical Components

The assumption that chemical components released from plastic materials are etiologically involved has been repudiated in various ways, as discussed earlier. Yet such chemicals may modify FB reactions through tissue irritation, cell damage, and the like, which may have an effect on neoplastic maturation and actual tumor incidence.

*8.2. Physicochemical Surface Properties*

503
FOREIGN
BODY
INDUCED
SARCOMAS

Several investigators have suggested (Bischoff and Bryson, 1964; Kordan, 1967) and attempted to demonstrate (Carter *et al.*, 1971; Andrews. 1972) that electrostatic charge or wettability may be of major etiological significance. Such physicochemical surface properties cannot be expected to relate directly to the tumorigenic key event, which occurs in cells distant from the implant surface. However, there is an influence on the FB reaction with regard to degree of fibrosis (Andrews, 1972) and macrophage activity (Carter *et al.*, 1971; Andrews, 1972), which would explain the observed effect on tumor incidence. This effect is weak and easily overpowered by other factors. As an example, hydrophilic and electropositive Millipore filters were shown to be either fully tumorigenic or nontumorigenic, the only variable being pore size within the narrow range of 0.1–0.22 $\mu$m (Karp *et al.*, 1973*b*).

## 8.3. Interruption of Cellular Contact or Communication

Tumor induction studies by means of Millipore filters (Merwin and Algire, 1959; Goldhaber, 1961, 1962; Zajdela, 1966) suggested that the interruption of cellular contact or communication may be of etiological importance (Oppenheimer *et al.*, 1959; Vasiliev *et al.*, 1962; Karp *et al.*, 1973*b*). This hypothesis received support from work on the role of intercellular messenger molecules in embryonal development (Grobstein and Dalton, 1957; Wessels, 1962; Saunders and Gasseling, 1963; Nordling *et al.*, 1971; Tarin, 1972*a,b*), epidermal wound healing (Mizuno and Fuggi, 1969), induction of bone formation (Büring and Urist, 1967; Urist *et al.*, 1967; Friedman *et al.*, 1968; Small *et al.*, 1970), and similar processes. Recent experiments have shown that physical interruption of contact has no bearing on FB tumorigenesis. Millipore filters with a thickness of 150 $\mu$m and a pore size of 0.22 $\mu$m seem to prevent direct contact of opposite cell layers even by cytoplasmic processes (Wartiovaara *et al.*, 1972; Karp *et al.*, 1973*b*), but are nevertheless completely nontumorigenic (Karp *et al.*, 1973*b*). Whether interference with intercellular communication is of any consequence remains an open question, although, again, the effect would be on the neoplastic maturation process, not on the initial tumorigenic key event in parent cells.

## 8.4. Tissue Anoxia and Insufficient Exchange of Metabolites

Tissue anoxia (Warburg, 1956) and insufficient exchange of metabolites have been incriminated as a major etiological factor by numerous investigators (Alexander, 1954; Mohr and Nothdurft, 1958; Alexander and Horning, 1959; Merwin and Algire, 1959; Oppenheimer *et al.*, 1959; Schabad, 1960; Goldhaber, 1961, 1962; Vasiliev *et al.*, 1962; Bates and Klein, 1966). The histology of FB reactions induced by tumorigenic solid films would support this hypothesis. It was shown that the distances between blood vessels and implant surface are mostly in the range of 200–300 $\mu$m (Johnson *et al.*, 1972), which corresponds to about 20 cell diameters. However, a direct etiological connection between insufficient vascularization of the tissue capsule and FB tumorigenicity was shown to be unlikely when it was found that capsules around tumorigenic Millipore filters with pore sizes of $\leqq 0.1$ $\mu$m are highly vascularized and that the capillaries are separated from the implant surface by not more than one to three cell diameters (Karp *et al.*, 1973*a*).

## 8.5. Virus

After various unsuccessful attempts (Hollmann, 1960; Nothdurft, 1960), virus particles have been detected in FB sarcomas. Johnson *et al.* (1973*a,b*) found intracisternal type-A particles in 12 of 17 sarcomas induced by plastic films in CBA/H and CBA/H-T6 mice, and immature type-C particles in all the sarcomas induced in AKR mice. The biological properties of these virus particles and their etiological significance in FB tumorigenesis have not been determined at this time. Preliminary biochemical investigations on FB sarcomas induced in CBA/H mice, including molecular hybridization attempts, were negative (Johnson *et al.*, 1973*a*).

## 8.6. Disturbance of Cellular Growth Regulation

Theoreticians of carcinogenesis generally agree that the basic cause of neoplasia lies in a disturbance of cellular growth regulation. Since neoplastic growth is a hereditary property throughout subsequent cell generations, the responsible aberration must be assumed to occur at the genetic–epigenetic–regulatory level of cellular growth control (Pasternak, 1970; Rabinowitz and Sachs, 1970; Tsanev and Sendov, 1971*a,b*; Yamamoto *et al.*, 1973). Knowledge concerning growth regulation in mammalian cells is still very limited, but it seems obvious that we are dealing with a complex multifactorial system. It must involve multiple functional units, each probably highly complex in itself, which are engaged in membrane interactions such as transport or contact inhibition, in intercellular communication, and in cell division and functional differentiation with numerous biochemical cascade reactions and switching mechanisms, all being subject to continuous checks and balances. A single error in any one of these "various sensitive points" (Tsanev and Sendov, 1971*a*) may conceivably lead to disorder of cellular growth regulation. Such errors may be manifold. They may involve genetic or regulatory molecules; they may be in the form of a genuine defect, a functional blockade, or an irreversible derepression; they may be spontaneous or induced by chemicals, ionizing radiation, or viruses. Significantly, errors occurring at the chromosomal level (Rabinowitz and Sachs, 1970; Yamamoto *et al.*, 1973) can be repaired by chromosomal reconstitution achieved through hybridization of neoplastic cells with normal ones (Weiss *et al.*, 1968; Harris *et al.*, 1969; Harris, 1971; Klein *et al.*, 1971; Azarnia and Loewenstein, 1973; Loewenstein, 1973). The demonstration of distinct latency categories in FB tumorigenesis (Brand *et al.*, 1971) and other forms of carcinogenesis (Iverson *et al.*, 1968; Turusov *et al.*, 1971) may be interpreted to reflect multiplicity of tumorigenic targets or events within the cellular growth regulation system.

## 9. References

ALEXANDER, P., 1954, The reactions of carcinogens with macromolecules, *Advan. Cancer Res.* **2**:1.

ALEXANDER, P., AND HORNING, E. S., 1959, Observations on the Oppenheimer method of inducing tumors by subcutaneous implantation of plastic films, in: *CIBA Foundation Symposium on Carcinogenesis*, pp. 24–26, London.

ALEXANDER, P., DUKES, C. E., AND MITCHLEY, B. C. V., 1960, Carcinogenic action of subcutaneously embedded plastic sponges, *A. R. Brit. Emp. Cancer Campaign* **38**:92.

ANDREWS, E. J., 1972, Possible importance of detergent in Millipore filter carcinogenesis, *J. Natl. Cancer Inst.* **48**:1251.

ASHLEY, D. J. B., 1969a, A male–female differential in tumour incidence, *Brit. J. Cancer* **23**:21.

ASHLEY, D. J. B., 1969b, Sex differences in the incidence of tumours at various sites, *Brit. J. Cancer* **23**:26.

AZARNIA, R., AND LOEWENSTEIN, W. R., 1973, Parallel correction of cancerous growth and of a genetic defect of cell-to-cell communication, *Nature (Lond.)* **214**:455.

BANERJEE, M. R., AND BATES, R. B., 1966, Prevalence of heteroploidy in plastic film–induced primary sarcomas, *Brit. J. Cancer* **20**:555.

BARNES, D. W. H., AND KHRUSCHCHOV, N. G., 1968, Fibroblasts in sterile inflammation: Study in mouse radiation chimaeras, *Nature (Lond.)* **218**:599.

BARNES, D. W., EVANS, E. P., AND LOUTIT, J. F., 1971, Local origin of fibroblasts deduced from sarcomas induced in chimaeras by implants of pliable disks, *Nature (Lond.)* **233**:267.

BASHEY, R. I., WOESSNER, J. F., JR., AND BOUCEK, R. J., 1964, Connective tissue development in subcutaneously implanted polyvinyl sponge. III. Ribonucleic acid changes during development, *Arch. Biochem. Biophys.* **104**:32.

BATES, R. B., AND KLEIN, M., 1966, Importance of a smooth surface in carcinogenesis by plastic film, *J. Natl. Cancer Inst.* **37**:145.

BAUER, K. H., 1963, *Das Krebsproblem, Kunststoffe*, pp. 379–384, Springer, Berlin.

BELL, E. B., AND SHAND, F. L., 1972, A search for lymphocyte-derived macrophages during xenogeneic graft-versus-host reactions induced by rat thoracic duct cells, *Immunology* **22**:537.

BENDITT, E. P., AND BENDITT, J. M., 1973, Evidence for a monoclonal origin of human atherosclerotic plaques, *Proc. Natl. Acad. Sci.* **70**:1753.

BERING, E. A., AND HANDLER, A. H., 1957, The production of tumors in hamsters by implantation of polyethylene film, *Cancer* **10**:414.

BERING, E. A., McLAURIN, R. L., LLOYD, J. B., AND INGRAHAM, F. D., 1955, The production of tumors in rats by the implantation of pure polyethylene, *Cancer Res.* **15**:300.

BIEDLER, J. L., 1962, Chromosomal patterns in chemically-induced tumors in mice, *Proc. Am. Assoc. Cancer Res.* **3**:304.

BISCHOFF, F., 1972, Organic polymer biocompatibility and toxicology, *Clin. Chem.* **18**:869.

BISCHOFF, F., AND BRYSON, G., 1964, Carcinogenesis through solid state surfaces, *Prog. Exp. Tumor Res.* **5**:85.

BRAND, K. G., 1970, Induction of sarcomas by subcutaneous implantation of plastics in mice, *Dermatol. Dig.* **9**:59.

BRAND, K. G., AND BRAND, I., 1973, Karzinogene Eigenschaften von Fremdkörper-Implantaten, *Fortschr. Med.* **91**:1181.

BRAND, K. G., AND BUOEN, L. C., 1968, Polymer tumorigenesis: Multiple preneoplastic clones in priority order with clonal inhibition, *Proc. Soc. Exp. Biol. Med.* **128**:1154.

BRAND, K. G., BUOEN, L. C., AND BRAND, I., 1967a, Premalignant cells in tumorigenesis induced by plastic film, *Nature (Lond.)* **213**:810.

BRAND, K. G., BUOEN, L. C., AND BRAND, I., 1967b, Carcinogenesis from polymer implants: New aspects from chromosomal and transplantation studies during premalignancy, *J. Natl. Cancer Inst.* **39**:663.

BRAND, K. G., BUOEN, L. C., AND BRAND, I., 1967c, Malignant transformation and maturation in non-dividing cells during polymer tumorigenesis, *Proc. Soc. Exp. Biol. Med.* **124**:675.

BRAND, K. G., BUOEN, L. C., AND BRAND, I., 1971, Foreign body tumorigenesis: Timing and location of preneoplastic events, *J. Natl. Cancer Inst.* **47**:829.

BRAND, K. G., BUOEN, L. C., AND BRAND, I., 1972, Antigen-deficient cell variants in preneoplastic foreign body reaction in mice, *J. Natl. Cancer Inst.* **49**:459.

BRAND, K. G., BUOEN, L. C., AND BRAND, I., 1973, Foreign body tumorigenesis in mice: Most probable number of originator cells, *J. Natl. Cancer Inst.* **51**:1071.

BRYSON, G., AND BISCHOFF, F., 1965, Polymer carcinogenesis, in: *Symposium on Polymer Chemistry*, American Chemical Society Western Regional Meeting, Los Angles.

BRYSON, G., AND BISCHOFF, F., 1967, Silicate-induced neoplasms, *Prog. Exp. Tumor Res.* **9**:77.

BRYSON, G., AND BISCHOFF, F., 1969, The limitations of safety testing, *Prog. Exp. Tumor Res.* **11**:100.

BUOEN, L. C., AND BRAND, K. G., 1968, Double-minute chromosomes in plastic film–induced sarcomas in mice, *Naturwissenschaften* **3**:135.

BÜRING, K., AND URIST, M. R., 1967, Transfilter bone induction, *Clin. Orthop.* **54**:235.

BURNS, W. A., KANHOUWA, S., TILLMAN, L., SAINI, N., AND HERRMANN, J. B., 1969, Fibrosarcoma occurring at the site of a plastic vascular graft, *Cancer* **29**:66.

CALNAN, J. S., 1970, Assessment of biological properties of implants before their clinical use, *Proc. Royal Soc. Med.* **63**:1115.

CARTER, R. L., 1969a, Early development of injection-site sarcomas in rats: A study of tumours induced by a rubber additive, *Brit. J. Cancer* **23**:408.

CARTER, R. L., 1969b, Early development of injection-site sarcomas in rats: A study of tumours induced by iron–dextran, *Brit. J. Cancer* **23**:559.

CARTER, R. L., 1970, Induced subcutaneous sarcomata: Their development and critical appraisal, in: *Metabolic Aspects of Food Safety* (F. J. C. Roe, ed.), pp. 569–591, Blackwell, Oxford.

CARTER, R. L., AND ROE, F. J. C., 1969, Induction of sarcomas in rats by solid and fragmented polyethylene: Experimental observations and clinical implications, *Brit. J. Cancer* **23**:401.

CARTER, R. L., BIRBECK, M. S. C., AND ROBERTS, J. D. B., 1970, Development of injection-site sarcomata in rats: A study of the early reactive changes evoked by a carcinogenic nitrosoquinoline compound, *Brit. J. Cancer* **24**:300.

CARTER, R. L., ROE, F. J. C., AND PETO, R., 1971, Tumor induction by plastic films: Attempt to correlate carcinogenic activity with certain physicochemical properties of the implant, *J. Natl. Cancer Inst.* **46**:1277.

CONTZEN, H., 1963, Die lokale Gewebereaktion auf implantierte Kunststoffe in Abhängigkeit von deren Form, *Langenbecks Arch. Klin. Chir.* **304**:922.

CORONEL, S., AND KERNEIS, J. P., 1948, Les resines acryliques intratissulaires, *Rev. Stomat. Paris* **49**:281.

CROCKER, D. J., MURAD, T. M., AND GEER, J. C., 1970, Role of the pericyte in wound healing, *Exp. Mol. Pathol.* **13**:51.

CRONKITE, E. P., BOND, V. P., FLIEDNER, T. M., AND KILLMANN, S. A., 1960, The use of tritiated thymidine in the study of haemopoietic cell proliferation, in: *CIBA Foundation Symposium: Haemopoiesis, Cell Production and Its Regulation* pp. 70–92, London.

DANISHEFSKY, I., OPPENHEIMER, E. T., WILLHITE, M., STOUT, A. P., AND FISHMAN, M. M., 1959, Biochemical changes during carcinogenesis by plastic films, *Cancer Res.* **19**:1234.

DAVIS, J. M. G., 1963, The ultrastructural changes that occur during the transformation of lung macrophages to giant cells and fibroblasts in experimental asbestosis, *Brit. J. Pathol.* **44**:568.

DAVIS, J. M. G., 1967, The effects of chrysotile asbestos dust on lung macrophages maintained in organ culture, *Brit. J. Exp. Pathol.* **48**:379.

DAVIS, J. M. G., 1970, The long term fibrogenic effects of chrysotile and crocidolite asbestos dust injected into the pleural cavity of experimental animals, *Brit. J. Exp. Pathol.* **51**:617.

DE CHOLNOKY, T., 1970, Augmentation mammaplasty: Survey of complications in 10,941 patients by 265 surgeons, *Plast. Reconstruct. Surg.* **45**:573.

DIZON, Q. S., AND SOUTHAM, C. M., 1968, Growth of human cancer cells in interscapular brown fats of rats, *Transplantation* **6**:351.

DOBBERSTEIN, J., 1960, Berliner Symposium über Fragen der Carcinogenese, *Abhandl. Deutsch. Akad. Wiss. Berl. Klasse Med.* **3**:98.

DOMINGO, E. O., AND WARREN, K. S., 1968, The inhibition of granuloma formation around *Schistosoma mansoni* eggs, *Am. J. Pathol.* **52**:613.

DUKE, H. N., AND VANE, J. R., 1968, An adverse effect of polyvinylchloride tubing used in extra-corporeal circulation, *Lancet* **2**:21.

DUKES, C. E., AND MITCHLEY, B. C. V., 1962, Polyvinyl sponge implants: Experimental and clinical observations, *Brit. J. Plast. Surg.* **15**:225.

DUTTON, J., 1959, Acrylic investment of intracranial aneurysms, *Brit. Med. J.* **2**:597.

FRANKS, L. M., AND COOPER, T. W., 1972, The origin of human embryo lung cells in culture: A comment on cell differentiation, *in vitro* growth and neoplasia, *Int. J. Cancer* **9**:19.

FRANKS, L. M., AND WILSON, P. D., 1970, "Spontaneous" neoplastic transformation *in vitro*: The ultrastructure of the tissue culture cell, *Europ. J. Cancer* **6**:517.

FRANKS, L. M. CHESTERMAN, F. C., AND ROWLATT, C., 1971, The structure of tumours derived from mouse cells after "spontaneous" transformation *in vitro, Brit. J. Cancer* **24**:843.

FRIEDMAN, B., HEIPLE, K. G., VESSELY, J. C., AND HANAOKA, H., 1968, Ultrastructural investigation of bone induction by an osteo-sarcoma using diffusion chambers, *Clin. Orthop.* **59**:39.

FRITZ, K. E., JARMOLYCH, J., AND DAOUD, A. S., 1970, Association of DNA synthesis and apparent dedifferentiation of aortic smooth muscle cells *in vitro, Exp. Mol. Pathol.* **12**:354.

FURST, A., AND HARO, R. T., 1969, A survey of metal carcinogenesis, *Prog. Exp. Tumor Res.* **12**:102.

GILLMAN, T., AND WRIGHT, L. J., 1966, Autoradiographic evidence suggesting *in vivo* transformation of some blood mononuclears in repair and fibrosis, *Nature (Lond.)* **209**:1086.

GOLDHABER, P., 1961, The influence of pore size on carcinogenicity of subcutaneously implanted Millipore filters, *Proc. Am. Assoc. Cancer Res.* **3**:228.

GOLDHABER, P., 1962, Further observations concerning the carcinogenicity of Millipore filters, *Proc. Am. Assoc. Cancer Res.* **3**:323.

GOLDMAN, A. S., AND WALKER, B. E., 1962, The origin of cells in the infiltrates found at the sites of foreign protein injection, *Lab. Invest.* **11**:808.

GRASSO, P., AND GOLDBERG, L., 1966, Subcutaneous sarcoma as an index of carcinogenic potency, *FD Cosmet. Toxicol.* **4**:297.

GROBSTEIN, C., AND DALTON, A. J., 1957, Kidney tubule induction in mouse metanephrogenic mesenchyme without cytoplasmic contact, *J. Exp. Zool.* **135**:57.

HADDOW, A., AND HORNING, E. S., 1960, On the carcinogenicity of an iron–dextran complex, *J. Natl. Cancer Inst.* **24**:109.

HARRIS, H., 1971, Cell fusion and the analysis of malignancy, *Proc. Royal Soc. Lond. Ser. B.* **179**:1.

HARRIS, H., MILLER, O. J., KLEIN, G., WORST, P., AND TACHIBANA, T., 1969, Suppression of malignancy by cell fusion, *Nature (Lond.)* **223**:363.

HELLSTRÖM, I., AND HELLSTRÖM, K. E., 1967, Cell-bound immunity to autologous and syngeneic mouse tumors induced by methylcholanthrene and plastic discs, *Science* **156**:981.

HELLSTRÖM, I., HELLSTRÖM, K. E., AND PIERCE, G. E., 1968, *In vitro* studies of immune reactions against autochthonous and syngeneic mouse tumors induced by methylcholanthrene and plastic discs, *Int. J. Cancer* **3**:467.

HIGURASHI, M., AND CONEN, P. E., 1971, Comparison of chromosomal behavior in cultured lymphocytes and fibroblasts from patients with chromosomal disorders and controls, *Cytogenetics* **10**:273.

HOLLMANN, M. K. H., 1960, Ultrastructure d'un sarcome du rat provoqué par implantation de polystyrène, *Bull. Assoc. Franc. Canc.* **47**(2):308.

HOOPES, J. E., EDGERTON, M. T., AND SHELLEY, W., 1967, Organic synthetics for augmentation mammaplasty: Their relation to breast cancer, *Plast. Reconstruct. Surg.* **39**:263.

HORN, K., PASTERNAK, G., AND GRAFFI, A., 1966, Experiments on the induction of tumor-specific resistance against isologous transplants of sarcomas induced by implantation of plastic pellets, *Arch. Immunol. Ther. Exp.* **14**:737.

HOWE, A., AND RASTELLI, G. C., 1969, Late deterioration of intracardiac ivalon sponge patches, *J. Thorac. Cardiovasc. Surg.* **58**:87.

HUEPER, W. C., 1959, Carcinogenic studies on water-soluble and -insoluble macromolecules, *Arch. Pathol.* **67**:589.

HUEPER, W. C., 1964, Cancer induction by polyurethan and polysilicone plastics, *J. Natl. Cancer Inst.* **33**:1005.

IVERSEN, U., IVERSEN, O. H., AND BJERKNES, R., 1968, A comparison of the tumourigenic effect of five graded doses of 3-methyl-cholanthrene applied to the skin of hairless mice at intervals of 3 or 14 days, *Acta Pathol. Microbiol. Scand.* **73**:502.

JOHNSON, F. B., 1965, *Studies on Polymer Implants in Humans: Plastics in Surgical Implants*, pp. 102–104, Special Technical Publication 386, American Society for Testing Materials.

JOHNSON, K. H., BUOEN, L. C., BRAND, I., AND BRAND, K. G., 1970, Polymer tumorigenesis: Clonal determination of histopathological characteristics during early preneoplasia; relationships to karyotype, mouse strain, and sex, *J. Natl. Cancer Inst.* **44**:785.

JOHNSON, K. H., GHOBRIAL, H. K. G., BUOEN, L. C., BRAND, I., AND BRAND, K. G., 1972, Foreign-body tumorigenesis in mice: Ultrastructure of the preneoplastic tissue reactions, *J. Natl. Cancer Inst.* **49**:1311.

JOHNSON, K. H., GHOBRIAL, H. K. G., BUOEN, L. C., BRAND, I., AND BRAND, K. G., 1973a, Intracisternal type A particles occurring in foreign body–induced sarcomas, *Cancer Res.* **33**:1165.

JOHNSON, K. H., GHOBRIAL, H. K. G., BUOEN, L. C., BRAND, I., AND BRAND, K. G., 1973b, Nonfibroblastic origin of foreign body sarcomas implicated by histologic and electron microscopic studies, *Cancer Res.* **33**:3139.

KANAZAWA, K., BIRBECK, M. S. C., CARTER, R. L., AND ROE, F. J. C., 1970, The migration of asbestos fibres from subcutaneous injection sites, *Brit. J. Cancer* **24**:96.

KARP, R. D., JOHNSON, K. H., BUOEN, L. C., BRAND, I., AND BRAND, K. G., 1973a, Foreign-body tumorigenesis: No requirement for tissue anoxia, *J. Natl. Cancer Inst.* **50**:1403.

KARP, R. D., JOHNSON, K. H., BUOEN, L. C., GHOBRIAL, H. K. G., BRAND, I., AND BRAND, K. G., 1973b, Tumorigenesis by Millipore filters in mice: Histology and ultrastructure of tissue reactions as related to pore size, *J. Natl. Cancer Inst.* **51**:1275.

KLÄRNER, P., 1962, Erzeugung von Sarkomen durch Fremdkörper aus Polymethacrylaten und Zusätzen, *Z. Krebsforsch.* **65**:99.

KLEIN, G., SJÖGREN, H. O., AND KLEIN, E., 1963, Demonstration of host resistance against sarcomas induced by implantation of cellophane films in isologous (syngeneic) recipients, *Cancer Res.* **23**:84.

KLEIN, G., BREGULA, U., WINER, F., AND HARRIS, H., 1971, The analysis of malignancy by cell fusion. I. Hybrids between tumor cells and L-cell derivatives, *J. Cell. Sci.* **8**:659.

KORDAN, H. A., 1967, Localized interfacial forces resulting from implanted plastics as possible physical factors involved in tumor formation, *J. Theoret. Biol.* **17**:1.

KOSUNEN, T. U., WAKSMAN, B. H., FLAX, M. H., AND TIHEN, W. S., 1963, Radioautographic study of cellular mechanisms in delayed hypersensitivity. I. Delayed reactions to tuberculin and purified proteins in the rat and guinea pig, *Immunology* **6**:276.

KRIPKE, M. L., AND WEISS, D. W., 1970, Studies on the immune responses of Balb/c mice during tumor induction by mineral oil, *Int. J. Cancer* **6**:422.

KUNTZ, R. E., CHEEVER, A. W., AND MYERS, B. J., 1972, Proliferative epithelial lesions of the urinary bladder of non-human primates infected with *Schistosoma haematobium*, *J. Natl. Cancer Inst.* **48**:223.

LANGVAD, E., 1968, Iron–dextran induction of distant tumours in mice, *Int. J. Cancer* **3**:415.

LEDER, L. D., 1967, The origin of blood monocytes and macrophages, *Blut* **16**:86.

LEININGER, R. I., 1965, *Changes in Properties of Plastics During Implantation: Plastics in surgical Implants*, pp. 71–76, Special Technical Publication 386, American Society for Testing Materials.

LOEWENSTEIN, W. R., 1973, Membrane junctions in growth and differentiation, *Fed. Proc.* **32**:60.

MARK, J., 1968, Relationships of chromosomal and pathological findings in Rous sarcoma virus–induced tumors in the mouse, *Int. J. Cancer* **3**:663.

MAROUDAS, N. G., O'NEILL, C. H., AND STANTON, M. F., 1973, Fibroblast anchorage in carcinogenesis by fibres, *Lancet* **1**:807.

MAXIMOW, A. A., 1927, Morphology of the mesenchymal reactions, *Arch. Pathol.* **4**:557.

MCDONALD, A. D., HARPER, A., EL ATTAR, O. A., AND MCDONALD, J. C., 1970, Epidemiology of primary malignant mesothelial tumors in Canada, *Cancer* **26**:914.

MCDOUGAL, J. S., AND AZAR, H. A., 1972, Tritiated proline in macrophages: *In vivo* and *in vitro* uptake by foreign-body granulomas, *Arch. Pathol.* **93**:13.

MERWIN, R. M., AND ALGIRE, G. H., 1959, Induction of plasma-cell neoplasms and fibrosarcomas in Balb/c mice carrying diffusion chambers, *Proc. Soc. Exp. Biol. Med.* **101**:437.

MILNE, J., 1969, Fifteen cases of pleural mesothelioma associated with occupational exposure to asbestos in Victoria, *Med. Z. Austral.* **2**:669.

MIZUNO, T., AND FUGII, T., 1969, Analysis of the two processes, wound repair and early changes in carcinogenesis, by the use of Millipore filter implanting: The possible role of heparin-like compound in cell interactions, *J. Fac. Sci. Univ. Tokyo* **11**:475 (Sect. IV).

MOHR, H. J., AND NOTHDURFT, H., 1958, Bindegewebskapseln um subcutan eingeheilte Fremdkörper und ihre Entartung zu Sarkomen, *Klin. Wschr.* **36**:493.

MURPHY, W. M., 1971, Tissue reaction of rats and guinea pigs to Co-Cr implants with different surface finishes, *Brit. J. Exp. Pathol.* **52**:353.

NOACK, W., 1970, Elektronenmikroskopische Untersuchungen über die Entstehung von Phagozyten und Fibroblasten auf peritonealen Implantaten, *Blut* **21**:35.

NORDLING, S., MIETTINEN, H., WARTIOVAARA, J., AND SAXEN, L., 1971, Transmission and spread of embryonic induction. I. Temporal relationships in transfilter induction of kidney tubules *in vitro, J. Embryol. Exp. Morphol.* **26**:231.

NOTHDURFT, H., 1955a, Die experimentelle Erzeugung von Sarkomen bei Ratten und Mäusen durch Implantation von Rundscheiben aus Gold, Silber, Platin oder Elfenbein, *Naturwissenschaften* **42**:71.

NOTHDURFT, H., 1955b, Über die Sarkomauslösung durch Fremdkörperimplantationen bei Ratten in abhängigkeit von der Form der Implantate, *Naturwissenschaften* **42**:106.

NOTHDURFT, H., 1960, Tumorerzeugung durch Fremdkörperimplantation, *Abhandl. Deutsch. Akad. Wiss. Berl. Klasse Med.* **3**:80.

NOTHDURFT, H., 1962, Unterschiedliche Ausbeuten an subcutanen Fremdkörpersarkomen der Ratte in Abhängigkeit von der Körperregion, *Naturwissenschaften* **49**:18.

OBERLING, C., 1960, Berliner Symposium über Fragen der Carcinogenese, *Abhandl. Deutsch. Akad. Wiss. Berl. Klasse Med.* **3**:98.

O'GARA, R. W., AND BROWN, J. M., 1967, Comparison of the carcinogenic actions of subcutaneous implants of iron and aluminum in rodents, *J. Natl. Cancer Inst.* **38**:947.

OLD, L. J., AND BOYSE, E. A., 1964, Immunology of experimental tumors, *Ann. Rev. Med.* **15**:167.

OPPENHEIMER, B. S., OPPENHEIMER, E. T., DANISHEFSKY, I., STOUT, A. P., AND EIRICH, F. R., 1955, Further studies of polymers as carcinogenic agents in animals, *Cancer Res.* **15**:333.

OPPENHEIMER, B. S., OPPENHEIMER, E. T., STOUT, A. P., WILLHITE, M., AND DANISHEFSKY, I., 1958, The latent period in carcinogenesis by plastics in rats and its relation to the precancerous stage, *Cancer* **11**:204.

OPPENHEIMER, B. S., OPPENHEIMER, E. T., STOUT, A. P., DANISHEFSKY, I., AND WILLHITE, M., 1959, Studies of the mechanism of carcinogenesis by plastic films, *Acta Unio Int. Contra Cancrum* **15**:659.

OPPENHEIMER, E. T., WILLHITE, M., STOUT, A. P., DANISHEFSKY, I., AND FISHMAN, M. M., 1964, A comparative study of the effects of imbedding cellophane and polystyrene films in rats, *Cancer Res.* **24**:379.

OTT, G., 1970, Fremdkörpersarkome, *Exp. Med. Pathol. Klin.* **32**:1.

PASTERNAK, C. A., 1970, Pathological Consequences: Cancer, in: *Biochemistry of Differentiation*, Interscience, New York.

POTT, F., AND FRIEDRICHS, K. H., 1972, Tumoren der Ratte nach i.p.-Injektion faserförmiger Stäube, *Naturwissenschaften* **57**:318.

PREHN, R. T., 1963, The role of immune mechanisms in the biology of chemically and physically induced tumors, in: *Conceptual Advances in Immunology and Oncology*, pp. 475–485, 16th Annual Symposium, New York.

RABINOWITZ, Z., AND SACHS, L., 1970, Control of the reversion of properties in transformed cells, *Nature (Lond.)* **225**:136.

RAYKHLIN, N. T., AND KOGAN, A. K., 1961, The development and malignant degeneration of the connective tissue capsules around plastic implants, *Probl. Oncol.* **7**:11.

RHODIN, J. A. G., 1968, Ultrastructure of mammalian venous capillaries, venules, and small collecting veins, *J. Ultrastruct. Res.* **25**:452.

RICHMOND, H. G., 1959, Induction of sarcoma in the rat by iron–dextran complex, *Brit. Med. J.* **1**:947.

RIGDON, R. H., 1973, Local reaction to polyurethane—A comparative study in the mouse, rat, and rabbit, *J. Biomed. Mater. Res.* **7**:79.

ROBERTS, G. H., 1970, Diffuse pleural mesothelioma: A clinical and pathological study, *Brit. J. Dis. Chest* **64**:201.

ROE, F. J. C., DUKES, C. E., AND MITCHLEY, B. C. V., 1967, Sarcomas at the site of implantation of polyvinyl plastic sponge: Incidence reduced by use of thin implants, *Biochem. Pharmacol.* **16**:647.

ROSS, R. EVERETT, N. B., AND TYLER, R., 1970, Wound healing and collagen formation. VI. The origin of the wound fibroblast studied in parabiosis, *J. Cell Biol.* **44**:645.

ROSSI, G. L., ALROY, J., AND RÖTHENMUND, S., 1973, Morphological studies of cultured swine aorta media explants, *Virchows Arch, Abt. B. Zellpathol.* **12**:133.

RUBIN, L. R., BROMBERG, B. E., AND WALDEN, R. H., 1971, Long term human reaction to synthetic plastics, *Surg. Gynecol. Obstet.* **132**:603.

RYAN, G. B., AND SPECTOR, W. G., 1969, Natural selection of long-lived macrophages in experimental granulomata, *J. Pathol.* **99**:139.

RYAN, G. B.,. AND SPECTOR, W. G., 1970, Macrophage turnover in inflamed connective tissue, *Proc. Royal Soc. Lond. Ser. B.* **175**:269.

SAAL, F., COLMERAUER, M. E. M., BRAYLAN, R. C., AND PASQUALINI, C. D., 1972, Tumor growth in allogeneic mice bearing a lucite cylinder, *J. Natl. Cancer Inst.* **49**:451.

SALYAMON, L. S., 1961, The role of inflammation in the mechanism of carcinogenic, co-carcinogenic and certain anti-carcinogenic effects, *Probl. Oncol.* **7**:44.

SAUNDERS, J. W., AND GASSELING, M. T., 1963, Trans-filter propagation of atypical ectoderm maintenance factor in the chick embryo wing bud, *Develop. Biol.* **7**:64.

SCHABAD, L., 1960, Berliner Symposium über Fragen der Carcinogenese, *Abhandl. Deutsch. Acad. Wiss. Berl. Klasse Med.* **3**:98.

SCHMITT, W., AND BENEKE, G., 1971, Das Bindegewebswachstum in subcutan implantierten Kunststoffschwämmchen bei der Ratte, *Virchows Arch, Abt. B. Zellpathol.* **9**:218.

SHAND, F. L., AND BELL, E. B., 1972, Studies on the distribution of macrophages derived from rat bone marrow cells in xenogeneic radiation chimaeras, *Immunology* **22**:549.

SHUBIK, P., SAFFIOTTI, U., LIJINSKY, W., PIETRA, G., RAPPAPORT, H., TOTH, B., RAHA, C. R., TOMATIS, L., FELDMAN, R., AND RAMAHI, H., 1962, Studies on toxicity of petroleum waxes, *Toxicol. Appl. Pharmacol.* **4**:1.

SJÖGREN, H. O., 1965, Transplantation methods as a tool for detection of tumor-specific antigens, *Prog. Exp. Tumor Res.* **6**:289.

SMALL, G. S., UPTON, L. G., AND HAYWARD, J. R., 1970, Bone induction studies with filter chambers, *J. Oral. Surg.* **28**:766.

SPECTOR, W. G., 1969, The granulomatous inflammatory exudate, *Int. Rev. Exp. Pathol.* **8**:1.

SPECTOR, W. G., AND LYKKE, A. W. J., 1966, The cellular evolution of inflammatory granulomata, *J. Pathol. Bacteriol.* **92**:163.

SPECTOR, W. G., AND RYAN, G. B., 1969, New evidence for the existence of long-lived macrophages, *Nature (Lond.)* **221**:860.

SPECTOR, W. G., AND WILLOUGHBY, D. A., 1968, The origin of mononuclear cells in chronic inflammation and tuberculin reactions in the rat, *J. Pathol. Bacteriol.* **96**:389.

SPECTOR, W. G., WALTERS, M. N. I., AND WILLOUGHBY, D. A., 1965, The origin of mononuclear cells in inflammatory exudates induced by fibrinogen, *J. Pathol. Bacteriol.* **90**:181.

SPECTOR, W. G., LYKKE, A. W. J., AND WILLOUGHBY, D. A., 1967, A quantitative study of leucocyte emigration in chronic inflammatory granulomata, *J. Pathol. Bacteriol.* **93**:101.

SPENCE, W. T., 1954, Form-fitting plastic cranioplasty, *J. Neurosurg.* **11**:219.

STANTON, M. F., AND WRENCH, C., 1972, Mechanisms of mesothelioma induction with asbestos and fibrous glass, *J. Natl. Cancer Inst.* **48**:797.

STINSON, N. E., 1964, The tissue reaction induced in rats and guinea pigs by polymethylmethacrylate (acrylic) and stainless steel (18/8/Mo), *Brit. J. Exp. Pathol.* **45**:21.

STOUT, A. P., 1960, Fibrous tumors of the soft tissues, *Minn. Med.* **43**:455.

STRAUMANN, F., AND PASCHKE, E., 1967, *Grundlagen der Alloplastik mit Metallen und Kunststoffen*, Thieme, Stuttgart.

SUTTON, J. S., AND WEISS, L., 1966, Transformation of monocytes in tissue culture into macrophages, epithelioid cells, and multinucleated giant cells, *J. Cell Biol.* **28**:303.

TARIN, D., 1972a, Tissue interactions in morphogenesis, morphostasis and carcinogenesis, *J. Theoret. Biol.* **34**:61.

TARIN, D., 1972b, Morphological studies on the mechanism of carcinogenesis, in: *Tissue Interactions in Carcinogenesis* (D. Tarin, ed.), pp. 227–289, Academic Press, London.

THOMASSEN, M. J., BUOEN, L. C., AND BRAND, K. G., 1975, Foreign body tumorigenesis: Number, distribution, and cell density of preneoplastic clones, *J. Natl. Cancer Inst.* (in press).

THOMPSON, R. J., AND ENTIN, S. D., 1969, Primary extraskeletal chondrosarcoma, *Cancer* **23**:936.

TOMATIS, L., 1963, Studies in subcutaneous carcinogenesis with implants of glass and teflon in mice, *Acta Unio Int. Contra Cancrum.* **19**:607.

TOMATIS, L., 1966, Subcutaneous carcinogenesis by $^{14}$C and $^{3}$H labelled polymethylmethacrylate films, *Tumori* **52**:165.

TSANEV, R., AND SENDOV, B., 1971a, An epigenetic mechanism for carcinogenesis, *Z. Krebsforsch.* **76**:299.

TSANEV, R., AND SENDOV, B., 1971b, Possible molecular mechanism for cell differentiation in multicellular organisms, *J. Theoret. Biol.* **30**:337.

TURUSOV, V., DAY, N., ANDRIANOV, L., AND JAIN, D., 1971, Influence of dose on skin tumors induced in mice by single application of 7,12-dimethylbenz(a)anthracene, *J. Natl. Cancer Inst.* **47**:105.

URIST, M. R., SILVERMAN, B. F., BÜRING, K., DUBUC, F. L., AND ROSENBERG, J. M., 1967, The bone induction principle, *Clin. Orthop.* **54**:243.

VAN WINKLE, W., 1967, The fibroblast in wound healing, *Surg. Gynecol. Obstet.* **124**:369.

VASILIEV, J. M., OLSHEVSKAJA, L. V., RAYKHLIN, N. T., AND IVANOVA, O. J., 1962, Comparative study of alterations induced by 7,12-dimethylbenz(a)anthracene and polymer films in the subcutaneous connective tissue of rats, *J. Natl. Cancer Inst.* **28**:515.

VIRENQUE, M., LEROUX, R., DELAUNAY, A., LASFARQUES, E., CORONEL, S., AND KERNEIS, J. P., 1947, Les resines acryliques en prothese et en biologie, *Presse Med.* **55**:736.

VOLKMAN, A., 1966, The origin and turnover of mononuclear cells in peritoneal exudates in rats, *J. Exp. Med.* **124**:241.

VOLKMAN, A., AND GOWANS, J. L., 1965a, The production of macrophages in the rat, *Brit. J. Exp. Pathol.* **46**:50.

VOLKMAN, A., AND GOWANS, J. L., 1965b, The origin of macrophages from the bone marrow in the rat, *Brit. J. Exp. Pathol.* **46**:62.

VON LICHTENBERG, F., SMITH, T. M., LUCIA, H. L., AND DOUGHTY, B. L., 1971, New model for schistosome granuloma formation using a soluble egg antigen and bentonite particles, *Nature (Lond.)* **229**:199.

WAGNER, J. C., AND BERRY, G., 1969, Mesotheliomas in rats following inoculation with asbestos, *Brit. J. Cancer* **23**:567.

WARBURG, O., 1956, On the origin of cancer cells, *Science* **123**:309.

WARTIOVAARA, J., LEHTONEN, E., NORDLING, S., AND SAXEN, L., 1972, Do membrane filters prevent cell contacts? *Nature (Lond.)* **238**:407.

WEISS, M. C., TODARO, J., AND GREEN, H., 1968, Properties of a hybrid between lines sensitive and insensitive to contact inhibition of cell division, *J. Cell. Physiol.* **71**:105.

WESSELS, N. K., 1962, Tissue interaction during skin histo-differentiation, *Develop. Biol.* **4**:87.

WILSON, P. D., AND FRANKS, L. M., 1972, The ultrastructure of tumours derived from spontaneously transformed tissue culture cells, *Brit. J. Concer* **26**:380.

WISSLER, R. W., 1967, The arterial medial cell, smooth muscle or multifunctional mesenchyme? *J. Atheroscler. Res.* **8**:201.

YAMAMOTO, T., RABINOWITZ, Z., AND SACHS, L., 1973, Identification of the chromosomes that control malignancy, *Nature New Biol.* **243**:247.

YOSIDA, T. H., IMAI, H. T., AND MORIWAKI, K., 1967, Cytogenetical and biochemical studies of 19 primary plasma cell neoplasms induced in Balb/c mice, *Ann. Rep. Natl. Inst. Genet. Japan* **18**:13.

ZAJDELA, F., 1966, Production de sarcomes souscutanes chez le rat au moyen de membranes cellulosiques de porosite connue, *Bull. Cancer* **53**:401.

ZOLLINGER, H. U., 1952, Experimentalle Erzeugung maligner Nierenkapseltumoren bei der Ratte durch Druckreiz, *Schweiz. Z. Pathol. Bakteriol.* **15**:666.

# Index